Methods in
Mammalian Reproduction

Contributors

Gary B. Anderson

Fuller W. Bazer

Staffan Bergström

Patsy K. Williams Boyce

Benjamin G. Brackett

Bruce M. Carlson

Arthur K. Champlin

Joseph C. Daniel, Jr.

W. Richard Dukelow

P. Eckstein

R. L. Gardner

Y.-C. Hsu

P. R. Hurst

Matthew H. Kaufman

S. P. Leibo

Carmen B. Lozzio

Jeffrey A. MacCabe

Robert W. McGaughey

Ralph R. Maurer

Peter Mazur

Finnie A. Murray

Anna Niemierko

Jolanta Opas

Marilyn B. Renfree

R. Michael Roberts

Anthony G. Sacco

D. C. Sharp, III

Michael I. Sherman

C. Alex Shivers

M. H. L. Snow

C. H. Tyndale-Biscoe

Jonathan Van Blerkom

R. G. Wales

Wesley K. Whitten

Methods in

Mammalian
Reproduction

EDITED BY

JOSEPH C. DANIEL, JR.

Department of Zoology
University of Tennessee
Knoxville, Tennessee

ACADEMIC PRESS
New York   San Francisco   London   1978
A Subsidiary of Harcourt Brace Jovanovich, Publishers

ACADEMIC PRESS, INC.
111 Fifth Avenue, New York, New York 10003

United Kingdom Edition published by
ACADEMIC PRESS, INC. (LONDON) LTD.
24/28 Oval Road, London NW1   7DX

Library of Congress Cataloging in Publication Data

Main entry under title:
Methods in mammalian reproduction.

    Includes bibliographies and index.
    1. Embryology--Mammals. 2. Mammals--Reproduc-
tion. 3. Embryology, Experimental--Technique.
I. Daniel, Joseph C.   [DNLM: 1. Mammals--
Embryology--Laboratory manuals. 2. Research--
Methods.   QS625 M592]
QL959.M48   599'.03   78-1820
ISBN 0-12-201850-8

Contents

v

7 Techniques for Separating Early Embryonic Tissues

M. H. L. Snow

8 Methods for the Preservation of Mammalian Embryos by Freezing

S. P. Leibo and Peter Mazur

9 Immunologic Inhibition of Development

Anthony G. Sacco and C. Alex Shivers

10 *In Vitro* Development of Whole Mouse Embryos beyond the Implantation Stage

Y.-C. Hsu

Contents

11 Implantation of Mouse Blastocysts *in Vitro*

Michael I. Sherman

12 Advances in Rabbit Embryo Culture

Ralph R. Maurer

13 Advances in Large Mammal Embryo Culture

Gary B. Anderson

14 Embryo Transfer in Large Domestic Mammals

Finnie A. Murray

15 Manipulation of Marsupial Embryos and Pouch Young

Marilyn B. Renfree and C. H. Tyndale-Biscoe

16 Experimentation Involving Primate Embryos

Benjamin G. Brackett

17 Transplanting and Explanting Organ Primordia

Jeffrey A. MacCabe

18 The Regeneration of Mammalian Limbs and Limb Tissues

Bruce M. Carlson

22 The Use of Amniocentesis in Prenatal Diagnosis

Carmen B. Lozzio

23 Collection and Analysis of Female Genital Tract Secretions

Fuller W. Bazer, R. Michael Roberts, and D. C. Sharp, III

24 Experimental Approaches for Elucidating the Antifertility Action of Intrauterine Devices in Monkeys and Rodents

P. Eckstein and P. R. Hurst

25 Surgical Induction of Endometriosis

Joseph C. Daniel, Jr. and Patsy K. Williams Boyce

Contents

List of Contributors

Numbers in parentheses indicate the pages in which the authors' contributions begin.

Gary B. Anderson (273), Department of Animal Science, University of California, Davis, California

Fuller W. Bazer (503), Animal Science Department, University of Florida, Gainesville, Florida

Staffan Bergström (419), Department of Obstetrics and Gynecology, University Hospital, Uppsala, Sweden

Patsy K. Williams Boyce (545), Department of Zoology, University of Tennessee, Knoxville, Tennessee

Benjamin G. Brackett (333), Department of Clinical Studies, School of Veterinary Medicine, and Department of Obstetrics and Gynecology, School of Medicine, University of Pennsylvania, Philadelphia, Pennsylvania

Bruce M. Carlson (377), Department of Anatomy, University of Michigan Medical School, Ann Arbor, Michigan

Arthur K. Champlin (403), Department of Biology, Colby College, Waterville, Maine

Joseph C. Daniel, Jr. (545), Department of Zoology, University of Tennessee, Knoxville, Tennessee

W. Richard Dukelow (437), Endocrine Research Unit, Michigan State University, East Lansing, Michigan

P. Eckstein (529), Department of Anatomy, Medical School, University of Birmingham, Birmingham, England

R. L. Gardner (137), Department of Zoology, University of Oxford, Oxford, England

Y.-C. Hsu (229), Laboratory of Mammalian Development and Oncogenesis, Department of Pathobiology, Johns Hopkins School of Hygiene and Public Health, Baltimore, Maryland

P. R. Hurst (529), Department of Anatomy, Medical School, The University of Birmingham, Birmingham, England

Matthew H. Kaufman (21), Department of Anatomy, University of Cambridge, Cambridge, England

S. P. Leibo (179), Biology Division, Oak Ridge National Laboratory, Oak Ridge, Tennessee

Carmen B. Lozzio (461), Birth Defects Evaluation Center, Memorial Research Center and Hospital, University of Tennessee, Knoxville, Tennessee

Jeffrey A. MacCabe (359), Department of Zoology, University of Tennessee, Knoxville, Tennessee

Robert W. McGaughey (1), Department of Zoology, Arizona State University, Tempe, Arizona

Ralph R. Maurer (259), United States Department of Agriculture, Agricultural Research Service, U.S. Meat Animal Research Center, Clay Center, Nebraska

Peter Mazur (179), Biology Division, Oak Ridge National Laboratory, Oak Ridge, Tennessee

Finnie A. Murray (285), Reproductive Physiology, Department of Animal Science, Ohio Agricultural Research and Development Center, Wooster, Ohio

Anna Niemierko (49), Laboratory of Experimental Embryology, Institute of Obstetrics and Gynecology, Medical Academy, Warsaw, Poland

Jolanta Opas (49), Department of Embryology, Zoological Institute, University of Warsaw, Warsaw, Poland

Marilyn B. Renfree (307), School of Environmental and Life Sciences, Murdoch University, Murdoch, Western Australia

R. Michael Roberts (503), Department of Biochemistry, University of Florida, Gainesville, Florida

Anthony G. Sacco (203), Department of Gynecology and Obstetrics, Wayne State University, School of Medicine, Detroit, Michigan

D. C. Sharp, III (503), Animal Science Department, University of Florida, Gainesville, Florida

Michael I. Sherman (247), Department of Cell Biology, Roche Institute of Molecular Biology, Nutley, New Jersey

C. Alex Shivers (203), Department of Zoology, University of Tennessee, Knoxville, Tennessee

M. H. L. Snow (167), MRC Mammalian Development Unit, University College London, London, England

C. H. Tyndale-Biscoe (307), Division of Wildlife Research, Commonwealth Scientific and Industrial Research Organization, Lyneham, Australia

Jonathan Van Blerkom (68), Department of Molecular, Cellular and Developmental Biology, University of Colorado, Boulder, Colorado

R. G. Wales (111), School of Veterinary Studies, Murdoch University, Murdoch, Western Australia

Wesley K. Whitten (403), The Jackson Laboratory, Bar Harbor, Maine

Preface

While the field of mammalian reproduction expands, as a research area, as a special subject in the curricula of many colleges and universities, and as a clinical specialty, so does the demand for more and better procedures and the need to be able to repeat them carefully and confirm previous findings. It is these needs which this book intends to serve.

The twenty-five chapters in "Methods in Mammalian Reproduction" present some of the latest techniques for manipulating, analyzing, observing, testing, and generally experimenting with mammalian mothers and their gametes and embryos, and give historical perspectives on the techniques. Although most of the chapters, as does most of the work in the field, focus on laboratory rodents and lagomorphs, there is also coverage of marsupials, domestic farm species, and primates including humans.

The reader will quickly note the inclusion of many chapters relating to microtechniques for manipulating or assaying various synthesizing activities and/or metabolic phenomena in oocytes or embryos. This reflects the current wave of interest in examining mammalian reproductive events in detail and with greater accuracy than was possible when this field of investigation was first emerging.

Mammalian reproduction involves an intimate relationship between mother and embryo, and the coverage of the book reflects this duality. The first eighteen chapters are arranged in an order which follows a developmental sequence from oocyte to fetal organs and the remaining seven chapters deal with the maternal side of the relationship.

The successful completion of this volume has resulted from the high level of cooperation and flexibility from the thirty-three contributing authors. As editor, I am most appreciative of the constructive and tolerant attitudes of the participants.

Joseph C. Daniel Jr.

1

In Vitro Oocyte Maturation

ROBERT W. McGAUGHEY

I. GENERAL INTRODUCTION

The gametogenic cells of female mammals enter meiotic prophase during the late stages of fetal development, and, in most species, primary oocytes reach the diplonema stage around the time of birth (Cowperthwaite, 1925; Freud, 1939; Borum, 1961; Jones and Krohn, 1961). In terms of progress through the later stages of meiosis, mammalian oocytes remain static, with their nuclei in the germinal vesicle configuration (i.e., late diplonema) until a few hours before they are ovulated. Such oocytes containing a germinal vesicle (Fig. 1A) can be called immature in the context of meiosis, while oocytes that have progressed to diakinesis (Fig. 1B), metaphase I and anaphase I (Fig. 1C) can be termed "maturing" oocytes. Oocytes that have completed the first meiotic reductional division progress through telophase I (Fig. 1D) to metaphase II, and are considered at this latter stage to be meiotically mature and prepared for ovulation and penetration by spermatozoa (Donahue, 1972). The nuclear process of oocyte

1

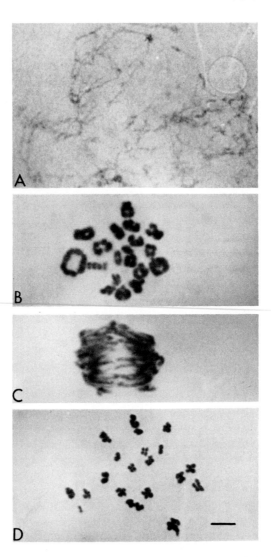

Fig. 1. The chromatin of air-dried porcine oocytes, stained with basic fuchsin. The "fibrous" chromatin of an oocyte at the germinal vesicle stage is shown in (A). In (B) the 19 bivalents of an oocyte at diakinesis are shown. Anaphase of the first meiotic division is shown in (C), and the 19 chromosomes of the second meiotic metaphase are shown in (D). Magnification of these photographs is × 1750. The bar represents 5.0 μm.

maturation, therefore, can be considered to include the meiotic stages of diakinesis through metaphase II. Completion of meiosis in the female mammalian gamete, however, occurs in most species only when the secondary oocyte is penetrated by a spermatozoon.

In addition to the chromosomal events which occur during oocyte maturation, the nucleus and cytoplasm of mammalian oocytes undergo changes including both morphology and metabolic function. Changes involving the oolemma, mitochondria, endoplasmic reticulum, Golgi complex, and nucleolus have been defined for maturing oocytes (Zamboni, 1972; Szollosi, 1972). The possible controls of energy metabolism by developing oocytes have been discussed by Biggers (1972), and recent studies have described some characteristics of RNA and protein synthesis during oocyte maturation (Wasserman and Letourneau, 1976; Rodman and Bachvarova, 1976; McGaughey and Van Blerkom, 1977; Van Blerkom and McGaughey, 1977).

The physiological significance of oocyte maturation is the preparation of "stored," immature follicular oocytes for release from the follicle at ovulation and for interaction with spermatozoa during fertilization. It therefore should be borne in mind that the overall process of oocyte maturation is a highly complex developmental sequence which by no means can be limited to the chromosomal events of condensation and division.

Many characteristics of oocyte maturation *in vivo*, including the chronology of meiotic stages, the influence of gonadotropins on maturation, and the descriptive ultrastructure of maturing oocytes have been carefully examined in several species (see Donahue, 1972, for review). However, due to the complexity of the follicular environment, it has not been possible to approach several questions related to the maturation of mammalian oocytes by examining the process *in vivo*. Obviously, oocytes enclosed within the ovarian follicle are not accessible to direct, continuous observation and experimental manipulation. In addition, it is not possible, with a system of oocyte maturation *in vivo*, to isolate oocytes from contact and interaction with the several cellular components of the intact ovarian follicle (i.e., granulosa and theca cells), or with the currently undefined components of the liquor folliculae (follicular fluid) which fills the follicular antrum. For these and other reasons, several investigators have isolated mammalian oocytes and have examined the process of oocyte maturation under conditions which are perhaps more amenable to experimental control and manipulation *in vitro*.

By applying culture methods to the study of oocyte maturation, it has been possible to examine the influence of follicular components, either singly or in combination, on the process (e.g., Thibault, 1972; Tsafriri and Channing, 1975a; McGaughey, 1975, 1977a) and to compare maturation *in vitro* to that occurring *in vivo*. Although it appears that, for most mammalian species, oocyte maturation takes place over approximately the same period of time both *in vivo* and *in vitro* (Table I), certain aspects of maturation *in vitro* have been found not to

TABLE I

Maturation of Porcine Oocytes _in Vivo_ and _in Vitro_[a]

		No. (%) of examined oocytes at each stage					
				Developing beyond the germinal vesicle stage			
Hours after HCG (_in vivo_)[b] or hours of culture (_in vitro_)[c]	Total oocytes examined (No. of gilts)	Remaining at the germinal vesicle stage		Total Diak-MII		Dividing AI-MII	
		No.	(%)	No.	(%)	No.	(%)
In vivo 26	87 (8)	49	(56)	38	(44)	3	(3)
In vitro 26–27.5	107 (7)	61	(57)	46	(43)	2	(2)
In vivo 28–30	129 (12)	35	(27)	94	(73)	0	—
In vitro 33–33.5	99 (6)	39	(39)	60	(61)	10	(10)
In vivo 34	63 (4)	1	(2)	62	(98)	26	(41)
In vitro 36–37	96 (8)	24	(25)	72	(75)	28	(29)
In vivo 38	99 (6)	3	(5)	63	(95)	44	(67)
In vivo 43	61 (5)	0	—	61	(100)	49	(80)
In vitro 42.5–43.5	147 (10)	40	(27)	107	(73)	82	(56)

[a] Oocytes examined as air-dried preparations.

[b] All females received an injection of HCG following a priming injection of PMS. Data in this table reflect the sequence of maturation _in vivo_ of oocytes from females entering estrus within 24 hours after the injection of HCG (R. W. McGaughey and C. Polge, unpublished observations).

[c] Immature oocytes were cultured in TC199 containing 1.0 mg of BSA/ml (McGaughey and Polge, 1971).

faithfully duplicate the developmental process _in vivo_. In addition to chromosomal and ultrastructural abnormalities observed in oocytes during or following maturation _in vitro_ (McGaughey and Polge, 1971; McGaughey, 1977a; Zamboni, 1972), the embryonic developmental capacity of oocytes matured _in vitro_ has been reported to be inferior to that of physiologically matured oocytes (Cross and Brinster, 1970; Thibault, 1972). Therefore, until more information is gathered from investigations of oocytes and their ability to mature _in vitro_, the maturation of isolated mammalian oocytes _in vitro_ must be considered to be an approximation of and not identical to oocyte maturation _in vivo_. An important challenge currently existing in the field of the developmental biology of mammalian oocytes is to delineate those molecular and morphological events that occur during maturation *in vivo*, but not *in vitro*. Such differences will be significant, not only to our understanding of the development of mammalian oocytes, but perhaps also to the interpretation of investigations of cultured cells in general.

The following technical descriptions for the study of oocyte maturation *in vitro* are directly related to the work on porcine oocytes carried out in the author's laboratory. The fundamental methodological approach should be applicable, with modifications, to the examination of oocytes from other mammalian species.

II. METHODS EMPLOYED IN THE CULTURE OF OOCYTES

A. Selection of Oocytes for Culture

1. Collection and Selection of Ovaries

The success of culture experiments will depend first upon the repeatable selection of a pool of immature oocytes, a given proportion of which are capable of maturing *in vitro*. When dealing with porcine reproductive tracts obtained from a commercial slaughterhouse, it is important to return the tracts to the laboratory in a reasonably short period of time following slaughter. Tracts are transported in a warm (i.e., 37°–38°C) thermos and arrive at the author's laboratory within 30–40 minutes after slaughter of the donor pigs.

By gross examination one can select ovaries whose largest follicles are preovulatory (i.e., follicular diameter between 6 and 10 mm), medium-sized (i.e., 3–5 mm), or small (i.e., 1.0–2.0 mm). In order to reduce the possible variation due to differences in oocyte quality between females, we use a single ovary from each of three or more tracts for the collection of oocytes from follicles of one of the above ranges of size for a given experiment. For two reasons, porcine oocytes from large follicles normally are not used for culture in this laboratory. In our experience, ovaries with preovulatory follicles are seldom encountered in batches of reproductive tracts obtained at slaughter, and it is not possible to determine whether or not oocytes from large follicles have been exposed to the ovulatory surge of endogenous luteinizing hormone.

2. Equipment for Oocyte Manipulations

The use of a temperature-controlled microscope hood, of the type described by Mintz (1971), may reduce the incidence of microbial contamination and will aid in the maintenance of a stable, warm environment during manipulation of the oocytes. In the author's laboratory, however, such a hood has not been found to be necessary for the elimination of contamination. The harvesting and manipulation of oocytes is carried out on a clean laboratory counter in a room in which the air circulation system has been turned off to reduce airborne dust. Watchglasses and other glassware containing culture medium and oocytes are placed on an histological warming plate (37°C) between steps of microscopic manipulation. Binocular dissecting microscopes of the "zoom" types (Bausch and Lomb), with lens systems allowing magnification in the range of 7.0–30 ×, and with transmitted illumination are employed in the manipulation of oocytes. All tools and glassware with which the liberated oocytes come in contact either are sterile, disposable types or are autoclaved prior to use.

3. Harvesting Follicular Oocytes

If the experiment dictates the use of porcine oocytes from large preovulatory follicles, the oocytes are collected by aspirating follicles by means of a 21-gauge hypodermic needle attached to a sterile, disposable syringe. The aspirated follicular contents are placed in a sterile watchglass, and the oocytes removed with a small-bore pipette under a dissecting microscope.

Porcine oocytes are harvested from medium-sized or small follicles by tearing the appropriate follicles with the tip of a sterile 18-gauge needle. During the harvesting procedure, the ovaries are in a large sterile watchglass (10.0 cm) to which 5–10 ml of culture medium (cf., Section II, B) has been added. As the follicles are torn, the ovaries are turned in the medium to allow the released oocytes to fall onto the floor of the watchglass. After the follicles from all ovaries have been torn, the ovaries are discarded, and the culture medium covering the liberated oocytes is replaced two to three times to remove debris and blood, which interfere with visualizing the harvested oocytes. A 10-cc disposable syringe, fitted with an 18-gauge needle, works well for removing the cloudy medium.

4. Classification of Oocytes

Oocytes are pipetted from the harvesting watchglass to a clean watchglass (5.0 cm) containing fresh culture medium. At this point, the collected oocytes can normally be separated into three categories, depending upon their general appearance and the density of granulosa cells surrounding them. In this laboratory, oocytes are grossly classified as "good" if they are well rounded and are completely surrounded by a dense layer of granulosa (corona) cells (Fig. 2A), "fair" if they are round and contain a nearly complete layer of surrounding cells (Fig. 2B), and "poor" if they are either abnormally shaped or have few or no surrounding granulosa cells (Fig. 2C). Oocytes of the first category usually represent approximately 25% of the total pool of oocytes harvested from small or medium-sized follicles and are considered to be the group most capable of maturation in vitro (McGaughey and Montgomery, 1977).

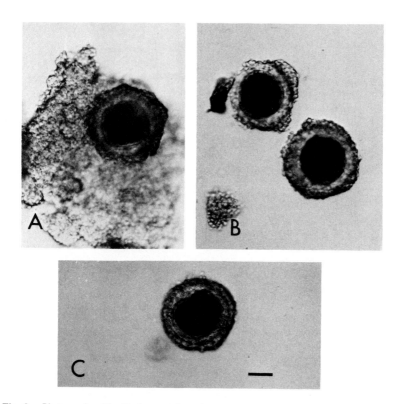

Fig. 2. Photographs of freshly harvested porcine oocytes, to represent the criteria used in selecting pools of "good" (A), "fair" (B), and "poor" (C) oocytes. The oocyte in (A) is completely surrounded by dense layers of granulosa; the oocytes in (B) are nearly completely surrounded by granulosa; and the oocyte in (C) not only has fewer surrounding granulosa cells but also is abnormally shaped. Magnification of these photographs is × 130. The bar represents 50 μm.

After the pool of good oocytes has been selected by carefully eliminating obviously degenerate or denuded oocytes, further selection of smaller groups of oocytes from the pool is carried out at low magnification (approximately 10 ×). This final selection of experimental and control groups of oocytes for culture is carried out at low magnification in order to randomize the distribution of oocytes from the pool among the various culture dishes. Groups of oocytes from each pool are air-dried (McGaughey and Polge, 1971) without culture in order to assess the configuration of their germinal vesicle chromatin and to make certain that no maturing oocytes were included within the pool. The germinal vesicle chromatin of uncultured porcine oocytes usually is in one of three configurations—fibrous or lampbrushlike (Fig. 1A), diffuse (Fig. 3A), or degenerate (Fig. 3B–D). The incidence of oocytes with fibrous germinal vesicle chromatin is highest in the good category; whereas the poor category contains

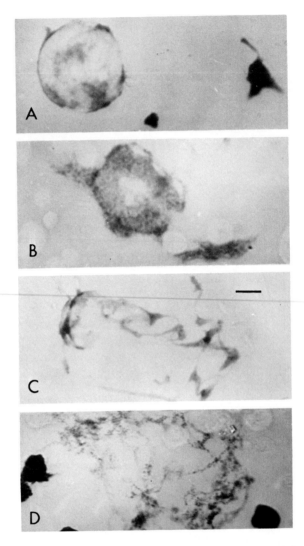

Fig. 3. The chromatin of air-dried immature porcine oocytes, stained with basic fuchsin. (A) represents the ''diffuse'' configuration of germinal vesicle chromatin, and (B–D) represent degenerate chromatin of germinal vesicles considered to be in the diffuse (B) and ''fibrous'' (C,D) configurations. Magnification of these photographs is × 1750. The bar represents 5.0 μm.

high incidences of oocytes in the diffuse and degenerate configurations (McGaughey and Montgomery, 1977).

5. *Removal of Granulosa Cells*

For experiments in which oocytes without surrounding granulosa cells are to be cultured, groups of oocytes are randomly selected from the above pool of good oocytes, and, after transfer to a fresh watchglass, are denuded by means of micropipettes. The micropipettes are either pulled by hand or by means of a microforge (e.g., DKI, Model 700C), so that their openings are approximately the diameter of the oocyte, as measured across the zona pellucida. Enzymatic removal of the tightly adhering granulosa cells has not yet been found to be satisfactory because of the possibility of enzymatic effects on the zona pellucida and on the oolemma.

B. Culture Media

1. *Complex Media*

The selection of culture media for studies of oocyte maturation *in vitro* will depend upon the intent of a particular investigation. For those studies in which oocyte maturation *in vitro* is employed merely for the production of secondary oocytes to be used in investigations of fertilization and later embryogenesis, it is perhaps justifiable to select a complex medium containing serum or other undefined supplements. Complex media, such as TC199 and F10, containing various concentrations of sera have been employed by some investigators in the study of oocyte maturation (e.g., Tsafriri and Channing, 1975a,b; Tsafriri *et al.*, 1976; Liebfried, 1976; Jagiello *et al.*, 1975). On the other hand, it is believed by the author that for those investigations designed to determine the developmental parameters involved in the maturation *in vitro* of isolated mammalian oocytes, culture media which are as nearly defined chemically as is currently possible should be used. Defined media may be classified either as complex or as minimal (e.g., Brinster's BMOC-3, or similar media) and usually are supplemented with a macromolecule such as BSA, dextran, or polyvinylpyrrolidone. The author has employed TC199, supplemented with BSA, in studies of the chronological sequence of porcine oocyte maturation (McGaughey and Polge, 1971; and Table I) and to examine the influence of porcine follicular fluid on the process of oocyte maturation (McGaughey, 1975).

2. *Minimal, Chemically Defined Media*

In order to determine some of the basic chemical requirements for the maturation of porcine oocytes, the author tested the ability of these cells to develop in BMOC-3 (Brinster, 1971), supplemented with 4.5 mg of BSA/ml (McGaughey,

TABLE II
Composition of Modified BMOC-3, Used for
Culturing Pig Oocytes

Component	Concentration (gm/liter)	
Sodium lactate	2.253	
Sodium pyruvate	0.056	
NaCl	5.012	
KCl	0.321	
CaCl$_2$	0.170	"Salt group"
KH$_2$PO$_4$	0.146	
MgSO$_4$ · 7 H$_2$O	0.264	
NaHCO$_3$	2.106	
Glucose	1.000	
Phenol red	0.0012 (1.2 ml)[a]	
Dextran T70	4.500	
Penicillin G	0.060[b]	
Streptomycin sulfate	0.050	

[a] Phenol red made up initially in distilled water at a concentration of 1 mg/ml.

[b] Activity equals 1669 units/mg.

1976, 1977a). It has been determined that in minimal medium (Table II), devoid of amino nitrogen and supplemented with dextran T70 (4.5 mg/ml), a sizable proportion of cultured porcine oocytes undergo maturation *in vitro* (Table III). The modified BMOC-3 shown in Table II is currently employed as the control culture medium for investigations of porcine oocyte maturation in the author's laboratory. Although at the present time the possible influence of all amino acids on porcine oocyte maturation has not been determined, it has been demonstrated that the four amino acids, found by Gwatkin and Haidri (1973) to improve the incidence of hamster oocyte maturation *in vitro*, are not required for the maturation of denuded porcine oocytes (McGaughey, 1977b).

    a. Preparation of Media.   The porcine oocyte culture medium (Table II) is made up by dissolving each of the salts individually, in the order listed. Care is taken to ensure complete solution of each salt before addition of the next one. The salts are dissolved in about 800 ml of deionized, glass-distilled water contained in a 1-liter graduated cylinder by mixing with a magnetic stir bar. The sugars and antibiotics are then added individually as described above, followed by addition of the phenol red and dextran T70. Again, complete solubilization of a component is allowed before addition of the next component. Sodium bicarbonate is added last, and while it dissolves, the total volume is adjusted to 1 liter by

TABLE III

Incidences of Maturation of Pig Oocytes Cultured in Media Containing Fluid from Large and Small Follicles

					Percentage of examined oocytes[c]		
					Remaining at the dictyate stage	Developing beyond dictyate stage	
				No. of oocytes examined		Total (Diak-MII)	Dividing (ANAI-MII)
Exp. No.	Oocytes cultured[a]	Hour of culture	Culture medium supplements[b]	(dishes)	$\bar{X}$ % ± SE	$\bar{X}$ % ± SE	$\bar{X}$ % ± SE
I	Intact	48	BSA, 35 mg/ml	51 (6)	42 1.5%	58 1.5%	44 1.0%
			BSA, 4.5 mg/ml	56 (6)	43 0.5%	57 0.5%	49 1.0%
			FF-L, 1:1	52 (6)	41 1.1%	59 1.1%	33 1.2%
			FF-L, 1:19	43 (5)	60 1.0%	40 1.0%	28 1.0%
II	Intact	48	BSA, 35 mg/ml	50 (6)	24 0.6%	75 0.6%	63 1.0%
			BSA, 4.5 mg/ml	55 (6)	31 0.5%	69 0.5%	60 0.6%
			FF-S, 1:1	51 (6)	33 1.9%	69 1.9%	38 0.8%
			FF-S, 1:19	51 (6)	69 1.3%	31 1.3%	20 1.1%
III	Intact	24	T 70, 4.5 mg/ml	71 (8)	35 0.8%	65 0.8%	23 0.4%
			FF-S, 1:1	31 (4)	32 0.9%	68 0.9%	16 0.2%
			FF-S, 1:9	39 (4)	33 0.4%	67 0.4%	33 0.6%
IV	Denuded	24	T 70, 4.5 mg/ml	73 (8)	71 1.1%	29 1.0%	6 0.2%
			FF-S, 1:1	34 (4)	60 0.9%	40 0.9%	6 0.6%
			FF-S, 1:9	40 (4)	55 0.6%	45 0.6%	9 1.0%

[a] Intact oocytes have adhering granulosa cells. Denuded refers to oocytes whose granulosa cells were mechanically removed by micropipetting.

[b] In Exp. I and II, two control media were used; containing either 35 mg or 4.5 mg of BSA/ml of BMOC-3. FF-L and FF-S are fluids from large (6.0–10 mm) and small (3.5–4.5 mm) follicles, respectively. The ratio 1:1, 1:9, and 1:19 refers to 1 part FF to 1, 9, and 19 parts of culture medium. In Exp. III and IV, culture medium consists of BMOC-3, which was modified as described in the text. T70 refers to dextran T70 added to culture media in Exp. III and IV.

[c] Group mean percentages ($\bar{X}$%) and SE were calculated after angular transformation of proportions for each culture dish (Snedecor and Cochran, 1967). Experimental groups within experiments, which are joined by a vertical line belong to the same statistical subset; those which are not belong to statistically different subsets ($p < 0.05$) according to Duncan's Multiple Ranges Test (Nie *et al.*, 1975). Mean percentages within groups may not add up to 100%, due to averaging (note SE ranges for mean values).

the addition of water. As soon as the sodium bicarbonate has dissolved, the solution is equilibrated by bubbling through it a mixture of 5% CO_2, 5% O_2, and 90% N_2. The correct indicator color for a properly equilibrated solution is light coral or salmon (pH 7.3–7.4). Immediately following the equilibration procedure the culture medium is passed through a Millipore filter (0.45 μm pore size), under positive pressure supplied by the compressed equilibration gas mixture. After filtration, the medium is poured into individual sterile glass bottles, leaving an air space of at least one-third of the bottle's total volume. A sterile Pasteur pipette, attached to the equilibration gas tank, is inserted into each bottle, and the gas mixture is bubbled through the solution for 2–3 minutes, after which the bottles are sealed. The bottles of medium are stored in a refrigerator at 5°–7°C until use. A 1-liter batch of medium is used up within 7–10 days, or is discarded after that period of storage. The culture medium is never frozen because of the possibility of precipitation of some of the salts.

b. Modification of Media. The composition of the culture medium can be modified, and certain supplements have been added to it under specific conditions. The osmolarity of the culture medium must be maintained within certain limits in order for its successful use with porcine oocytes (McGaughey, 1976). If osmotically active components are removed or added to the medium, the concentration of the whole "salt group" (cf., Table II) should be raised or lowered, proportionately for each salt, to adjust the calculated osmolarity of the medium to the control level (i.e., 285 mOsM).

Undefined heterogeneous solutions, such as serum or follicular fluid, can also be added to the culture medium. In this laboratory, these solutions are added to sterilized culture medium at the desired concentration, and the mixture is immediately filtered for use by means of a Millipore filter (0.45 μm pore size) with a syringe adaptor.

When steroids are to be added to the culture media, they must be added aseptically, since Millipore filters will absorb these molecules. We dissolve steroids in benzene or ethanol to make stock solutions of desired concentration. An aliquot of the stock solution is allowed to dry in the bottom of a sterile glass bottle, and filtered culture medium is then added to give the appropriate final concentration. The medium is slowly stirred for 6 hours or overnight at 4°C to dissolve the steroid (McGaughey, 1977a). Steroid-supplemented media prepared in this way have been found to be as free of microbial contamination as is control medium.

C. Culture Procedure

The selected pool of good oocytes is usually broken down into groups of 10. Normally, with 3–5 ovaries we are able to obtain sufficiently large pools to form 6–10 groups, each with 10 oocytes.

In a typical experimental replicate, each control or experimental culture group will contain two or more dishes of oocytes. An individual culture dish (Falcon, No. 1008) routinely contains 0.5 ml of the appropriate culture medium for a particular control or experimental group. After addition of media to the culture dishes, they are placed in a vacuum desiccator (16-cm diameter) which is humidified by filling the bottom compartment with water. The desiccator is attached to the tank containing 5% CO_2, 5% O_2, and 90% N_2, and allowed to equilibrate for 2 minutes. During the time that oocytes are being harvested and selected, the equilibrated culture dishes are stored in the sealed desiccator which is kept in an incubator maintained at 37.5°C.

Since the harvesting and selecting procedure is routinely performed in control culture medium (Table II), control groups of oocytes are pipetted directly into equilibrated culture dishes containing control medium. Experimental groups of oocytes are washed 2 times in 1.0-ml aliquots of test media (i.e., containing supplements or deficiencies) before they are pipetted into their appropriate dishes containing a particular test medium.

Culture dishes are replaced in the vacuum desiccator, which is then gassed, sealed, and replaced in the incubator. Increased pressure within the desiccator, due to heating and expansion of the equilibration gas mixture, is relieved by opening a stopcock in the top of the desiccator twice, at 10-minute intervals after the start of incubation.

Depending upon the experimental design, porcine oocytes in our laboratory are normally cultured for periods of 24, 33–35, or 48 hours. The shorter culture periods are used in studies to determine the incidence of oocytes that will begin the maturation process under various conditions; whereas the longer culture intervals are employed to obtain information on the requirements of oocytes for development through the later stages of oocyte maturation, particularly the first meiotic division.

D. Examination of Cultured Oocytes

The end point of an oocyte culture experiment is dictated by the intent of an individual investigation, and, in this laboratory, includes cytogenic analysis, ultrastructural examination, and/or molecular analysis. In those investigations in which molecular or ultrastructural analyses are performed on cultured oocytes, representative oocytes are also air-dried for cytogenetic examination in order to assess the incidence of nuclear maturation within the analyzed groups of cultured oocytes.

1. Cytogenetic Examination

The air-drying procedure for examination of oocyte chromatin has been published previously for mouse (McGaughey, and Chang, 1969) and porcine oocytes (McGaughey and Polge, 1971), and it will not be described in detail here. In summary, the oocytes are treated in hypotonic sodium citrate (1%, w/v in water), fixed on microscope slides in ethanolic acetic acid (1 part glacial acetic acid : 3 parts absolute ethanol), allowed to air-dry, stained in basic fuchsin (0.5%, w/v, in water), and mounted under cover slips in Euparol. Generally, the oocytes from an individual culture dish (routinely 10 oocytes) are air-dried on a single slide.

Microscopic examination of air-dried oocytes is performed on a Leitz phase contrast microscope with attachments for 35-mm photography. The examinations are done with an oil-immersion lens at a magnification of 1000 ×. For each microscope slide, each oocyte is classified either as having remained at the germinal vesicle stage, or as having developed beyond the germinal vesicle stage. For the latter category, oocytes are further classified as having reached or completed the first meiotic division (anaphase I to metaphase II). For each slide of oocytes (i.e., one culture dish), the proportion of the total oocytes on the slide which is in each of the above categories is calculated and recorded. The proportionate data are transformed to angles (arcsin $\sqrt{p}$; where p is an individual proportion), using corrections for zero, $p = 1/4 \, n,$ where n is the number of oocytes on the slide, and 100% values, $p = (n-1/4)/n,$ according to Snedecor and Cochran (1967). The angular data are punched on computer cards and processed by the SPSS Oneway Program (Nie *et al.*, 1975), making use of the Duncan Multiple Ranges Test to determine statistical differences among experimental and control groups. Each experimental or control group consists of data from four or more replicate culture dishes (McGaughey, 1977a), and the Oneway Program performs testing for homogeneity of the variances among experimental and control groups.

2. Ultrastructural and Molecular Examination

In experiments in which the ultrastructure of cultured oocytes is to be examined, groups of porcine oocytes are cultured as described in the previous section, but they are fixed for electron microscopy after intervals of culture (McGaughey, 1977c). The primary fixative used in this laboratory is that of Ito and Karnovsky (1968), which includes glutaraldehyde, paraformaldehyde, and picric acid, dissolved in phosphate buffer (Millonig, 1961). Because of the high osmolarity of the above fixative, oocytes are first placed in a solution consisting of 25% (v/v) fixative and 75% (v/v) culture medium. After 10 minutes, additional fixative is added to increase the concentration to 50% fixative; and, after an additional 10 minutes, the oocytes are transferred to 100% fixative. Fixation is continued for an additional 40–60 minutes, after which the oocytes are washed in buffer, postfixed in OsO_4, and dehydrated. Flat embedding is carried out either in Epon or in mixtures of Epon and Araldite. Sectioning is performed with an MT-2 ultramicrotome, and the grids are observed in a Phillips EM300 electron microscope.

Recently, porcine oocytes have been examined for their capacity to synthesize proteins during varied intervals of maturation *in vitro* (McGaughey and Van Blerkom, 1977). The details of applying high-resolution two-dimensional electrophoresis (O'Farrell, 1975) to mammalian embryos are given in a subsequent chapter (Van Blerkom), and basically the same methods are applied in the examination of oocytes.

III. SPECIAL APPLICATIONS

An area of current interest in the field of mammalian oocyte maturation is related to the follicular factors which may be inhibitory to this process *in vivo*. It has been suggested that porcine follicular fluid contains a small molecular weight component that acts to inhibit oocyte maturation (Tsafriri *et al.*, 1976). This reported inhibition has not been confirmed in another study of porcine and bovine follicular fluids (Leibfried, 1976), and data from our laboratory indicate that porcine follicular fluid, diluted in minimal defined medium, does not inhibit the maturation of porcine oocytes in comparison to control oocytes cultured in defined medium (Table III). It is possible that constituents of follicular fluid interact with some component of an undefined, complex culture medium, of the type employed by Tsafriri *et al.* (1976), to cause inhibition of oocyte maturation. It is clear that the question of follicular fluid inhibitory constituents requires further study.

One obvious requirement of a physiological inhibitor of oocyte maturation is that it must act reversibly. In studies of inhibitory substances related to oocyte maturation, experimental groups must be included to determine whether the inhibited oocytes are capable of maturational development after their removal from the inhibitory influence. Such reversible inhibition of oocyte maturation has been demonstrated with estradiol-17β (McGaughey, 1977a). In addition to demonstrating the reversible nature of a steroid inhibitor, the subsequent maturation of mammalian oocytes *in vitro*, after removal from an inhibitory culture medium, indicates that the oocytes remain viable during culture in the inhibitory medium.

Two additional criteria for establishing viability of cultured porcine oocytes have been employed. Ultrastructural examination has been carried out to determine whether oocytes maintain their fine structural integrity during maturation *in vitro* (Fig. 4A,B). In addition, two-dimensional polyacrylamide gel electrophoresis has been employed (McGaughey and Van Blerkom, 1977; Van Blerkom and McGaughey, 1977) to determine the capacity of cultured porcine and rabbit oocytes for synthesis of proteins. Not only are porcine oocytes capable of producing large numbers of polypeptides during maturation *in vitro*, but the patterns of synthesis in these oocytes undergo specific, progressive changes during maturation (Figs. 5,6).

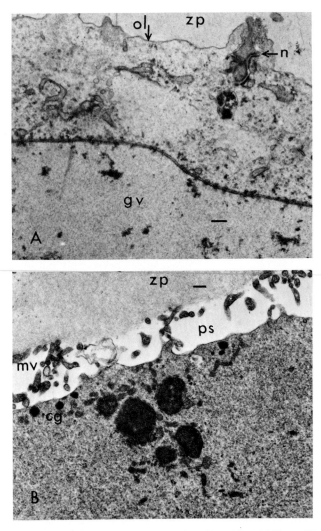

Fig. 4. Electron micrographs of porcine oocytes after 0 hours (A) and 24 hours (B) of culture. It is seen that the zona pellucida (zp) is in contact with the oolemma (ol) of the uncultured oocyte, but that a perivitelline space (ps) has formed in the oocyte undergoing maturation *in vitro*. The oolemma of the uncultured oocyte is relatively smooth compared with that of the cultured oocyte which exhibits large numbers of microvilli (mv). Many nexuslike junctional complexes (n) between the oocyte and granulosa–cell processes are observed in uncultured oocytes. The ooplasm of cultured oocytes is much denser than is that of uncultured oocytes, and cortical granules (cg) can be observed inside the oolemma. The germinal vesicle is designated gv. The bars represent 0.1 μm.

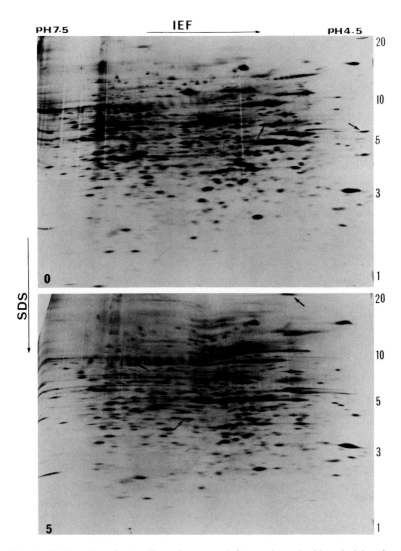

Fig. 5. Photographs of autoradiographs prepared from polyacrylamide gel slabs after two-dimensional electrophoresis of porcine oocytes. The first dimension, isoelectric focusing, is represented by IEF, and the second dimension by SDS. The figure represents a comparison of the polypeptide synthetic patterns of porcine oocytes after 0 hours (above) and 5 hours (below) of culture in minimal, defined medium. The numbers along the right side of the figure refer to molecular weight ($\times 10^4$). The arrows represent major polypeptides, which either appear or disappear between 0 hours and 5 hours of culture. (From McGaughey and Van Blerkom, 1977.)

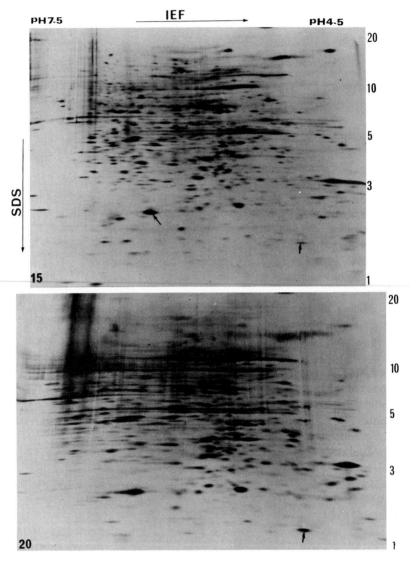

Fig. 6. The patterns of polypeptide synthesis of porcine oocytes after culture for 15 hours (above) or 20 hours (below). See Fig. 5 for additional explanation of this figure. (From McGaughey and Van Blerkom, 1977.)

IV. SUMMARY

The methods described in this chapter can be employed in studies of the physiological controls involved in mammalian oocyte maturation, as well as in investigations of the developmental characteristics of maturing mammalian oocytes. In order to draw meaningful conclusions from such studies, freshly obtained oocytes must be employed, and they must be carefully selected in order to avoid degenerate (i.e., atretic) oocytes. A wide variety of culture media can be employed in studies of oocyte maturation *in vitro;* however, this author believes that the use of minimal, defined medium will allow for the clearest interpretations of data from many experimental designs. In order to evaluate the influence of various culture conditions on mammalian oocytes, cytogenetic, ultrastructural and molecular analyses should be performed on the cultured oocytes, as described in this chapter.

ACKNOWLEDGMENT

The work reported in this chapter was supported in part by Research Grant NIH HD 06532, and by the Arizona State University Faculty Grant-in-Aid program.

REFERENCES

Biggers, J. D. (1972). *In* "Oogenesis" (J. D. Biggers and A. W. Schuetz, eds.), pp. 241–252. Univ. Park Press, Baltimore, Maryland.

Borum, K. (1961). *Exp. Cell Res.* **24**, 495–507.

Brinster, R. L. (1971). *In* "Methods in Mammalian Embryology" (J. C. Daniel, Jr., ed.), pp. 215–227. Freeman, San Francisco, California.

Cowperthwaite, M. H. (1925). *Am. J. Anat.* **36**, 69–89.

Cross, P. C., and Brinster, R. L. (1970). *Biol. Reprod.* **3**, 298–307.

Donahue, R. P. (1972). *In* "Oogenesis" (J. O. Biggers and A. W. Schuetz, eds.), pp. 413–438. Univ. Park Press, Baltimore, Maryland.

Freud, J. (1939). *Acta Brevia Neerl. Physiol., Pharmacol., Microbiol.* **9**, 202–204.

Gwatkin, R. B. L., and Haidri, A. A. (1973). *Exp. Cell Res.* **76**, 1–7.

Ito, S., and Karnovsky, M. J. (1968). *J. Cell Biol.* **39**, 168–169.

Jagiello, G., Ducayen, M., Miller, W., Graffeo, J., and Fang, J. (1975). *J. Reprod. Fertil.* **43**, 9–22.

Jones, E. C., and Krohn, P. T. (1961). *J. Endocrinol.* **21**, 469–495.

Leibfried, J. (1976). *9th Annu. Meet., Soc. Study Reprod.* Abstract No. 121.

McGaughey, R. W. (1975). *Biol. Reprod.* **13**, 147–153.

McGaughey, R. W. (1976). *9th Annu. Meet., Soc. Study Reprod.* Abstract No. 122.

McGaughey, R. W. (1977a). *Endocrinology* **100**, 39–45.

McGaughey, R. W. (1977b). The ultrastructure of porcine oocytes during maturation *in vitro*. (In preparation.)

2

The Experimental Production of Mammalian Parthenogenetic Embryos

MATTHEW H. KAUFMAN

I. INTRODUCTION

Parthenogenesis has been defined as the production of an embryo, with or without eventual development into an adult, from a female gamete in the absence of any contribution from a male gamete (modified after Beatty, 1957). Interest in the production of mammalian parthenogenetic embryos was initiated in the 1930's and early 1940's with the experiments of Pincus and his co-workers with rabbit eggs. Further studies on rabbit and rodent eggs were reported by Thibault in the 1940's, by Austin and Braden and also by Chang in the 1950's, and more recently by Graham and Tarkowski in the 1970's. A complete review of the literature in the field of mammalian parthenogenesis will not be given, but extensive background information on the subject has been provided by Beatty (1957, 1967, 1972), Austin (1961), Austin and Walton (1960), Tarkowski, (1971, 1975), Graham (1974), and Kaufman (1975a). A few of the more important recent contributions in this area of research are also indicated in the relevant sections of the text. In this chapter, emphasis is placed largely on the methodology of activation and production of parthenogenetic mouse embryos. The mechanisms of action of the various stimulating agents, and other aspects of early development, are dealt with only briefly. The importance of this material in providing a new approach to investigating problems associated with early mammalian development are indicated, and some future lines of research are suggested.

II. CULTURE METHODS RELEVANT TO *IN VITRO* PARTHENOGENETIC ACTIVATION

A. Choice of Medium

Krebs-Ringer bicarbonate or Tyrode's solution supplemented with bovine serum albumin, with lactate, pyruvate, and glucose as energy sources have been found adequate for parthenogenetic activation by most workers. The main advantage of this type of medium is that it has a known chemical composition, which probably facilitates biochemical analysis on embryos. These media can also maintain preimplantation development to the blastocyst stage *in vitro* of certain strains of activated eggs that are not subject to the "2-cell block." The addition of serum and the use of more complex biologic media are not essential and may give a greater variability in results, and may indeed be detrimental in this system.

Protein-free stock solutions of embryo culture medium should be prepared at weekly or at most 2- to 3-weekly intervals. Lactate and pyruvate are essential energy substrates, and pyruvate is labile and undergoes spontaneous decarboxylation in dilute solution. Glucose is also generally added to culture media and may help to improve the developmental potential of the activated embryos, especially for prolonged culture of activated 1-cell eggs to the blastocyst stage, as well as serving as an additional energy substrate. A detailed study of the energy requirements of preimplantation mouse embryos has been given by Biggers (1971) and Whittingham (1971). A few of the defined embryo culture media that have been successfully used in various *in vitro* parthenogenetic activation studies are Whittingham's medium (Whittingham, 1971—favored by Kaufman), modifications of White's medium (see Graham, 1970), and Whitten's medium (Whitten, 1971—favored by Graham).

Details of methods for the preparation of culture media are to be found in many sources, but reference should be made to the papers by Whitten and Biggers (1968), Biggers *et al.* (1971), and Whittingham (1971). The latter two papers also provide information on routine preimplantation embryo culture work, which are equally suitable for parthenogenetic studies. For most purposes, particularly where long-term embryo culture is contemplated, a McIntosh and Fildes pattern anaerobic jar gassed with humidified 5% CO_2 in air, or 5% CO_2, 5% O_2, 90% N_2, and incubated at 37°C, is adequate. When frequent observations on embryos in culture are required, such as in studies on the entry of embryos into the first cleavage division (Kaufman, 1973a,b), a continuous-flow incubation chamber is preferable, but not absolutely essential.

When only a limited amount of technical assistance is available, it is probably safer to use disposable plastic petri dishes, which are specifically recommended for tissue culture work (e.g., Falcon plastic petri dishes, Cat. No. 3002), rather than embryologic watchglasses or glass petri dishes if these items cannot be washed to the high standard which is essential for reliable embryo culture work. Eggs and embryos are cultured in drops of medium under light paraffin oil according to the method originally described by Brinster (1963).

B. Choice of Animals

The activation frequency achieved depends as much on the strain of mice employed, whether they are inbred or randomly bred or F_1 hybrids, as on the culture conditions or the type of stimulus applied to eggs *in situ*. It is also possible to obtain parthenogenetic activation of some mutant strains of mice (e.g., Bpa, see Phillips and Kaufman, 1974). High rates of activation and development may also be achieved when oocytes isolated from females that are heterozygous for particular translocations are activated (e.g., T6/+, see Kaufman and Sachs, 1975). Eggs isolated from XO mice are also readily activated (M. H. Kaufman, unpublished).

There seems little evidence for impaired preimplantation development in haploid and diploid parthenogenetic embryos that may possess an additional X chromosome or autosome, or a segment of one or other of these chromosomes. Equally, these genetically unbalanced parthenogenetic embryos appear to be capable of development beyond implantation, but generally die shortly thereafter. Haploid embryos that lack complete autosomes or segments of autosomes probably die during the preimplantation period, but they are capable of development at least up to the 2- or 4-cell stage (Kaufman and Sachs, 1975).

Graham and Deussen (1974) and Iles *et al.* (1975) have shown that the effect of strain variation alone is sufficient to account for striking differences in response of eggs of the same postovulatory age to similar *in vitro* "activating" conditions (see Tarkowski, 1975, for detailed discussion on the effect of genetic constitution on induced parthenogenesis). The original literature should be consulted for details of strain of mice employed, as this may indicate the types of parthenogenones induced, and the activation frequency which might be expected under a given set of circumstances. This should serve only as a very approximate guide, as some variation in this kind of study is to be expected between different laboratories.

F_1 hybrids have been found to be most suitable, especially when the maternal strain is C57BL. Whitten and Biggers (1968) demonstrated that fertilized embryos from various F_1 hybrids were capable of development from the 1-cell stage to the blastocyst *in vitro*. Similar high rates of development of *in vitro* activated eggs have recently been reliably achieved with (C57BL × CBA)F_1 and (C57BL × CBA-T6T6)F_1 hybrid eggs (Kaufman and Sachs, 1975, 1976).

Unfortunately, for most other stocks of mice, development in culture usually ceases after the first cleavage division, which normally occurs about 12–20 hours following activation. Development progresses to the 2-cell stage for all types of parthenogenones except those that undergo "immediate cleavage" or "delayed cleavage" (the "delayed immediate cleavage" described by Graham, 1971), which normally cleave to the 4-cell stage by this time. Further development of these eggs is achieved only when activated eggs are transferred to the ampullary region of the oviduct of a pseudo-pregnant recipient (for details, see Tarkowski, 1959). A convenient timing schedule for these procedures, normally used by this author, is as follows: spontaneously ovulating females are mated to vasectomized males on the afternoon or evening before the activation experiment is to be carried out; females are checked the next morning for evidence of mating, and oviduct transfers carried out early in the afternoon of finding the vaginal plug, that is on day 1 of pseudopregnancy. Uterine transfers of morulae or blastocysts are usually carried out in the morning or afternoon of day 3 of pseudopregnancy. Activation is normally carried out between 8:00 and 9:00 A M and pronuclear eggs selected at about 2:00 P M for immediate transfer to recipients. Batches of between 5 and 10 or more activated eggs, depending on the availability of activated eggs and recipients, are transferred to the oviducts of lightly anesthetized recipients. The anesthetic usually used for this procedure is tribromoethanol (Avertin:Winthrop). The standard dose of a freshly prepared 1.2% solution of Avertin dissolved in 0.9% NaCl is 0.02 ml Avertin/gm body weight. Other workers advocate Nembutal or ether anesthesia. As it is likely that all anesthetics are capable of inducing a proportion of the recipient's own eggs to develop parthenogenetically (Kaufman, 1975b), it may be advisable in certain critical experiments to use genetic or biochemical markers for one or other stock of mice (e.g., see Kaufman and Sachs, 1975). It is well to be aware that this factor may complicate, for example, interpretation of implantation rates not only in parthenogenetic studies, but also where fertilized embryos are transferred under similar circumstances. This complication does not arise when embryos are transferred to day 3 recipients, as the recipient's own eggs are no longer capable of being activated parthenogenetically.

III. ISOLATION OF EGGS FROM SUPEROVULATED AND SPONTANEOUSLY OVULATING FEMALES

A. Superovulation

The main advantage of superovulation is that large synchronous populations of eggs can be obtained at the convenience of the experimenter, and that the time of ovulation can be accurately assessed to within about an hour. However, there are often considerable variations in the response of different strains of mice to superovulation treatment (see Gates, 1971, for discussion). It will almost certainly be necessary to try different hormone regimens when untested stocks are to be employed. The injection of 1–5 or even 10 IU PMSG followed 48 hours later by 1–5 or 10 IU HCG will usually provide large numbers of eggs, and receptive females which will mate with sterile or fertile males if this is required. While one hormone regimen may induce the ovulation of particularly large numbers of eggs, another, usually smaller, dose may synchronize estrus and encourage a higher proportion of the hormonally induced population to mate. Ovulation occurs in most strains between 11 and 12 hours after the HCG injection for superovulation, and the time of the HCG injection provides a very useful baseline for most *in vitro* and *in vivo* studies. Some strains of mice respond poorly to exogenous hormone treatment, and, in these cases, eggs should be obtained from spontaneously ovulating females.

Some controversy exists over the supposed inferiority of superovulated compared to spontaneously ovulated eggs (see Elbling, 1973). However, most authorities consider that the general convenience and availability of large numbers of eggs that can usually be obtained following superovulation probably far outweighs the possible detrimental effect of the hormone treatment. The poorer pregnancy outcome in superovulated females is attributed either to "crowding effects" within the uterus, or to hormonal imbalance. For *in vitro* parthenogenetic studies, however, 1-cell eggs are normally isolated from the ampullary region of the oviduct into embryo culture medium.

B. Spontaneous Ovulation

Spontaneously ovulating mice at a suitable stage of the estrous cycle can be selected by vaginal inspection using the criteria outlined by Champlin *et al.*, (1973). This technique is usually extremely reliable, and normally well over half the females selected on the afternoon or evening of proestrous ovulate that night. While fewer eggs are generally obtained from spontaneously ovulating females, only the very occasional degenerating or fragmented egg is normally found within the cumulus mass. This, however, has to be balanced with the advantages of superovulation outlined above.

When oocytes are isolated from spontaneously ovulating females, it is essential to note the mid-dark point of the lighting schedule in the animal room in which the mice are normally kept, as this gives a reasonable indication of the time of ovulation (Braden, 1957). This, in addition, provides a convenient baseline value for certain timing studies (see Kaufman, 1975b).

IV. REACTION OF EGGS TO PARTHENOGENETIC STIMULATION

Most mammalian eggs are ovulated at metaphase of meiosis II, and these only complete second meiosis if activated by appropriate stimuli. Under normal conditions *in vivo*, the activation stimulus is provided by the fertilizing spermatozoon, but it seems likely that a series of biochemical events which closely resemble this type of activation can be induced by a wide range of stimuli. Not only is meiosis resumed in this case, but, under optimal conditions, parthenogenetic embryonic development may proceed well beyond implantation, possibly even to the birth of viable offspring.

Following parthenogenetic activation eggs progress along different developmental routes, depending on whether the second polar body had been extruded or not, whether cytokinesis results in the production of blastomeres of equal or unequal volume, and on whether haploid or diploid nuclei are formed at the various meiotic divisions (Beatty, 1957, 1967). The different routes of early development are illustrated in Fig. 1.

At the completion of second meiosis, which usually occurs within about 2–3 hours of activation, second polar body extrusion normally occurs. Under certain experimental conditions, this may be the commonest type of reaction seen. If, instead of extruding the second polar body, the egg divides into two equal blastomeres, this is referred to as "immediate cleavage" (Braden and Austin, 1954a). If cytokinesis does not occur at the completion of second meiosis, either two haploid pronuclei or a single diploid pronucleus develops within about 4–5 hours of activation.

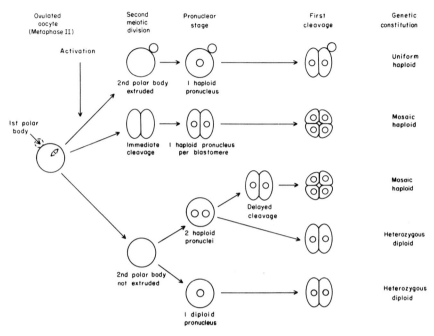

Fig. 1. Possible routes of development and genetic constitution of parthenogenetically activated eggs. (From Kaufman and Sachs, 1976.)

Confusion may arise in certain strains of mice in determining the different types of parthenogenones induced due to the persistence of the first polar body. In some strains, the first polar body disperses or lyses soon after ovulation, whereas in others it may persist for many hours and, thus, may be confused with the second polar body. When the first and second polar bodies are both present, they are usually morphologically quite dissimilar in appearance, the cytoplasm of the second polar body looking the healthier of the two.

Pronucleus formation usually commences within a few hours of the completion of meiosis II. The incidence of the different types of parthenogenones observed at this time depends on the strain of mouse employed, the postovulatory age of the oocyte at the time of activation, the culture conditions at and during the first few hours following activation, and, to an extent, the type of stimulation employed.

Under normal conditions, the single pronucleus, or two pronuclei that form contain either the exact haploid, or diploid number of chromosomes. Unequal chromosome segregation may occur, for example, as a result of nondisjunction or chromosome lagging. The incidence of these events probably varies from strain to strain, or may result from the experimental conditions at the time of activation. The oocyte may extrude small cytoplasmic fragments, or one or many subnuclei may be formed in addition to the presence of one or more "pronuclei." Subnuclei usually contain one or several chromosomes, so that when these are present the egg is likely to have an aneuploid karyotype. Most of these anomalous events are probably due to suboptimal conditions at or following activation.

Only in the immediate cleavage and delayed cleavage types of eggs are the two chromosome sets genetically dissimilar as a result of crossing-over events at meiosis I. Here, the two blastomeres give rise to two genetically different clones of cells, and this has accordingly been termed mosaic haploid development (Kaufman and Sachs, 1976). When a single haploid pronucleus forms following second polar body extrusion, a single clone of cells results, and this has been termed uniform haploid development. When a single diploid pronucleus forms, or the contents of two haploid pronuclei amalgamate at the first cleavage metaphase, the resultant embryo will be homozygous at some loci and heterozygous at others. The extent of homozygosity or heterozygosity will be dependent on the chiasma frequency. Uniform diploid parthenogenetic development would only occur in embryos with two haploid or a single diploid pronucleus in the unlikely event that the chiasma frequency was zero. This type of embryo may, however, be induced experimentally when the first cleavage division of uniform haploid embryos is inhibited.

V. EFFECT OF POSTOVULATORY AGING OF THE OOCYTE ON THE ACTIVATION FREQUENCY AND TYPES OF PARTHENOGENONES INDUCED

Detailed observations on the effect of the postovulatory age of the oocyte at the time of activation (usually referred to as hours after spontaneous ovulation, or hours after the HCG injection for superovulation— ovulation occurs about 11–12 hours after HCG) have been presented by Kaufman (1973c). This study demonstrated that the activation rate tended to rise with an increase in the postovulatory age of oocytes. Thus, when oocytes were released from the oviduct at 14 hours after HCG into culture medium containing hyaluronidase and the cumulus-denuded eggs transferred to enzyme-free medium 5–10 minutes later, no eggs were activated. At 16, 18, and 20 hours after HCG, an increasing proportion of oocytes became activated, reaching a maximum of between 75 and 85% at 18–20 hours after HCG (see Fig. 2). The majority of the stimuli which are capable of activating oocytes *in vitro* show a similar type of response. A similar pattern has also been observed when oocytes are stimulated *in situ* with Avertin anesthesia (Kaufman, 1975b). However, when eggs are stimulated *in situ* by an electric shock, or *in vitro* by heat shock, activation of more recently ovulated eggs (up to and including HCG + 16

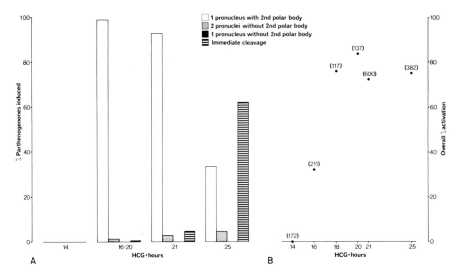

Fig. 2. Effect of postovulatory aging of the oocyte on (A) the incidence of the various types of parthenogenones induced and (B) the activation frequency. Eggs from (C57BL × A₂G)F₁ female mice were examined at approximately 6–8 hours after hyaluronidase treatment, and the total number examined in each group given in parentheses. (Data from Kaufman, 1973c; Kaufman and Surani, 1974.)

hours) may be achieved, though the incidence of fragmentation, and atresia is often quite high. If eggs are stimulated beyond about 13 hours after ovulation has occurred (beyond HCG + 25 hours), an increased incidence of fragmentation and atresia is to be expected beyond that normally found when eggs within the range HCG + 18–24 are activated. A slight increase in the proportion of apparently healthy pronuclear eggs which fail to progress beyond the first cleavage division may also be observed.

In addition, a different pattern is usually seen in the incidence of the various types of parthenogenones induced when eggs are activated at different times after ovulation. This is probably related to the migration of the second meiotic spindle from the periphery to the center of the egg, which tends to occur with postovulatory aging of the oocyte (see Szollosi, 1971). This central migration probably explains the high incidence of immediate cleavage and the slight but significant increase in the number of eggs observed in which one of two pronuclei form in the absence of second polar body extrusion. Reducing the osmolarity of the culture medium immediately after activation (Graham and Deussen, 1974; Kaufman and Surani, 1974) and activating eggs in medium lacking calcium and/or magnesium ions (Kaufman et al., 1977; Surani and Kaufman, 1977) are other methods of altering the incidence of the various types of parthenogenones induced.

Further observations on the effect of aging on the activation frequency have been reported by Kaufman (1975a), who treated batches of freshly ovulated (HCG + 14.5–15.0 hours) and more aged (C57BL × $A_2G)F_1$ eggs (HCG + 21.5–22.0 hours) for 10–15 minutes with 0.15% pronase in phosphate-buffered saline. Half of the eggs had been pretreated with hyaluronidase to remove cumulus cells. In the earlier time group, no activation occurred, whereas in the later time group very high rates of activation were observed (98–99%). A single pronucleus developed following second polar body extrusion in the majority of the activated eggs.

The general observation that oocytes tend to be more readily activated with increased postovulatory aging is probably also related to changes in the metabolism of the egg. The cumulative effect of these aging changes appears to be inversely related to the ease with which eggs may undergo normal monospermic fertilization and is presumably also related to the increased incidence of abnormal fertilization seen with gamete aging (Marston and Chang, 1964; Austin, 1970).

VI. BASIC TECHNIQUES

The basic techniques that have been employed recently for inducing mouse oocytes to develop parthenogenetically may for convenience be divided into two major groups, depending on whether oocytes are (a) isolated from the oviduct and stimulated *in vitro*, or (b) stimulated *in situ* within the oviduct of an anesthetized animal (*in vivo* techniques).

A. *In Vitro* Activation

1. *Stimulation Induced by Handling Alone When Oocytes Are Released into Standard Embryo Culture Medium*

In many strains of mice, the stimuli involved in handling oocytes during their isolation from the oviduct and release into suitable embryo culture medium may be sufficient to induce a high proportion of eggs to initiate parthenogenetic development. The factors involved when oocytes are stimulated by handling alone may include mild mechanical disturbance of the vitelline membrane, or possibly chemical stimulation such as may result from a change in the pH, temperature, or even chemical composition of their microenvironment. The proportion of eggs that may become activated under these circumstances varies considerably and seems largely to depend on the strain involved and on the postovulatory age of the oocyte at the time of activation. This latter factor will not only influence the overall activation frequency, but it will also tend to modify the proportionate incidence of the different types of parthenogenones observed.

A similar type of response is usually observed when activation is induced by handling or following enzyme stimulation, though the activation frequency tends to be higher when oocytes are stimulated in the presence of hyaluronidase. Thus, about 45–65% of oocytes from several strains of mice isolated at about 18–19 hours after HCG became activated in response to handling alone (Kaufman and Surani, 1974; Kaufman et al., 1977; M. H. Kaufman, unpublished), compared to an activation frequency of 70–75% when eggs from similar strains were activated in the presence of hyaluronidase.

2. The Effect of Releasing Oocytes into Medium Lacking Calcium and/or Magnesium Ions

The chemical composition of the culture medium appears to be one of the major factors which can influence not only the activation frequency, but also the incidence of the different types of parthenogenones (Surani and Kaufman, 1977). The type of response obtained when cumulus masses from (C57BL $\times$ A$_2$G)F$_1$ hybrid mice isolated at about 18 hours after the HCG injection for superovulation were released into standard embryo culture medium (Whittingham, 1971) lacking Ca^{2+} and/or Mg^{2+} is presented in Fig. 3. The eggs were examined about 5 hours after the cumulus masses had been released into the various culture media. To facilitate observation on oocytes at this time, the cumulus masses were incubated for 5–10 minutes in medium containing hyaluronidase to denude the eggs of adherent follicle cells. The activation frequency and the incidence of the various types of parthenogenones could then be assessed.

When eggs were cultured in medium lacking calcium and magnesium, the activation frequency was similar to that observed in the control group (standard medium) and in the medium lacking calcium alone. A considerably higher activation frequency was observed when eggs were cultured in medium lacking magnesium alone, but the explanation for this finding is not immediately apparent. In standard medium and medium lacking Ca^{2+} and/or Mg^{2+}, the incidence of the various types of parthenogenones obtained varied considerably (see Fig. 3).

In the control group, the majority of the activated eggs developed a single haploid pronucleus following second polar body extrusion, whereas in the Ca^{2+} and Mg^{2+}-free medium as well as in the medium lacking Ca^{2+} alone, only a small proportion of the eggs were of this type. A corresponding increase was observed in the eggs which either failed to extrude a polar body (i.e., those which developed either two haploid or a single diploid pronucleus) or those which underwent immediate cleavage. In the medium in which Ca^{2+} was present but Mg^{2+} absent, an intermediate response was obtained.

When (C57BL $\times$ CBA)F$_1$ eggs which had been activated in medium lacking Ca^{2+} and Mg^{2+} were retained in culture for up to 100 hours in standard medium, a moderate proportion of the haploid and diploid parthenogenones developed to the blastocyst stage. Highest rates of development were observed in the 2-pronuclear type where about 50–60% of the eggs developed to the blastocyst

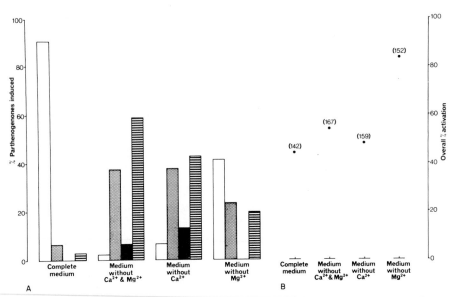

Fig. 3. (A) Incidence of different types of parthenogenones induced and (B) activation rate when eggs were activated in complete medium, and medium lacking Ca^{2+} and/or Mg^{2+}. Cumulus masses from (C57BL × A_2G)F_1 female mice were released into various media at 18 hours after HCG, and observations made 5–6 hours later. Coding for different routes of development following activation same as for Fig. 2. (Data from Surani and Kaufman, 1977.)

stage *in vitro* (Kaufman *et al.*, 1977; M. H. Kaufman, unpublished). These diploid parthenogenetic blastocysts were transferred to a single uterine horn of day 3 pseudopregnant recipients previously mated to vasectomized males. The recipients were bilaterally ovariectomized immediately after transfer of blastocysts and thereafter maintained on exogenous steroid hormones. After an initial hormone-free period of 2 days, recipients were maintained for 4 days on 1 mg progesterone daily, during which time blastocysts presumably enter into quiescence. Implantation was initiated by injecting 20 ng estradiol along with progesterone for 3 days, and, thereafter, pregnancy was maintained with 8 ng estradiol and 1.6 mg progesterone daily per female.

Implantation commenced about 24 hours after the initial injection of estradiol, which is equivalent to about day 5 of pregnancy, and recipients were killed at intervals between the 6th and 11th day of "pregnancy". About 80% of the transferred blastocysts implanted, 35–40% developed to the egg cylinder stage (see Fig. 4), and 25% to somite embryos. All implantation sites up to day 9 were immediately fixed in Bouin's solution and examined histologically. After day 8 of "pregnancy," embryos were dissected from the uterus and examined under a dissecting microscope. The two most advanced embryos obtained were at the

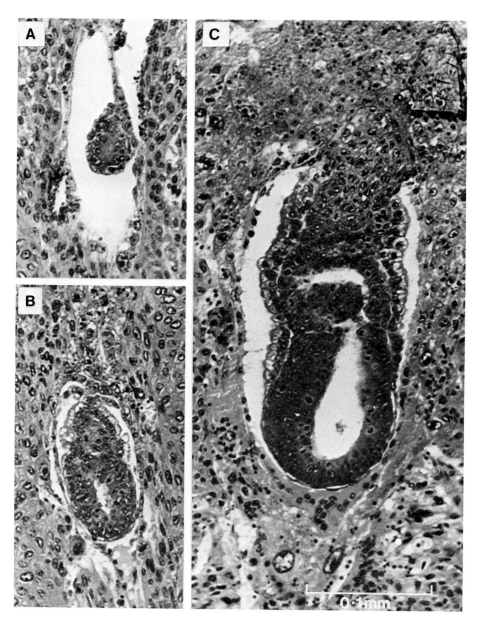

Fig. 4. Different stages of early postimplantation development of diploid (2-pronuclear type) parthenogenetic embryos following the transfer of (C57BL × CBA)F$_1$ blastocysts to the uteri of pseudopregnant recipients. Egg cylinder stages approximately equivalent to days (A) 5, (B) 6, and (C) 7 of gestation. The scale bar represents 0.1 mm and is the same for all three embryos.

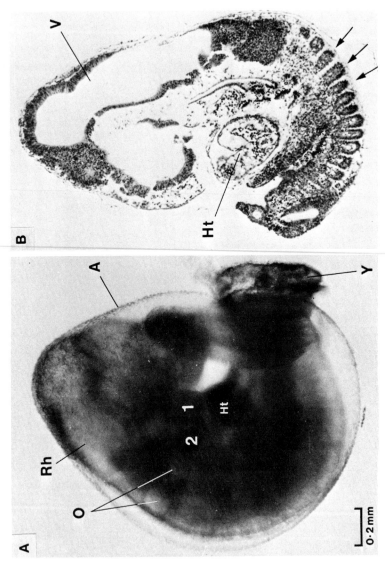

Fig. 5. (A) Parthenogenetic mouse embryo with about 25 somites photographed within its amnion, unfixed preparation. (B) Near-sagittal section of embryo in (A) showing large number of well-formed somites (arrowed). Embryo fixed in Bouin's solution about 4 hours after isolation from the uterus. Scale bar represents 0.2 mm. 1 and 2, First and second branchial bars: O, otic vesicle; Ht, heart; Rh, rhombencephalon with fourth ventricle; A, amnion; Y, yolk sac; V, fourth ventricle. (From Kaufman *et al.*, 1977.)

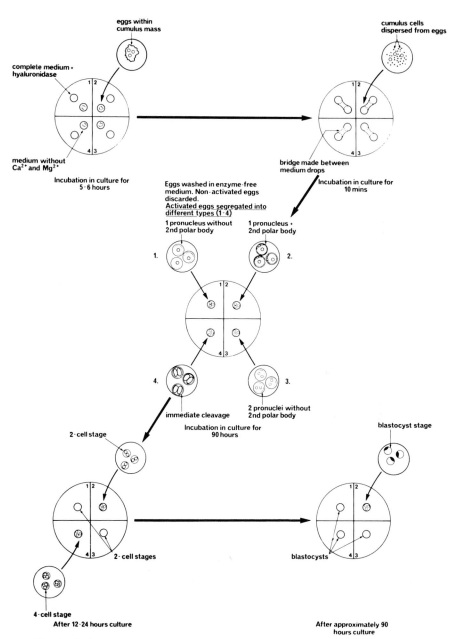

Fig. 6. Basic technique for obtaining complete development *in vitro* to the blastocyst stage following activation of eggs in medium lacking Ca^{2+} and Mg^{2+}. Approximate timing of the different stages is indicated.

forelimb-bud stage on the 11th day of "pregnancy"; both had about 25 somites and were apparently healthy with beating hearts and a good yolk sac circulation at the time of isolation from the uterus. These embryos were later fixed for histology (see Fig. 5). Development of presumptive haploid embryos to the advanced egg cylinder stage has also been achieved using a similar experimental approach (Kaufman, 1978). Because of the effectiveness of this activation technique, the various *in vitro* stages involved are illustrated diagrammatically in Fig. 6.

The activation induced by handling described here is not comparable to, and should not be confused with, spontaneous activation. This phenomenon occurs only infrequently in the mouse but quite commonly in the hamster (Austin, 1956; Yanagimachi and Chang, 1961; Longo, 1974). However, in the hamster spontaneous development has not been observed to progress beyond the 2-cell stage, though studies in which hamster oocytes *in situ* were stimulated by electric shock treatment demonstrated that parthenogenetic development to the blastocyst stage could be achieved in this species (Kaufman *et al.*, 1975).

3. Hyaluronidase Activation

Graham (1970) demonstrated that a high proportion of mouse oocytes could be activated *in vitro* if they were incubated in culture medium containing hyaluronidase for a sufficient time to denude the oocytes of adherent cumulus cells. Mouse oocytes were released into simple embryo culture medium kept initially at 5°C, and hyaluronidase crystals were added until a final concentration of about 100 IU/ml of the enzyme was present. After about 5 minutes, the cumulus-free eggs were isolated; washed several times in enzyme-free medium; then cultured at 37°C under 5% CO_2, 5% O_2, 90% N_2 for varying periods of time. A proportion of the activated eggs developed to the morula and blastocyst stage, but, as the parthenogenones had not been segregated into their various types at the pronuclear stage, the developmental potential of the individual types could not be assessed.

The basic technique may be simplified by the prior addition of hyaluronidase to the embryo culture medium to achieve a final concentration of between 100 and 300 IU/ml. Secondly, the period of incubation in hyaluronidase medium may be carried out at 37°C in either the same gas mixture employed by Graham, or under 5% CO_2, 95% air (see Kaufman, 1973c). The concentration of hyaluronidase in the medium and the duration of exposure to this enzyme do not appear to be critical. In various studies (M. H. Kaufman, unpublished observations), exposure for about 10 minutes (range 5–20 minutes) has usually resulted in high rates of activation. Eggs should be washed once or twice in enzyme-free medium before transfer to drops of similar medium under light paraffin oil for long-term culture. When activation is carried out as described above, second polar body extrusion usually occurs within about 2–3 hours, and pronuclear formation within about 4–5 hours. Entry of parthenogenones into the first cleavage division occurs at about 12–14 hours after activation. Mitosis in the haploids lasts about 2½ hours compared with about 2 hours in fertilized eggs of the same strain (Kaufman, 1973b). However, it is likely that the exact timing of these events will vary slightly from one strain of mouse to another.

When oocytes from a single source were activated by the two techniques outlined in this section, similar rates of activation were obtained (see Graham and Deussen, 1974).

4. Effect of Culture of Cumulus-Denuded Oocytes in Hypo- and Hypertonic Medium Directly after Hyaluronidase Treatment

The osmolarity of the medium in which eggs are cultured during the first few hours following activation plays an important part in influencing the incidence of the different types of parthenogenones obtained and may also, in some strains, influence the activation frequency. The pattern of activation obtained in one series of experiments when hyaluronidase-treated oocytes were cultured for 2¼ hours in media whose measured osmolarity ranged between 0.168 and 0.402 OsM (Kaufman and Surani, 1974) is illustrated in Fig. 7. In this study, hypotonicity was achieved by diluting the culture medium with distilled water (see Graham, 1971, 1972) and hypertonicity by the addition of solid sodium

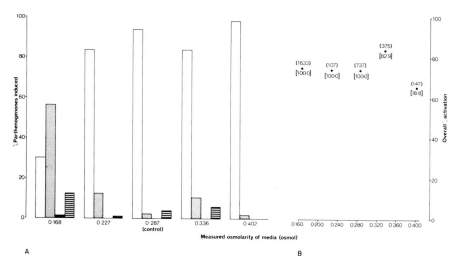

Fig. 7. Effect of incubation for 2¼ hours in media of different osmolarities directly after hyaluronidase activation on (A) the incidence of the various types of parthenogenones induced, and (B) the activation frequency. Eggs from (C57BL × A₂G)F₁ female mice were isolated at 20–21 hours after HCG and observations made 6–8 hours later. The total number of eggs examined in each group is given in parentheses, and the cleavage rate at 24 hours in brackets. Coding for different routes of development same as for Fig. 2. (Data from Kaufman and Surani, 1974.)

chloride to the medium. Little difference was observed in the overall activation frequency between the control and the experimental treatment groups. In similar studies by Graham and Deussen (1974), an increase in the activation frequency, compared to control levels, was observed in some strains of mice when eggs were cultured in hypotonic media. It is unclear whether these differences were due to strain variation or differences in experimental technique.

As may be seen from Fig. 7, the most obvious effect of culturing eggs in low osmolar medium (0.168 OsM) was to increase the incidence of 2-pronuclear eggs from about 3% to 56% of the activated population. A moderate increase was also seen in the incidence of eggs undergoing immediate cleavage. An intermediate effect was observed when eggs were cultured in 0.227-OsM medium.

Apart from the slight effect on the incidence of the different types of parthenogenones induced when oocytes were cultured in hypertonic media compared with the control pattern, the main effect appeared to be on development. All of the activated oocytes in the control and low osmolar series developed to the 2-cell stage in culture compared with 83% and 19% of the activated eggs cultured in 0.336- and 0.402-OsM medium, respectively.

Culturing eggs in hypotonic (0.168 OsM) medium does not appear to have a detrimental influence on their pre- or early postimplantation development as 50–56% of the 2-pronuclear type successfully implanted following transfer at the pronuclear stage to the oviducts of suitable recipients (Kaufman and Gardner, 1974). When similar eggs were isolated on day 4, 59% of these diploid parthenogenones appeared to be morphologically normal morulae or blastocysts.

5. The Effect of Heat Shock

Two recent studies have investigated the effect of heat shock on mouse oocytes *in vitro*. In the first study (Komar, 1973), excised oviducts containing superovulated (HCG + 14.5–17.5 hours), and spontaneously ovulated ova from "A" strain and Swiss Albino females were subjected to a heat shock of 43°–45.5°C lasting for 5–10 minutes. The excised oviducts were placed in a test tube containing 0.5 ml Ringer's solution, and the tube was immersed in a thermostatically controlled water bath set at various temperatures between 43° and 45.5°C for 5, 7½, or 10 minutes. The oviducts were then transferred to medium and retained in culture for either 5–10 hours to assess the activation rate, or for 4 days to assess their development potential. Highest rates of activation were observed (57.0%) when oviducts were maintained at 44°–44.5°C, although 37.7% of the activated eggs contained subnuclei. Slightly higher rates of activation were observed when eggs were exposed to temperatures ranging from 43°–45.5°C for 5 minutes compared to groups heated for 7½ or 10 minutes. At all temperatures tested, haploid eggs predominated over diploid. After 4 days in organ culture, 15.4% of the heat-treated eggs that were recovered had developed to the morula or blastocyst stage, compared with 57.4% of fertilized eggs cultured under similar conditions. As only 5.8% of the eggs recovered in the parthenogenetic series, and 30.7% of the eggs in the fertilized series had developed to the blastocyst stage by this time, it suggests that the culture conditions employed were suboptimal.

In a more recent study, Balakier and Tarkowski (1976), using a similar technique to that employed by Komar (1973), activated superovulated Swiss Albino and C57BL/10 eggs and spontaneously ovulated A strain eggs *in vitro* by a heat shock of 44°C for 5 or 7½ minutes. After the heat shock, eggs with the cumulus mass intact were isolated from the oviducts and cultured in Whitten's medium (Whitten, 1971) containing 10 μg/ml of Cytochalasin B for 5–8 hours. The cumulus cells were then removed with hyaluronidase and the eggs transferred to Cytochalasin-free medium for a further period of 1–4 hours. The activation frequency was then assessed. In a control series activated in the absence of Cytochalasin B, and in an experimental group cultured in the presence of this agent, about 70% of Swiss Albino eggs were successfully activated. About 40% of C57BL and 90% of A strain eggs were also activated in the presence of Cytochalasin B. This agent suppressed second polar body extrusion in over 90% of the activated eggs, with the majority containing two pronuclei. The development potential of these eggs was assessed following their transfer to the oviducts of pseudopregnant recipients. Two healthy looking egg cylinders were found on the 8th and 9th days of gestation out of a total of 41 implants. Both embryos appeared to be retarded and were at a stage characteristic for the 7th day of normal gestation.

This second study indicates that under optimal conditions heat shock *in vitro* is an effective means of obtaining parthenogenetic development beyond implantation. This study also demonstrates the value of Cytochalasin B for inhibiting early cleavage. This agent had previously been shown to be effective in inhibiting the second cleavage division of fertilized eggs, with the production of tetraploid embryos (Snow, 1973). In the present context, it is likely that this agent may provide one means of inhibiting the first cleavage division of uniform haploid embryos with the production of homozygous as opposed to heterozygous diploid embryos.

6. Activation Induced by Ionophore

Steinhardt and Epel (1974) demonstrated that exposure of sea urchin eggs to the divalent ionophore A23187 induced a cortical reaction indistinguishable from that initiated by sperm. This event was associated with elevation of the "fertilization membrane," a respiratory burst, an increase in protein and DNA synthesis, and typical plasma membrane conductance changes. Subsequent studies with sea urchin, *Xenopus*, and hamster oocytes (Steinhardt *et al.*, 1974) demonstrated that the ionophore was capable of inducing activation in all three species.

A 5 mM stock solution of A23187 was prepared in dimethyl sulfoxide and stored in the dark. When the stock solution was diluted for use with oocytes, continuous stirring was required to ensure good mixing, since the ionophore is insoluble in water and some precipitation tends to occur. Final concentrations of the ionophore are, therefore, maximum estimates.

Hamster eggs were isolated from randomly bred superovulated females at 15–17 hours after HCG. The eggs were freed from cumulus cells by treatment for 15 minutes with 0.1% hyaluronidase (300 IU/ml), then rinsed thoroughly in Ca^{2+}- and Mg^{2+}-free culture medium in which the albumin was replaced with 0.2% polyvinylpyrrolidone, and the pH adjusted to 7.3. Highest rates of activation were achieved when oocytes were exposed to a 3-μM concentration of the ionophore in Ca^{2+}- and Mg^{2+}-free medium throughout the incubation period. Continuous exposure to concentrations above 10 μM were detrimental to the eggs. Brief exposure to 3- to 10-μM concentrations of the ionophore (2 minutes), followed by culture in Ca^{2+} and Mg^{2+}-free medium was also effective. The majority of eggs showed cortical granule breakdown within 30 minutes, and well-developed pronuclei were formed within 2 hours. However, protein synthesis was not maintained, mitosis was delayed, and cleavage, if it took place, was abnormal (Steinhardt and Epel, 1974; Steinhardt et al., 1974).

To date, no information has been published on the effect of the ionophore on mouse eggs in culture. Pretreatment with hyaluronidase to remove cumulus cells would be less acceptable in this species, where this enzyme is capable of inducing high rates of activation in the absence of the ionophore. However, this would not apply to recently ovulated eggs (HCG + 12–14 hours), which are usually resistant to stimulation by this enzyme.

B. *In Vivo* Activation

Various experimental techniques have been employed which are capable of inducing mouse eggs to develop parthenogenetically *in situ*, within the oviduct of the anesthetized animal. The two activation methods which have so far been most rigorously investigated are (1) electric shock applied to the eggs within the ampullary region of the oviduct of anesthetized animals (Tarkowski *et al.*, 1970), and (2) the use of anesthesia alone, without surgical intervention (Kaufman, 1975b). A third method has also been employed, namely, heat shock to the eggs within the exteriorized oviduct of anesthetized mice (Braden and Austin, 1954a). This approach gave reasonable rates of activation, but little further information is available on this technique beyond the original description. Indirect information is, however, available on its effect on the oocyte from experiments which investigated the effect of heat shock applied to eggs shortly after mating (Braden and Austin, 1954b).

Under certain experimental conditions, the anesthesia necessary to carry out the first and third techniques indicated above may complement the stimuli involved in electric shock or heat shock treatment. Similarly, in electric shock treatment, local heating of the tissues may play a role in the activation process. These factors complicate interpretation of the findings and assessment of the underlying mechanisms involved.

1. Electric Shock

Tarkowski *et al.* (1970) were the first to report the successful use of electric shock stimulation to activate mouse eggs *in situ*. Eggs within the ampullary region of the oviduct were stimulated by a single electric shock produced from an 8-μF capacitor charged through a rectifier from an ac source of 30, 40, or 50 V, with an automatic "charge–discharge" switch. The oviducts were brought to the exterior through a dorsolateral incision, and the current was passed across the ampullary region using the tips of two steel needles as electrodes. All females were anesthetized with Nembutal (0.01 ml/gm body weight of a 6 mg/ml solution).

Groups of mice from the A, CBA-p, and CBA-T6T6 inbred strains were anesthetized with Nembutal either at 14–16 hours after the HCG injection for superovulation, or between 8:00 AM and 11:00 AM in the case of spontaneously ovulating females. Mice were examined 4–10 hours after electric stimulation to assess the immediate effects of this procedure, and at daily intervals until the 10th day of pregnancy (day of finding vaginal plug = day 1 of pregnancy). In preliminary experiments, operations were performed unilaterally to assess any influence of the anesthetic, but, as no eggs from the control oviducts showed signs of activation, later operations were performed bilaterally. The results of this and a further similar series of experiments have been described in great detail by Witkowska (1973a,b). All of the types of parthenogenones illustrated in Fig. 1 were observed. In addition, in about 8–10% of the activated eggs second polar body extrusion failed to occur, and more than two nuclei were seen (presumed to be subnuclei).

The activation rate in the spontaneously ovulated eggs was about 50%, compared with approximately 40% in the superovulated group, with the majority of the activated eggs developing a single haploid pronucleus following second polar body extrusion. The incidence of degenerated, nonactivated, and activated classes was related to the voltage used, with the highest activation frequency occurring when a 40-V shock was applied. With a stronger current, the number of degenerated eggs increased, while the number of nonactivated eggs decreased. Rates of implantation were relatively high, especially in the spontaneously ovulating A-strain females, where between a quarter and a third of the activated eggs survived until implantation. When results from the three strains of mice and experiments using different voltages are pooled, the implantation rate for the whole series was about 0.7 implantations per horn.

Twelve out of 19 of the implantation sites examined on days 6 and 7 contained egg-cylinder stage embryos, but the mortality increased rapidly when implants were examined on the 8th through 10th days of pregnancy. On the 9th day, a single healthy egg-cylinder embryo was found out of a total of 81 implants examined, and on the 10th day a single morphologically normal 8-somite embryo was found out of 16 implants examined (data from Table 3, Witkowska, 1973b).

The main advantage of this technique is that, under optimal conditions, moderate rates of postimplantation development, at least to the egg-cylinder stage, may be expected to occur when relatively freshly ovulated eggs are stimulated by an electric shock. Its main limitation is that it does not allow an assessment of the development potential of different types of parthenogenetic embryos to be made, as a mixed population of haploid and diploid embryos are induced.

This technique, with suitable modifications (up to 20 or 25 50-V shocks may be required) was found to be effective in stimulating hamster eggs to develop to the morula and blastocyst stage (Kaufman et al., 1975), though it is likely that local heating of the tissues may have influenced the outcome of these experiments. In a previous study, Gwatkin et al. (1973) demonstrated that the cortical granules in electrically stimulated hamster eggs disappeared rapidly after the stimulus was applied and that the zona reaction was also induced.

Studies on spontaneous and induced parthenogenetic activation suggest that there may be considerable variation in the incidence of cortical granule breakdown under different in vivo and in vitro conditions (spontaneous activation in the hamster, see Austin, 1956; Longo, 1974; cold-shock-induced activation in rabbit eggs, see Flechon and Thibault, 1964; Longo, 1975; hyaluronidase-induced activation in mouse eggs, see Solter et al., 1974), and that it would be inappropriate at this stage to draw general conclusions from the results obtained with one technique or from a single species.

Mintz and Gearhart (1973) demonstrated that parthenogenetic embryos induced by electric stimulation showed a response in the time taken to dissolve the zona pellucida with a dilute pronase solution intermediate between that seen in unfertilized and fertilized eggs. However, the significance of these observations on the development potential of parthenogenones remains to be established.

2. Effect of Anesthesia

Various authors have demonstrated that rodent eggs may be induced to develop parthenogenetically in situ when intact animals are anesthetized after ovulation has occurred. Thus, rat eggs have been activated parthenogenetically with ether (Thibault, 1949; Austin and Braden, 1954), chloroform, ethyl chloride, ethyl alcohol, paraldehyde, nitrous oxide, and intraperitoneal (ip) Nembutal (Austin and Braden, 1954), and mouse eggs with ether (Braden and Austin, 1954a) and ip Avertin (Kaufman, 1975b). Apart from the study with Avertin, where postimplantation development was obtained, previous workers had only reported the occasional development of these eggs as far as the 2- or 4-cell stage. While only the Avertin experiments will be discussed in detail here, it seems likely that a range of anesthetics given at an appropriate time after ovulation are probably also capable of inducing mouse eggs to develop parthenogenetically beyond implantation.

In a recent study (Kaufman, 1975b), spontaneously ovulating and superovulated (C57BL $\times$ A$_2$G)F$_1$ hybrid mice were killed about 24 hours after anesthesia with tribromoethanol (Avertin: Winthrop, dose 0.02 ml/gm body weight of a freshly prepared 1.2% solution of Avertin dissolved in 0.9% saline). In both groups of females, an increasing activation frequency was observed when anesthesia was carried out at about 6.5, 9, and 13 hours after ovulation, reaching a maximum of about 46%. No activation was induced when females were anesthetized at about 4 hours after ovulation, 7% were activated at 6.5 hours, and 17% at 9 hours after ovulation. Both the activation rate and the incidence of the various types of parthenogenones induced was related to the postovulatory age of eggs at the time of anesthesia, and a pattern of response was observed similar to that seen when mouse eggs were activated *in vitro* by handling alone, or following activation with hyaluronidase (Kaufman and Surani, 1974).

In a spontaneously ovulating group of females anesthetized about 13 hours after ovulation, approximately 13% of all the eggs ovulated, or 27% of all the eggs activated, survived until implantation. Preliminary studies had demonstrated that the majority of the eggs activated in this time group were undergoing immediate cleavage, so that it is likely that most of the embryos which implanted were haploid in origin.

3. Effect of Heat Shock

Braden and Austin (1954a) observed that about 50% of spontaneously ovulated mouse eggs had initiated parthenogenetic development when these were examined 4–5 hours after heat shock had been applied to the oviduct *in situ*. Mice were anesthetized with Nembutal about 8–12 hours after ovulation, a dorsolateral incision made in the body wall, and the ovaries and oviducts brought to the exterior and immersed for 5–10 minutes in a water bath maintained at 44–45°C. Most of the activated eggs developed a single haploid pronucleus following extrusion of the second polar body. A few eggs underwent immediate cleavage, and a single egg developed two pronuclei in the absence of a second polar body. A few 2- and 4-cell eggs were isolated 48–70 hours after heat-shock stimulation.

In a similar study, Braden and Austin (1954b) investigated the effect of hot shock applied to eggs 3 hours after mating. This increased the incidence of polyspermy (dispermy) from 0.3% to 3.8%, and of eggs exhibiting suppression of second polar body formation from 0.5% to 12.4%. This study also confirmed earlier observations of Fischberg and Beatty (1952) that triploidy could result from dispermy or from suppression of second polar body formation (digyny). In Fischberg and Beatty's (1952) series, a single 6-cell haploid egg was isolated which was probably parthenogenetic in origin.

C. Microsurgical Methods for Obtaining Nonparthenogenetic Haploid Embryos

Two promising experimental techniques have recently been described which allow a limited degree of haploid development to be initiated. Both methods require a considerable degree of microsurgical skill and have yet to be fully evaluated. Modlinski (1975) has obtained haploid embryonic development to the blastocyst stage following the microsurgical removal of one pronucleus from fertilized mouse eggs, while Tarkowski and Rossant (1976) have also obtained advanced preimplantation development when fertilized 1-cell eggs were bisected and transferred to the oviducts of suitable recipients following the insertion of these fragments into empty zonae pellucida.

Attempts have also been made (Graham, 1970) to produce chimeras by the aggregation of parthenogenetic and fertilized 8-cell embryos and morulae, and survival to term of definite chimeric individuals by this means has recently been reported by Stevens *et al.* (1977). When the inner cell masses of diploid parthenogenones were inserted microsurgically into intact fertilized blastocysts that were subsequently transferred to pseudopregnant recipients, the development to term of chimeric embryos with contributions from parthenogenetically-derived and fertilized cells was also successfully achieved (Surani, Barton, and Kaufman, 1977).

D. Parthenogenetically Derived Spontaneous Ovarian Tumors in LT Strain Mice

Another potential source of parthenogenetic cells is the LT strain of mice, which has a high incidence of spontaneous parthenogenetic development of ovarian oocytes to apparently normal egg cylinder or primitive streak stage embryos (Stevens and Varnum, 1974; Stevens, 1975). Subsequent growth of parthenogenones is disorganized, and both teratomas and teratocarcinomas are often found in the ovaries of these mice. Spontaneously activated eggs may also be recovered from the oviduct and uterus in this strain, and were used in the experiments of Stevens *et al.* (1977) described above.

VII. CONCLUSIONS

With the availability of experimental methods which give high rates of parthenogenetic activation, and, in some cases, development beyond implantation, it seems likely that rapid advances in our understanding of the activation process and the factors which influence early mammalian development can be expected within the next few years. Even the limited advances that have been achieved in the few months prior to the writing of this chapter have necessitated a radical reevaluation of the importance of certain embryologic and genetic factors which were generally thought to play an essential role in controlling mammalian embryonic development. For example, it is almost certain that we will have to reexamine our ideas as to the precise role of sperm and the importance of X chromosome activity in development (Kaufman et al., 1978).

While a high proportion of mouse parthenogenones undoubtedly die in the early postimplantation period possibly as a result of intrinsic deficiencies within the embryonic genome, the recent demonstration that a few parthenogenetic mouse embryos were capable of surviving at least to the forelimb-bud stage (Kaufman *et al.*, 1977) suggests that improved methods of activation and greater control over the hormonal status of the recipient may allow a higher proportion of embryos to survive beyond implantation, possibly even to term.

While there have been several attempts to obtain parthenogenetic cell lines from the "growths" which develop when parthenogenetic embryos are transferred to ectopic sites (Graham, 1970; Iles *et al.*, 1975), the establishment of a stable haploid mammalian cell line has yet to be achieved. However, the apparently normal morphology of the somite-stage diploid parthenogenetic embryos recently described by Kaufman *et al.* (1977, and unpublished observations), coupled with the considerable range of cell types identified in the growths described above, and the observations of Van Blerkom and Runner (1976), which suggest that parthenogenetic blastocysts are similar at the ultrastructural level to normal fertilized blastocysts, are all extremely encouraging signs.

Parthenogenetic embryos would be particularly valuable in the analysis of many early developmental processes, as they would allow the complex events which take place at activation, during the pre- and early postimplantation period, and during morphogenesis and organogenesis in haploid and diploid parthenogenones to be compared with similar events in fertilized embryos. The availability in the near future of haploid and diploid mammalian parthenogenetic cell lines will also be of great value for studies in developmental biology, genetics, and carcinogenesis.

It is hoped that the methods described in this chapter for achieving high rates of activation and advanced parthenogenetic development will encourage embryologists, geneticists, and biochemists to avail themselves of this potentially extremely valuable but largely unexploited source of material.

ACKNOWLEDGMENT

The author's techniques described in this chapter have largely been developed under grants from the Ford Foundation to Professor C. R. Austin.

.REFERENCES

Austin, C. R. (1956). *Exp. Cell Res.* **10**, 533–540.

Austin, C. R. (1961). "The Mammalian Egg." Blackwell, Oxford.

Austin, C. R. (1970). *J. Reprod. Fertil., Suppl.* **12**, 39–53.

Austin, C. R., and Braden, A. W. H. (1954). *Aust. J. Biol. Sci.* **7**, 195–210.

Austin, C. R., and Walton, A. (1960). *In* "Marshall's Physiology of Reproduction" (A. S. Parkes, ed.), Vol. 1, Part 2. Longmans, Green, New York.

Balakier, H., and Tarkowski, A. K. (1976). *J. Embryol. Exp. Morphol.* **35**, 25–39.

Beatty, R. A. (1957). "Parthenogenesis and Polyploidy in Mammalian Development." Cambridge Univ. Press, London and New York.

Beatty, R. A. (1967). *In* "Fertilization" (C. B. Metz and A. Monroy, eds.), Vol. 1, pp. 413–440. Academic Press, New York.

Beatty, R. A. (1972). *In* "Oogenesis" (J. D. Biggers and A. W. Schuetz, eds.), pp. 277–299. Univ. Park Press, Baltimore, Maryland.

Biggers, J. D. (1971). *J. Reprod. Fertil., Suppl.* **14**, 41–54.

Biggers, J. D., Whitten, W. K., and Whittingham, D. G. (1971). *In* "Methods in Mammalian Embryology" (J. C. Daniel, Jr., ed.), pp. 86–116. Freeman, San Francisco, California.

Braden, A. W. H. (1957). *J. Exp. Biol.* **34**, 177–188.

Braden, A. W. H., and Austin, C. R. (1954a). *Exp. Cell Res.* **7**, 277–280.

Braden, A. W. H., and Austin, C. R. (1954b). *Aust. J. Biol. Sci.* **7**, 552–565.

Brinster, R. L. (1963). *Exp. Cell Res.* **32**, 205–208.

Champlin, A. K., Dorr, D. L., and Gates, A. H. (1973). *Biol. Reprod.* **8**, 491–494.

Elbling, L. (1973). *Nature (London)* **246**, 37–39.

Fischberg, M., and Beatty, R. A. (1952). *J. Genet.* **50**, 455–470.

Flechon, J. E., and Thibault, C. (1964). *J. Microsc. (Paris)* **3**, 34.

Gates, A. H. (1971). *In* "Methods in Mammalian Embryology" (J. C. Daniel, Jr., ed.), pp. 64–75. Freeman, San Francisco, California.

Graham, C. F. (1970). *Nature (London)* **226**, 165–167.

Graham, C. F. (1971). *Adv. Biosci.* **6**, 87–97.

Graham, C. F. (1972). *Adv. Biosci.* **8**, 263–277.

Graham, C. F. (1974). *Biol. Rev. Cambridge Philos. Soc.* **49**, 399–422.

Graham, C. F., and Deussen, Z. A. (1974). *J. Embryol. Exp. Morphol.* **31**, 497–512.

Gwatkin, R. B. L., Williams, D. T., Hartmann, J. F., and Kniazuk, M. (1973). *J. Reprod. Fertil.* **32**, 259–265.

Iles, S. A., McBurney, M. W., Bramwell, S. R., Deussen, Z. A., and Graham, C. F. (1975). *J. Embryol. Exp. Morphol.* **34**, 387–405.

Kaufman, M. H. (1973a). *J. Cell Sci.* **12**, 799–808.

Kaufman, M. H. (1973b). *J. Cell Sci.* **13**, 553–566.

Kaufman, M. H. (1973c). *Nature (London)* **242**, 475–476.

Kaufman, M. H. (1975a). *In* "The Early Development of Mammals" (M. Balls and A. E. Wild, eds.), pp. 25–44. Cambridge Univ. Press, London and New York.

Kaufman, M. H. (1975b). *J. Embryol. Exp. Morphol.* **33**, 941–946.

Kaufman, M. H. (1978). *J. Embryol. Exp. Morphol.* (In press.)

Kaufman, M. H., and Gardner, R. L. (1974). *J. Embryol. Exp. Morphol.* **31**, 635–642.

Kaufman, M. H., and Sachs, L. (1975). *J. Embryol. Exp. Morphol.* **34**, 645–655.

Kaufman, M. H., and Sachs, L. (1976). *J. Embryol. Exp. Morphol.* **35**, 179–190.

Kaufman, M. H., and Surani, M. A. H. (1974). *J. Embryol. Exp. Morphol.* **31**, 513–526.

Kaufman, M. H., Huberman, E., and Sachs, L. (1975). *Nature (London)* **254**, 694–695.

Kaufman, M. H., Barton, S. C., and Surani, M. A. H. (1977). *Nature (London)* **265**, 53–55.

Kaufman, M. H., Guc-Cubrilo, M., and Lyon, M. F. (1978). *Nature (London)* (In press.)

Komar, A. (1973). *J. Reprod. Fertil.* **35**, 433–443.

Longo, F. J. (1974). *Anat. Rec.* **179**, 27–56.

Longo, F. J. (1975). *J. Exp. Zool.* **192**, 87–112.

Marston, J. H., and Chang, M. C. (1964). *J. Exp. Zool.* **155**, 237–252.

Mintz, B., and Gearhart, J. D. (1973). *Dev. Biol.* **31**, 178–184.

Modlinski, J. A. (1975). *J. Embryol. Exp. Morphol.* **33**, 897–905.

Phillips, R. J. S., and Kaufman, M. H. (1974). *Genet. Res.* **24**, 27–41.

Snow, M. H. L. (1973). *Nature (London)* **244**, 513–515.

Solter, D., Biczysko, W., Graham, C., Pienkowski, M., and Koprowski, H. (1974). *J. Exp. Zool.* **188**, 1–23.

Steinhardt, R. A., and Epel, D. (1974). *Proc. Natl. Acad. Sci. U.S.A.* **71**, 1915–1919.

Steinhardt, R. A., Epel, D., Carroll, E. J., and Yanagimachi, R. (1974). *Nature (London)* **252**, 41–43.

Stevens, L. C. (1975). *Sym. Soc. Dev. Biol.* **33**, 93–106.

Stevens, L. C., and Varnum, D. S. (1974). *Dev. Biol.* **37**, 369–380.

Stevens, L. C., Varnum, D. S., and Eicher, E. M. (1977). *Nature (London)* **269**, 515–517.

Surani, M. A. H., and Kaufman, M. H. (1977). *Dev. Biol.* **59**, 86–90.

Surani, M. A. H., Barton, S. C., and Kaufman, M. H. (1977). *Nature (London)* **270**, 601–603.

Szollosi, D. (1971). *Am. J. Anat.* **130**, 209–226.

Tarkowski, A. K. (1959). *Acta Theriol.* **2**, 251–267.

Tarkowski, A. K. (1971). *J. Reprod. Fertil.,Supp.* **14**, 31–39.

Tarkowski, A. K. (1975). *Symp. Soc. Dev. Biol.* **33**, 107–129.

Tarkowski, A. K., and Rossant, J. (1976). *Nature (London)* **259**, 663–665.

Tarkowski, A. K., Witkowska, A., and Nowicka, J. (1970). *Nature (London)* **226**, 162–165.

Thibault, C. (1949). *Ann. Sci. Nat., Zool. Biol. Anim.* [*11*] **11**, 133–219.

Van Blerkom, J., and Runner, M. N. (1976). *J. Exp. Zool.* **196**, 113–124.

Whitten, W. K. (1971). *Adv. Biosci.* **6**, 129–139.

Whitten, W. K., and Biggers, J. D. (1968). *J. Reprod. Fertil.* **17**, 399–401.

Whittingham, D. G. (1971). *J. Reprod. Fertil., Suppl.* **14**, 7–21.

Witkowska, A. (1973a). *J. Embryol. Exp. Morphol.* **30**, 519–545.

Witkowska, A. (1973b). *J. Embryol. Exp. Morphol.* **30**, 547–560.

Yanagimachi, R., and Chang, M. C. (1961). *J. Exp. Zool.* **148**, 185–203.

Manipulation of Ploidy in the Mouse

ANNA NIEMIERKO AND JOLANTA OPAS

Studies of the development of haploid and polyploid embryos can contribute to the understanding of the mechanisms of normal embryonic development. Since spontaneous polyploidy in mammals is rare, attempts to produce polyploidy experimentally have been undertaken for a long time (for review of older literature, see Beatty, 1957, 1972), but it has not been until quite recently that real progress has been made in this field. It is now possible to obtain routinely haploid, triploid, tetraploid, and $2n/4n$ mosaic blastocysts, at least in the mouse.* In fact, the mouse is the most convenient experimental animal for

*Most of the methods described in this chapter have been developed in the laboratory of Prof. A. K. Tarkowski, to whom the authors are most grateful.

producing haploidy and polyploidy because *in vitro* techniques, which are essential in manipulating of egg ploidy, have been developed primarily for mouse eggs.

If not stated otherwise, standard techniques of egg recovery and handling of culture *in vitro* are followed. In all the methods described in this chapter, experimental treatment is applied to the eggs *in vitro*, after which the eggs may be either cultured *in vitro* (see Biggers *et al.*, 1971) or transplanted to recipients (see Tarkowski, 1971).

Two general comments are to be made before going into details. First, all the methods concerned require that at the time of treatment the eggs are in a precisely defined stage. Since timing is given in this chapter for a few strains only, it is necessary that the experiments be preceded by timing of the desired stage in the strain one works with. Second, determination of ploidy at the one-cell stage is not always accurate. For example, the tripronucleate state may sometimes be transient and the egg develops into a diploid or haplodiploid mosaic embryo. One must remember, therefore, that karyological analysis is the only way to prove ploidy of the embryo. For karyological analysis of preimplantation stages, the methods of Tarkowski (1966) or Fujimoto *et al.* (1975), and of postimplantation stages the method of Evans *et al.* (1972) are advised.

I. HAPLOIDY

Haploid parthenogenetic embryos have been experimentally produced and studied for some years (see Chapter 2 by Kaufman). Obtaining haploid embryos from fertilized, pronucleate eggs offers somewhat different opportunities: (1) one deals with "normal" cytoplasm which had undergone all physiological changes in the course of fertilization; (2) one can obtain androgenetic haploid embryos, which makes it possible to study the role of a male-derived genome, especially that with Y chromosome, in development.

In this chapter, two microsurgical methods of obtaining haploid embryos from fertilized eggs will be described.

A. Microsurgical Removal of One Pronucleus*

Modliński (1975) has developed a method of removal of one pronucleus from the fertilized mouse egg. Among somewhat different variants of his method, the one in which the pronucleus is destroyed by removing the nuclear membrane seems the most promising. It involves the use of a very thin pipette (1 μm in diameter) which improves the survival rate of operated eggs (up to 50% as

---

*We are indebted to Dr. J. A. Modliński for his consultation in preparing this section.

opposed to about 30% in eggs enucleated by removal of the whole pronucleus). The embryos developed from operated eggs are haploid when examined karyologically. Up to 40% of the haploid eggs which survive the operation develop to the 5th day.

1. Obtaining Eggs

The early pronuclear stage is the most convenient for these experiments because in this stage both pronuclei are located near the egg surface where they are clearly visible. It is possible to distinguish the male from the female pronucleus on the basis of their relative position and size, the female pronucleus being closer to the second polar body and smaller than the male one.

If the eggs are collected from spontaneously ovulating females kept under a 16-hour light/8-hour dark cycle centered on midnight, the optimal time for operation is between 10:00 A.M. and 1:00 P.M. Eggs can be also collected from delayed controlled matings as described in Section II,A,1,a. These reach the proper stage 6–7 hours after mating.

2. Microsurgical Procedure

The eggs, after being released from cumulus cells with hyaluronidase, are placed in groups of four to eight in a drop of culture medium. The drop is laid on the bottom of the chamber (for instance, a slide with a well), filled with liquid paraffin. The choice of culture medium is not of crucial importance, but it is convenient to use a phosphate-buffered medium (Whittingham and Wales, 1969), which does not change pH in contact with air. Two instruments are introduced into the chamber: a wide mouth-controlled pipette used for holding the egg and a micropipette (1 μm in diameter) for removing the nuclear membrane. Schematic representation of the system is shown in Fig. 1. Details of preparation of pipettes are not given here, as they are sufficiently described by Lin (1971).

The instruments are fixed onto a mechanical micromanipulator (for example,

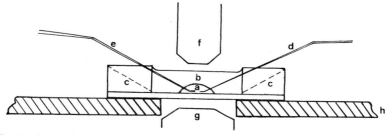

Fig. 1. Schematic representation of the operation chamber and the tools for enucleation of mouse eggs: (a) drop of medium containing eggs; (b) liquid paraffin; (c) chamber; (d) micropipette; (e) mouth-controlled pipette for holding the egg; (f) objective 16 ×; (g) condenser; (h) microscope stage. (Courtesy of Dr. J. A. Modliński.)

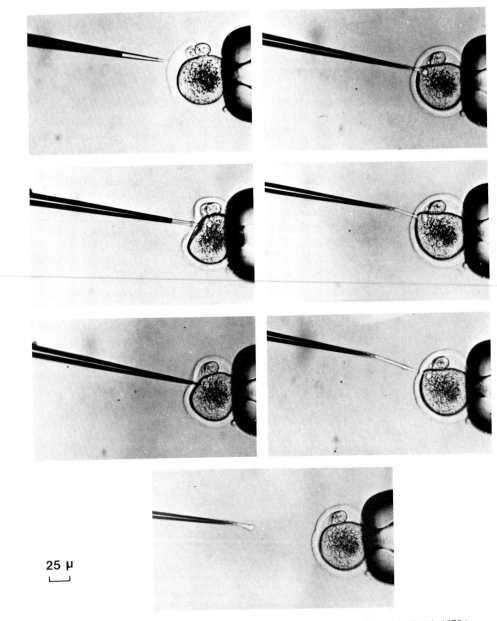

25 μ

Fig. 2.   Enucleation of mouse egg by removal of nuclear membrane. (From Modliński, 1975.)

Carl Zeiss, Jena) connected with a microscope (for example, NfpK, Carl Zeiss, Jena). The micropipette is connected by a Teflon tube with an extraction and injection syringe (for example, of de Fonbrune type, Beaudouin). The whole system, except the very tip of the micropipette, is filled with liquid paraffin.

After the egg has been immobilized by a mouth-controlled pipette, the micropipette is inserted into the egg so that its tip lies close to one pronucleus. The pronuclear membrane is then aspirated to the tip of the micropipette and drawn out of the egg. The membrane is quite elastic and becomes a long protrusion filled with the content of the pronucleus, which does not rupture until the moment when tightly packed nucleoli "cork" the opening in the egg. The sequence of events is shown in Fig. 2. The nucleoli disappear within 15 minutes after the operation. It is better to perform the operation at room temperature rather than at 37°C, as mechanical resistance of eggs seems higher at lower temperatures. If an egg is going to degenerate, it usually does so within 10–15 minutes after operation. Eggs that survive this period very rarely degenerate later.

B. Bisection of Fertilized Eggs

This method, as opposed to the former one, does not require sophisticated devices or prolonged training. Eggs are cut into halves with a glass needle operated by hand. Fifty to 100% of eggs survive operation, and up to 29% of halves developed into blastocysts *in vitro* (Tarkowski, 1977). It seems worthwhile to call attention to two implications of producing haploid embryos by bisection. First, this method offers unique opportunity to produce simultaneously andro- and gynogenetic haploid embryos derived from the same egg. Second, egg halves have a normal nucleocytoplasmic ratio, thus being comparable with normal diploid eggs in this respect.

1. Obtaining Eggs

Eggs from spontaneous or induced ovulation may be used, but the first source is recommended, as egg halves from spontaneously ovulated eggs develop much better. Bisection may be performed throughout the whole 1-cell stage, but it is convenient to use eggs with big, clearly visible pronuclei. In F_1 (C57 × CBA/H) females mated to CBA-T6T6 males, such eggs are obtained between 3:00 and 5:00 PM. Cumuli oophori are removed by hyaluronidase and zonae pellucida are dissolved by pronase.

2. Bisection

The operation is performed under dissecting microscope (magnification about 50 times). It is convenient to maintain a low temperature, about 4°C, with the help of a cool stage during the operation. If this is not possible, the petri dish should be precooled in a refrigerator.

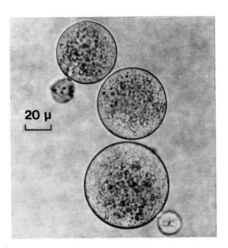

Fig. 3. Egg-halves produced by bisection of fertilized egg. Intact zona-free egg shown for comparison. (Courtesy of Prof. A. K. Tarkowski.)

Cold phosphate-buffered salt solution with 0.1% bovine serum albumin is added to a petri dish covered with 1% agar in 0.6% NaC1, and a group of 5–10 eggs is placed there. Glass needles of a width equal to one-third to one-fourth of the egg diameter should be prepared; these can be easily made by hand over a microburner. The tip of the glass needle is lightly touched to the agar near an egg, and the needle is pressed down so that it squashes the egg between the pronuclei. Complete separation of halves (Fig. 3) may be achieved in this way, but often the halves remain connected by the cytoplasmic bridge. In the latter case, separation is achieved by repeating the operation or by vigorous pipetting.

After separation, the halves may be cultured *in vitro* or may be transplanted to empty zonae pellucida and transferred to recipients (Tarkowski and Rossant, 1976). Transplantation to the zona pellucida (Rossant, 1975) is a sophisticated manipulation, however, and its description is beyond the scope of this chapter.

II. TRIPLOIDY

Both digynic and dispermic triploidy in mammals can be induced experimentally. Attempts to induce dispermic triploidy are summarized by Bedford (1971), who also described successful production of triploidy in the rabbit (Bomsel-Helmreich, 1965) and in the rat (Piko and Bomsel-Helmreich, 1960). For an extensive review on triploidy in the rabbit, see Bomsel-Helmreich (1971).

Digynic triploidy in the mouse is produced by applying experimental agents at the time of the second polar body extrusion, which leads to the incorporation of the second polar body nucleus into the egg as the third pronucleus.

A. Induction of Triploidy by Cytochalasin B (CB)

When applied to the oocytes *in vitro* at 5–10 μg/ml concentration, CB inhibits cytokinesis of the second maturation division. Oocytes fertilized *in vivo* and then treated with CB *in vitro*, as well as those fertilized *in vitro* in the presence of CB, become triploid in a high percentage.

1. Oocytes Fertilized in Vivo

The method yields up to 80% of tripronucleate eggs among fertilized ones, 30–50% of which develop into morulae and blastocysts, and the latter are able to implant (Niemierko, 1975).

a. Obtaining Eggs. Spontaneously ovulated eggs fertilized in delayed and controlled matings are used. When working with delayed matings, the light/dark cycle should be properly adjusted to minimize the interval between ovulation and mating, as the fertilization rate decreases with the postovulatory age of eggs. Mice kept under a 16-hour light/8 hour dark cycle centered on midnight were placed with males at 7:00 A.M. and checked for vaginal plugs every 20–30 minutes until 10:00 A.M.

In A females mated to A males, eggs may be subjected to CB between 2.5 and 3.5 hours postcoitum. By manipulation of the interval between mating and subjecting the eggs to CB within this range, varying proportions of diploid, presumably triploid, and unfertilized eggs can be obtained. When the interval is short, all fertilized eggs become tripronucleate, but many remain unfertilized. When the interval is long, all eggs are fertilized, but many of them are diploid. All three groups coexist when the interval is intermediate.

b. Preparation of CB Medium. To prepare the medium containing 5 or 10 μg of CB/ml, 0.5 ml or 1 ml of the stock CB solution is added to 100 ml of culture medium [for example, Whitten's medium (Whitten, 1971)]. The stock solution of CB is obtained by dissolving 10 mg CB in 10 ml of dimethylsulfoxide (DMSO).

c. Experimental Procedure. The most convenient method of treating the eggs with CB is as follows: (1) the fallopian tube is placed in a drop of CB medium under liquid paraffin; (2) the eggs in cumulus oophorus are released by piercing the ampulla with a needle; (3) the empty fallopian tube is removed from the drop. As penetration of CB into the eggs is not impaired by the presence of cumulus cells, they are left intact. Culture of eggs in CB medium should last 5–7 hours. When the culture period is shorter than 5 hours, many eggs undergo surface changes after transferring them to CB-free medium.

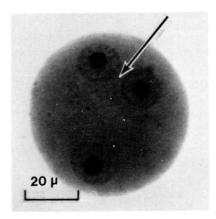

Fig. 4.   Tripronucleate egg produced by CB treatment. Pronuclei lie close to the egg surface. Arrow indicates two female pronuclei. Permanent preparation. (From Niemierko, 1975.)

d. Classification of Eggs.   After 5–7 hours of culture, fertilized eggs are surrounded by few cumulus cells as opposed to unfertilized ones which have compact cumulus. A drop of hyaluronidase is added to the culture drop to remove cumulus cells so that the eggs become clearly visible.

Since the eggs transferred from CB medium to pure medium react by surface wrinkling which lasts 0.5–1 hour, it is recommended that presumed ploidy be determined in CB medium. Classification of eggs is not difficult because the pronuclei occupy a characteristic position; they lie immediately underneath the egg surface (Fig. 4). Thus, even in the eggs with nontransparent cytoplasm, the number of pronuclei and the presence of the second polar body can be determined. For preliminary classification, the examination of eggs under a dissecting microscope is sufficient, but examination under an inverted microscope will allow more accurate observation.

Before transplantation or other manipulation, a thorough washing of eggs in CB-free medium is necessary.

2. Oocytes Fertilized in Vitro

Niemierko and Komar (1976) developed a method of inducing triploidy in eggs exposed to CB during fertilization *in vitro*. Since in this technique mating is not included and ovulation is induced hormonally, it is possible to collect a large number of eggs for each experiment. As much as 80–90% of tripronucleate eggs are obtained among fertilized ones.

a. Fertilization Medium with CB.   The composition of the medium is shown in Table I (after Toyoda *et al.*, 1971). Fresh medium should be prepared every week. CB is added to this medium according to the procedure given in

TABLE I

Composition of the Medium for *In Vitro* Fertilization
of Mouse Eggs[a]

Component	Amount (gm/liter)	mM
NaCl	6.976	119.37
KCl	0.356	4.78
$CaCl_2 \cdot 2 H_2O$	0.251	1.71
KH_2PO_4	0.162	1.19
$MgSO_4 \cdot 7 H_2O$	0.293	1.19
$NaHCO_3$	2.106	25.07
Na pyruvate	0.110	1.00
Glucose	1.000	5.56
Bovine albumin	4.000	
Streptomycin sulfate	0.050	
Penicillin potassium	0.075	

[a]Toyoda et al., 1971.

Section II,A,1,b. The concentration of CB applied is also 5 μg/ml. At this concentration, CB does not impair penetration of eggs by sperm. Higher concentration (10 μg/ml) decreases the fertilization rate.

b. Obtaining Eggs. Females are induced to ovulate by ip injection of 5 IU each of PMSG and HCG given 48 hours apart. The eggs are collected between 13 and 16 hours post-HCG. The highest fertilization rate is usually obtained when eggs are harvested 13 hours post-HCG. The eggs are released from the oviducts in the same way as described in Section II,A,1,c. Eggs from up to 10 females are placed in 0.4 ml of CB medium under liquid paraffin.

c. Obtaining Sperm. The suspension of sperm is prepared by suspending a dense mass of sperm, squeezed from the cauda epididymis and vas deferens of an adult male, in 0.4 ml of CB-free medium under liquid paraffin. The sperm suspension is then incubated for 15 minutes at 37°C to become homogenous. Stirring of the suspension should be avoided because this damages sperm. It is advisable to prepare separate sperm suspensions from two to three individuals and to choose the one showing least signs of agglutination (homogenous, whitish, opalescent). When 0.04 ml of this suspension are added to the drop containing eggs, the final concentration of spermatozoa is close to the optimal one, which is 2200–2500/mm³.

d. Classification of Eggs. The number of pronuclei and the presence of the second polar body are determined 7 hours after the introduction of sperm suspension into the culture drop containing eggs. The procedure and precautions are the same as in Section II,A,1,d, except that the eggs, after the addition of hyaluronidase, should be transferred to another drop of CB medium because the large number of follicular cells in the first drop makes observation difficult.

B. Obtaining Triploids and Haplodiploid Mosaics by Means of a "Flat Drop"

By exposing eggs to severe flattening at the time of the second maturation division, one can suppress the second polar body extrusion; a certain number of these eggs give rise to triploids and haplodiploid mosaics (A. Niemierko, unpublished observations).

Cumulus-free eggs that show the presence of a cytoplasmic bulge heralding the second polar body (see Fig. 5A) are placed in a small drop of culture medium under liquid paraffin. Most of the medium is removed with a very fine pipette, the diameter of which precludes sucking up the eggs. During this procedure, in some eggs, cytoplasm flows through the slit in the zona pellucida left by the sperm (Fig. 5B), but this outflow is soon inhibited by the pressure of the flattening drop. The eggs are cultured in flat drops for 2 hours. During this period, up to 60% of eggs show presence of three pronuclei. At the end of culture, a cleavage furrow progressing up to one-third of egg diameter appears in some eggs (Fig. 6). These eggs will further become $n/2n$ mosaics. Subsequently, the medium is very slowly introduced into the flat drop by means of a thin pipette. The speed of the medium inflow should be under control—if it is too high, the eggs adhere to the paraffin and may be lost. After the medium is added so that the drop is restored, eggs should be cultured for 1 hour, because the tripronucleate state in most eggs is only transitory. About 5% of tripronucleate eggs extrude the second polar

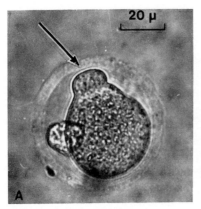
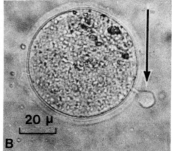

Fig. 5.   (A) An egg with a cytoplasmic bulge heralding the second polar body (arrow); (B) The same egg in a "flat drop." Cytoplasmic fragment indicated by an arrow.

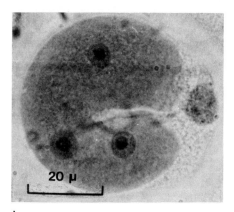

Fig. 6. An egg after 1.5 hours in a "flat drop." A cleavage furrow has begun to form. Permanent preparation.

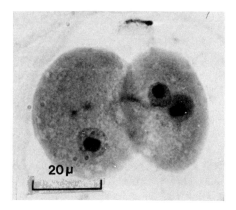

Fig. 7. Haplodiploid mosaic egg after 2 hours in a "flat drop" and 1 hour in restored drop. Permanent preparation.

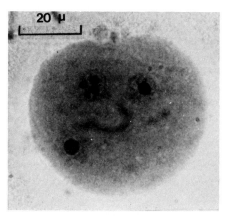

Fig. 8. Tripronucleate egg produced by a "flat-drop" method; 2 hours in a flat drop and 1 hour in restored drop. Permanent preparation.

body. Thirty percent undergo immediate cleavage and become haplodiploid mosaics. The "blastomeres" of these eggs are usually of different size (Fig. 7). Eventually, 25% of eggs remain tripronucleate (Fig. 8). All types of eggs can attain morula stage after 3 days in the oviduct; further development has not been investigated.

C. Induction of Triploidy by Strong Osmotic Shock

This method is based on the observation that pronucleate mouse eggs subjected to short-lasting strong osmotic shock (distilled water) incorporate the second polar body in 30–60% of the treated eggs, giving rise to digynic triploid eggs. Of such eggs, 30–50% develop into blastocysts, and the blastocysts are able to implant (Opas, 1977). Though slightly less effective than CB treatment, this method gives the advantage of extreme simplicity.

1. Obtaining Eggs

A wide range of pronuclear stages can be used, but the efficiency varies according to the stage. Eggs with very small pronuclei yield about 30% of tripronucleate eggs, whereas those with bigger pronuclei yield up to 60%. Eggs with very big, closely apposed pronuclei should be avoided, however, because a nucleus of the second polar body may not complete DNA synthesis and contribute in the first cleavage, even if the second polar body has been incorporated.

When using F_1 (C57 × CBA/H) females mated to CBA-T6T6 males eggs are recovered between 9:00 AM and 12:00 noon (spontaneous ovulation) or 18–20 hours post-HCG (induced ovulation). Cumuli oophori are removed by hyaluronidase, and the eggs are pooled in a drop of culture medium. If all or even some of the eggs are in too early a stage, they can be cultured for some time before the experiment.

2. Distilled Water Treatment

It is convenient to prepare a petri dish half filled with liquid paraffin and to put drops of distilled water and culture medium as follows: first row, water; second and third rows, medium; fourth row, water, etc. Eggs are placed individually in drops of distilled water. Medium introduced with the eggs should be removed. During treatment, eggs are continuously examined under dissecting microscope: swelling of all eggs and bursting of cytoplasm from some eggs will occur. Outflowing cytoplasm forms round-shaped "cytoplasmic fragments." These may sporadically contain a pronucleus. If any egg becomes "transparent" during water shock (which precedes lysis), it is immediately transferred to the culture medium, no matter how long it was treated. "Healthy looking" eggs are treated for 5–6 minutes. Before removing an egg, some medium is poured around it to stop the osmotic reaction. Eggs and their cytoplasmic fragments, if such have been formed, are individually placed in drops of culture medium in the second row, and, after they attain their normal appearance, which takes a few minutes, they are transferred to drops of medium in the third row for the whole culture period.

3. Selection of Presumably Triploid Eggs

The eggs should be cultured for about an hour. During this period, the eggs which are going to "reextrude" the second polar body, will do so. Preliminary classification may be performed under a dissecting microscope; eggs without the second polar body and with no pronucleus in the cytoplasmic fragment, if there are such, are chosen. These eggs are further examined under an inverted microscope for the presence of three pronuclei.

D. Induction of Triploidy by Mild Osmotic Shock

Before "the distilled water method" was invented, effects of slightly changed osmolarity on fertilized mouse eggs had been investigated (A. Niemierko, unpublished observations). Eggs from induced ovulation and delayed matings (2.5–3 hours postcoitum and 16–17 hours post-HCG) were placed in White's medium (Knowland and Graham, 1972) made hypertonic with extra NaCl added to 350–436 mOsM, or in hypotonic medium (Whitten's medium: distilled water, 3 : 2) for 1–3 hours and then cultured for 2 hours in normal medium. Fifty percent of the eggs were tripronucleate after such treatment. Development of these eggs has not been investigated, however.

Duration of treatment is a limiting factor in the method described; when cultured longer than 1 hour in experimental medium, some eggs begin to degenerate.

III. TETRAPLOIDY

In 1971, Graham applied a Sendai virus-induced fusion technique to obtain tetraploid mouse embryos. He fused pairs of 1-cell eggs or pairs of blastomeres from the two-cell stage. Such 4n heterokaryons developed into blastocysts in vitro, but postimplantation development was limited to formation of trophoblastic giant cells. This fusion technique, despite its technical limitations, had been the only way routinely to produce tetraploidy in the mouse until the application of CB to induce this anomaly has been invented. These are the limitations: (1) it is necessary to remove the zona pellucida before virus treatment, which implies that the fused eggs cannot be transplanted to recipients before at least 2 days of culture in vitro; (2) each pair of eggs or blastomeres has to be treated individually; (3) Sendai virus easily damages eggs or blastomeres and often impairs their viability.

Consequently, the duration of treatment and the concentration of virus must be precisely adjusted every time. Since the CB method avoids these difficulties, the fusion technique, while invaluable in the research of nucleocytoplasmic interactions, has lost some of its value as a tool for inducing tetraploidy.

The method of inducing tetraploidy with CB consists in blocking the second cleavage. As this method has been devised independently in two laboratories (Snow, 1973; Tarkowski *et al.*, 1977), somewhat different experimental procedures have been worked out. The differences are nonessential, however, and it is a matter only of convenience which of the two ways should be chosen.

A. CB Treatment of Spontaneously Ovulated Eggs

This procedure, developed by Snow (1973), permits blockage of the second cleavage in 100% of treated eggs. About 40% of these eggs develop into blastocysts when cultured *in vitro*, and, after transplantation to recipients, the blastocysts are able to implant (Snow, 1973, 1975). Very rarely, diploid or $2n/4n$ mosaic embryos appear among presumed tetraploid embryos.

This procedure requires that the experiments are performed at a precisely defined time of the day, i.e., when spontaneously ovulated eggs begin the second cleavage. When mice are kept under natural diurnal cycle, this occurs in the evening or at night of the second day of pregnancy. Presence of few 3- and 4-cell eggs among recovered eggs indicates that the moment has been properly chosen.

In Q strain, eggs were obtained between 5:00 and 6:00 P.M. and cultured in CB medium (10 μg/ml) until 6:00 A.M. the following day. On removal from CB medium, all eggs were at the two-cell stage with two nuclei in each blastomere, i.e., presumably tetraploid. However, 10–15% of the eggs did not cleave and 20–25% of the eggs were delayed in their next cleavage when cultured in CB-free medium. This indicates that, if the eggs are to be transplanted to recipients, the selection of presumably tetraploid embryos should be performed after some hours of culture in CB-free medium.

B. CB Treatment of Eggs from Induced Ovulation

The procedure, developed by Tarkowski *et al.* (1977) yields above 50% of presumably tetraploid embryos and about 20% of $2n/4n$ mosaic embryos. About 80% of tetraploids reach the blastocyst stage *in vitro*, and the blastocysts are able to implant. Single diploid and $2n/4n$ mosaics appear among presumed tetraploids. Preimplantation development of $2n/4n$ mosaic embryos do not differ from that of control diploid embryos, and $2n/4n$ mosaic blastocysts are able to implant.

1. Obtaining Eggs

By adjusting the time of hormone injections, it is possible to obtain eggs in the desired stage at any time of the day. We usually start the experiments in the morning so that the eggs, after 5 hours of culture in CB medium and 2 hours of culture in CB-free medium, may be transplanted to recipients on the same day. Alternatively, the eggs may be left in culture (CB-free medium) until they resume the next cleavage i.e., until the morning of the next day. In F_1(C57 × CBA/H) females mated to A males, the second cleavage begins between 47 and 49 hours post-HCG.

2. Experimental Procedure

About one-third of the 2-celled eggs are cultured in pure medium or medium with DMSO as a control. The remaining ones, as well as 3-cell and 4-cell stage eggs, are cultured in CB medium (10 μg/ml). Eggs are inspected every hour until all control eggs reach the 4-cell stage (3–9 hours, usually about 5 hours). Experimental eggs, after thorough washing, are then transferred to CB-free medium.

3. Selection of Presumably 4n and 2n/4n Mosaic Eggs

Some CB-treated eggs retain their smooth appearance in pure medium (Figs. 9 and 10), but many undergo violent surface changes which resemble fragmentation (Fig. 10). In such "fragmented" form the eggs persist for some hours, after which they become smooth, becoming 2-celled (probably 4n), 3-celled (probably 2n/4n mosaic), or 4-celled (probably diploid). This is why at least 2 hours of culture in pure medium are necessary after CB treatment before segregation of eggs is carried out.

Eggs that were 2-celled before treatment and smooth after it are expected to be 4n. Eggs that were 3-celled upon placement in CB medium remain such after treatment (presumed mosaic) or become 2-celled (presumed 4n). Eggs which were at the 4-cell stage on placing them in CB medium remain unchanged (diploid) or become 3-celled (presumed mosaic).

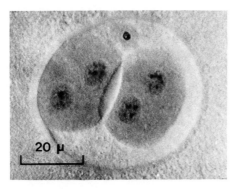

Fig. 9. Tetraploid egg produced by CB method. Permanent preparation.

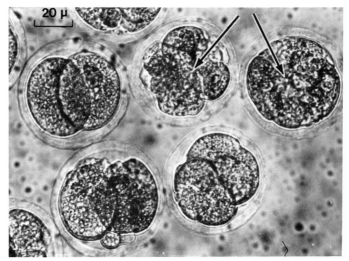

Fig. 10.   A group of 2-cell eggs treated with CB for 5 hours and then cultured 1 hour in CB free medium. Some eggs remain smooth, others undergo serious surface changes (arrows).

It is also possible to select the eggs after culturing them *in vitro* overnight. By the next morning diploid eggs reach the 8-cell stage, presumed mosaics—the 6-cell stage, and presumed tetraploids—the 4-cell stage. There is a danger, however, that some slowly dividing diploid eggs are hidden among the two latter groups.

REFERENCES

Beatty, R. A. (1957). "Parthenogenesis and Polyploidy in Mammalian Development." Cambridge Univ. Press, London and New York.

Beatty, R. A. (1972). *In* "Oogenesis" (J. D. Biggers and A. W. Schuetz, eds.), pp. 277–299. Univ. Park Press, Baltimore, Maryland.

Bedford, J. M. (1971). *In* "Methods in Mammalian Embryology" (J. C. Daniel, Jr., ed), pp. 37–63. Freeman, San Francisco, California.

Biggers, J. D., Whitten, W. K., and Whittingham, D. G. (1971). *In* "Methods in Mammalian Embryology" (J. C. Daniel, Jr., ed.), pp. 86–116. Freeman, San Francisco, California.

Bomsel-Helmreich, O. (1965). *Preimplantation Stages Pregnancy, Ciba Found. Symp., (1965)* pp. 246–267.

Bomsel-Helmreich, O. (1971). *Adv. Biosci.* **6,** 381–402.

Evans, E. P., Burteñshaw, M. D., and Ford, C. E. (1972). *Stain Technol.* **47,** 229–234.

Fujimoto, S., Passantino, T. J., Koenczoel, I., and Segal, S. J. (1975). *Cytologia* **40,** 469–475.

Graham, C. F. (1971). *Acta Endocrinol. (Copenhagen), Suppl.* **153,** 154–165.

Knowland, J., and Graham, C. (1972). *J. Embryol. Exp. Morphol.* **27,** 167–176.

Lin, T. P. (1971). *In* "Methods in Mammalian Embryology" (J. C. Daniel, Jr., ed.), pp. 157–171. Freeman, San Francisco, California.

Modliński, J. A. (1975). *J. Embryol. Exp. Morphol.* **33**, 897–905.

Niemierko, A. (1975). *J. Embryol. Exp. Morphol.* **34**, 279–289.

Niemierko, A., and Komar, A. (1976). *J. Reprod. Fertil.* **48**, 279–284.

Opas, J. (1977). *J. Embryol. Exp. Morphol.* **37**, 65–77.

Piko, L., and Bomsel-Helmreich, O. (1960). *Nature (London)* **186**, 737–739.

Rossant, J. (1975). *J. Embryol. Exp. Morphol.* **33**, 991–1001.

Snow, M. H. L. (1973). *Nature (London)* **244**, 513–515.

Snow, M. H. L. (1975). *J. Embryol. Exp. Morphol.* **34**, 707–721.

Tarkowski, A. K. (1966). *Cytogenetics* **5**, 394–400.

Tarkowski, A. K. (1971). *In* "Methods in Mammalian Embryology" (J. C. Daniel, Jr., ed.), pp. 172–185. Freeman, San Francisco, California.

Tarkowski, A. K. (1977). *J. Embryol. Exp. Morphol.* **38**, 187–202.

Tarkowski, A. K., and Rossant, J. (1976). *Nature (London)* **259**, 663–665.

Tarkowski, A. K., Witkowska, A., and Opas, J. (1977). *J. Embryol. Exp. Morphol.* **41**, 47–64.

Toyoda, Y., Yokoyama, M., and Hosi, T. (1971). *Jpn. J. Anim. Reprod.* **16**, 147–151.

Whitten, W. K. (1971). *Adv. Biosci.* **6**, 129–141.

Whittingham, D. G., and Wales, R. G. (1969). *Aust. J. Biol. Sci.* **22**, 1065–1068.

4

Methods for the High-Resolution Analysis of Protein Synthesis: Applications to Studies of Early Mammalian Development

JONATHAN VAN BLERKOM

I. GENERAL INTRODUCTION

The electrophoretic separation of proteins on polyacrylamide gels (PAGE) is one of the most direct and incisive methods available for the analysis of protein synthesis during development. The migration of proteins in an electric field (electrophoresis) is a function of both the physical and chemical properties of the molecules. Typically, electrophoresis involves one of the following properties of proteins: (1) molecular weight (sodium dodecyl sulfate electrophoresis, SDS-PAGE), (2) isoelectric point (isoelectric focusing electrophoresis, IEF), and (3) differences in the net mobilities of proteins in an electric field caused by size or charge (isotachophoresis). Either singly (one-dimensional electrophoresis) or in combination (multidimensional electrophoresis), these properties have been exploited in both the separation and chemical identification of proteins and polypeptides. Since it is not the intention of this review to discuss in detail the physical and chemical basis of electrophoresis, the readers' attention is directed to the excellent contributions of Maurer (1971) and Drysdale (1975) for this necessary information. However, it is the purpose of this chapter to acquaint embryologists, reproductive physiologists, and developmental biologists in general with recent advances in protein electrophoresis, and is specifically oriented to those investigators with limited experience in this area of analysis.

Due to limitations of space, only two electrophoretic techniques are discussed. However, Table I lists several methods and describes their applicability to special types of experimental analyses and should be consulted by those whose requirements do not fit within the scope of the methods presented here. The one-(SDS-PAGE) and two-dimensional procedures (IEF and SDS-PAGE) discussed in this chapter are routinely employed in our laboratory and, of the several methods currently available, have proved to be the most consistent in offering high resolution and, more importantly, reproducibility. In addition, throughout the text problems in both construction of gels and interpretation of electrophoretic patterns are illustrated. The problems discussed are by no means an exhaustive list but are, in our experience, the most commonly encountered. In studies of many developing systems, one major restriction on the kinds of analyses performed is the availability of sufficient quantities of material; this restriction is

TABLE I
**Current Two-Dimensional Polyacrylamide Gel Systems Useful in the
Electrophoretic Analysis of Protein Synthesis**

Developed by	First dimension	Second dimension	Application
Ames and Nikaido (1976)	IEF[a]	SDS[b]	Putative membrane proteins
Kaltschmidt and Wittman (1970)	Urea	Urea	Ribosomal proteins
Klose (1975)	IEF	SDS	General cellular proteins
O'Farrell (1975)	IEF	SDS	General cellular proteins with pI between pH 4 and 8
Scheele (1975)	IEF	SDS	General cellular proteins
Woodland, H.R., and Adamson (1977)	Urea	SDS	Histones

[a] IEF, isoelectricfocusing electrophoresis.
[b] SDS, sodium dodecyl sulfate electrophoresis.

traditionally acute in early mammalian embryogenesis. To this end, techniques and procedures are described which will permit the analysis of protein synthetic patterns in comparatively minimal amounts of material.

II. ELECTROPHORESIS IN SDS-POLYACRYLAMIDE GRADIENT SLAB GELS

In a polyacrylamide gel system containing SDS and 2-mercaptoethanol, most proteins migrate in an electric field as a function of their molecular weight (Shapiro et al., 1967; Shapiro and Maizel, 1969). Under the denaturing conditions of this system, hydrogen and hydrophobic bonds are disrupted by SDS and disulfide linkages are destroyed by 2-mercaptoethanol. Consequently, many enzymes and complex proteins composed of subunits of different molecular weights are broken down into component polypeptides. Under denaturing conditions, therefore, an inverse linear relationship exists between the relative migration distance of a protein (polypeptide) and the log of its molecular weight. The presence of the detergent SDS and the resultant formation of micellar complexes with proteins appears to minimize negative charge differences on the proteins such that most proteins migrate as anions. In a one-dimensional, SDS gel separation, proteins are ultimately resolved as a series of bands (either by protein staining or by autoradiography; Fig. 4). It must be emphasized that each band is most likely composed of several different species of polypeptides which share the same approximate molecular weight. Thus, until proved otherwise by the investigator, it seems most prudent to assume that each band is likely to be a complex mixture of different proteins.

The use of a single slab gel which permits the side-by-side comparison of numerous samples electrophoresed under identical conditions has obvious analytical advantages over the more traditional cylindrical gels. The incorporation of a gradient of acrylamide in the construction of a slab gel offers high resolution and definition of proteins across the entire molecular weight range of the gel. During the electrophoretic separation of proteins in the most commonly used polyacrylamide gels (between 7 and 12% acrylamide in nongradient systems), relatively low molecular weight proteins tend to diffuse with time, resulting in broad, fuzzy bands at the lower regions of the gel. The application of a gradient of acrylamide introduces the concept of sieving or pore-limiting electrophoresis in which the spaces (pores) in the polyacrylamide matrix through which proteins pass get smaller as the concentration of acrylamide increases. Since the rate of migration of a protein in a gradient system decreases with time, a protein of a particular size will eventually reach its pore limit, at which point further movement is restricted. Thus, the final position of a protein in the gradient will be determined by pore size, as well as by the size of the protein, and gel bands of increased sharpness and definition will be obtained. Although several different types of gradients may be constructed, the most commonly used are linear and exponential acrylamide gradients. The construction and applications of these two particular types of gradients are discussed below. The discontinuous SDS-glycine-Tris buffer system described in the following section was introduced by Laemmli (1970) and consists of the Ornstein (1964) and Davis (1964) stacking

TABLE II
Proteins Useful for the Molecular Weight Calibration
of SDS-Polyacrylamide-Gradient Slab Gels

Protein	Molecular weight
Cytochrome *c*	11,700
Ribonuclease A	14,700
Chymotrypsinogen A	25,500
Rabbit muscle β-tropomyosin	33,000
Rabbit muscle α-tropomyosin	37,000
Rabbit muscle actin	43,000
Ovalbumin	45,000
Rabbit muscle tubulin	47,000
Glutamate dehydrogenase (subunit)	53,000
Catalase (subunit)	60,000
Bovine serum albumin	67,000
σ subunit, *E. Coli* RNA polymerase	85,000–95,000
Phosphorylase A	94,000
β subunit, *E. coli* RNA polymerase	145,000–155,000
β' subunit, *E. coli* RNA polymerase	150,000–165,000
Rabbit muscle myosin	212,000

system with the addition of SDS. The molecular calibration (distribution) of the gels involves the numerous "standard" proteins listed in Table II.

A. Reagents

1. Acrylamide (electrophoresis grade, Eastman Kodak)
2. Bisacrylamide (Eastman Kodak)
3. N, N, N', N - tetramethylethylenediamine (TEMED, Eastman Kodak)
4. Sodium dodecyl sulfate (SDS, highest purity is essential, SDS from British Drug House, BDH, is suggested and is available in the United States from Gallard-Schlesinger)
5. Tris (hydroxymethyl)aminomethane (Trizma-base, Sigma Chemical Co.)
6. Ammonium persulfate (reagent grade)
7. Glycine (reagent grade, Eastman Kodak)
8. Bromophenol blue
9. Glycerol

B. Stock Solutions

1. 30% (w/v) acrylamide and 0.8% bisacrylamide
2. Lower gel buffer: 1.5 M Tris, 0.4% SDS, add HCl to pH 8.8 at 23°C
3. Upper gel buffer: 0.5 M Tris and 0.4% SDS, add HCl to pH 6.8 at 23°C
4. 80% Glycerol
5. 10% Ammonuim persulfate (made fresh)
6. Electrophoresis running buffer (electrode buffer): 0.025 M Tris (Trizma base), 0.192 M glycine, 0.1% SDS, pH approximately 8.3; *Do not titrate this buffer with HCl, NaOH, or add any salt*
7. Sample buffer: 10% (w/v) glycerol, 5% (v/v) 2-mercaptoethanol, 0.0625 M Tris, add HCL to pH 6.8 at 23°C, 2–3.6% SDS (w/v)
8. 0.1% Bromophenol blue solution

Electrophoresis running buffer is stored at room temperature and the ammonium persulfate stock is made fresh. All other stocks and reagents are stored at 5°C and remain stable for several months.

C. Apparatus

The Plexiglas electrophoresis tanks described in the following were modified from a design originally introduced by Studier (1973).

1. Glass slab gel plates: The dimensions and appearance of the notched and unnotched plates which make one slab gel unit are illustrated in Figs. 1 and 2.

2. Electrophoresis gel tanks: The appearance and dimensions of these Plexiglas tanks are shown in Fig. 2.

3. Gradient makers: Linear or exponential gradients are formed by standard, two-chambered gradient makers which are commercially available (Buchler Instruments). It is suggested that for the best possible reproducibility, several slab gels are cast at the same time if numerous samples are to be compared. In this case, gradient makers with approximately 40-ml capacities per chamber and multiple exit ports are required.

4. Teflon well formers: Teflon well formers permit the side-by-side comparison of numerous samples and are machined from a single piece of Teflon. The dimensions of a well former that allows the electrophoresis of 13 samples is illustrated in Fig. 1.

5. Latex rubber spacers: Glass plates are assembled with spacers along the bottom and side edges. The spacers are composed of strips of latex rubber, 16 × 6 × 0.8 mm.

6. Magnetic stirrer

7. Peristaltic, multichannel pump.

D. Assembly of Slab Gel Plates

The components of a single gel unit are illustrated in Fig. 1. Glass plates must be absolutely clean and free of dust for best results. In our laboratory, glass plates are soaked overnight in Chemsolve (Mallinkrodt Chemical Co.), rinsed extensively with tap water, then with deionized water and finally, soaked for 15 minutes in 95% ethanol. Glass plates are stored in closed containers. To assemble a slab gel unit, a thin film (approximately 2 mm wide) of petroleum jelly is applied by hand to the bottom and side edges of both the notched and unnotched plates (see Fig. 1). Latex strips, which have been previously wiped clean and coated with a very thin film of jelly, are layered on the bottom and side edges of one of the glass plates. The two plates are then joined and 1-inch binder

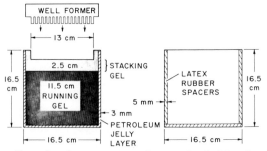

Fig. 1. Diagram illustrating the components of a completed slab gel unit for either one-dimensional SDS-gradient PAGE or as the second dimension in two-dimensional PAGE.

clamps are applied. The appearance of the completed gel unit is illustrated in Fig. 2. Extreme care must be taken to prevent contamination of the internal surfaces of the plates either by fingerprints or leakage from the latex rubber (which indicates that too much jelly has been applied). Contamination of interior surfaces will prevent the proper polymerization of the acrylamide. The assembled units are then covered with a plastic wrap and may be stored for several days. Upon prolonged storage, however, the water tightness of the units should be checked prior to the pouring of the acrylamide gels. After removal of water and assurance of a tight seal, all lint and dust must be eliminated from the interior of the gel unit.

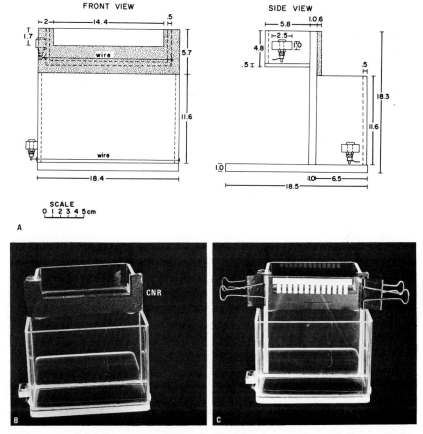

Fig. 2. (A) Dimensions and construction of a Plexiglas electrophoresis tank required for slab gels. (B) Photograph of a completed gel tank. The rubber used to seal the gel unit is composed of closed-cell neoprene (CNR). (C) Photograph of an electrophoresis tank containing a completed slab gel unit. The horizontal mark on the gel plate indicates the boundary between the stacking and running gels.

E. Construction of Polyacrylamide Gradient Slab Gels: Choice of Gradients

The determination of whether linear or exponential gels are to be constructed depends in part upon the proteins of interest. For most purposes, linear gradients offer sharp resolution of proteins between approximately 10,000 and 200,000 daltons. However, if the investigator is concerned with relatively low or relatively high molecular weight proteins, varying types of exponential gradient gels may be of more use and yield more detailed information. Figure 4 compares the same sample of rabbit blastocyst protein electrophoresed on either 8–15% linear, or 8–15% exponential gradient gels. In the linear gradient, approximately 60% of the entire gel is composed of bands with molecular weights below approximately 45,000 daltons, while in the exponential gel approximately 45% of the gel contains bands below 45,000 daltons. Thus, with various exponential gradient gels, the investigator may achieve sharp resolution across the entire gel and may separate to a greater or lesser degree proteins within certain molecular weight ranges. As long as the conditions of construction are kept rigorously constant, the reproducibility of band position from one gel to the next will be faithfully maintained.

F. Casting of an 8–15% Linear Gradient Polyacrylamide Slab Gel

Solutions for One Gel
Dense Solution (15% acrylamide)
1. 2.7 ml Lower gel buffer stock
2. 2.7 ml 80% Glycerol stock
3. 5.3 ml 30% Acrylamide stock
4. 20 μl 10% Ammonium persulfate stock
Light Solution (8% acrylamide)
1. 2.7 ml Lower gel buffer stock
2. 5.3 ml 3x Distilled water
3. 2.7 ml 30% Acrylamide stock
4. 20 μl 10% Ammonium persulfate stock

The two solutions are degassed for 1 minute in 125-ml filter flasks and immediately following degassing, 5 μl of TEMED is added to each flask. With the gradient maker, peristaltic pump and slab gel unit set up as illustrated in Fig. 3, 9.5 ml of the dense solution are added to the front chamber, and 9.5 ml of the light solution are added to the rear chamber. Although a peristaltic pump is not necessarily essential, it is quite useful in maintaining a constant flow rate. With the stir bar in the front chamber rotating at a medium speed, the stopcock

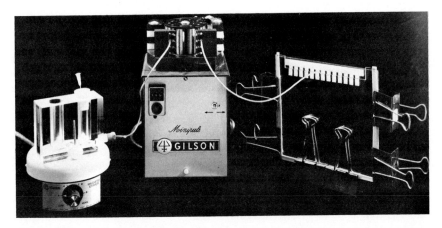

Fig. 3. Photograph of the apparatus used in the construction of an SDS-gradient, polyacrylamide slab gel. The gradient former is set up to pour an exponential gradient. The hypodermic needle is withdrawn prior to the pouring of the gel as described in the text. The Teflon well former is included in the photograph to show its usual depth after the stacking gel is applied, but it is not present during the construction of the running gel.

separating the two chambers is opened and a slight pressure is applied (by hand) to the rear chamber to ensure the flow of the light solution into the front chamber. At this point, the pump is turned on and the gradient is poured into the top of the gel unit (with the tube from the pump in the middle of the plate). A flow rate of approximately 3 ml/minute seems to be optimal. The flow from the gradient maker is stopped when the level of acrylamide solution reaches 1 inch below the base of the notch (see Fig. 1). After the gradient is poured, the gel solution is gently overlaid with distilled water sprayed from an atomizer or applied with a syringe. Only a few millimeters of overlay is required, and care should be taken to minimize any mixing between the gel solution and the overlay. The gels are allowed to stand until a sharp, straight boundary is observed (approximately 20 minutes, with polymerization beginning at the lower portion of the gel). When an interface is clearly established, the water and unpolymerized acrylamide are removed by aspiration and replaced with several milliliters of lower gel buffer which has been previously diluted fourfold with distilled water. In any event, the gels should *not stand* for more than 1 hour after the interface is first observed (i.e., during water overlay). The gels are covered with plastic wrap and allowed to "age" for between 12 and 16 hours before the stacking gel is applied (see below). For optimal reproducibility, gels should age for the same period of time since within limits, the degree of completion of the polymerization process is a function of time.

G. Construction of an 8–15% Exponential Gradient SDS Polyacrylamide Slab Gel

The same solutions described for linear gradients apply to the construction of exponential gradients. However, 2 times the volume of the light solution is prepared. In order to generate an exponential gradient of acrylamide, the volume of the dense solution must be kept constant during the pouring of the gel. The conditions and procedures used to produce the exponential gradient gel pattern illustrated in Fig. 4 are as follows: 6 ml of the dense solution (15%) of acrylamide are placed in the front chamber, while 16 ml of the light solution (8%) are placed in the rear chamber. With both chambers isolated from each other, a silicon stopper containing a large-gauge needle is inserted into the front chamber. The needle is used to relieve the pressure produced when the stopper is pushed into the chamber and is subsequently withdrawn. The filled gradient maker is placed on a magnetic stirring device, the two chambers are connected, and the contents of the front chamber gently stirred, and finally withdrawn at approximately 3 ml/minute either by a peristaltic pump or by gravity flow (Fig. 3). During the pouring of the gel, the volume of the front chamber remains constant at 6 ml and is continuously diluted by the incoming solution from the rear chamber. This produces an exponentially decreasing gradient of acrylamide. Subsequent overlaying and aging of the gel are identical to linear gradient gels. The shape of the exponential gradient may be varied by altering the volume of dense acrylamide loaded into the front chamber. For certain molecular weight separations, higher or lower volumes may be preferable and should be examined by the investigator. The following formula may be conveniently used to calculate the acrylamide concentration at any point in the gel:

$$A_c = (A_i - A_f)e \; (V/D_p) + A_f$$

where A_c is the acrylamide concentration $\times$ 100, at a distance in centimeters (c) from the bottom of the gel; A_i is the initial acrylamide concentration in the front chamber (dense) $\times$ 100; A_f is the acrylamide concentration in the rear chamber (light) $\times$ 100; V is the total volume of the gel; D is the length of the gel in centimeters; p is the pool size (i.e., milliliters in the front chamber); $e = 2.718$. Gradients using ranges of acrylamide other than those shown here may be constructed by altering the proportions of the solutions listed above.

H. Preparation of the Stacking Gel

Fundamentally, "stacking" is the isotachophoretic separation of proteins in a large-pore (4.5% acrylamide) polyacrylamide gel in which different proteins in a mixture stack on top of each other in order of their respective net mobilities. In the stacking gel, proteins are located between a leading ion (chloride) and a trailing ion (glycinate) and, with the application of an electric field, the proteins concentrate into narrow and sharp zones or discs. In the running or separating gel (i.e., the actual gradient gel), these discs are further separated from each other, thus producing the characteristic banding pattern of one dimensional gels. Since the stacking gel is critical for obtaining high resolution, care must be taken to make certain that the pH of the upper gel buffer is 6.8. In addition, the presence of chloride ions in the electrophoresis running buffer (electrode buffer) will upset localization of leading and trailing ions and will result in improper stacking of proteins. Therefore, this buffer must never be titrated with *HCl*. For a detailed discussion of the physical and chemical basis of stacking, the reader's attention is directed to Maurer (1971).

Solutions for One Stacking Gel
1. 1.25 ml Upper gel buffer stock
2. 3.00 ml Distilled water
3. 0.75 ml 30% Acrylamide stock
4. 15 μl 10% Ammonium persulfate stock

This mixture is degassed in a 50 ml filter flask. The overlay is removed from the surface of the slab gel by aspiration. Five microliters of TEMED are added to this mixture and 0.5 ml of the solution are added to the surface of the slab gel. This solution is washed over the surface by rocking the gel unit and is then removed. A Teflon well former is inserted between the two plates, and the remainder of the stacking gel solution is added until it covers the individual partitions of the well former (Figs. 1 and 3). Extreme care should be taken to prevent small bubbles from forming under the individual partitions of the well former, and, of course, all dust or particles should be prevented from entering this solution. After polymerization the well former is carefully removed (about 30 minutes) and any unpolymerized acrylamide is taken out with a narrow-bore needle. The wells are rinsed several times with electrophoresis running buffer, and the completed slab gel is ready for sample loading and electrophoresis. For optimal results, electrophoresis should begin shortly after the stacking gel has polymerized.

I. Preparation of Samples and Electrophoresis

Although protein bands may be visualized by staining with Coomassie brilliant blue (Schwartz Mann Chemical Co.), a pattern of higher resolution and detail may be obtained by autoradiography (see below) of samples labeled with radioactive amino acids. The electrophoretic patterns presented in this chapter are mostly derived from autoradiographs. For embryos and oocytes, (see Chapter 1 by McGaughey), proteins were labeled with high specific activity [^{35}S-1]methionine (New England Nuclear, 450–500 Ci/mmole) under conditions described elsewhere (Van Blerkom and Manes, 1974; Van Blerkom and Brockway, 1975a,b; Van Blerkom et al., 1976; McGaughey and Van Blerkom, 1977; Van Blerkom, 1977). ^{14}C-labeled amino acids may also be used although, in general, the specific activity of the samples (cpm/μg) is usually lower than with [^{35}S-1]methionine. Following isotopic labeling of tissues, the samples are transferred to 1-ml tubes, and all extraneous fluid is removed. To this sample is added approximately 25–50 μl of sample buffer containing SDS and 2-mercaptoethanol. The tubes are sealed with parafilm and placed in a boiling water bath for approximately 1 minute. For some tissues, nucleic acids and carbohydrates may form a rather viscous material in the sample buffer. This material may be withdrawn with a glass needle. If the samples prove difficult to solubilize, several cycles of freezing and thawing sometimes overcomes this problem. Samples in powder form may also be dissolved in this solution. Trichloroacetic acid (TCA)-precipitated material (after removal of TCA), immunoprecipitated samples, ammonium sulfate fractions, and molecular weight standards (Table II) may be readily electrophoresed in this system after a suitable final volume of liquid is obtained (by lyophilization, etc.). The SDS, 2-mercaptoethanol buffer may be diluted with liquid samples (i.e., tissue fractions, gradient fractions, etc.) between one- and twofold without any appreciable loss of resolution, although the smaller the final volume the more convenient it is to work with. As a general guide, 10 μl of sample may be added to between 30 and 40 μl of sample buffer. For most preparations, it is usually not necessary to remove salts by dialysis before mixing with sample buffer. It is also important not to load an "excessive" amount of protein onto the gels, since overloading will distort the bands and reduce resolution considerably. For autoradiography, it is usually best to maximize the amount of label and minimize the amount of protein in which the label is contained. Concentrations up to 50–60 μg may be loaded for protein staining or where low incorporation is a factor (however, for the latter problem, see section on fluorography). The investigator should attempt to vary the concentration of protein, assess resolution, and then derive a figure which offers the best "compromise" between sharp, definitive protein patterns and the amount of sample required. Samples in the SDS–2-mercaptoethanol buffer may be stored between $-20°$ and $-70°$C, although prolonged storage of several months should be avoided—especially when the samples are highly radioactive (i.e., to prevent radioautolysis).

When samples are ready for electrophoresis, the bottom latex rubber strip of the slab gel unit is removed, as is all electrophoresis running buffer contained in the wells of the stacking gel. In wells which contain no samples, approximately 25 μl of sample buffer should be loaded. Samples for electrophoresis should be heated in a boiling water bath for 30 seconds to insure complete lysis (i.e., in addition to any previous treatment) and when cool, loaded into the wells. After all wells are loaded, electrophoresis running buffer is carefully applied to each well until the wells are completely filled. Care should be taken to prevent mixing between the samples and electrophoresis running buffer. A sharp interface should exist between the sample buffer and electrophoresis running buffer. Carefully, the loaded slab gel is transferred to the gel tank, placed with the notched plate towards the "closed-cell neoprene rubber," and secured with two 1-inch binder clamps (see Fig. 2). It is important to keep the slab gel unit level during all manipulations in order to prevent spillover from one well to the next. For this reason, it is best to keep the total volume in each well (i.e., of sample) below 50 μl. Both upper and lower reservoirs are filled with electrophoresis running buffer. Several drops of bromophenol blue stock solution are added to the upper gel reservoir until the running buffer is pale blue in color (tracking dye). Since air bubbles will be trapped between the glass plates at the lower end of the gel, they are conveniently removed (along with any excess petroleum jelly) with a stream of electrophoresis running buffer ejected from a syringe connected to a cannula which is bent upwards at the tip. With the positive terminal connected to the lower reservoir and the negative terminal connected to the upper chamber, the gel is electrophoresed at a constant current of between 15 and 20 mA until the blue tracking dye reaches the bottom of the gel (between 4 and 6 hours, depending upon current and age of electrode buffer). Several gel tanks may be run in parallel with the current set at between 15 and 20 mA per gel tank. Following electrophoresis, gels may be either stained for protein or prepared for autoradiography.

J. Fixing, Staining, and Autoradiography of Slab Gels

Solutions and Apparatus
1. Pyrex dishes
2. 50% TCA
3. 50% TCA containing 0.1% Coomassie brilliant blue
4. 7% Acetic acid
5. Slab gel dryer (available commercially from Hoeffer Scientific or BioRad Biochem. Co.)

Following electrophoresis, the gel units are removed from the tanks, the rubber spacers gently pulled out, and the two glass plates carefully pried apart with a spatula. The gels are fragile at this point and should be handled from the lower edge of the gel (i.e., the region containing the heavy acrylamide concentration). If electrophoretic bands are to be visualized by staining, the stacking gel may be removed, and the remaining running gel placed into a solution of 0.1% Coomassie brilliant blue in 50% TCA for 30 minutes, making certain that the gel is completely submerged during staining as acrylamide slab gels have a tendency to float in 50% TCA, which results in incomplete fixation and staining

of the protein bands. Gels are destained overnight in 7% acetic acid. (This is
done to remove TCA and to promote proper drying of the gel). After gels have
remained in acetic acid for a sufficient length of time, they are transferred to a
bath of distilled water for 1 minute, in order to remove any surface acid. Gels are
then carefully placed on plastic wrap, covered with a sheet of moist Whatman
3MM filter paper or dialysis tubing, and then positioned on a gel dryer.

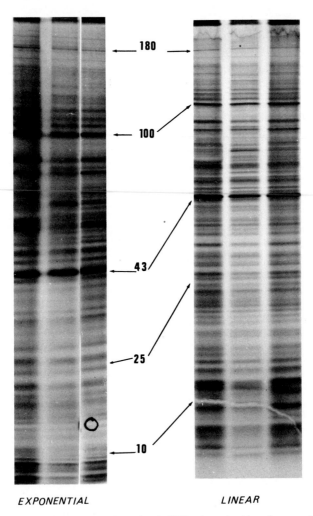

EXPONENTIAL   LINEAR

Fig. 4. Autoradiographs of one-dimensional, SDS-polyacrylamide gels comparing the separation of [^{35}S-1]methionine-labeled rabbit blastocyst proteins electrophoresed in either exponential or
linear gradients as described in the text. The crack in the linear gradient gel occurred during drying.
Approximate molecular weights ($\times$ 10^{-3}) are indicated in the center of the figure.

Gels are dried under heat (250-watt infrared lamps) and under vacuum (from either a good mechanical pump or aspirator).

Perhaps the most frustrating aspect of this entire process is to have a slab gel crack during drying. Gels will crack into pieces of varying size if they are removed from the dryer before drying is complete (Fig. 4). In addition, a constant vacuum must be applied, since any major variation in the vacuum will cause the gels to crack (the gels are under considerable stress during drying). Even if a small portion of the gel has not dried completely, it may serve as a nucleus for crack formation when the gel is removed from the dryer. On the other hand, if gels are dried for too long and/or under too much heat (the gel surface should feel moderately warm, not extremely hot), the gels will become quite brittle, and numerous hairline cracks may develop. Under optimal conditions, it should take approximately 45 minutes to dry one slab gel prepared in the manner described here. Close attention must be paid to the drying of acrylamide gradient gels—this point cannot be too strongly emphasized. If a mechanical vacuum pump is employed, the hot vapor from the gel should first pass through a chamber containing a drying agent (the chamber is usually embedded in ice) and then through a large cold trap (Dry Ice–ethanol bath is most effective) before entering the pump. Untreated, hot acetic acid vapors will eventually erode the metal vanes of the pump even if the vacuum pump oil is changed frequently.

Following drying, gels (still attached to filter paper or dialysis tubing) are stapled to cardboard to retard curling. For autoradiography, dried gels may be exposed to Kodak no-screen medical X-ray film (type NS2T) or its equivalent. The duration of exposure is a function of the amount of incorporated counts applied to each well. Typically, 50,000 cpm/well requires between 7 and 10 days for complete resolution of the autoradiographic bands, although some bands may be detected after as few as 1 or 2 days of exposure. Where extremely low levels of incorporation are a problem, fluorography may replace autoradiography (see Section IV,A).

K. Important Procedural Aspects to Reemphasize

1. Acrylamide is a potential neurotoxin and the handling of acrylamide in both powder and liquid forms should be done with the utmost caution.

2. The pH of the upper gel buffer must be 6.8, while that of the lower gel buffer must be 8.8 at 23°C.

3. Only SDS of the highest quality should be used.

4. The electrophoresis running buffer (electrode buffer) should not be titrated with either HCL or NaOH. If titration is necessary (and only if the pH varies greatly from approximately 8.3), either glycine or Tris (Trizma-base) should be used.

5. Remove all trapped air bubbles from below the Teflon well formers during the preparation of the stacking gel.

6. Make certain that no air spaces are present between the stacking and running gel (i.e., the actual gradient gel) nor between the plates at the lower edge of the gel unit.

7. Dry gels under constant vacuum and moderate heat (maximum 250 W/gel) until the surface feels smooth, even, and hard. Do not leave gels drying for prolonged lengths of time.

III. ELECTROPHORESIS IN TWO-DIMENSIONAL POLYACRYLAMIDE GELS

The application of high resolution, two-dimensional polyacrylamide gel electrophoresis offers the potential for an enormous expansion in the ability to study translational products and programs during development (McGaughey and Van Blerkom, 1977; Van Blerkom and Manes, 1977; Van Blerkom, 1977; Van Blerkom and McGaughey, 1978a, 1978b). The two-dimensional system described in this section was developed by Patrick O'Farrell (1975) and represents a very significant advance in the direct visualization of cellular protein synthetic activity. Other two-dimensional systems which may have particular applications to certain types of analyses are listed in Table I. In the present system, proteins are first separated according to their isoelectric points (pI) in cylindrical, polyacrylamide gels (isoelectric focusing electrophoresis, IEF). In the second dimension, proteins are separated further according to molecular weight in the SDS-polyacrylamide gradient system described in the previous section. Proteins are resolved in the first dimension as a series of bands (Fig. 4), whereas in the second dimension, protein components of the individual bands separate into a series of spots (see Figs. 6–12), each of which usually represents a single polypeptide species.

Fundamentally, IEF is an equilibrium method for separating amphoteric molecules according to their isoelectric points by electrophoresis in a stable gradient which increases progressively from anode to cathode. Such a gradient is established by the electrolysis of carrier ampholytes in a polyacrylamide gel matrix. Ampholytes are aliphatic polyaminopolycarboxylic acids synthesized in the reaction between acrylic acid and an aqueous solution of different polyethylene polyamines. A mixture of carrier ampholytes which migrates in an electric field and has the *potential* of producing a pH gradient from approximately 3.5 to 10 may contain as many as 360 species of ampholytes which range in MW from 300 to greater than 1000 daltons (Latner, 1975). The physicochemical basis of isoelectric focusing electrophoresis is quite simple:

A protein or other amphoteric molecule introduced into the pH gradient below its pI will be positively charged and be repelled by the anode. As it moves into regions of higher pH it will lose its positive charge and gain negative charge, e.g., through deprotonation of carboxyl or amine functions. Eventually, it will reach a pH region at which its net electrical charge is zero (pI). Should it diffuse away from its pI, it will develop a net charge and be repelled back towards its pI. Thus, by counteracting backdiffusion with an appropriate electrical field, the protein will reach an equilibrium position and so be concentrated, or focused, at its pI. By this means, different proteins can be segregated into narrow zones in the same pH gradient (Drysdale, 1975).

The combination of IEF and SDS-gradient-PAGE has resulted in the resolution of nearly 1600 individual polypeptide species derived from a rat liver hepatoma cell line (O'Farrell and O'Farrell, 1977). In the autoradiographs of two-dimensional gels presented in this chapter (as well as in those by R. W. McGaughey), at least several hundred polypeptide species are readily visualized.

A. Preparation of Samples for Two-Dimensional Gel Electrophoresis

The composition of the two-dimensional lysis buffer is as follows:

1. 9.5 M urea (ultrapure, Schwarz-Mann)
2. 5% 2-Mercaptoethanol
3. 2% Carrier ampholytes comprised of 1.6% ampholines, pH 5–7 (LKB), 0.4% ampholines, pH 3.5–10 (LKB), *or* 0.4% pHisolytes, pH 2–10 (Brinkmann). Ampholytes are used as supplied (i.e., 40% w/v)
4. *2% (w/v) Nonidet P-40 (Imperial Shell or Particle Data Laboratory)*

This solution is stored as 1-ml aliquots at $-70°C$, and will remain stable for several months.

In our experience, most problems of poor resolution in the second dimension are traceable to the preparation of samples for electrophoresis in the first dimension. It is critical, therefore, that in the two-dimensional system described here sample preparation must receive careful attention. The following description is derived from the types of analyses routinely done in our laboratory, and may be modified by the investigator to fit particular requirements. Oocytes, preimplantation embryos, or fetal tissues are placed in 1-ml test tubes, and all excess fluid is completely withdrawn. For embryos which contain relatively large amounts of blastocoelic fluid, such as the rabbit, this fluid is removed (as is the zona pellucida) and the embryonic tissues transferred to lysis buffer and prepared as described below. After suitable concentration, blastocoelic fluid may also be analysed. Approximately 30 μl of lysis buffer is added to the tissue/embryo samples and the progress of lysis is monitored under a dissecting microscope. In 1-ml test tubes sealed with Parafilm, lysis should be fairly complete at room temperature within 1 minute. If lysis is not complete, however, samples may be frozen and thawed for several cycles and/or disrupted in a tissue homogenizer. During the thawing step, it is important that the water bath be below 35°C and that the samples be removed immediately when the ice has melted. The exposure to warm water should be minimized in order to prevent the chemical modification of proteins that may alter their electrophoretic mobilities in this system. If samples still prove difficult to solubilize completely, then sonication is sometimes helpful (see O'Farrell, 1975, for a detailed discussion of both the artifactual chemical modification of proteins and procedures used for sonication of samples). After lysis is complete, samples are stored at $-70°C$ and electrophoresed as soon as possible.

For the optimal separation of proteins in the isoelectric focusing dimension, it is essential that the concentration of urea in the lysis buffer not be below 9.5 M after the addition of sample. The dilution of urea below this molarity may result in poor resolution and/or incomplete separation of proteins during isoelectric focusing electrophoresis. Consequently, if the samples being analyzed will constitute appreciable volume (such as blastocoelic or other embryonic fluids), either of the following two procedures may be employed: (1) the increase in volume of a known amount of lysis buffer after the addition of sample is measured, and crystalline urea is added to bring the solution to 9.5 M; or (2) after lysis is complete, it is often easier to add several small crystals of urea to the lysis buffer until the crystallization of the urea seems imminent. For a volume of 30 μl, only a few crystals of urea are required. If the urea crystallizes, the samples may be heated in warm water for only the period of time required for the urea to return to solution. These samples may be either stored at $-70°C$ or loaded directly onto the first dimension gel tubes with a warm 50–100 μl syringe (to prevent crystallization of urea in the syringe during loading). The urea in these particular samples may crystallize in the gel tubes after loading, but this will not adversely affect either electrophoresis or resolution. In our laboratory, generally 27 μl of sample is applied to the first dimension, with the remaining 3 μl used for determining incorporation of radioactivity into acid (TCA)-precipitable material.

The presence of a nonionic detergent (NP-40) in the lysis buffer presents a special problem in the determination of the amount of acid insoluble radioactivity in a sample. The addition of TCA to a solution of NP-40 causes the detergent to separate into a different phase that can pass through a Millipore filter and carry protein with it, thus presenting the potential for an inaccurate determination of incorporated radioactivity. To avoid this problem, the following procedure, developed by O'Farrell and O'Farrell (1977), is used: to 0.5 ml of water is added one drop of 0.2% bovine serum albumin, between 1 and 3 μl of sample (in lysis buffer), and 0.5 ml of 10% TCA. The solution will immediately become opaque, and the precipitate is allowed to form at room temperature for 20 minutes. The precipitate is collected on Millipore filters with subsequent washes of 5% TCA. Since the number of proteins detected in this two-dimensional system depends in part upon the specific activity of the samples, it is again important for the investigator to maximize incorporation and minimize the amount of material subject to electrophoresis. Typically, less than 10 μg of protein are contained in the 27 μl of sample applied to the first dimension gel; however, as many as 100 μg of protein may be loaded, although a considerable reduction in resolution in the second dimension should be anticipated.

B. Construction of the First Dimension or Isoelectric Focusing Gel

*Solutions**

1. Acrylamide stock: 28.38% acrylamide and 1.62% bisacrylamide. This stock should not be confused with the acrylamide stock used in the construction of slab gels
2. 10% w/v NP-40 (diluted with distilled water)
3. 40% Ampholytes stock (these are available commercially as 40% w/v solutions: pH 5–7 from LKB, pH 3.5–10 from LKB or pH 2–10 from Brinkman)
4. *N, N, N', N*–Tetramethylethylenediamine (TEMED)
5. 10% Ammonium persulfate (made fresh)
6. Urea (Schwarz-Mann, Ultrapure)
7. 0.01 *M* H$_3$PO$_4$ (made from a 1 *M* stock)
8. 0.02 *M NaOH* (degassed and stored under vacuum at room temperature)
9. Gel overlay solution: 8 *M* urea (stored as 1-ml aliquots at −70°C)
10. Sample overlay solution: 9 *M* urea, 0.8% ampholytes, pH 5–7, 0.2% pH 3.5–10 or pH 2–10, stored as 1-ml aliquots at −70°C

C. Apparatus

1. Pyrex tubes, 2.5 mm (i.d.) × 130 mm
2. Cylindrical gel polymerization rack (Buchler Instruments)
3. Cylindrical electrophoresis gel tank (Savant Instruments)
4. Gel-loading syringe; 5-ml syringe fitted with a 22-gauge, 6-inch needle
5. Power supply capable of providing a constant voltage output of 1000 Volts and a constant current output of 100 mA or greater (Instrumentation Specialists, ISCO)

To make enough gel mixture for approximately 10 gels, the following solution is prepared.

1. 5.5 gm Urea
2. 1.33 ml Acrylamide stock
3. 2.0 ml 10% NP-40
4. 1.95 ml H$_2$O

*Stored at 4°C unless noted.

5. 0.4 ml Ampholytes, pH 5–7; 0.1 ml Ampholytes, pH 3.5–10 or 2–10
6. 7 μl 10% Ammonium persulfate

If the investigator chooses to use the expanded range ampholytes, pH 2–10, then both the lysis buffer and the sample overlay solution should contain the same ranges. In order to maximize consistency of the protein patterns, large quantities of this solution (without ammonium persulfate and TEMED) may be prepared in advance as aliquots and stored at −70°C. Each aliquot of the gel solution is thawed at room temperature and then TEMED and ammonium persulfate are added as above.

Prior to the formulation of the first dimension gel mixture, as many cylindrical gel tubes as required are prepared (10 ml of gel mix is sufficient to prepare approximately 16 gels). One end of the 130-mm tubes is sealed with Parafilm and placed in a gel polymerization rack. It is critical that these tubes be absolutely clean! Cylindrical gel tubes are routinely cleaned by soaking in chromic acid, rinsing in water, soaking in a saturated solution of KOH in ethanol, followed by extensive rinsing in deionized water, treatment with 100% ethanol and, finally, by air-drying. If gel tubes are not absolutely clean, the isoelectric focusing gel may not adhere properly to the walls of the tube and may result in poor separation of proteins during electrophoresis.

After the gel tubes have been prepared, the components of the first dimension gel are added to a 125-ml vacuum flask and swirled in a 37°C water bath until all crystals of urea are dissolved. The solution is briefly evacuated and 5 μl of TEMED are added. This solution is then immediately loaded into a 5-ml syringe (gel-loading syringe), and the tubes are filled with the tip of the hypodermic placed at the bottom of the tube and gradually withdrawn as the gel mix fills up the tube. The gel tubes are filled to within 5 mm of the top. However, if samples significantly in excess of approximately 25 μl are to be loaded (i.e., if they contain large amounts of material), then gels may be filled to within 15 mm of the top. It is absolutely essential that, for optimal reproducibility between different gel samples, all gel tubes be filled to precisely the same level. After the tubes are filled, the bottom portion is tapped in order to remove trapped air bubbles. If large bubbles have been trapped, then the level of gel mix may be reduced once the bubble has reached the surface, and additional gel mix must be added to bring the volume to the proper level. The gel mixture is overlaid with 8 M urea (gel overlay solution), the tubes covered with plastic wrap, and the gels allowed to polymerize for between 1 and 2 hours.

Following polymerization, all overlay and unpolymerized acrylamide are carefully removed from the surface of the gel and replaced with 25 μl of lysis buffer. The remaining portion of the gel tubes is filled with distilled water, and care is taken to prevent mixing of the lysis buffer and the water. The gel tubes are again covered with plastic wrap and allowed to stand for an additional 1–2 hours in order to equilibrate the surface of the gel with ampholytes and detergent. After this period of time has elapsed, the lysis buffer/water overlay is removed, and 25 μl of fresh lysis buffer is added. The Parafilm seal is removed, and the gel tubes are placed in a cylindrical gel electrophoresis tank. The remaining portion of the gel tubes is filled with degassed 0.02 M NaOH, again taking care not to mix the two phases. The lower reservoir of the gel tank is completely filled with 0.01 M H_3PO_4, and degassed 0.02 M NaOH is added to fill the upper reservoir. At this point, the gels are ready for prerunning. The prerun step is required to remove ammonium persulfate, TEMED, and isocyanate (formed from the decomposition of urea) from the gel prior to the actual electrophoresis of the sample(s). The prerun schedule is as follows: with the anode on the bottom and cathode on the top, the gels are prerun for 15 minutes at 200 V, 30 minutes at 300 V, and 30 minutes at 400 V at constant voltage.

Following the prerun, the upper reservoir solution is discarded, and all fluid on the surface of the gels is removed by aspiration. At this stage, samples are thawed (or heated if the urea is crystalline at room temperature) and then loaded onto the surface of the gel either with a microsyringe or an Eppendorf micropipette (or equivalent). After the samples are loaded, 10 μl of sample overlay solution (9.0 M urea plus ampholytes and NP-40) are carefully layered on the samples. This solution should float on the lysis buffer, and this step should be monitored closely to ensure the existence of two phases. If the sample overlay solution does not float, then the concentration of the urea in the lysis buffer (plus sample) is below 9.5 M urea and should be corrected immediately. The remaining portion of the gel tubes and the upper reservoir are completely filled with degassed 0.02 M NaOH (Fig. 5B). The actual running time of the first dimension gel may be varied to fit the schedule of the investigator, although the total number of volt hours (the product of the time and voltage) must be kept uniform from one run to the next in order to obtain optimal reproducibility. In our laboratory, the first dimension is electrophoresed for a total of 6400 V hours. This figure includes a total of 400 V hours for the prerun, 400 V for 13 hours, followed by a final pulse of 800 V for 1 hour (to sharpen the bands). As recommended by O'Farrell (1975), the total volt hours of electrophoresis should total more than 5000 and less than 10,000, while the final voltage should be a minimum of 400 V. Bands will become distorted if the first dimension gels are electrophoresed at too high a voltage. Following IEF, gels are either prepared for storage or for electrophoresis in the second dimension.

D. Equilibration of IEF Gels for Storage or for Electrophoresis in the Second Dimension

Following the completion of electrophoresis, the cylindrical gels are removed from the gel tubes by means of a short piece of Tygon tubing, one end of which is connected to a 5-ml syringe filled with water and the other to the upper end of the gel tube. The gels are carefully extruded into 15-ml plastic, screw cap test tubes by gently applying pressure to the syringe. The test tubes are filled with 10 ml of the SDS-sample buffer used for preparing samples for SDS-slab gel electrophoresis (see Section I,B). The gels must be removed slowly and with care, since a too rapid rate of extrusion may cause the gels to break. Special care must be taken when the upper 1.5–2 cm of the gel (the basic region) is removed, since a constriction forms in this region during IEF and the gel becomes quite fragile; in addition, this constriction may be used as a marker to note the basic portion of the gel. The tubes are placed in a rotator or shaker (tube rotator, BioQuest Laboratories, BBL), and the gels are equilibrated with the SDS sample buffer for 1 hour. If gels are to be stored, then after 1 hour, the SDS sample buffer is removed through a small piece of fine-mesh stainless steel screen placed over the opening of the tube. If radioactive protein has been electrophoresed, some protein may be eluted from the gel during equilibration, and, consequently, the sample buffer should be treated as contaminated waste. Five milliliters of fresh sample buffer are added, the tubes placed on their sides, and the gels are stored at −70°C. Although electrophoresis in the second dimension should be carried out as soon as possible, these gels are stable for several months. If storage is not required, then 10 ml of fresh sample buffer are added, and the gels are equilibrated for an additional hour. During the final hour of equilibration, the stacking gel is applied to SDS-slab gels which should have been prepared between 12 and 16 hours previously (as described in the section on one-dimensional slab gels). For gels which have been stored, after thawing, an additional 5 ml of sample buffer is added, and the gels are equilibrated for an additional hour.

E. Electrophoresis in the Second Dimension

Solutions

    1. All reagents listed in Section II, F. For gradient slab gels
    2. 1% Agarose dissolved in SDS sample buffer (stored at −70°C in 1 ml aliquots)

With some modification, the same apparatus required to cast SDS-gradient slab gels is employed in the second dimension of this procedure. Three types of glass plates may be used to form the second-dimension gel unit: (1) the most convenient form is two beveled plates (45° bevel), one of which has a rectangular back plate attached at the top of one of the beveled plates with silicone cement (Fig. 5A, design introduced by O'Farrell, 1975). When the two plates are joined with the proper rubber spacers in place, the groove formed between the bevels will accomodate the cylindrical first-dimension gel; (2) one plate may be beveled and the back plate may be the unnotched plate illustrated in Figs. 1 and 5C; (3) alternatively, the one-dimensional slab gel unit may be set at a 45° angle and

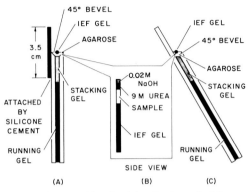

Fig. 5. Two designs for the assembly of a slab gel unit required for two-dimensional gel electrophoresis (after O'Farrell, 1975). (A) Both plates have a 45° bevel which when joined form a groove into which the IEF gel is placed. In addition, a rectangular glass plate is cemented onto one of the beveled plates to form a back plate. (B) The appearance of the first dimension, isoelectric-focusing gel prior to electrophoresis. (C) In this design, one plate has a bevel while the back plate is the unnotched gel plate illustrated in Fig. 1.

the first dimension gel applied. However, in our experience, the first-dimension gel has a slight tendency to separate from the stacking gel during electrophoresis, and either design (1) or (2) is recommended. Although beveled glass plates are commercially available (BioRad), they may be readily constructed in a machine shop.

A second modification in the two-dimensional system involves the stacking gel. Instead of placing a Teflon well former in the stacking gel, a strip of Teflon (130 × 0.8 × 20 mm) is inserted to approximately 2 mm below the base of the notch (design 3) or beveled edges (designs 1 or 2). The first-dimension gel is applied after polymerization of the stacking gel (about 30 minutes) and after all excess fluid and unpolymerized acrylamide have been removed from the surface of the stacking gel. The first-dimension gel is placed on a clean piece of Parafilm and is aligned parallel to one of the edges. Excess sample buffer is withdrawn from the vicinity of the gel with filter paper, and the basic region of the gel (which has a constriction) is noted for later reference. Prior to layering the IEF gel on the stacking gel, the 1% agarose solution should be completely melted (in a hot water bath). With the IEF gel aligned parallel to one edge of the Parafilm, 1 ml of the agarose solution is pipetted into the groove (or notch, with plates at a 45° angle), and the IEF gel is immediately transferred into the groove by simply sliding the gel off the Parafilm. It is extremely important to make absolutely certain that no small air bubbles have been trapped between the first dimension gel and the agarose bed. If air bubbles are visible after the agarose has gelled, the IEF gel/agarose bed may be removed, the IEF gel separated from the agarose bed and the entire process carefully repeated. After the gel has been transferred, a light coat of agarose may be applied to the exposed surface of the IEF gel; however, this step is optional. The agarose is allowed to gel for about 5 minutes, the rubber spacer sealing the bottom of the glass plates is removed, and the gel unit is transferred to an electrophoresis tank. At this point, electrophoresis follows the steps described in the section on one-dimensional SDS-gradient slab gels. Following electrophoresis at constant current, the slab gel is separated from the stacking/IEF gel, and a small notch is placed in the region of the gel, which should contain the more basic proteins. Fixing, staining, drying, and autoradiography follow procedures previously described.

F. Determination of pH in the First Dimension and Calibration of Molecular Weight Distribution in the Second Dimension

In order to determine the relative pH distribution across the isoelectric focusing gel, a gel containing only 25 μl of lysis buffer is included in the run. After isoelectric focusing is completed, the gel is extruded from the tube and cut into 5-mm segments. These segments are placed in 0.5 ml of deionized water which has been extensively degassed, the mixture is shaken for 1 hour at room temperature (in sealed vials), after which time the pH is quickly measured. Since some proteins may be modified under the denaturing conditions of the lysis buffer and electrophoresis, the presence of a protein in a particular pH range should be interpreted only as a relative or approximate indication of the pI.

If the SDS-polyacrylamide gradient slab gels are prepared uniformly, then it is usually not necessary to calibrate molecular weight distribution for each set of gels. The molecular weight calibration of the slab gels is very straightforward. Approximately 5 μg each of proteins with both known molecular weights and spanning molecular weights between approximately 10,000 and 200,000 daltons, or greater, are added to 1 ml of one-dimensional SDS-sample buffer. During the heating of this solution in a boiling water bath, 1% agarose is added, and this mixture is used as the agarose bed upon which one of the IEF gels is placed. After electrophoresis in the second dimension, the slab gels are stained with Coomassie brilliant blue, and the various proteins will appear as lines across the gel. After staining, the gels may be prepared for autoradiography, and the approximate molecular weight of a particular polypeptide may be estimated by comparing its position to that of a protein of known molecular weight. Proteins which may be used for molecular weight determinations are listed in Table II. As was described for one dimensional SDS-slab gels, considerably greater resolution is routinely obtained by autoradiography rather than by protein staining with Coomassie brilliant blue. This observation also applies to the two-dimensional procedure. Various two-dimensional gel patterns of both stained gels and autoradiographs are shown in Figs. 6–12.

IV. SPECIAL APPLICATIONS

A. Fluorography

Inherent in most studies involving the direct biochemical visualization of synthetic processes occurring during early mammalian development is the relatively large amounts of material required. This problem is especially acute in studies of protein synthesis during oocyte maturation (McGaughey and Van Blerkom, 1977) and during the preimplantation development of intact (Epstein and Smith, 1974; Van Blerkom and Manes, 1974, 1977; Van Blerkom and Brockway, 1975a,b; Van Blerkom, 1977) and the microdissected embryos (Van Blerkom et al., 1976), where the availability of embryonic material is frequently a limiting factor. Although some microelectrophoretic techniques have been described (Petzoldt, 1972, 1975), these procedures generally offer poor resolution. Since the resolution of proteins and polypeptides by autoradiography is usually superior to protein staining, techniques that amplify the radioactivity of proteins are particularly useful when only low levels of incorporation are obtained. The combination of scintillation autoradiography (fluorography) and high resolution one- and two-dimensional electrophoresis permits the detection of proteins and polypeptides from embryonic samples in which the level of incorporated radioactivity is extremely low. In the system introduced by Bonner and Laskey (1974), β particles from either ^3H or $^{35}S/^{14}C$ will interact with a scintillant (2,5-diphenyloxazole, PPO), resulting in the emission of light which in turn will cause a local blackening on the X-ray film. An approximate hundredfold amplification is obtained with ^3H, while a tenfold increase is observed with $^{14}C/^{35}S$ (Bonner and Laskey, 1974). In our laboratory, the combination of two-dimensional electrophoresis and fluorography has permitted the detection of several hundred polypeptide species from a single preimplantation mouse embryo when the level of incorporated radioactivity was on the order of a few hundred counts per minute (Figs. 6 and 7).

Solutions and Apparatus

1. Pyrex dishes (8 inches $\times$ 13 inches)
2. Dimethyl sulfoxide (DMSO)
3. 2,5-Diphenyloxazole (PPO)
4. Stock solution of 20% (w/v) PPO in DMSO
5. Medium-powered electronic photographic flash unit (Honeywell, Vivitar)
6. Wratten No. 22 filter (Kodak)
7. Kodak X-Omat R Film, type XR/5 (also distributed as type RP/R54) or equivalent

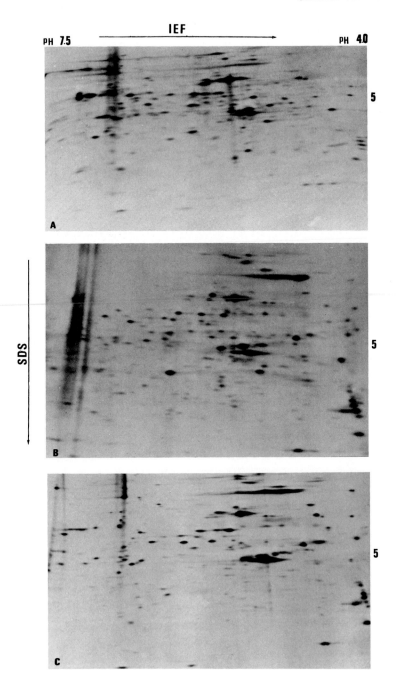

The fluorographic amplification of radioactive proteins contained within one- or two-dimensional slab gels is accomplished as follows. After electrophoresis, the slab gels are fixed in 50% TCA and washed overnight in 7% acetic acid as previously described. The gels are then placed in approximately 300 ml of DMSO, the Pyrex dishes covered with plastic wrap, and then gently rocked on a platform shaker for 30 minutes. After this time, the DMSO is replaced with 300 ml of fresh DMSO and the dehydration process continued for an additional 30 minutes. The DMSO may be reused several times and is stored in the presence of a dehydrant (molecular sieves, 4–8 mesh, Fisher Biochemical). After dehydration, the slab gels are transferred to several hundred milliliters of 20% PPO/ DMSO stock, the dishes covered, and the gels gently rocked in this solution for 3–4 hours. During infiltration with PPO, the gels will shrink considerably. After infiltration, the gels are transferred to several liters of 7% acetic acid containing 1% glycerol (which helps to prevent cracking during drying). Since PPO will precipitate in aqueous solutions, the gels immediately turn white, and during several hours in acetic acid, will expand to nearly their original dimensions. After expansion, gels are dried under vacuum and under heat as previously described. The stock solution of PPO/DMSO may be replenished by determining the amount of PPO incorporated by each slab gel.

One major disadvantage in the application of fluorography to the analysis of complex one- and two-dimensional protein patterns is a nonlinear film response, i.e., film images produced by fluorography may not be true representations of the actual distribution of radioactivity in the gel (Laskey and Mills, 1975). Although this is frequently useful in qualitative studies, it introduces the potential for serious error in quantitative analyses. However, preexposure of the X-ray film to a single flash of light hypersensitizes the film, greatly increases the efficiency of the fluorographic process, and, more importantly, after preexposure, the density of the fluorographic image is corrected to linearity, such that the

---

Fig. 6. High resolution, two-dimensional fluorographs of [^{35}S-1]methionine-labeled mouse embryos. (A) Fluorograph of a single parthenogenetic mouse morula. Approximately 1000 cpm were applied, with an exposure time of 2 months on preflashed film stored at $-70°C$. (B) Fluorograph of a single, normal mouse morula containing approximately 1500 cpm and exposed at $-70°C$ for 2 months on unflashed film. (C) Fluorograph of a single early mouse blastocyst containing approximately 2000 cpm and exposed to unflashed film at $-70°C$ for 2 months. Differences in relative spot position between (A), (B) and (C) resulted from the fact that the samples in (A) and in (B)/(C) were electrophoresed at very different times and under somewhat different conditions. Comparisons of polypeptides may be readily made between (B) and (C), and with more difficulty, between (A) and (B)/(C). The first dimension was isoelectric-focusing electrophoresis (IEF) between approximately pH 4 and 7.5. The second dimension was electrophoresis on 8–15% linear gradient, sodium dodecyl sulfate, polyacrylamide slab gels (SDS). Approximate molecular weights ($\times$ 10^{-4}) are given on the far right.

IEF

pH 7.5   pH 4.0

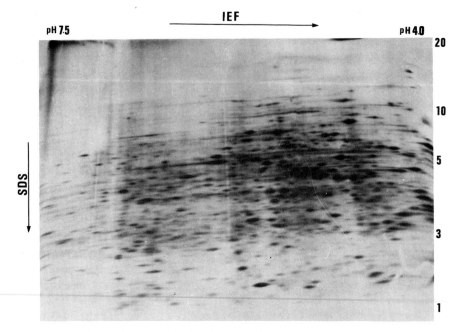

SDS

20

10

5

3

1

Fig. 7. High resolution, two-dimensional fluorograph of a single early rabbit blastocyst labeled with ^{3}H-amino acids. This particular sample contained approximately 300,000 cpm, and was exposed at $-70°C$ to unflashed X-ray film for 1 hour. This sample was treated with both RNase and DNase prior to the addition of lysis buffer. The emulsion on the X-ray film required for fluorography is very soft when wet and is easily scratched (fine line in the relatively acidic region of the fluorograph). Approximate molecular weights ($\times 10^{-4}$) are given on the far right.

density of an electrophoretic band or spot is proportional to the amount of radioactivity which produced it (Laskey and Mills, 1975). It should be reemphasized that fluorography requires a special type of X-ray emulsion film such as in Kodak X-Omat R Film (XR/5) or Kodak RP Royal X-Omat Film (RP/R54).

The hypersensitization process involves the exposure of X-ray film to a single flash of light. To hypersensitize Royal X-Omat film, a single sheet of film is placed between 50 and 80 cm from a moderate-powered, electronic flash unit. Taped to the window of the flash are a sheet of filter paper (to diffuse light) and a Wratten No. 22 filter (or No. 21 filter if a low-powered flash is used, Laskey and Mills, 1975). The unit is activated to produce a 1-msec flash. After flashing, the dried, PPO infiltrated slab gel is exposed to the film and stored at $-70°C$. For both autoradiography and fluorography, the film/gel unit is contained between two pieces of particle board which are held together tightly by four 1-inch binder clamps. Although hypersensitized film may be stored at room temperature (22°C) during exposure, storage at $-70°C$ produces superior results, and, as noted by

Laskey and Mills (1975), when fluorographs are exposed at room temperature, the relative increase in sensitivity due to preexposure is greater than for unflashed film stored at $-70°C$ but is less sensitive than for preflashed film stored at $-70°C$. If a $-70°C$ freezer is not available, preflashed films may be exposed to gels at room temperature or for optimal results, in Dry Ice.

One important parameter of preexposure which must be determined by the investigator is the distance (in centimeters) between the film and the flash unit. Clearly, as the flash unit is moved closer to the film, a background of increasing density (fog) will result. With too high a background, some of the bands or spots that contain comparatively low levels of radioactivity may not be distinguished above the blackened background. Thus, a compromise between sensitivity (signal) and a tolerable increase in background (noise) is determined by varying the distance between film and flash, followed by immediate development. The increase in the density of the flashed film (i.e., above background) is measured in a densitometer. Laskey and Mills (1975) reported that preexposure of film to an increase in absorbance of 0.15 O.D. resulted in a completely linear relationship between fluorographic image absorbance and the amount of radioactivity (3H or ^{14}C) (for exposures stored at $-70°C$). Our experience has indicated that an optical density (O.D.) increase of 0.2, O.D. is most satisfactory. However, the investigator should attempt to obtain a range of O.D.s in order to determine which optical density produces linearity. This is especially true since the age of the film (as well as the manufacturer) and the type of flash will vary between individual investigators. In our experience, a distance of 70 cm. from a medium powered flash (Vivitar, model 252) offers both optimal signal to noise ratio and an increase in the optical density of fresh film of 0.2. An additional parameter that is more readily controlled is the natural darkening of the film due to aging and exposure to environmental radiation during storage. Fluorographic emulsions are quite sensitive to natural radiation and upon prolonged storage, unexposed film will darken appreciably after development. The investigator should determine the background density before preexposure and rotate film stocks regularly (every 2 months).

Finally, fluorography will permit the detection of proteins in samples containing extremely low levels of incorporated radioactivity in a significantly shorter time than by autoradiography. In addition, low-energy β particles emitted by ^3H cannot be detected by conventional autoradiography, and, consequently, fluorography is very useful for these samples. Although fluorography decreases exposure time, it will not necessarily increase the resolving power (sensitivity) of either one- or two-dimensional gel electrophoretic procedures. Protein bands or spots containing ^{14}C or ^{35}S which would not be detected by long-term autoradiography will probably remain undetected by fluorography—even with preexposure and prolonged storage at $-70°C$. However, with these limitations in mind, the combination of high-resolution gel electrophoresis and fluorography provides the

TABLE III

Approximate Exposure Times for Optimal Resolution of Proteins or Polypeptides by Either Autoradiography or Fluorography following Either One- or Two-Dimensional Polyacrylamide Gel Electrophoresis[a]

Incorporated radio-activity (cpm)	Autoradiography		Fluorography			
	First dimension	Second dimension	First dimension		Second dimension	
	$^{14}C/^{35}S$	$^{14}C/^{35}S$	^{3}H	$^{14}C/^{35}S$	^{3}H	$^{14}C/^{35}S$
100	F	F	3 Weeks, or F.T.G. 1.5 weeks	2–3 Months, or F.T.G. 1 month	2–3 Months	> 3 months
1000	2–3 Months, or F, 3 weeks, or F.T.G., 1.5 weeks	F	1–2 Days	3 Weeks, or F.T.G. 1 week	2–3 Weeks	2–3 Months
10,000	3 Weeks, or F	2–3 Months, or F	< 1 Day	2 Days	5 Days	2–3 Weeks
100,000	1–2 Days	2–3 Weeks	< 1 Hour	< 1 Day, or A	1 Hour	1 Day
1,000,000	< 1 Day	5 Days	< 1 Hour	A	< 1 Hour	< 1 Hour, or A

[a] F, Fluorography recommended; F.T.G., fluorography combined with ultrathin gels; A, autoradiography recommended.

investigator with a powerful tool to examine the protein synthetic activities of single embryos, parts of embryos or individual cells (Figs. 6 and 7), to mention several possibilities. Table III presents comparative exposure times required for full resolution of bands or spots utilizing either fluorography or autoradiography. It should be noted that bands or spots may be observed after much shorter exposure times, and that the times indicated in Table III are only approximate but useful guides for obtaining optimal sensitivity from the electrophoretic systems. For a more detailed discussion of the physical basis of fluorography and preexposure, the readers' attention is directed to the articles of Bonner and Laskey (1974) and of Laskey and Mills (1975).

B. Determination of the "Purity" of Enzymes and Other Proteins

In many biochemical studies, a major criterion of the "purity" of an isolated protein (enzyme) is the presence of a single band on a one-dimensional polyacrylamide gel. However, as mentioned previously, the actual number of protein species that could comprise a single band is usually unknown. This may even be true when a "highly purified" protein appears as a single band after electrophoresis (Van Blerkom and Manes, 1977). Two-dimensional electrophoretic procedures are particularly useful in determining the actual purity of an isolated enzyme or other cellular protein. The two-dimensional patterns of stained gels presented in Figs. 8A and B illustrate this point.

Figure 8A shows the two-dimensional pattern of rabbit muscle actin prepared in our laboratory. In a one-dimensional, SDS gradient slab gel, only three bands were evident: (1) the actin band which was heavily stained with Coomassie brilliant blue, and (2) two minor bands located below actin and which were thought to be α and β tropomyosin. However, the two-dimensional separation not only confirmed the presence of tropomyosin, but indicated the existence of an additional component (arrow, Fig. 8A) below actin. This spot is likely an autolytic fragment of actin which, due to its apparent molecular weight, was not differentiated from the putative tropomyosin bands by one-dimensional electrophoresis. Figure 8B illustrates the purity of rabbit muscle lactate dehydrogenase (LDH, E. C. 1.1.1.27) prepared in our laboratory by affinity chromatography. Not only are the two major subunits of LDH present at their expected molecular weights and approximate isoelectric points (36,000 daltons, pI 4.5–4.8), but an additional component is evident (arrow).

Other studies in which it was originally thought that a single electrophoretic band indicated the presence of a single species of protein (after fractionation and purification) have revealed varying degrees of contamination by other protein species. Both fluorography and autoradiography may be applied to such analyses. In addition, the purity of antibody preparations are easily tested by

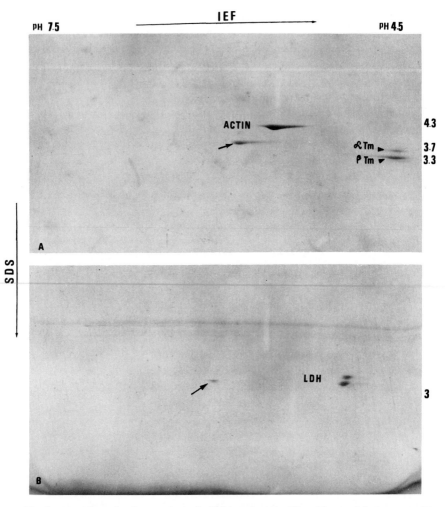

Fig. 8. Two-dimensional separations of rabbit muscle actin (A) and lactate dehydrogenase (B) stained with Coomassie brilliant blue. Components resolved in (A) include actin, α- and β-tropomyosin, and, an additional polypeptide (arrow), which may be an autolytic fragment of actin. The purity of a preparation of lactate dehydrogenase (LDH) is illustrated in (B). Approximate molecular weights ($\times 10^{-4}$) are given on the far right.

immunoprecipitation followed by two-dimensional electrophoresis of the im-
munoprecipitate.

C. Ultrathin Gels

An additional procedure which in our experience has been very useful in
studies involving minute amounts of embryonic material combines
autoradiography/fluorography and one- and two-dimensional PAGE in ultrathin
slab gels. By reducing the thickness of the slab gel from approximately 1 mm to 0.3
mm or less, not only will a few micrograms of protein usually be detected by
staining, but the resultant reduction in self-absorption will permit the detection of
radioactive proteins in samples containing approximately 100 cpm by one- dimensional SDS-PAGE. The construction of ultrathin gels is not unusually difficult,
although special modifications to the design and construction of the gel are
required. The basic slab gel unit is indentical to the unit described in the section on one-dimensional slab gels (Figs. 1 and 3). However, in place of latex
rubber spacers, Teflon or rubber strips approximately 0.3 mm (or less) in
thickness are inserted. No petroleum jelly layer is required to seal the gel plates.
Well formers are machined from pieces of 0.2-mm Teflon. Due to the thin-
ness of the gels, heating effects of electrophoresis are reduced. Consequently,
samples may be electrophoresed at higher currents (25–30 mA), resulting in
both an increase in the sharpness of the bands and a reduction in the time required for electrophoresis (about 1 hour). Since at the higher currents, electrophoretic bands will be sharper throughout the molecular weight range of the gel,
a gradient of acrylamide is not necessary. In our laboratory, a single acrylamide
concentration of between 10 and 12% offers optimal resolution.

1. Solutions: Lower (Running) Gel
      10% gel
   1. 2.7 ml Lower gel buffer
   2. 4.65 ml 80% Glycerol Stock
   3. 3.35 ml 30% Acrylamide stock
   4. 10 μl 10% Ammonium persulfate stock
      12% gel
   1. 2.7 ml Lower gel buffer
   2. 4.0 ml 80% Glycerol stock
   3. 4.0 ml 30% Acrylamide stock
   4. 10 μl 10% Ammonium persulfate stock

After either of the above solutions has been extensively degassed, 2–3 μl of
TEMED is added. Five milliliters of the solution are slowly withdrawn by a
syringe, with care taken to prevent any air from entering the syringe. A 6-inch
28-gauge needle is attached, and 0.5 ml of the acrylamide solution is ejected in

order to remove trapped air. It is critical that no air remain trapped in either the syringe or the hypodermic needle. The tip of the needle is inserted between the two glass plates at the lower portion of the gel unit and the acrylamide solution is introduced at a moderate rate until it reaches a level approximately 1 inch from the base of the notch (as previously described). Air bubbles trapped between the glass plates may be removed with the hypodermic needle. The gel is immediately overlayed with distilled water (from a hypodermic syringe), taking care to avoid mixing between the water and gel solution. Alternatively, a 0.2 mm Teflon strip is placed on the surface of the gel solution to ensure a sharp interface, free of irregularities. After a sharp interface is observed (about 20 minutes), water (and Teflon strip) and unpolymerized acrylamide are removed and replaced with gel-overlay solution (fourfold dilution of lower gel buffer). Ultrathin slab gels are allowed to polymerize for about 6 hours before the stacking gel is applied. The components of the stacking gel are the same as described in the section on one-dimensional SDS gradient gels with the exception that the concentration of ammonium persulfate is reduced from 15–7 μl for the thin gels.

After polymerization, all overlay solution and unpolymerized acrylamide are removed from the surface of the gel. A well former (0.1–0.2 mm thick Teflon) is inserted between the glass plates and the stacking gel solution is slowly and carefully added, making certain that no small air bubbles are trapped by the well former. The stacking gel is allowed to polymerize for 1 hour. Since the partitions forming the wells are extremely fragile, the well former is slowly lifted out. The wells are rinsed with electrophoresis running buffer (electrode buffer), the lower Teflon or rubber spacer removed, and the samples applied (10–15 μl). From this point, electrophoresis follows procedures previously described with the exception that (1) samples are electrophoresed at a constant current of 20–25 mA, and (2) the time required for the dye front to reach the bottom of the gel is approximately 1 hour.

Following electrophoresis, the Teflon spacers are removed and the glass plates carefully separated. The slab gel will usually remain attached to one of the plates, and the entire gel/plate is transferred to 50% TCA. During fixation, the gel is removed from the glass plate. Since ultrathin gels are easily torn, any direct handling of the gel should be avoided. In our experience, a large stainless steel screen is most useful in transferring gels between solutions. Fixation or staining in either 50% TCA or TCA/Coomassie brilliant blue is accomplished in approximately 10–15 minutes. For fluorography, the times required for dehydration in DMSO and infiltration by PPO are reduced by approximately 50% or more. Drying of ultrathin gels under heat and under vacuum is usually complete in about 20 minutes.

The one major problem which tends to arise in this procedure is the entrapment of air during the pouring of the gels. Although this may result from the incomplete removal of air from the hypodermic syringe, it is more frequently associated with the cleanliness of the glass plates. If trapped air bubbles seem to be a recurrent problem, then during the cleaning of the plates, a final soak in a wetting agent such as Photo-flo (Kodak) will generally prevent the formation of air bubbles during the pouring and polymerization of the gel.

It is also of interest to note that two-dimensional separations of proteins may be accomplished on ultrathin gels. The first dimension, or isoelectric focusing gel is constructed as previously described (Section III,B), but in a 100 μl micropipet (Corning) with an appropriate reduction in size and volume. The total volume of the sample should not exceed approximately 5 μl and the volume of the sample overlay should be between 3 and 5 μl. The gel tubes are placed in a standard electrophoresis tank with sufficient modification of the gaskets which separate the chambers. A total running time (including pre-run) of between 3500 and 4000 volt hours offers optimal separation of proteins according to isoelectric point. Although the polymerized gels can usually be extruded from the micropipets with slight pressure, if their removal proves difficult, treatment of the washed micropipets with a wetting agent (such as Kodak Photo-Flo, or its equivalent) usually eliminates this problem. Of course the tubes must be absolutely dry before the gel solution is poured.

The second dimension slab gel is constructed as described above in either of the three plate forms shown in Fig. 5. However, it is critical that before the agarose bed is applied, a sharp surface is established above the stacking gel. A strip of Teflon, approximately 0.2 mm in thickness and absolutely free of irregularities is most convenient for this purpose or a water overlay may also be used. An irregular surface above the stacking gel usually results in severe horizontal rippling of the polypeptides separated in the second dimension. The first dimension microgel is not unusually difficult to handle and is applied to the agarose layer (approximately 0.3 ml of agarose) as described in Section III, E. With ultrathin gels and fluorography, approximately 500 cpm of incorporated ^{3}H is resolved into between 250 and 350 spots after an exposure period (at $-70°C$) of 5–6 weeks. However, for the detection of ^{14}C or ^{35}S, autoradiography, rather than fluorography, of thin, two-dimensional gels is generally sufficient.

V. PROBLEMS OF RESOLUTION AND INTERPRETATION

When unexpectedly poor resolution has been obtained after one- or two-dimensional electrophoresis, the interpretation and analysis of protein polypeptide patterns are usually quite difficult. Some of the more common examples of poor resolution that we have encountered are illustrated in Figs. 9–12, and, in the following discussion, their probable origin is considered. For two-dimensional electrophoresis, other frequent causes of poor resolution have been described in detail by O'Farrell (1975).

Horizontal streaking of the relatively high molecular weight proteins, as is evident in Figs. 9A and 9B, usually occurs during IEF and may result from either an insufficient concentration of urea in the lysis buffer after the addition of sample or from the presence of nucleic acids. Measures to ensure proper urea concentrations have been presented in this chapter. Streaking due to nucleic acids may be minimized or eliminated by exposure of samples to RNase and DNase or frequently, by the inclusion of 0.1% SDS in the IEF lysis buffer. SDS binds to proteins with a high binding constant, but will come off and form mixed micelles with NP-40, which during IEF will migrate to the acidic end of the gel. Neither the separation or resolution of proteins during IEF is usually affected by the addition of SDS to the lysis buffer. Samples containing SDS should not be heated above 25°C as prolonged exposures to higher temperatures may result in artifactual generation of multiple spots (see below).

An important characteristic of the two-dimensional electrophoretic system described in this chapter is the separation of some polypeptide species into a series of multiple spots (see arrows, Figs. 9A and B). Although most polypeptide species are resolved in the second dimension as a single spot, some proteins which exhibit charge and/or size heterogeneity separate as a distinct series of spots. The generation of multiple spots may be a consequence of the (1) artifactual chemical modification of proteins during preparation for IEF, or (2) may be an indication of the biochemical composition of the protein. Artifactual generation of multiple spots may result from prolonged storage of samples (even as a lyophilyzed powder), heating of samples at too high a temperature, or from the decomposition of urea and resultant production of isocyanate. Careful attention to these parameters should eliminate or reduce the possibility of producing artifactual modifications of proteins. Artifactual charge heterogeneity of a single protein species is usually recognizable as a distinct series of spots with the same approximate molecular weight (O'Farrell, 1975).

Modifications to the carbohydrate moiety of a glycoprotein could produce heterogeneity in both the charge and size of the molecule and would be resolved in the SDS dimension as a series of multiple, diagonal spots. The chemical modification of proteins, especially involving the carbohydrate portion of glycoproteins, may be a normal developmental characteristic of the tissue being analyzed, and would be expected to occur *in vivo*. It is suspected that the series of multiple spots indicated in Figs. 9A and B are derived, in fact, from glycoproteins, since (1) extreme care was taken to avoid artifactual modification during sample preparation, and (2) these series of spots were consistently and reproducibly observed in numerous samples of maturing porcine oocytes (Fig. 9A) and early rabbit blastocysts (Fig. 9B) prepared for electrophoresis at very different times. Clearly, more rigorous evidence must be accumulated before a chemical composition may be assigned to a particular set of polypeptide spots. However, the appearance of multiple diagonal spots, such as those illustrated here, suggests that out of a complex electrophoretic pattern, there are potential candidates suitable for additional investigation.

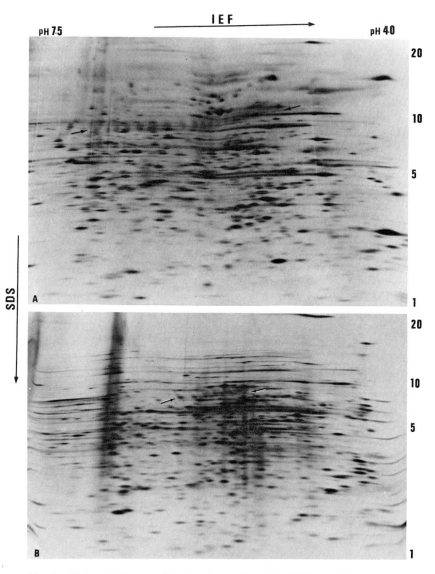

Fig. 9. High-resolution, two-dimensional autoradiographs of [^{35}S-1]methionine-labeled (A) porcine oocytes between the germinal vesicle stage and metaphase I and (B) early rabbit blastocysts. The porcine sample contained approximately 200,000 cpm and 50 oocytes, while the blastocyst sample contained 1 million cpm derived from 15 embryos. Arrows denote multiple, diagonal spots that may indicate the presence of a glycoprotein in that region. Approximate molecular weights ($\times$ 10^{-4}) are given on the far right.

Figure 10 compares the autoradiographic patterns of early (Fig. 10A) and late (Fig. 10B) day 4 mouse blastocysts and illustrates how the separation of polypeptides in the SDS dimension is distorted by the presence of a small air bubble trapped in the agarose gel (Fig. 10B). A similar distortion is observed in one-dimensional SDS-PAGE patterns if bubbles are present beneath the Teflon well former (see, for example, Fig. 2, Van Blerkom and Brockway, 1975b). Small air bubbles trapped in the agarose bed may frequently be undetected, and, consequently, this portion of the second dimension gel must be carefully inspected. In addition, these particular samples contained no SDS, nor were they treated with nucleases. This probably accounts for the streaking of some polypeptides located at the basic region of the gel.

The severe horizontal streaking illustrated in Fig. 11A was caused by an insufficient concentration of urea in the lysis buffer/sample mixture. During the preparation of the IEF gel for electrophoresis, the 9.0 M urea overlay solution was observed to sink rapidly through the sample. Other examples of severe streaking involving both high and low molecular weight polypeptides usually were traceable to a final concentration of urea in the samples considerably below 9.5 M. Streaking of this nature is most often eliminated by the addition of crystalline urea, as previously described. The extreme distortion of the polypeptide patterns evident in Fig. 11B resulted from the presence of air bubbles in the interface between the stacking and running gels. If polymerization of the stacking gel is not complete, air bubbles may form at the interface, with obvious consequences for resolution. These small bubbles may frequently remain undetected, especially if several gels are being electrophoresed simultaneously. A second source of this type of distortion is due to incomplete contact between the IEF gel and the agarose bed, which during electrophoresis may result in the first dimension gel actually separating from the agarose. This problem originates when the IEF gel is placed upon a partially cooled/gelled agarose bed. The transfer of the IEF gel to agarose must be accomplished quickly, and the agarose must be in a liquid state when the transfer is completed. If it is observed that contact between agarose and the IEF gel is incomplete, the IEF gel/agarose bed may be removed, separated from each other, and the procedure for applying the IEF gel repeated. The dense vertical smears located at the basic portion of the autoradiographs shown in Fig. 11 likely result from the precipitation of nucleic acids by the more basic ampholytes. Treatment of similar samples with RNase and DNase eliminated this type of smearing.

The presence of small air bubbles in the running gel is another source of poor resolution. The slight distortion of the polypeptide patterns shown in Fig. 12A was caused by a small air bubble located approximately 1 cm from the upper surface of the running gel. The extensive vertical streaking which is evident in Fig. 12B was due to the incomplete removal of dust and other debris from the surface of the running gel prior to the application of the stacking gel mixture.

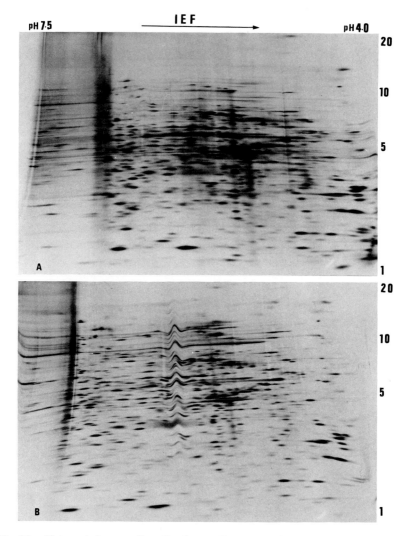

Fig. 10. High-resolution, two-dimensional autoradiographs of [^{35}S-1]methionine-labeled early (A) and late (B) blastocyst-stage mouse embryos. These samples were not treated with nucleases. The distortion of the patterns evident in (B) resulted from the presence of a small air bubble trapped in the agarose bed. Approximately 100,000 cpm were applied to (A) and 75,000 cpm applied to (B). Approximate molecular weights ($\times$ 10^{-4}) are given on the far right.

IEF

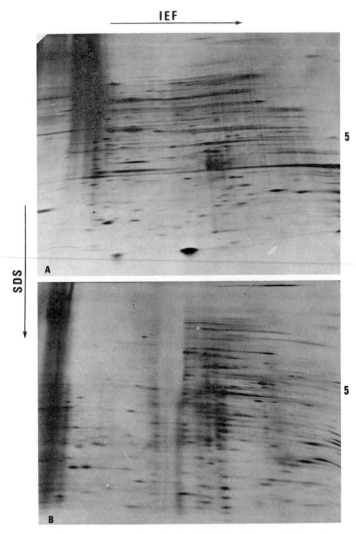

Fig. 11. Two-dimensional autoradiographic patterns of ^{35}S-labeled rabbit oocytes indicating the consequences for resolution of (A) too little urea in the lysis buffer after sample addition, and (B) the presence of air bubbles in the interface between the running and stacking gels. The same type of distortion shown in (B) also results from incomplete contact between the IEF gel and the agarose bed. The intense vertical smearing at the basic region of the gel probably resulted from the precipitation of nucleic acids by the more basic ampholytes.

IEF

pH 7·5 → pH 4·0

SDS

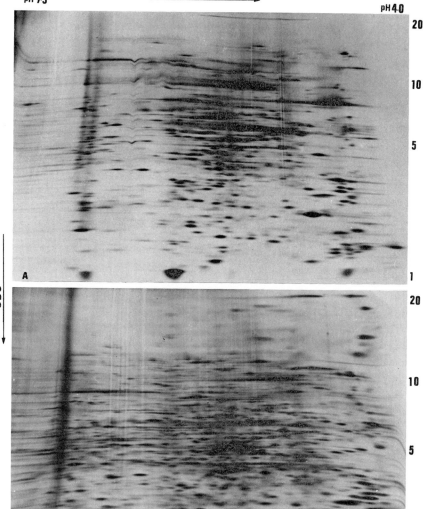

Fig. 12. High-resolution, two-dimensional autoradiographs of [^{35}S-1]methionine-labeled (A) rabbit morulae and (B) late rabbit blastocysts. The distortion in the patterns in (A) was caused by a small air bubble trapped in the running gel. The extreme vertical streaking in (B) was due to the presence of dust and small fragments of glass (from a Pasteur pipette) which were not completely removed from the surface of the running gel prior to the addition of the stacking gel. Approximately 200,000 cpm were applied in (A) and 1 million cpm in (B). Approximate molecular weights ($\times 10^{-4}$) are given on the far right.

Had this gel been stained with Coomassie brilliant blue, the vertical lines would have appeared as dark blue streaks. For optimal resolution with both one-dimensional SDS-slab gels, it is essential that the interface between the running and stacking gels be absolutely free of contamination. In this regard, glass Pasteur pipettes are not recommended for either aspiration or transfer of fluids (gel mixtures or samples), since the tips of these pipettes tend to fragment into minute pieces of glass, which are then both difficult to observe and remove.

The types of problems discussed above are by no means a complete account of the factors which could result in less than optimal resolution. For example, the chemical composition of the samples being analyzed may present particular difficulties which should be considered in the actual preparation of samples for electrophoresis (Helenius and Simons, 1975). However, since both one- and two-dimensional procedures require numerous steps, the most critical aspects are attention to detail and awareness at each step of the potential for introducing conditions that may ultimately make interpretation difficult or reduce the relatively enormous resolving power of these techniques.

VI. NOTE ADDED IN PROOF

Since this chapter was completed in late 1966, O'Farrell et al. (1977) have developed a high resolution, two-dimensional electrophoretic system for the separation of acidic and basic proteins (histones and ribosomal proteins). In conjunction with the standard two-dimensional system described in this chapter, the application of a second electrophoretic system provides a significant expansion in the range of cellular proteins which may now be resolved.

ACKNOWLEDGMENTS

It was the intent of this chapter to provide a complete and "self-contained" description of the various methods currently in use in the high-resolution analysis of protein synthesis and also, to discuss how these methods may be employed in the study of mammalian reproduction and development. This chapter was designed especially for the investigator with limited experience in the application of electrophoretic techniques. Consequently, because some of the methods presented here have been developed by other investigators, there is necessarily some overlap between the descriptions in this chapter and their published works and the reader would profit by consulting these works. I would especially like to thank Dr. Patrick O'Farrell for his numerous suggestions dating back over a period of many years. I would also like to thank Scott Panter and Hobart Bell for their helpful suggestions in the preparation of this manuscript. The work reported here was supported by a grant from the National Institutes of Health, United States Public Health Service (HD-04274) and by a fellowship from the European Molecular Biology Organization.

REFERENCES

Ames, G. F. L., and Nikaido, K. (1976). *Biochemistry* **15**, 616–623.
Bonner, W. M., and Laskey, R. A. (1974). *Eur. J. Biochem.* **46**, 83–88.
Davis, B. J. (1964). *Ann. N.Y. Acad. Sci.* **121**, 404–427.
Drysdale, J. W. (1975). *In* "Methods of Protein Separation" (N. Catsimpoolas, ed.), pp. 93–126. Plenum, New York.
Epstein, C. J., and Smith, S. A. (1974). *Dev. Biol.* **40**, 233–244.
Helenius, A., and Simons, K. (1975). *Biochim. Biophys. Acta* **415**, 29–79.
Kaltschmidt, E., and Wittman, H. G. (1970). *Anal. Biochem.* **36**, 401–417.
Klose, J. (1975). *Humangenetik* **26**, 231–243.
Laemmli, U. K. (1970). *Nature (London)* **227**, 680–685.
Laskey, R. A., and Mills, A. D. (1975). *Eur. J. Biochem.* **56**, 335–341.
Latner, A. L. (1975). *Adv. Clin. Chem.* **17**, 193–250.
McGaughey, R. W., and Van Blerkom, J. (1977). *Dev. Biol.* **56**, 241–254.
Maurer, H. R. (1971). "Disc Electrophoresis and Related Techniques of Polyacrylamide Gel Electrophoresis." de Gruyter, Berlin.
O'Farrell, P. H. (1975). *J. Biol. Chem.* **250**, 4007–4021.
O'Farrell, P. H., and O'Farrell, P. A. (1977). *In* "Methods in Cell Biology," (D. M. Prescott, G. Stein, J. Stein, G. J. Kleinsmith, eds.), Vol. 16, pp. 407–420. Academic Press, New York.
O'Farrell, P. Z., Goodman, H. M., and O'Farrell, P. H. (1977). *Cell* **12**, 1133–1142.
Ornstein, L. (1964). *Ann. N.Y. Acad. Sci.* **121**, 321–349.
Petzoldt, U. (1972). *Cytobiologie* **6**, 473–475.
Petzoldt, U. (1975). *Cytobiologie* **11**, 490–493.
Scheele, G. A. (1975). *J. Biol. Chem.* **250**, 5375–5385.
Shapiro, A. L., and Maizel, J. V. (1969). *Anal. Biochem.* **29**, 505–514.
Shapiro, A. L., Vinuela, E., and Maizel, J. V. (1967). *Biochem. Biophys. Res. Commun.* **28**, 815–820.
Studier, F. W. (1973). *J. Mol. Biol.* **79**, 237–248.
Van Blerkom, J. (1977). *In* "Immunobiology of the Gametes" pp. 187–206. (M. H. Johnson and M. Edidin, eds.). Cambridge Univ. Press, London and New York.
Van Blerkom, J., and Brockway, G. (1975a). *Dev. Biol.* **44**, 148–157.
Van Blerkom, J., and Brockway, G. (1975b). *Dev. Biol.* **46**, 446–451.
Van Blerkom, J., and Manes, C. (1974). *Dev. Biol.* **40**, 40–51.
Van Blerkom, J., and Manes, C. (1977). *In* "Concepts in Early Mammalian Development" (M. I. Sherman, ed.). MIT Press, Cambridge, Massachusetts, pp. 37–94.
Van Blerkom, J., and McGaughey, R. W. (1978a). *Dev. Biol.* **63**, 139–150.
Van Blerkom, J., and McGaughey, R. W. (1978b). *Dev. Biol.* **63**, 151–164.
Van Blerkom, J., Barton, S., and Johnson, M. H. (1976). *Nature (London)* **259**, 319–321.
Woodland, H. R., and Adamson, E. D. (1977). *Devel. Biol.* **57**, 118–135.

5

Microtechniques with Preimplantation Embryos

R. G. WALES

Because of the limited amount of biologic material available, almost any study of the biochemistry of the mammalian embryo utilizes microtechniques in one form or another. Measurement of oxygen consumption requires micromanometric techniques (Mills and Brinster, 1967; Fridhandler, 1971). Studies of the uptake and utilization of substrates and precursors have utilized isotopically labeled substrates and a variety of microtechniques to isolate and fractionate the embryos. Likewise, the activity of enzymes in embryos has been measured using microadaptations of standard procedures for enzyme analysis (Brinster, 1971).

Few quantitative measurements of intracellular metabolites have been made in mammalian embryos. Lowenstein and Cohen (1964) estimated dry weight and the proportions of lipid and protein in mouse embryos. Total protein (Brinster, 1967; Schiffner and Speilmann, 1976), glycogen (Stern and Biggers, 1968; Snyder et al., 1971; Ozias and Stern, 1973), adenyl nucleotides (Quinn and

Wales, 1971; Epstein and Daentl, 1971; Ginsberg and Hillman, 1973), nucleic acids (Reamer, 1963; Olds *et al.*, 1973), and total NAD (Kuwahara and Chaykin, 1973) have been measured in embryos by various microtechniques. In most of these assays, the sensitivity was such that the measurements could only be performed on groups of embryos. More recently, certain metabolic intermediates have been assayed in single embryos (Barbehenn *et al.*, 1974; Wales, 1974), using enzymatic cycling techniques. Such methods have the advantage of conserving embryos, assessing individual variability, and allowing a large number of assays to be performed on a limited amount of biologic material. Furthermore, they can be adapted to measure a wide range of metabolites. It is the purpose of this chapter to describe in some detail the application of the methodology of enzymatic cycling to the assay of these metabolites and to comment on its possible use in the study of mammalian embryology.

I. GENERAL CONSIDERATIONS

The assays are based on the techniques developed by Dr. Oliver H. Lowry and his co-workers at Washington University School of Medicine over the last decade or more. For further information on the general laboratory procedures associated with these techniques, the reader is referred to the recent book by Lowry and Passonneau (1972) entitled *A Flexible System of Enzymatic Analysis*.

The methods depend upon enzymatic assays of metabolites in which pyridine nucleotides act as the oxidizing or reducing agents for the specific enzyme system. Providing that conditions for the assay are chosen such that the enzyme reaction proceeds to completion, then the amount of nucleotide reduced or oxidized in the reaction will be equal on a molar basis to the amount of metabolite present. Thus, measurement of the conversion of nucleotide at the completion of the enzymatic reaction can be used to assay the level of metabolite present. The reduced nucleotides (NADH and NADPH) have an absorption band with a peak at 340 nm. Some of the absorbed light is reemitted as fluorescence at 460 nm, and this can be measured with great accuracy in a fluorometer. With standard spectrophotometric equipment, reduced nucleotide concentrations in the range 10–100 μM can be measured accurately. Fluorometry offers a tenfold increase in sensitivity and is the method of choice where small amounts of metabolite are to be assayed.

Thus, in a direct fluorometric assay of a metabolite, using conventional equipment with a 1 ml final reaction volume, the smallest amount of metabolite that can be measured is in the vicinity of $0.1–1.0 \times 10^{-9}$ mole. However, in a single mammalian preimplantation embryo, the metabolites measured to date lie in the range $10^{-13}–10^{-15}$ mole, far below the range of sensitivity of the direct one-step assay technique involving the reduction or oxidation of nucleotide and the measurement of (1) the reduced nucleotide formed in the reaction, or (2) the fall in concentration of the reduced form where the reaction involves the oxidation of the pyridine nucleotide.

Measurement of the levels of metabolites in single embryos has been made possible by linking the enzymatic assay techniques to an amplification step referred to as enzymatic cycling (Lowry *et al.*, 1961a). The cycling system consists of two enzymatically catalyzed reactions, one of which oxidizes nucleotide, the other causing its reduction as shown below.

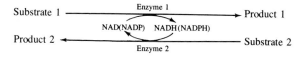

Thus the reduced or oxidized nucleotide produced in an enzymatic assay can be shuttled through these two reactions, the nucleotide being alternately reduced and oxidized during the cycling. If the conditions of the cycle are such that the amount of nucleotide is rate limiting, then the amount of product formed is directly proportional to the amount of nucleotide present. By varying the level of substrates and enzymes for the cycling reactions, the rate of cycling and, thus, the degree of amplification can be controlled. With optimum conditions, it is possible to obtain considerable amplification (up to 20,000- to 30,000-fold) and an equivalent increase in the sensitivity of the overall assay. The final step in such an assay depends on the enzymatic measurement of one of the products of the cycling reaction leading to the reduction of nucleotide which can be measured fluorometrically. This step is often referred to as the "indicator reaction."

The initial enzyme reaction produces from the metabolite to be measured an equimolar amount of either reduced or oxidized nucleotide from the appropriate nucleotide added to the reaction mixture, normally added in excess to ensure completion of the reaction. Prior to the cycling reaction, it is necessary to remove unreacted nucleotide so that only the nucleotide which has reacted in the initial step remains. Nucleotide can be destroyed due to the instability of the oxidized and reduced forms to alkaline and acidic conditions, respectively (Lowry *et al.*, 1961b). Thus, when the initial reaction results in the reduction of nucleotide, the excess oxidized form of the nucleotide that had been added to the reaction to bring about its completion can be completely destroyed, without affecting the reduced form produced by the enzymatic reaction, by adjusting the pH of the reaction mixture to approximately 12.0, and heating at 80°C for 20 minutes. Conversely, where the product of the reaction is oxidized nucleotide, the excess reduced form added to the reaction mixture can be destroyed, without affecting the oxidized product, by adjusting the pH to approximately 2.0, and heating as above. After either of these procedures, the pH can be readjusted to neutrality and the cycling reactions carried out on the nucleotide products of the initial reaction.

As stated above, the cycling reaction can produce a 20,000- to 30,000-fold increase in the sensitivity of the assay procedure and allow the measurement of 10^{-13}–10^{-14} mole of metabolite. This level of sensitivity is sufficient for the assay of some metabolites in single embryos. However, the level of other metabolites in preimplantation embryos is of the order of 10^{-15} mole, and a further increase in sensitivity is necessary to allow their assay in individual embryos. This increase in sensitivity can be achieved after the indicator step by conversion of the nucleotide product of the indicator reaction to a strongly fluorescent compound (alkaline enhancement of fluorescence). Following cycling, one of the products of the cycling reaction is assayed in the usual way, resulting in the reduction of pyridine nucleotide. After the excess oxidized nucleotide has been removed by acid or alkali, the reduced nucleotide formed in the indicator reaction can be converted to the highly fluorescent product by heating the reaction mixture in the presence of strong alkali. This causes a five- to tenfold increase in fluorescence over that of the nucleotide and allows measurement of small amounts of cycling product to be achieved. However, care must be exercised in this procedure, as both oxidized and reduced forms of the nucleotide produce a fluorescent product under these conditions. Thus, it is essential that all unreacted nucleotide remaining from the indicator reaction is destroyed, as incomplete destruction would lead to spuriously high fluorescence values.

II. BASIS OF TECHNIQUE

The basic steps for the assay of metabolites in embryos are listed below.

Step 1. Carry out the specific enzymatic reaction for the particular metabolite. This results in the oxidation or reduction of pyridine nucleotide.

Step 2. Destroy unreacted nucleotide in the assay reaction of step 1.

Step 3. Cycle reacted nucleotide from step 1 to build up product.

Step 4. Terminate the cycling reaction.

Step 5. Assay a product of the cycling reaction by enzymatic means leading to the production of reduced nucleotide.

Step 6.(a) Where the particular metabolite is present at the level of 10^{-13} to 10^{-14} mole, sufficient reduced nucleotide is formed in step 5 to allow its direct measurement in a fluorometer. (b) Where the particular metabolite is present at a level below 10^{-14} mole, insufficient reduced nucleotide is formed in step 5 for accurate measurement by native fluorescence, and the following steps are necessary.

Step 7. Destroy unreacted oxidized nucleotide from step 5 under controlled conditions.

Step 8. Convert reduced nucleotide produced in step 5 to a highly fluorescent product by heating in strong alkali (alkaline enhancement).

Step 9. Measure the fluorescent product in a fluorometer.

For such assays, it is necessary to include blanks and standards covering the expected range of the metabolite in the samples. These are carried through the procedure in exactly the same way as the samples and are used (1) to assess the contribution of background fluorescence and (2) to calibrate the assay. The factors listed below need to be considered in performing the steps as outlined above.

Step 1. Specific Enzymatic Reaction

The specific reaction should be carried out in as small a volume as practicable to decrease the fluorescence of the blank and to maintain a sufficiently high concentration of the metabolite to be assayed. Prior to undertaking this microassay, it is normal to carry out preliminary studies of the specific reaction on a macroscale in a standard fluorometer tube. In this way, optimal conditions for the reaction can be checked. Once this procedure has been carried out, the volume can be scaled down while maintaining the concentration of reactants in the mixture.

Typically, when measuring metabolites in embryos at the level of 10^{-13}–10^{-15} mole, the final volume for the initial specific reaction is of the order of 200–250 nl. Working with these small volumes presents a number of problems.

a. Evaporation. Evaporation is controlled by performing all analyses under oil. For the assay, the oil (60% light mineral oil, 40% hexadecane) is pipetted into small wells drilled in a Teflon rack. Full details of the Teflon oil well racks and their use are given by Lowry and Passonneau (1972). Flat-bottomed wells are drilled in a Teflon block approximately 4 mm thick. Each well is drilled sufficiently deep so that the bottom of the well is translucent and can be illuminated by the substage light of a microscope. The small volumes used in the assays are pipetted directly into the oil in the wells while viewing through a binocular dissecting microscope.

b. Surface Inactivation of Enzymes. In the small volumes used in the specific reaction, the ratio of surface to volume is high; under these conditions, the addition of bovine serum albumin helps to stabilize the enzymes and protect them against surface inactivation.

c. Electrostatic Charge. Considerable electrostatic charge can build up on droplets in the oil wells during pipetting, causing difficulty in ensuring coalescence of droplets during the assay. Thus, during all additions to oil wells, it is necessary to suspend a small metal strip impregnated with a radioactive source (e.g., radium-226) in order to dissipate the electrostatic charge. This metal strip is suspended over the well on a flexible arm and is coated with 20–30 μCi of the radionuclide.

d. Accurate Pipetting. Constriction pipettes of the Lang–Levy type are used for the addition of small volumes of reagents. While constriction pipettes of this kind are readily available commercially in larger sizes (commonly down to 2 μl), pipettes delivering volumes in the nanoliter range are not easily obtainable. It is, therefore, common for workers carrying out these microassays to construct their own pipettes. Details for the construction and calibration of these pipettes are given by Lowry and Passonneau (1972).

Pipettes used for the addition of reagents to oil wells must be fine tipped for effective use. They are constructed of quartz, as it is easier to fabricate a pipette of the right proportions using quartz than Pyrex glass, and the final product is sturdier. The final steps in construction are carried out using a microtorch while viewing through a dissection microscope.

Step 2. Destruction of Unreacted Nucleotide

After allowing sufficient time for completion of the specific enzyme reaction, the enzymes are inactivated, and the unreacted nucleotide remaining in the drop is destroyed. The time required for the initial reaction is calculated from the preliminary studies of the reaction carried out in a volume of 1 ml.

Where the initial reaction leads to the formation of reduced pyridine nucleotide, the drop in the oil well is made alkaline by addition of a small volume of 0.15 N NaOH (approximately 50–80 nl). In assays causing oxidation of the cofactor, the drop in the oil well is acidified by the addition of 0.15 N HCl. After the addition of either acid or alkali to all reaction wells in the Teflon block, the block is placed in an 80°C incubator for 20 minutes to destroy unreacted nucleotide. Both of these procedures also cause denaturation of enzymes added for the initial reaction.

Step 3. Cycling Reaction

After destruction of unreacted nucleotide in step 2, the reacted nucleotide can be amplified by the enzymatic cycling reaction. Prior to carrying out the cycling reaction, it is necessary to neutralize the drops in the oil well. This can be done in a number of ways. A simple procedure is to add an appropriate amount of NaOH or HCl to neutralize the acid or alkali added in step 2. However, considerable care must be taken with pipetting to ensure exact neutralization. If excess acid or alkali is added, there is a risk of destruction of some of the reacted nucleotide. A safer procedure is to add the appropriate amount of Tris base or Tris-HCl to the drop in the oil well to form Tris buffer at approximately pH 8.0. Under these circumstances, minor errors in pipetting will have little effect on the final pH of the resultant mixture. A third alternative is to adjust the pH of the cycling reagent such that when it is added to the drop in the oil well, the final pH of the mixture is at the optimum for the cycling reaction. If this procedure is used, care must be exercised to ensure that the pH of the cycling reagent is not such as to have a detrimental effect on its constituents prior to addition to the drop. However, where it is necessary to keep the volume of the reaction to a minimum at all stages, this latter alternative is an advantage. In addition, it eliminates one pipetting step from the overall assay.

There are many enzyme pairs which can be coupled in the cycling reaction, and the choice of the appropriate enzymes depends on several factors such as kinetics of the reaction, pH optimum of the enzymes, inhibition by product or substrate, and the ease of product assay. At present, the following cycling reactions are used for amplification of NAD (NADH) and NADP (NADPH).

a. NAD (NADH) Cycle.   This cycle was described by Kato et $al.$ (1973), and consists of the following reactions:

$$NAD^+ + ethanol \rightarrow NADH + acetaldehyde + H^+ \tag{1}$$

$$NADH + oxaloacetate \rightarrow NAD^+ + malate \tag{2}$$

Reaction 1 is catalyzed by the enzyme alcohol dehydrogenase, while reaction 2 is catalyzed by malate dehydrogenase. Prior to use, the enzymes must be treated with charcoal to remove nucleotide in order to reduce blank values (see Kato et $al.$, 1973). Even after this treatment, it is advisable to keep the volume of the cycling reagent as small as possible, particularly where high sensitivity is required, in order to minimize blank values.

b. NADP (NADPH) Cycle.   This cycle is described in detail by Lowry and Passonneau (1972), and consists of the following reactions.

$$NADP^+ + glucose\text{-}6\text{-}P \rightarrow NADPH + 6\text{-}P\text{-}gluconolactone + H^+ \tag{1}$$

$$NADPH + \alpha\text{-}ketoglutarate + NH_4^+ \rightarrow NADP^+ + glutamate \tag{2}$$

Reaction 1 is catalyzed by glucose-6-phosphate dehydrogenase, and the second by glutamate dehydrogenase. Variations in the cycling rate can be obtained by adjusting the conditions, such as enzyme levels and time of cycling. Under optimal conditions, cycling rates of 15,000–35,000/hour may be anticipated. As a preliminary step, the cycling reactions can be studied on a macroscale to determine optimum conditions and cycling rates before use in the microanalysis. In the microanalyses, it is wise to keep the volume of the cycling mixture sufficiently low to ensure that nucleotide concentrations are in the range 10^{-7}–10^{-9} mole. This helps to keep blank values in the overall reaction low. In assays of metabolites in embryos, it is normal to add 1–3 μl of the appropriate cycling reagent to the drop in the oil well and allow cycling to continue for 60 minutes. However, the conditions for the cycle reaction need to be varied, depending on the anticipated level of the metabolite in the embryo and, thus, the nucleotide concentration in the drop after the initial specific enzyme reaction. If the nucleotide concentration is high, the rate of cycling may not remain directly proportional to the nucleotide concentration. In addition, under these conditions or when the volume of cycling reagent is low, the substrate for the cycling reaction may become exhausted, leading to a premature termination of the reaction.

The NAD (NADH) cycle has an optimum temperature in the range 25°–30°C (see Kato *et al.*, 1973) and cycling is usually carried out at room temperature. On the other hand, the NAD (NADPH) cycle has a temperature coefficient of 7.7% per degree between 25° and 38°C (Lowry *et al.*, 1961a) and to obtain high cycling rates, samples are incubated at 37°C during the cycling reaction.

Step 4. Termination of Cyling

The cycling reaction is allowed to proceed for the time required to produce the required degree of amplification. The cycling reaction is then terminated by the addition of alkali and heating the Teflon block at 80°C for 20 minutes.

Step 5. Indicator Reaction

In the NAD cycle, the malate formed as a product of the cycle is assayed, using malate dehydrogenase:

$$\text{Malate} + \text{NAD}^+ \rightarrow \text{oxaloacetate} + \text{NADH} + \text{H}^+$$

In the case of the NADP cycle, the 6-P-gluconolactone formed as a product of the cycle is assayed. The 6-P-gluconolactone is converted quantitatively to 6-P-gluconate during step 4 and 6-P-gluconate is assayed using 6-P-gluconate dehydrogenase:

$$\text{6-P-gluconate} + \text{NADP} \rightarrow \text{ribulose-5-P} + \text{CO}_2 + \text{NADPH} + \text{H}^+$$

Step 6. Indicator Step

a. Direct Measurement of Indicator Step. Where the indicator step yields 0.2–2×10^{-9} mole of reduced nucleotide (i.e., where 10^{-14}–10^{-13} mole of the metabolite was present in the embryo, and a cycling rate of 20,000 was achieved), the fluorescence of reduced nucleotide so formed can be read directly in a fluorometer, using standard fluorometer tubes. When this is to be carried out, 1 ml aliquots of indicator reagent can be pipetted into fluorometer tubes, and appropriate aliquots of the drops in the oil wells transferred to these tubes at the completion of step 5. After mixing and allowing the reaction to reach completion, the fluorescence of the reduced nucleotide can be measured directly. Alternatively, 10 μl aliquots of an appropriate indicator reagent may be added to the drops in the oil well. At the completion of the reaction, a sufficiently large aliquot of the reaction mixture is transferred to fluorometer tubes containing 1 ml of water. This second procedure, although adding an extra pipetting step to the overall procedure, may be useful where the indicator reagent shows a high background fluorescence.

b. Indicator Step for Low Levels of Metabolite. Where metabolites are present in the femtomole range (10^{-15} mole), insufficient product is formed even under optimum conditions of cycling to allow direct measurement of the reduced nucleotide formed in the indicator step. Further steps to enhance the native fluorescence of the nucleotide are necessary. When this is to be done, the indicator reaction must be carried out in a small volume in the oil well. The precise volume of indicator reagent added to the well after step 5 will depend on the metabolite to be assayed, and the particular problems related to the level of blank fluorescence encountered in the assay and may vary from 1 to 10 μl. In all cases, the concentration of reactants in the indicator reagent must be chosen to ensure completion of the reaction during the period of incubation in the oil well.

Step 7. *Destruction of Unreacted Nucleotide*

As both oxidized and reduced nucleotide will produce fluorescent products when heated in strong alkali, it is necessary to remove oxidized nucleotide remaining at the completion of the indicator step. This is accomplished by heating at alkaline pH, but the conditions must be controlled to ensure total destruction of the unreacted nucleotide without causing any formation of a fluorescent product due to the alkaline conditions. This is done after completion of step 6b above by transferring an aliquot of the drop in the oil wells (usually 80–90% of total volume) to fluorometer tubes containing 50 μl of 0.5 M phosphate buffer pH 12. Heating these tubes at 60°C for 15 minutes completely destroys the oxidized nucleotide without production of any highly fluorescent product.

Step 8. *Alkaline Enhancement*

This can be achieved by adding 1 ml of 6 N NaOH containing 0.03% H_2O_2 to the fluorometer tube and heating at 60°C for 15 minutes. The reduced nucleotide is oxidized by the H_2O_2, and the alkali converts the oxidized nucleotide to a highly fluorescent product. The fluorescent product is light sensitive, and difficulty can be experienced during reading due to fading in the light beam of the fluorometer. Fading can be minimized by the addition of 10 mM imidazole to the NaOH/H_2O_2 reagent. Alternatively, it can be overcome by adopting the following procedure. Following step 7 above, 100 μl of 9 N NaOH containing 0.045% H_2O_2 is added to the 50 μl in the fluorometer tube. After heating, water is added to give 1 ml final volume for reading in the fluorometer.

Step 9. Fluorometer Reading

The fluorescent product has its emission spectral peak at 460 nm. All tubes must be at room temperature before reading due to the temperature coefficient of the fluorescence.

III. PREPARATION OF EMBRYOS FOR ANALYSIS

The preceding section outlines the general procedures and reactions associated with the measurement of metabolic products in single embryos. Before proceeding to consider the details of the specific assays that have been carried out in embryos, it is appropriate to consider the preparation of embryos for assay.

In assaying metabolites in embryos, the experimental worker may be interested in (1) the changes in the levels of the metabolite within the embryo during an experimental manipulation while the embryo is cultured *in vitro*. (2) The level of a metabolite *in vivo*, i.e., the actual state of the metabolite while the embryo is present in the environment of the maternal reproductive tract.

Measurement of metabolites in cultured embryos is relatively simple, and estimates can be obtained under these conditions which reflect the true levels of the metabolite in the living embryo with a high degree of confidence. We shall consider the preparation of embryos for assay under these conditions before examining the problems associated with the determination of the concentration of metabolites in embryos resident in the maternal reproductive tract.

In order that the assay of a metabolite will be representative of the situation during the normal life of a cell or tissue, the enzyme systems that may alter the level of the particular metabolite must be inactivated rapidly, and the tissue must be preserved in such a way that no destruction of the metabolite occurs during storage. Inactivation is usually brought about by rapidly freezing the tissue, usually in liquid nitrogen. In the intact animal, there is a lag time between death of the animal, and consequent cessation of blood supply to the tissue, and the inactivation of enzyme activity by freezing. This lag time is critical when attempting to estimate the normal level of metabolites in living tissue. In the case of embryos cultured *in vitro*, the problem is minimal as the tissue volume is so small that almost instantaneous freezing of the sample can be anticipated. Following rapid freezing, the embryos are freeze-dried for storage and subsequent analysis.

Preimplanation embryos that have been flushed from the reproductive tracts of pregnant animals with culture medium can be frozen by transfer to a microscope slide and immersion in liquid nitrogen. It is unlikely that significant changes in the levels of metabolite will occur as long as the transfer is rapid, and no evaporation occurs while the embryos are on the slide prior to freezing. The transfer is accomplished by sucking up the required numbers of embryos from the culture dish with a fine Pasteur pipette and pipetting them onto a microscope slide, together with a small quantity of medium. The slide is then fully immersed in a bath of liquid nitrogen. The only real precaution to be taken during this operation is to ensure that an appropriate volume of medium is transferred with the embryos. If the volume of medium is too great, the embryos tend to become dislodged from the slide during the subsequent freeze-drying procedure. If too little medium surrounds the embryos at the time of freezing, the embryos adhere closely to the slide during subsequent freeze-drying and are difficult to dislodge from the slide for transfer to oil wells. In practice, the embryos are quickly transferred to the slide and excess medium withdrawn so that the embryos are just covered by fluid when frozen. This procedure can be accomplished in about 5 seconds. Following freezing in liquid nitrogen, the embryos can be stored for some time in a −80°C cabinet prior to drying.

While the preparation of embryos described above would be expected to provide samples that would reflect the metabolic state of the embryos at the time of sampling from the culture medium, it is far more difficult to obtain a preparation which one can be sure reflects the state of the metabolites in embryos *in vivo*. The recovery of embryos from the female tract of laboratory animals normally involves the sacrifice of the animal, removal of the appropriate area of the reproductive tract, and flushing of the embryos from the tract with culture medium. Even under favorable conditions of recovery, a period of 1–2 minutes must elapse between death of the animal and final freezing of the embryos by the methods described above. However, as the preimplantation embryo lies free in the lumen of the reproductive tract, the short sojourn in the tract after blood supply has ceased may have only minor effects on the environment. In addition, the use of flushing media whose composition reflects that of reproductive tract secretions should minimize changes in the recovered embryos. Even with these considerations, the concentration of metabolites measured can only be taken as a reflection of the *in vivo* levels and cannot be accepted with a high degree of confidence as being truly representative of the levels *in vivo*. A possible alternative that would more closely indicate true levels would be to freeze the reproductive tract while the blood supply was intact and undertake subsequent recovery of embryos from the reproductive tract. This would be a time-consuming procedure and has not been attempted to date.

Freeze-drying and subsequent low-temperature storage of samples increases the stability of metabolites and allows safe storage for long periods without breakdown of labile compounds or leaching of metabolites from cells into the surroundings. By using this process, it is possible to freeze-dry several embryos on the one slide, and, when analyses are required, the slide can be returned to room temperature, one embryo transferred to the oil well for assay, and the remainder re-stored for future use, perhaps a year or more later.

To freeze-dry the samples, the slides containing the frozen embryos are transferred to holders and loaded into vacuum tubes (see Lowry and Passonneau, 1972). This whole procedure is carried out below $-20°C$, taking care that all holders and glassware have been adequately precooled. The vacuum tube is then transferred to a freezer cabinet maintained at $-35°C$ and subjected to a vacuum equivalent to 0.01 mm of Hg for 16–18 hours. A dry ice trap is used to condense the moisture from the sample. At the completion of the drying period, the tube is allowed to return to room temperature while evacuation is continued. The vacuum tubes containing the dried samples can then be stored at $-20°C$ under vacuum. Lower temperatures for storage may be necessary where very labile compounds are to be assayed.

For the analysis of freeze-dried embryos, the evacuated vacuum tubes containing the embryos are removed from the $-20°C$ freezing compartment and allowed to return to room temperature while the vacuum is maintained. Once returned to room temperature, the vacuum can be released, slides removed, and the required embryos transferred to oil wells. All transfers are carried out in a room at $25°C$ and 50% humidity to prevent deterioration of the dried samples during the process. Following transfer of the required number of embryos, the remainder of the dried samples on the slides are returned to the vacuum tubes, evacuated, and stored at $-20°C$ for subsequent use.

At the commencement of an assay and while the vacuum tubes are warming to room temperature, wells in the Teflon blocks are filled with oil and a 50- to 80 μl drop of acid or alkali pipetted into each well. Where the initial specific reaction results in the reduction of pyridine nucleotide, the samples are transferred to drops of 0.02 N HCl. Heating of the samples in the drops prior to the assay destroys endogenous reduced nucleotide and tissue enzymes. Where oxidized nucleotide is the product of the specific reaction, the initial heating is carried out in NaOH, rather than acid.

The details of the methods and equipment used to transfer dried specimens to the oil wells for assay are given in Lowry and Passonneau (1972). Embryos dried on the microscope slides as described above are easily identified, embedded in a crystalline mesh of dried medium when viewed under the microscope. If the correct amount of medium was present during freezing, the embryos are undistorted and can be easily picked out of the medium with a simple instrument made by gluing a short length of hair into a handle. The embryos are then transferred to a tissue holder and subsequently added to the drop in the oil well. This final transfer is made with the aid of a quartz fiber glued into the end of a glass handle. While observing under the binocular microscope, the dried embryo is picked up on the end of the quartz fiber to which it adheres. On entering the oil in the well, the dried embryo detaches from the fiber and begins to sink. While keeping the sample in focus under the microscope, it is directed with the tip of the quartz fiber until it enters the aqueous drop in the well and dissolves.

IV. SPECIFIC ASSAYS OF METABOLITES IN EMBRYOS

A number of assays of metabolites have been carried out in single mouse embryos. These include some intermediates of the glycolytic and tricarboxylic acid cycles as well as ATP, AMP, P_i, and the pyridine nucleotides themselves. Results of some of these assays have been recorded (Barbehenn *et al.*, 1974, 1978; Wales, 1974).

The specific reactions involved in these assays and the conditions required to gain sufficient sensitivity to carry out the assays on single embryos will be described in the following paragraphs.

A. TCA Cycle Intermediates

The levels of citrate, isocitrate, malate, and α-ketoglutarate have been measured in single preimplantation mouse embryos, using enzymatic cycling techniques (Barbehenn *et al.*, 1974, 1978). The experimental conditions employed while carrying out the initial specific reactions for the measurement of each of these metabolites are given in Table I. There are considerable differences between metabolites in the amount present in embryos. Thus, it is necessary to vary the sensitivity of the assay procedure, depending on the metabolite and to some extent on the stage of development of the embryo.

1. Citrate

The levels of citrate are relatively high in preimplantation mouse embryos (2–8 $\times$ 10^{-13} mole), and, thus, only a moderate cycling rate is necessary for its assay. In addition, sufficient product is produced during the cycle to allow direct fluorometric measurement without alkaline enhancement. The steps in a citrate assay in such embryos are described below. It should be noted, however, that the sensitivity of the assay can be increased by either increasing the cycling rate or by the use of alkaline enhancement. Thus, measurement of levels in the range of 10^{-15}–10^{-14} mole could be achieved using protocols similar to those used for α-ketoglutarate described later in this chapter.

The measurement of citrate depends on the following specific reactions.

$$\text{Citrate} \xrightarrow[\text{lyase}]{\text{citrate}} \text{oxaloacetate} + \text{acetate}$$

$$\text{Oxaloacetate} + \text{NADH} + \text{H}^+ \xrightarrow[\text{dehydrogenase}]{\text{malate}} \text{malate} + \text{NAD}^+$$

TABLE I

Conditions for the Enzymatic Assay of TCA Cycle Intermediates in Preimplantation Mouse Embryos Prior to Amplification by Enzymatic Cycling

Metabolite (range of standards)	Buffer	Enzymes	Other components of assay mixture	Volume of reactants (nl)	Incubation time (minutes)
Citrate ($1-15 \times 10^{-13}$ mole)	Tris-HCl ($100~\mu M$, pH 7.6)	Malate dehydrogenase (0.3 μg/ml) Citrate lyase (3 μg/ml)	NADH (20 μM—use 4 μM at early developmental stages) $ZnCl_2$ (33 μM) Ascorbic acid (1.3 mM)	240	20
Malate ($4-16 \times 10^{-14}$ mole)	2-Amino-2-methyl-1-propanol-HCl (50 mM, pH 9.8)	Malate dehydrogenase (14 μg/ml) Glutamate-oxaloacetate transaminase (3 μg/ml)	NAD (50 μM) Glutamate (1 mM) Bovine serum albumin (0.25 mg/ml)	240	10
Isocitrate ($3-22 \times 10^{-15}$ mole)	Tris-HCl (90 mM, pH 8.0)	Isocitrate dehydrogenase (glycerol solution, 2 μg/ml)	NADP (9 μM) $MgCl_2$ (100 μM) Bovine serum albumin (0.25 mg/ml)	240	30
α-Ketoglutarate ($4-32 \times 10^{-15}$ mole)	Imidazole-acetate (85 mM, pH 6.9)	Glutamate dehydrogenase (glycerol solution, 10 μg/ml)	NADH (1 μM) Ammonium acetate (20 mM) ADP (100 μM) Ascorbic acid (2 mM) Bovine serum albumin (0.25 mg/ml)	160	20

The steps in the assay are as follows:

Step 1. Add embryos to 80 nl of 0.05 N NaOH in the oil wells of a Teflon block.

Step 2. Heat block to 80°C for 20 minutes to destroy endogenous enzymes and oxidized nucleotide, the latter being the product of the specific reaction.

Step 3. Add 80 nl of 0.1 M Tris-HCl to return pH of drop to approximately 8.0.

Step 4. Add 80 nl of reagent containing: 300 mM Tris-HCl buffer (pH 7.4), 60 mM NADH, 100 μM ZnCl$_2$, 4 mM ascorbic acid, 1 μg/ml malate dehydrogenase, 9 μg/ml citrate lyase.

After addition to the oil well, the final concentration of reactants will be as given in Table I at a final volume of 240 nl. The divalent metal ion is added to protect the enzyme, citrate lyase, while ascorbic acid prevents the spontaneous oxidation of NADH (see Lowry and Passonneau, 1972). As commerical preparations of bovine serum albumin contain citrate, it is not added to the reagent for this assay.

Step 5. Allow the reaction to proceed 20 minutes at 20°C.

Step 6. Add 80 nl of 0.5 N HCl and heat the drops at 80°C for 20 minutes to destroy unreacted NADH.

Step 7. Add 6 μl of NAD cycling reagent which contains 100 mM Tris-HCl buffer, pH 8.1, 300 mM ethanol, 6 mM oxaloacetate, 2 mM mercaptoethanol, 0.02% bovine serum albumin, 10μg/ml malate dehydrogenase, 100 μg/ml alcohol dehydrogenase.

This reagent gives approximately 10,000 cycles in 60 minutes at 20°C. The level of oxaloacetate is important, as it is inhibitory to the reaction and must be kept as low as possible consistent with the level of metabolite being measured. Thus, with mouse blastocysts, where citrate levels are high (up to 10^{-12} mole), it may be necessary to increase the concentration of oxaloacetate to avoid total utilization of this substrate during the cycling.

Step 8. Add 3.5 μl of 0.2 N NaOH to the drop and heat at 80°C for 15 minutes.

Step 9. Withdraw 6 μl of the drop from the oil well, and add to 1.0 ml of indicator reagent in a fluorometer tube in order to measure malate formed during cycling. The enzyme reactions for the measurement of malate are given below:

$$\text{Malate} + \text{NAD}^+ \xrightarrow[\text{dehydrogenase}]{\text{malate}} \text{oxaloacetate} + \text{NADH} + \text{H}^+$$

$$\text{Oxaloacetate} + \text{glutamate} \xrightarrow[\text{transaminase}]{\text{glutamate-oxaloacetate}} \text{aspartate} + \alpha\text{-ketoglutarate}$$

The composition of the indicator reagent is: 20 mM 2-amino-2-methyl-1-propanol-HCl buffer (pH 9.8), 1 mM glutamate, 50 μM NAD, 10 μg/ml malate dehydrogenase, 2 μg/ml glutamate-oxaloacetate transaminase.

Step 10. Incubate the tubes 25 minutes at 20°C to complete the reaction and measure NADH formed in a fluorometer against citrate standards taken through the whole procedure with the samples.

2. Malate

The specific enzyme reactions for the measurement of malate are the same as described in step 9 above. The expected level of malate in preimplantation mouse embryos is in the vicinity of 5×10^{-14} mole, and the increase in sensitivity over that for citrate is gained by increasing amplification during cycling. A summary of the steps in the assay follows below.

Step 1. Add samples to 80 nl of 0.05 N HCl and heat at 80°C for 20 minutes.

Step 2. Neutralize by adding 80 nl of 0.1 M Tris base. In all assays, this step can be omitted where it is advisable to keep volumes to a minimum. In such a situation, the reagent added in the next step has its buffer composition adjusted so that when it is added to the acidic samples above, final pH is 9.8.

Step 3. Add 80 nl of enzyme reagent to give final concentration of reactants as detailed in Table I, and allow the reaction to proceed 20 minutes.

Step 4. Add 80 nl of 0.5 N NaOH and heat at 80°C for 20 minutes.

Step 5. Add 3 μl of NAD cycle reagent. This reagent is essentially the same as that used for citrate, except that the oxaloacetate concentration is reduced to 2 mM and the amounts of enzymes increased to 30 μg/ml malate dehydrogenase and 300 μg/ml alcohol dehydrogenase. Under these conditions, a cycling rate of up to 25,000/hour can be anticipated.

Step 6. After 1 hour, add 6 μl of 0.1 N NaOH, heat at 80°C for 20 minutes, cool, and take a 6-μl aliquot for the indicator reaction as described for citrate.

3. Isocitrate

The measurement of isocitrate depends on the following specific reaction.

$$\text{Isocitrate} + NADP^+ \xrightarrow[\text{dehydrogenase}]{\text{isocitrate}} \alpha\text{-ketoglutarate} + CO_2 + NADPH + H^+$$

The assay of this substrate in embryos differs in two major respects from the preceding assays: (1) NADP is the cofactor, and so a NADP cycle is used. (2) Isocitrate is present in embryos at the 10^{-15} mole range, and alkaline enhancement is necessary after the indicator step to produce sufficient fluorescence for measurement. In such an assay, it is advisable to keep volumes to a minimum to reduce fluorescent blank values.

Step 1 and 2. Treat samples as for steps 1 and 2 of malate assay.

Step 3. Add 80 nl of enzyme reagent to give the concentration of reactant as detailed in Table I. Allow to react 30 minutes.

Step 4. Add 80 nl of 0.5 N NaOH and heat at 80°C for 30 minutes.

Step 5. Neutralize samples with 80 nl of Tris-acetate buffer (pH 8.0). Add 1 μl of NADP cycling reagent containing: 100 mM Tris-acetate buffer (pH 8.0), 5 mM α-ketoglutarate, 5 mM glucose-6-P, 10 mM ammonium acetate, 100 μM ADP, 50 μg/ml glucose-6-P dehydrogenase, 200 μg/ml glutamate dehydrogenase.

The enzyme glucose-6-P dehydrogenase is inhibited by sulfate ions. Thus prior to use this enzyme, if supplied commercially as a suspension in ammonium sulfate, must be centrifuged and resuspended in 2 M ammonium acetate. ADP is added to the reagent to stabilize this enzyme. Glutamate dehydrogenase is used as a solution in glycerol.

Step 7. Incubate 1 hour at 37°C.

Step 8. Add 500 nl of 0.2 N NaOH and heat at 80°C for 20 minutes.

Step 9. Neutralize to pH 8.0 by adding 200 nl of 1 N Tris-HCl.

Step 10. Add 6 μl of indicator reagent and incubate 30 minutes: 40 mM Tris-HCl buffer (pH 8.0), 100 μM EDTA, 30 mM ammonium acetate, 5 mM MgCl$_2$, 300 μM NADP, 0.03% bovine serum albumin, 5 μg/ml 6-P-gluconate dehydrogenase.

Step 11. Transfer 6 μl to fluorometer tube containing 50 μl of phosphate buffer (pH 12) and heat 15 minutes at 60°C.

Step 12. Cool and add 100 μl of 9 N NaOH containing 0.045% H$_2$O$_2$ and mix immediately.

Step 13. Heat 10 minutes at 60°C, add 1 ml H$_2$O to the fluorometer tube, mix, and read in a fluorometer.

With the isocitrate assay as described above, a 25,000-fold amplification can be achieved during cycling. Coupled with a five- to sevenfold amplification in the final alkaline enhancement step, a total amplification of 150,000-fold can be expected, allowing the assay of the metabolite in the femtomole range.

4. α-Ketoglutarate

This metabolite is assayed by the reaction:

$$\alpha\text{-Ketoglutarate} + NH_4^+ + NADH \xrightarrow[\text{dehydrogenase}]{\text{glutamate}} \text{glutamate} + NAD^+$$

The amount of α-ketoglutarate in mouse embryos is of the order of 1×10^{-14} mole. At this level it is possible, by taking precautions to maintain a low level of blank fluorescence (e.g., by keeping volumes as low as possible at all steps in the assay), to measure this metabolite without the use of the final alkaline enhancement step used for the isocitrate assay. The analytical steps to make this possible are described below. It should be noted that coupling to the alkaline enhancement of fluorescence, while increasing the complexity of the assay, would extend its sensitivity, should the level of this metabolite be lower in the embryos of other mammalian species.

Step 1. Heat samples in 50 nl of alkali.

Step 2. Add 50 nl of reagent to give the conditions for the specific enzyme reaction as detailed in Table 1.

Step 3. At completion of the specific reaction, add 80 nl of 0.5 N HCl and heat at 80°C for 20 minutes.

Step 4. Neutralize with 80 nl of 1.0 M tris base.

Step 5. Add 250 nl of NAD cycle reagent. In this case, the stock cycle is made up with double the final concentration of reagents so that after the addition to the neutralized drops above, the appropriate concentration of reagents is present to produce maximum rates of cycling.

Step 6. At the end of the cycling period, add 3 μl of 0.1 N NaOH, and after a further period of heating take an aliquot of 3 μl for the indicator reaction. Alternatively, the indicator step can be carried out in the oil well by following steps 8 and 9 for the isocitrate assay and adding 6 μl of the appropriate indicator reagent. At the completion of the reaction, 6 μl can be transferred to a fluorometer tube containing 1 ml water for reading in the fluorometer. However, this latter procedure appears to have little practical value in reducing blank values of the samples, and the extra steps involved seem justified only where alkaline enhancement of fluorescence is needed to increase sensitivity.

B. Glycolytic Intermediates

The glycolytic intermediates, glucose-6-phosphate, frucose 1, 6-diphosphate, and fructose 6-phosphate have been measured in preimplantation mouse embryos by Barbehenn (1974). The experimental conditions for the initial reaction are given in Table II.

1. Glucose 6-Phosphate

The assay of glucose 6-phosphate depends on the reaction.

$$\text{Glucose-6-P} + \text{NADP}^+ + \xrightarrow[\text{dehydrogenase}]{\text{glucose-6-P}} \text{6-P-gluconolactone} + \text{NADPH}^+ + \text{H}^+$$

Levels of this metabolite in freshly collected mouse embryos lie in the range of 8×10^{-15} mole at the 2-cell stage to approximately four times this value at the blastocyst stage. However, the levels of this metabolite, like those of many other metabolic intermediates, can fall to much lower values during incubation in substrate-free media. Barbehenn (1974), therefore, has described a procedure for measuring levels as low as 2×10^{-15} mole, using cycling followed by alkaline enhancement after the indicator step similar to those described above for the isocitrate assay. A 200,000-fold amplification is obtained and during the assay, all volumes are kept small to minimize blank values. This is achieved by:

1. Adding samples to 50 nl of 0.01 N HCl, followed by the addition of 50 nl of reagent to give the desired concentration of reactants for the specific reaction.

TABLE II
Conditions for the Enzymatic Assay of Glycolytic Intermediates in Preimplantation Mouse Embryos Prior to Amplification by Enzymatic Cycling

Metabolite (range of standards)	Buffer	Enzymes	Other components of assay mixture	Volume of reactants (nl)	Incubation time (minutes)
Glucose 6-phosphate ($2–12 \times 10^{-15}$ mole)	Tris-HCl ($50\ mM$, pH 8.1)	Glucose-6-P-dehydrogenase ($0.15\ \mu g/ml$)	NADP ($15\ \mu M$) Bovine serum albumin ($0.4\ mg/ml$) Dithiothreitol ($100\ \mu M$)	100	20
Fructose-1,6-phosphate plus triose-P ($2–5 \times 10^{-15}$ mole)	Imidazole-HCl ($50\ mM$, pH 7.5)	Aldolase ($10\ \mu g/ml$) Triose-P-isomerase ($1\ \mu g/ml$) Glyceraldehye-P-dehydrogenase ($50\ \mu g/ml$)	NAD ($25\ \mu M$) $Na_2\ HAsO_4$ ($1\ mM$) EDTA ($1\ mM$) Mercaptoethanol ($2\ mM$) Bovine serum albumin ($0.2\ mg/ml$)	100	25
Fructose 6-phosphate ($1.5–3 \times 10^{-14}$ mole)	Imidazole-HCl ($50\ mM$, pH 7.5)	Aldolase ($0.5\ \mu g/ml$) Triose-P-isomerase ($1\ \mu g/ml$) Glyceraldehyde-P-dehydrogenase ($12\ \mu g/ml$) Phosphofructokinase ($0.5\ \mu g/ml$)	NAD ($28\ \mu M$) $Na_2\ HAsO_4$ ($1\ mM$) EDTA ($1\ mM$) Mercaptoethanol ($2\ mM$) $MgCl_2$ ($2\ mM$) ATP ($50\ mM$) Bovine serum albumin ($0.2\ mg/ml$)	160	10

These steps are essentially the same as those described for the assay of
α-ketoglutarate above.

2. Destroying excess NADP by adding 50 nl of 0.15 N NaOH and heating.

3. Adding 500 nl of NADP cycling reagent to the above.

4. Terminating the cycle by the addition of 100 nl of 0.3 N NaOH and
heating at 80°C for 20 minutes.

5. Completing the indicator step in the oil well by the addition of 1 μl of
indicator reagent after the above step.

6. Transferring 1 μl at the completion of the indicator step to 50 μl of
phosphate buffer in a fluorometer tube for the alkaline enhancement steps.

2. Fructose 1, 6-Diphosphate

The assay depends on the following enzyme reactions:

$$\text{Fructose-1,6-P} \xrightarrow{\text{aldolase}} \text{dihydroxyacetone-P} + \text{glyceraldehyde-P}$$

$$\text{Dihydroxyacetone-P} \xrightarrow[\text{isomerase}]{\text{triose-P}} \text{glyceraldehyde-P}$$

$$\text{Glyceraldehyde-P} + \text{NAD}^+ \xrightarrow[\text{dehydrogenase}]{\text{glyceraldehyde-P}} \text{3-P-glycerate} + \text{NADH} + \text{H}^+$$

These reactions will measure the triose-P in the embryo, as well as fructose
diphosphate. Thus, to determine the true amounts of fructose diphosphate it
would be necessary to correct the values obtained in this assay by subtraction of
the triose-P values. Theoretically, these could be obtained by employing the
latter two reactions in the above assay. However, the values for fructose diphosphate plus triose-P are very low in embryos (of the order of $5–10 \times 10^{-16}$ mole),
and, as yet, triose-P values have not been determined. The levels of triose-P in
adult tissues are low compared to fructose diphosphate. If the same holds for
embryonic tissue, the correction would be small, and the measurement of
triose-P in embryos would be well below the level of sensitivity of the present
methods. In general, the steps in the assay follow those described above for
isocitrate and α-ketoglutarate.

Step 1. Add samples to 50 nl of 0.02 N HCl and heat 20 minutes at 80°C.

Step 2. Add 50 nl of reagent to give conditions shown in Table II for the
specific enzyme assay.

Step 3. Add 50 nl 0.3 N NaOH at the completion of the above reaction and
heat 20 minutes at 80°C.

Step 4. Add 2 μl NAD cycling reagent. This reagent has the same composition as that used for the malate assay and gives approximately 25,000 cycles in
60 minutes at 25°C.

Step 5. Terminate cycle with 100 nl 1 N NaOH and heat 20 minutes at
80°C.

Step 6. Add 1 μl indicator reagent and react 25 minutes.

Step 7. Take 2 μl from drop, add to 50 μl of phosphate buffer (pH 12) in a fluorometer tube and proceed with alkaline enhancement steps.

3. Fructose 6-Phosphate

Barbehenn (1974) has also described a method for measuring fructose-6-P in embryos based on the reactions below:

$$\text{Fructose-6-P} + \text{ATP} \xrightarrow{\text{P-fructokinase}} \text{Fructose-1,6-P} + \text{ADP}$$

$$\text{Fructose-1,6-P} \xrightarrow{\text{aldolase}} \text{dihydroxyacetone-P} + \text{glyceraldehyde-P}$$

$$\text{Dihydroxyacetone-P} \xrightarrow[\text{isomerase}]{\text{triose-P}} \text{glyceraldehyde-P}$$

$$\text{Glyceraldehyde-P} + \text{NAD}^+ \xrightarrow[\text{dehydrogenase}]{\text{glyceraldehyde-P}} \text{3-P-glycerate} + \text{NADH} + \text{H}^+$$

Because this procedure utilizes the enzyme reactions used for the assay of fructose-1, 6-P, it is necessary to correct fructose-6-P values for the levels of fructose diphosphate obtained using the assay described in the last section. To date, this correction has been made by performing these assays on separate embryos collected under similar conditions. True estimates of fructose-6-P in individual embryos would need both assays to be carried out on the one embryo. Theoretically, this should be possible by taking separate aliquots after the initial heating of the sample in 0.02 N HCl. However, the levels of these metabolites (at least those of fructose diphosphate) are close to the limit of sensitivity of the assay procedures as described here, and technical difficulties have so far precluded an assay of both metabolites in the same embryo.

The details of the method are similar to those already described. After heating in acid, the specific reaction is carried out in 160 nl final volume with the concentration of reactants as shown in Table II. One microliter of NAD cycling reagent is used, and cycling is terminated after 60 minutes by the addition of 5 μl of 0.15 N NaOH. After heating, 3.5 μl is transferred into 1 ml of indicator reagent to measure malate formed by direct fluorometry. If necessary, the sensitivity could be increased by use of alkaline enhancement of fluorescence, providing the contribution of blank fluorescence can be maintained at a low level.

C. Other Compounds Assayed by Cycling Techniques

1. Endogenous Nucleotides

NAD, NADH, NADP, and NADPH can be measured in embryos using the cycling techniques described above. The analytical procedures are simple and involve cycling of the endogenous nucleotide. However, Barbehenn (1974) has indicated that substantial losses of NADPH can occur during storage and handling of embryos. Therefore, special precautions are necessary in the preparation of embryos to ensure values obtained are representative of the *in vivo* situation.

The initial steps for the measurement of nucleotides are as follows:

1. NAD or NADP—add embryos to 50 nl of $0.02 N$ HCl and heat at 80°C to destroy endogenous NADH or NADPH and enzymes.

2. NADH or NADPH—add embryos to $0.02 N$ NaOH and heat to destroy oxidized nucleotide and enzymes.

3. Total NAD (NADH) or NADP (NADPH)—add embryos to 50 nl of Tris-HCl buffer (pH 8.0).

After this initial step, the remaining nucleotide is cycled, using $0.5-1.0 \mu l$ of the appropriate cycling reagent. After cycling for 60 minutes, the reaction is terminated by the addition of NaOH and heating for 20 minutes at 80°C. The appropriate indicator reaction is then carried out to measure the product of the cycling reaction. In the case of NAD and NADH, sufficient endogenous nucleotide is present in embryos to allow this reaction to be carried out in fluorometer tubes and fluorescence of the formed NADH measured directly in a fluorometer. For NADP and NADPH, it is necessary to use alkaline enhancement of fluorescence to gain sufficient sensitivity to measure the levels of these metabolites in single embryos.

2. Inorganic Phosphate

A method for the measurement of inorganic phosphate (P_i) using cycling techniques (Lowry and Passonneau, 1972) has been adapted to measure P_i in single embryos. It depends on the reactions shown below:

$$\text{Glycogen} + P_i \xrightarrow{\text{phosphorylase a}} \text{Glucose-1-P}$$

$$\text{Glucose-1-P} \xrightarrow{\text{P-glucomutase}} \text{Glucose-6-P}$$

$$\text{Glucose-6-P} + \text{NADP} \xrightarrow[\text{dehydrogenase}]{\text{glucose-6-P}} \text{6-P gluconolactone} + \text{NADPH} + H^+$$

The special precautions required to avoid contamination with inorganic phosphate and so keep blank values low in the assay are detailed by Lowry and Passonneau (1972). This is especially important when attempting to measure very small amounts of P_i, as in mammalian embryos (of the order of 8×10^{-15} mole/embryo). The multienzyme reactions used to measure inorganic phosphate will also produce NADPH from glucose-6-P (reaction 3 above). Thus, it is necessary to destroy glucose-6-P before carrying out the assay. This is achieved by heating the samples in $0.05 N$ NaOH at 95°C for 30 minutes in the first step of the procedure. The protocols for the assay are as follows:

Step 1. Add samples to 80 nl of 0.05 N NaOH and heat at 95°C for 30 minutes.

Step 2. Add 80 nl of reagent to carry out the specific enzymatic steps described above. The concentration and preparation of reagents have been described by Lowry and Passonneau (1972).

Step 3. After completion of the specific enzyme reaction (30 minutes), add 80 nl of 0.5 N NaOH to the drop and heat at 60°C for 20 minutes.

Step 4. Add 6.0 μl of NADP cycling reagent and incubate 60 minutes at 37°C.

Step 5. Add 3.5 μl of 0.2 N NaOH to terminate cycle. After heating 20 minutes at 60°C, 10 μl are withdrawn for the indicator reaction, which is carried out in fluorometer tubes for direct measurement in a fluorometer.

3. AMP

Barbehenn *et al.* (1976) have described an assay for 5′-AMP based on the reactions used in the phosphate assay above. Lowry *et al.* (1964) observed that in the initial enzyme reaction used in the phosphate assay, the activity of phosphorylase a is related to AMP concentration when glycogen and P_i are present at low levels. Thus, unlike the methods described above, this assay depends on the rate of reaction, and, therefore, the timing of the initial enzyme reaction is critical. At the same time, an advantage of the method is that some amplification occurs in the first step, and the yield of NADPH can be increased by increasing the time of reaction.

In the assay, the samples are treated initially in the same way as for inorganic phosphate. Next, the specific reagent is added. This reagent has all the components present for the reaction except inorganic phosphate (see Barbehenn *et al.*, 1976, for composition). The reaction is started by adding 100 nl of 0.9 mM P_i at specific times to each of the drops, and the reaction is terminated 20 minutes later by the addition of 100 nl of 0.15 N NaOH followed by heating 25 minutes at 80°C. The NADPH formed in the reaction is cycled 60 minutes at 37°C by the addition of 1.5 μl NADP cycling reagent. At the completion to the cycling (60 minutes at 37°C), NaOH is added and the indicator reaction is carried out on an aliquot transferred to a fluorometer tube.

4. ATP

Barbehenn (1974) has measured the levels of ATP in single embryos using enzymatic cycling. The assay depends on the following reactions:

$$\text{ATP} + \text{glucose} \xrightarrow{\text{hexokinase}} \text{glucose-6-P} + \text{ADP}$$

$$\text{Glucose-6-P} + \text{NADP}^+ \xrightarrow[\text{dehydrogenase}]{\text{glucose-6-P}} \text{6-P-gluconate} + \text{NADPH} + \text{H}^+$$

As in the preceding two assays, the endogenous glucose-6-P has to be destroyed in the initial step by heating the samples in 50 nl of 0.05 N NaOH at 95°C for 30 minutes. As the levels of ATP in embryos fall in the range $2–12 \times 10^{-13}$ mole, there is not as great a necessity to keep volumes as small as those used in some of the preceding assays. In the procedure described by Barbehenn (1974), the specific reaction is carried out in a final volume of 400 nl, using reaction conditions essentially as described by Lowry and Passonneau (1972). After the reaction, the unreacted NADP is removed by adding 5 μl of 0.05 N NaOH and heating for 25 minutes at 80°C. The cycling was carried out in fluorometer tubes by adding an aliquot from the oil-well drop to 50 μl of NADP cycling reagent in the tube. After incubating at 37°C for 60 minutes, the product of the cycling reaction is assayed by adding 1 ml of the appropriate indicator reagent and measuring the NADPH formed directly in a fluorometer.

D. Application of the Assay Procedures

The preceding sections describe a number of assay procedures that have been adapted to measure the level of specific metabolites in embryos. It is no doubt obvious to the reader that these procedures can be varied to suit the particular samples to be analyzed. Thus, the assay of citrate described here is that which is appropriate for the levels of this metabolite in mouse preimplantation embryos. If the amount of this metabolite in the embryos of other species was lower, the sensitivity of the assay could be increased 100-fold by increasing the rate of cycling and using alkaline enhancement of fluorescence as described for some of the other metabolites. Under these circumstances, it would be necessary to carry out preliminary studies to choose conditions which would reduce blank fluorescence so that the increase in fluorescence due to the lowest level of metabolites being measured would be significantly above that of the blank.

Even greater sensitivity could be obtained by using a second cycling step after the initial cycle, a procedure known as double cycling (Lowry and Passonneau, 1972). Theoretically, this procedure should allow the measurement of metabolites in the 10^{-18} mole range. The main problem involved in such assays is the very small volumes required for the initial steps (1 nl or less), and, while it is not, as yet, in general use as a practical procedure, it has enormous potential as a further development of these techniques.

The assays described in this chapter were adapted to measure metabolites in mouse embryos in order to study control points in the metabolic pathways of developing preimplantation embryos (Barbehenn et al., 1974). However, they should be considered only as samples of the types of assays which can be performed. Lowry and Passonneau (1972) describe 36 metabolite assays, all of which could be modified for analysis of single embryos. Furthermore, it should be emphasized that the use of these methods is not restricted even to these metabolites. Any substance that can be linked either directly or indirectly to an enzyme system resulting in the oxidation or reduction of pyridine nucleotides can be measured in this way. Equally, the methods can be used for measuring the activity of enzymes (Brinster, 1971).

By adopting the techniques described by Lowry and Passonneau (1972) for the dissection of frozen-dried specimens and their weighing, using a quartz fiber fishpole balance, it should be possible to analyze cells or cell aggregates both in pre- and postimplantation embryos, and, in so doing, to study biochemical parameters associated with early differentiation.

REFERENCES

Barbehenn, E. K. (1974). Ph.D. Thesis, Washington University, St. Louis, Missouri.
Barbehenn, E. K., Wales, R. G., and Lowry, O. H. (1974). *Proc. Natl. Acad. Sci. U.S.A.* **71**, 1056–1060.
Barbehenn, E. K., Wales, R. G., and Lowry, O. H. (1978). *J. Embryol. Exp. Morph.* (In press.)
Barbehenn, E. K., Law, M. M.-Y., Brown, J. G., and Lowry, O. H. (1976). *Anal. Biochem.* **70**, 554–562.
Brinster, R. L. (1967). *J. Reprod. Fertil.* **13**, 413–420.
Brinster, R. L. (1971). *In* "Methods in Mammalian Embryology" (J. C. Daniel, ed.), pp. 215–227. Freeman, San Francisco, California.
Epstein, C. J., and Daentl, D. L. (1971). *Dev. Biol.* **26**, 517–524.
Fridhandler, L. (1971). *In* "Methods in Mammalian Embryology" (J. C. Daniel, ed.), pp. 268–277. Freeman, San Francisco, California.
Ginsberg, L., and Hillman, N. (1973). *J. Embryol. Exp. Morphol.* **30**, 267–282.
Kato, T., Berger, S. J., Carter, J. A., and Lowry, O. H. (1973). *Anal. Biochem.* **53**, 86–97.
Kuwahara, M., and Chaykin, S. (1973). *J. Biol. Chem.* **248**, 5095–5099.
Lowenstein, J. E., and Cohen, A. I. (1964). *J. Embryol. Exp. Morphol.* **12**, 113–121.
Lowry, O. H., and Passonneau, J. V. (1972). "A Flexible System of Enzymatic Analysis." Academic Press, New York.
Lowry, O. H., Passonneau, J. V., Schulz, D. W., and Rock, M. K. (1961a). *J. Biol. Chem.* **236**, 2746–2755.
Lowry, O. H., Passonneau, J. V., and Rock, M. K. (1961b). *J. Biol. Chem.* **236**, 2756–2759.
Lowry, O. H., Schulz, D. W., and Passonneau, J. V. (1964). *J. Biol. Chem.* **239**, 1947–1953.
Mills, R. M., and Brinster, R. L. (1967). *Exp. Cell Res.* **47**, 337–344.
Olds, P. J., Stern, S., and Biggers, J. D. (1973). *J. Exp. Zool.* **186**, 39–46.
Ozias, C. B., and Stern, S. (1973). *Biol. Reprod.* **8**, 467–472.
Quinn, P. J., and Wales, R. G. (1971). *J. Reprod. Fertil.* **25**, 133–135.
Reamer, G. R. (1963). Ph.D. Thesis, Boston University, Boston, Massachusetts.
Schiffner, J., and Spielmann, H. (1976). *J. Reprod. Fertil.* **47**, 145–147.
Snyder, R. E., Weitlauf, H. M., and Nelson, S. R. (1971). *Biol. Reprod.* **5**, 314–318.
Stern, S., and Biggers, J. D. (1968). *J. Exp. Zool.* **168**, 61–66.
Wales, R. G. (1974). *Proc. Aust. Biochem. Soc.* **7**, 28.

6

Production of Chimeras by Injecting Cells or Tissue into the Blastocyst

R. L. GARDNER

I. INTRODUCTION

Analysis of metazoan organisms composed of two or more genetically distinct populations of cells has illuminated a number of hitherto elusive aspects of development, principally in insects and mammals (Nesbitt and Gartler, 1971; Hotta and Benzer, 1973; Mintz, 1974; Crick and Lawrence, 1975; Gardner and Papaioannou, 1975; McLaren, 1976; Gehring, 1977). Increasing awareness of the value of such organisms suggests that they will be exploited even more extensively in future.

The most common cause of natural mosaicism in eutherian mammals is attributable to the phenomenon of X chromosome inactivation (Lyon, 1974). However, although X inactivation mosaics have been employed in a variety of investigations, their usefulness is restricted by several factors. Thus, mosaicism is limited to loci exhibiting polymorphism that are either carried on the X chromosome or translocated to it. Also, representation of the two cell populations in tissues tends to be balanced; potentially informative cases of extremely unequal contributions are rare. This may reflect the presence of a fairly high number of cells when inactivation takes place (Nesbitt, 1971; Fialkow, 1973). Finally, it is uncertain when inactivation occurs during development, and whether it does so at the same stage in all tissues (Gardner and Lyon, 1971; Gardner, 1974; Deol and Whitten, 1972). Radiation-induced genetic mosaics or mosaics produced by hypermutable genes have been studied to a limited extent in mammals (Russell, 1964; Melvold, 1971), but are comparatively rare.

Viviparity in mammals predisposes situations in which cells derived from more than one zygote coexist in an individual. However, whole body or "primary chimerism" (Ford, 1969), which is of potentially greatest value, is also a rather rare natural phenomenon (reviewed by Benirschke, 1970; McLaren, 1976). Nicholas and Hall (1942) appear to have been the first to try to produce primary chimeras experimentally by aggregating pairs of denuded 1-cell rat eggs in order to study regulation. However, success was not verified by use of genetic markers, and the authors made no comment on the wider implications of this approach. Full credit is undoubtedly due to Tarkowski (1961) and to Mintz (1962), both for first producing unequivocal chimeras by embryo aggregation, and for drawing attention to the experimental possibilities they offered. The technique is discussed in detail by Mintz (1971). Briefly, it entails coculture of pairs of morulae denuded of their zonae until they form single integrated embryos that can be transplanted to the uteri of pseudopregnant mice. A proportion of the resulting offspring contain cells derived from both embryos in many or all organs and tissues. The nature and extent of genotypic differences between embryonic cells combined thus is limited only by the genetic polymorphism of the species and is, therefore, virtually inexhaustible.

The author sought to extend the scope of this approach by devising a means of injecting cells or pieces of tissue into more advanced, blastocyst-stage mouse embryos (Gardner, 1968, 1971). This technique requires considerable investment, both of money in purchasing sophisticated microsurgical equipment, and of time in acquiring proficiency in its use. Therefore, before embarking on technical details, it is worth examining its advantages in some detail.

If one's aim is simply to produce individuals whose tissues are composed of cells possessing specific genotypic differences, embryo aggregation is obviously the method of choice. Nevertheless, it is perhaps worth noting that a number of laboratories have experienced greater difficulty in routine production of chimeras by this method than its procedural simplicity might lead one to expect. This is most probably due to the sensitivity of cleavage-stage embryos to *in vitro* conditions (Bowman and McLaren, 1970).

Aggregation occurs most readily in midcleavage around the 8-cell stage. Although morphologically normal blastocysts have been obtained following pairing of late morulae (Mintz, 1965), early and late morulae (Stern and Wilson, 1972), and even with early blastocysts (Stern and Wilson, 1972), more advanced blastocysts have been aggregated only after treatment with versene (Stern, 1972). Production of chimeric conceptuses or offspring has not been demonstrated for these later-stage aggregates. Interspecific aggregations between matched cleavage stages of mouse with rat or bank-vole have also yielded blastocysts (Mulnard, 1973; Stern, 1973; Zeilmaker, 1973; Mystkowska, 1975). However, they degenerate or lose cells of the foreign species soon after implantation in the mouse uterus (Mystkowska, 1975; Rossant, 1976). Successful aggregation of cells from later embryos with morulae has been achieved only with inner cell masses (ICMs). Here, despite integration of the donor tissue, the rate of implantation of composite blastocysts was inexplicably low (Rossant, 1975). Attempts to produce chimeras by aggregating embryonal carcinoma or other cells with morulae has met with no success whatever (Mintz *et al.*, 1975; C. Babinet, personal communication). Successful exploitation of the aggregation method, therefore, seems to be restricted to nearly synchronous embryos of the same species at a stage of development prior to determination of the ICM and trophectoderm. Since three quarters or more cells in the blastocyst contribute exclusively to extraembryonic tissues, it is perhaps not surprising that at least 20% of offspring do not exhibit chimerism (McLaren, 1976).

The blastocyst is a remarkably resilient stage of development in the mouse, and can tolerate prolonged *in vitro* manipulation far better than earlier preimplantation embryos (Gardner, 1971; Gardner and Johnson, 1972). While fairly strong mutual cell adhesion is an essential prerequisite for embryo aggregation, it is probably less important for blastocyst injection. Once transplanted, donor cells are physically trapped in the contracting blastocoel or ICM, and their incorporation is encouraged by shortly returning the blastocysts to the physiologically regulated environment of the uterus. Hence, there is virtually no restriction on the type of cell whose capacity for integration and colonization is to be tested.

Another advantage of the injection method is that it is possible to exert control over the distribution of chimerism by choice of the type of cell or tissue injected into blastocysts or trophectodermal vesicles. This is invaluable in attempts to define the anatomical focus of action of lethal genes (Papaioannou and Gardner, 1976), and in studying cell lineages in the normal embryo (Gardner and Papaioannou, 1975; Gardner and Rossant, 1976, also unpublished data). Selective distribution of chimerism also appears to be important in producing interspecific chimeras. Chimeric fetuses can be obtained routinely by injecting rat isolated

ICMs into mouse blastocysts (Gardner and Johnson, 1973), whereas, as indicated earlier, composite blastocysts formed by aggregating rat and mouse morulae degenerate around the time of implantation (Rossant, 1976). Success of the former procedure is probably related to the fact that it ensures that the trophectoderm is of the same species as the uterine foster mother. The virtues of interspecific chimeras are discussed elsewhere (Gardner and Johnson, 1975).

Perhaps the most important advantage is that extensive chimerism can be obtained in 25% or more conceptuses and offspring after injecting single cells into blastocysts (Gardner, 1971, also unpublished data). This enables critical appraisal of the status of individual cells by following their clonal history *in vivo*. Clonal analysis has already been used to investigate the time of X chromosome inactivation (Gardner and Lyon, 1971; Gardner, 1974), and the potency of ICM and embryonal carcinoma cells (Gardner and Papaioannou, 1975; Gardner and Rossant, 1976; Illmensee and Mintz, 1976). A virtue of this particular way of producing chimeras is that it imposes minimal demands for size regulation on the embryo. The number of ICM cells is increased by approximately 6%, as opposed to more than 100% when pairs of cleaving eggs are aggregated (Buehr and McLaren, 1974). Although size regulation takes place shortly after implantation, its mechanism remains obscure (Buehr and McLaren, 1974). This inevitably introduces a measure of uncertainty when extrapolating from results based on aggregation chimeras to standard mice (see Gardner, 1977, for more detailed discussion of this point).

Finally, in species like the rabbit where retention of the zona is necessary for implantation, one has no choice but to inject cells through it (Gardner and Munro, 1974; Moustafa, 1974).

The above survey highlights the greater versatility of blastocyst injection, as opposed to morula aggregation, as a means of producing mammalian chimeras. The range of cell types that can colonize the blastocyst has yet to be explored. Apart from embryonal carcinoma cells (Mintz *et al.*, 1975; Papaioannou *et al.*, 1975) whose developmental status is obscure (Sherman and Solter, 1975), few other postblastocyst cells have been employed. The most advanced donor embryo whose cells have yielded unequivocal chimerism is 6½ day postcoitum (p.c.) (J. Rossant, unpublished data). Moustafa and Brinster (1972a) claimed success with unspecified cells from 8½ day p.c. donor embryos, though the results are somewhat equivocal, and have been criticized on several grounds (Mintz, 1974).

The preimplanted blastocyst is at present the most advanced host embryo that will develop normally following reimplantation *in utero*. Hence, use of more advanced donors necessitates greater chronological asynchrony between injected cells and host embryos. An attempt has been made to overcome this problem by injecting cells directly into 8½-day p.c. conceptuses *in utero*. Preliminary evidence of induction of hemopoietic chimeras has been obtained by this method

(Weissman *et al.*, 1977). However, its potential is limited by the need to inoculate rather large numbers of cells, and by the fact that they usually end up in the yolk cavity. Therefore, only migratory cells such as hemopoietic stem cells, primordial germ cells, and, possibly, neural crest cells are likely to colonize the fetus.

II. OUTLINE OF THE APPROACH

The method of injecting cells into the mouse blastocyst described below was developed over a period of several years with the following considerations in mind:
    1. Minimizing damage to both host embryo and donor cells,
    2. Achieving accurate placement of the transplanted cells,
    3. Minimizing the time required for each injection. Micromanipulation demands sustained concentration. Hence, the longer it takes to perform a series of injections, the greater the fatigue and likelihood of careless mistakes. Furthermore, donor cells may be affected adversely by prolonged isolation.

Moustafa and Brinster (1972b) published a ''simple'' technique in which the blastocyst is held by suction on the tip of one glass micropipette while the cells to be injected are forced into the blastocoel with a second beveled pipette. This technique had been rejected at an early stage by the present author because, as Moustafa and Brinster indeed acknowledge, good beveled pipettes are difficult to make and can be used for injection of only one or two embryos before blockage with debris necessitates their replacement. Also, the technique cannot be used to transplant isolated inner cell masses (ICMs) or other pieces of tissue.

The approach adopted finally is to use three siliconized glass microneedles to make a triangular hole in the trophectoderm opposite the ICM, through which a smooth-tipped pipette or clump of cells may be readily inserted into the blastocoelic cavity. The blastocyst is immobilized during the operation by suction applied to the embryonic pole through a second pipette. Hence, five microinstruments, each capable of being moved independently, have to be set up so that the tips of four lie on one side of the blastocyst and the fifth on the opposite side (Fig. 1). The following account proceeds from the choice and assembly of the necessary apparatus, via the preparation and setting up of each microinstrument, to the actual injection procedure. The text has been supplemented with figures wherever these seemed necessary or informative. Furthermore, emphasis has been placed on explaining less self-evident points of design and execution, and on highlighting the more common problems and mistakes. While being firmly convinced that the general approach to be described is the most efficient solution to the problem of injecting cells into the blastocyst, the author would be the last to deny that it could be improved in detail. This I leave to those

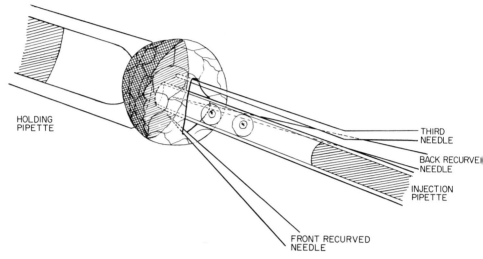

HOLDING
PIPETTE

THIRD
NEEDLE

BACK RECURVED
NEEDLE

INJECTION
PIPETTE

FRONT RECURVED
NEEDLE

Fig. 1.   Diagrammatic representation of cell injection into the blastocyst as it might appear when viewed obliquely from the above right to show the deployment of the five micro-instrument tips.

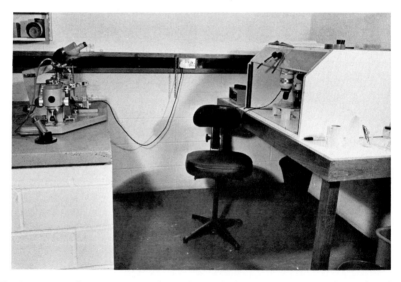

Fig. 2.   A convenient arrangement of the micromanipulation assembly in relation to the culture hood used to prepare blastocysts and cells for the injection operation.

with greater mechanical ingenuity. Meanwhile, the technique is presented as a reliable and versatile way of inducing chimerism at the blastocyst stage, which requires minimal modification of commercially available equipment.

Additional information on the principles and practice of micromanipulation, including solutions to the problem of vibration, may be found in a number of articles (e.g., De Fonbrune, 1949; Chambers and Kopac, 1950; Kopac, 1964). A block of reinforced concrete set away from the wall on top of two brick piers has proved an adequate table for the micromanipulator assembly in the author's laboratory. A culture hood containing a stereobinocular dissecting microscope is needed for recovery and preparation of blastocysts and cells, and for loading the manipulation chambers. Arrangement of the table or bench carrying the hood close to the manipulation table as shown in Fig. 2 enables the experimenter to shift from one to the other by rotating a swivel chair. The equipment for preparation of the glass micro-instruments should be located in a quiet corner that is free from drafts.

III. MICROMANIPULATION SYSTEM

This consists essentially of a Leitz micromanipulator assembly with minor modifications and additional items (Fig. 3A and B). Several makes of manipulator were tested initially, but the Leitz units proved to be most readily adapted for present purposes. A description of the design and mode of operation has been published (Kopac, 1964), and can also be obtained from the manufacturers. Briefly, precise horizontal movements free from backlash are produced by operating a single guide lever or joystick which moves a ball against a pair of sliding plates. The size of the circular field of movement can be adjusted to that of the microscope field by simply adjusting the height of the equator of the ball relative to the plates (Fig. 4). Four micro-instruments can be mounted on the assembly by fitting a double instrument head to each micromanipulator unit. The double heads each carry three knurled screw controls enabling back and forward movement of one instrument, and lateral plus vertical adjustment of the other (Fig. 5). However, though adequate for mutual prealignment of a pair of instruments, these controls are not, without modification, suitable for moving them independently during micromanipulation. This is because it is virtually impossible to turn the small screws without causing gross lateral displacement of the entire instrument head. This problem can be overcome quite simply by attaching light metal arms to the screw controls as shown in Fig. 5. By gently pushing such arms from the side with a finger, rather than gripping them, precise controlled movement of one or other instrument can be produced without difficulty. As described in detail later, the double instrument head on the left Leitz unit carries a pair of recurved microneedles whose sharp tips are initially apposed. It is the arm

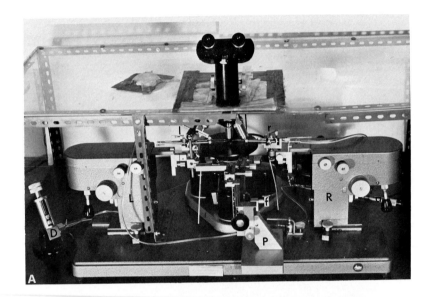

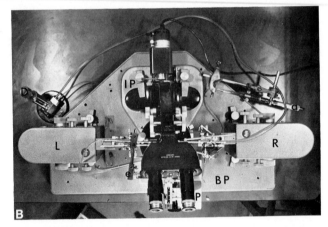

Fig. 3. Views of the author's micromanipulation assembly: (A) from the front and (B) from above, to show arrangement of the principal components. Key to abbreviations: a, Agla micrometer syringe connected to blastocyst holding pipette. It is attached to the manipulator base plate by means of a threaded vertical bar and retort clamps. B P, Leitz micromanipulator baseplate; D, De Fonbrune suction and force pump connected to injection pipette; e, extension arm that connects Prior manipulator with Leitz single instrument head; f, remote fine focus control of Leitz Laborlux microscope; IP, intermediate plate with screw clamps for securing Laborlux microscope to Leitz base plate; L, left Leitz manipulator unit; 1, left Leitz double instrument head; P, Prior manipulator unit attached to the front of the Leitz base plate; R, right Leitz manipulator unit; r, right Letiz double instrument head.

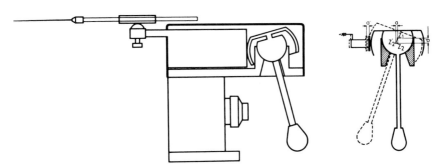

Fig. 4. Diagram illustrating the mode of operation of the guide lever or joystick of the Leitz micromanipulator. Movement of the micro-instruments in the two coordinates of the horizontal plane is controlled by the joystick. Movement of the joystick is transmitted to the sliding plates, and thence to the micro-instruments via a spherical segment. Thus, if the joystick is moved from its starting position to that indicated by the dashed lines, the center (Z_2) of the outer spherical segment will be displaced opposite the center point (Z_1) of the inner spherical segment through the distance a, and the plate and instruments through a similar distance. The joystick and instruments move in the same direction. The position of Z_2 can be changed along the longitudinal axis of the joystick relative to the fixed center point Z_1 of the inner spherical shell. This changes the position of the effective lever arm, so that reduction ratios from 1 : 1/16 to 1 : 1/800 can be set continuously. [Reproduced by kind permission of E. Leitz (Instruments) Ltd., Luton, England.]

attached to the lateral (''scissor action'') screw control that is used to make a slit in the trophectoderm once the needletips have been inserted into the blastocoel by means of the joystick control. The right hand Leitz unit carries the third blunt needle together with the injection pipette. In this case, exact control of the back-and-forth movement is needed to move the pipette into the blastocoel through the hole made by the three needles.

A third micromanipulator unit is required for positioning the fifth instrument, the blastocyst holding pipette. This can be a relatively simple device whose essential features are capacity for movement in three planes, compactness, and ease of attachment to the Leitz baseplate. A Prior right-hand manipulator plus stand (Fig. 3 A and B) meets these requirements admirably (see Table I for a detailed list of equipment). A right-angled metal extension arm carrying a Leitz single instrument head is needed to bring the holding pipette into correct alignment over the left Leitz manipulator unit (Fig. 3, A and B). This is a straightforward task for the laboratory workshop, as is attachment of arms to the Leitz double instrument heads.

Two micro-injectors are needed, one for immobilizing the blastocyst, and the second for cell or tissue injection. The device supplied by Leitz or an Agla micrometer syringe (Wellcome) with a metal spring or elastic band fitted to the plunger are suitable for the former purpose. The rather more sophisticated all-

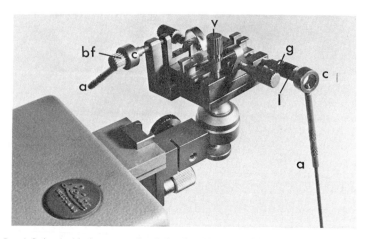

Fig. 5. A Leitz double instrument head showing the three knurled screw controls that enable independent back-and-forth (bf) movement of one micro-instrument and lateral (l) plus vertical (v) movement of the other. These controls can be operated efficiently during microsurgery by adopting the simple modification illustrated in the figure. A light metal arm (a) is threaded through a small brass collar (c) which fits loosely over the knurled head of a movement control screw. The collar is held on the screw head by projection of the proximal end of the arm into the groove (g). When the arm is unscrewed slightly, the collar will remain stationary under its weight, enabling the micro-instrument to be prealigned by turning the knurled screw. When the arm is screwed in tightly against the base of the groove, the collar is thereby locked on the knurled screw head. Very precise small displacements of one instrument relative to the other can then be produced by gently pushing the arm from one or other side. Such modification is essential for the lateral screw control on the double head of the left Leitz manipulator, since this movement is needed to part the recurved needles when making a slit in the trophectoderm. Providing a relatively long downward extending arm is used, the hand operating it can be rested on the manipulation base plate. A shorter arm attached to the back-and-forth movement of the double head on the right Leitz manipulator is also needed to move the injection pipette into the blastocoel past the third needle. Though the remaining independent movements are not required during microsurgery, occasional slight readjustments that may be necessary during a series of operations are facilitated by having arms locked to them also. The arms must not be too heavy; otherwise, they will keep returning to a downward position. Application of heavy-duty grease to the threads of the knurled screws will overcome any slight tendency of an arm to move spontaneously.

metal De Fonbrune suction and force pump (Beaudouin, Paris) is strongly recommended for handling cells. It can withstand higher pressures than injectors made from glass syringes, and enables exceedingly fine volume control. Providing it is set up correctly, and the flange on the plunger locked between the two retaining nuts, a cell can be held completely stationary in a fine micropipette indefinitely.

There is considerable diversity of opinion in the microsurgical literature regarding the most effective way of transmitting volume changes in an injector to

TABLE I

Inventory of Special Apparatus and Materials Recommended for Blastocyst Injection

Available from E. Leitz, Wetzlar, West Germany

1. Left and right micromanipulator units with clamps and baseplate.
2. Laborlux binocular microscope with fixed stage, image-erected optics,[a] remote fine focus, and intermediate plate plus clamps for attachment to micromanipulation baseplate. Microscope should be fitted with long working distance bright-field condenser, Periplan G.F. × 12.5 oculars, and × 10 plus × 25 objective lenses.
3. Two double instrument heads (one for each Leitz manipulator) and a single instrument head for attachment to third (Prior) manipulator unit.
4. At least six instrument holding tubes (one for each of the five microinstruments and a sixth for use with the microforge).
5. Six Puliv (oil-filled) manipulation chambers (interior height 3 mm). Supply of cover slips for chambers.
6. Leitz capillary tubing of approximately 1 mm overall diameter (supplied in batches of 100 lengths). A generous length of spare washer tubing for instrument holding tubes plus several spare brass washers.
7. A De Fonbrune microforge (available from Beaudouin, Paris, France).
8. A De Fonbrune suction and force pump (available from Beaudouin, Paris, France).
9. An Agla micrometer syringe outfit (Wellcome, Beckenham, England).
10. A Prior right-hand manipulator plus stand (Prior, Bishop's Stortford, England).
11. A gravity or electromagnetically operated electrode puller (various makes available).
12. Repelcote siliconizing agent (Hopkin & Williams, Chadwell Heath, England).
13. Nontoxic heavy grade liquid paraffin oil. Vaseline (various sources).
14. Thick-walled flexible translucent plastic tubing (i.d. approximately 2.5 mm) for connecting injectors to instrument holding tubes (various sources including E. Leitz).
15. Ocular graticule and micrometer calibration slide for use with microforge (various sources).

[a] Leitz ceased making such optics recently so that they can only be obtained second-hand. As far as the author is aware the only other microscope with such optics plus fixed stage is the ERGAVAL supplied by Carl Zeiss of Jena.

the micropipette. This concerns, for example, both the type of fluid and the amount of air in the system. Obviously, the most satisfactory solution for a particular individual can only be found by experimentation. The author prefers to have filtered heavy-grade paraffin oil throughout the system, and to exclude air altogether. The latter requires care, particularly in the case of the De Fonbrune injector in which enclosed air cannot be seen. The cylinder of this injector should be filled through one nozzle by slowly raising the plunger to its full extent. The cylinder is then rotated so that it communicates with the outlet nozzle that is connected by thick-walled plastic transparent tubing to a Leitz instrument holding tube. It is turned upside down so that the outlet nozzle is uppermost and held thus for a few seconds before depressing the plunger and emptying the injector of oil. This enables air to rise to the outlet nozzle and be expelled ahead of a column of paraffin oil. The entire cycle should be repeated until all air bubbles are driven out of the distal end of the instrument holder.

Both injectors are connected to instrument holding tubes by thick-walled flexible tubing. The advantage of using translucent plastic tubing for this purpose is that air bubbles are readily seen. The tubing should be long enough to allow each injector to be placed on the opposite side of the manipulator assembly to the instrument holder with which it connects. This enables each injector to be operated with one hand while the corresponding pipette is being maneuvered by the other. The joints at each end of the connector tubing can be made secure by binding them with wire. Finally, it is important to ensure that the tubing is well clear of the microscope lamp; otherwise, local heating will lead to uncontrolled expansion of the oil contained therein.

The final component of the assembly is a microscope. This should be a compound binocular rather than a dissecting microscope, and the Leitz Laborlux is undoubtedly the one of choice. It is designed specifically for use with the Leitz micromanipulators, and attaches to the baseplate via an intermediate plate and two screw clamps. It possesses several features of particular value for microsurgical work. First, the stage is fixed, both coarse- and fine-focus controls moving the turret. Second, a band-driven remote fine focus that obviates the need to grope behind the manipulators in order to refocus is available (Fig. 3A). Finally, until recently, an adaptor was available to provide image-erected optics (but see footnote to Table I). This is an enormous asset when attempting to maneuver five micro-instruments, particularly for the beginner.

Bright-field optics are essential, especially for working with blastocysts in hanging drops in the Leitz (Puliv) oil-filled manipulation chambers. Both a long-working distance condenser and objective lenses are needed for the same reason. An overall magnification of approximately × 100 is suitable for the initial arrangement of microinstruments and immobilization of the blastocyst. Higher magnification is required for the injection operation, the precise value being a compromise between two conflicting needs. Success of the operation depends critically on exact positioning of the embryos and instruments in the same plane. This may be achieved by increasing the magnification so that the depth of focus is correspondingly reduced. However, the size of the microscope field thereby is diminished and, as will be clear later, it is important to be able to see more than just the tips of the instruments throughout the operation. The author uses a pair of wide-field 12.5 × oculars in conjunction with a × 10 objective for the lower magnification, and with a × 25 objective for the higher.

Economic considerations may necessitate adaptation of other less suitable microscopes for use with the micromanipulator assembly. A colleague has found that it is possible to perform cell injections using a microscope with stage focusing and which lacks erected optics. Nevertheless, those planning to embark on extensive microsurgical work are urged to obtain a microscope of appropriate design (also see Kopac, 1964). Finally, whatever type is adopted, its stage should be stripped of mechanical movements and other projections that are likely to prove hazardous for setting up and aligning delicate micro-instruments.

IV. EQUIPMENT FOR MAKING GLASS MICRO-INSTRUMENTS

Essential items include a microforge and an electrode puller. So far as I am aware, the microforge designed by De Fonbrune is the only one available commercially that has the necessary versatility for making the variously shaped instruments required for this technique. This includes a facility for directing controlled jets of air towards the tip of the filament to allow localized heating. One filament holder should be fitted with platinum wire of approximately 0.3-mm diameter (*the thick filament*), and the other with 0.05- to 0.10-mm diameter wire (*the thin filament*). The filaments should be V shaped, and the apex of the thin one flattened out as much as possible by careful hammering. The microscope should be adapted to give an overall magnification of × 100 and fitted with a calibrated ocular micrometer. (The microscope is supplied with × 7 objective and × 5 ocular lenses. These are readily replaced by a × 10 objective and ocular on the old monocular model, but the new binocular microscope presents a problem for which I can suggest no immediate solution).

There are a number of different makes of electrode puller available commercially. Electromagnetically or gravity-operated devices with a straight pull are most suitable. Most types may have to be modified slightly because Leitz capillary is approximately two-thirds the diameter of standard microelectrode capillary. It is advisable to modify the puller rather than enlarge the captive nuts and brass washers of the Leitz instrument tubes to take the standard capillary. The floor to ceiling height of the manipulation chambers is only 3 mm. Therefore, using capillary of greater diameter will complicate the task of making instruments that fit into it. Finally, one needs both a standard Bunsen burner and a microburner made from Pyrex glass tubing or an abbreviated all-metal hypodermic needle (Chambers and Kopac, 1950), together with a pair of strong forceps for pulling capillary tubing by hand.

V. PREPARATION OF THE MICRO-INSTRUMENTS

A very detailed account of use of the De Fonbrune microforge can be found in a monograph on micromanipulative technique by its inventor (De Fonbrune, 1949). A précis of the relevant sections of this somewhat scarce publication is provided in a manual supplied with the apparatus. Details of design of the instruments needed for blastocyst injection will perhaps be made clearer by

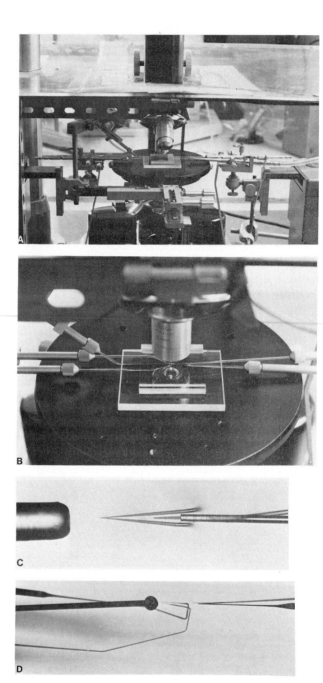

Fig. 6

considering briefly their arrangement on the micromanipulator assembly. The instrument tube carrying the blastocyst holding pipette is located by means of the extension arm on the Prior manipulator above the left Leitz unit. The pipette itself is bent proximally to its taper so that its distal end runs approximately horizontally to the right between the two instruments carried on the Leitz unit. It therefore is used to immobilize the blastocyst from the left so that the three needles and injection pipette must approach from the right. This means that the tips of the two instruments held on the left Leitz unit have to be recurved. It has been found most convenient to make these the pair of needles used to slit the trophectoderm, which are referred to hereafter as the recurved needles. The head on the right Leitz unit carries an injection pipette in its front position and the third needle behind it. Reference to Figs. 1 and 6 will hopefully make the arrangement clear. All instruments are normally prepared from the capillary tubing supplied by Leitz.

A. Micropipettes

There are two general points worth noting. First, the ratio of the internal diameter (i.d.) to overall diameter (o.d.) of glass tubing remains constant if it is pulled under optimal conditions, but decreases otherwise. Second, due to refraction of light, it is not possible to measure the true i.d. of a cylindrical capillary by viewing it from the side. This can be gauged only by viewing it end-on. This problem may be overcome by preparing a calibration curve as shown in Fig. 7, from which the o.d. corresponding to the desired i.d. can readily be found. It is important to appreciate, however, that such a graph is valid only for tubing whose diametric ratio is uniform, and which is pulled under optimal conditions of tension and temperature. Capillary that is pulled manually over a microburner flame tends to show much greater variation in thickness of its wall. This matters little for holding pipettes, but is critical in the case of those used for cell injection.

Holding pipettes are pulled by hand, since a long gradual taper is most easily obtained in this way. One end of a length of cleaned capillary is softened by rotation with the aid of forceps over a microburner flame. It is then pulled after withdrawal from the flame to yield a taper of at least 2–2.5 cm and a tip o.d. of

Fig. 6. The design and alignment of the five microinstruments used for blastocyst injections. (A) General view from the front to show the arrangement of the instruments on their instrument heads. An empty manipulation chamber is in position. (B) Close up of (A) from above. (C) View down the microscope at lower operating magnification to show correct alignment of the microinstrument tips. The third needle runs above the injection pipette, though presence of paraffin oil in the latter obscures this in the photograph. (D) A crude glass model to illustrate the basic shapes and arrangement of the three microneedles (lighter glass) and two pipettes (darker glass). (Details such as relative dimensions and tip characteristics of needles are inexact.)

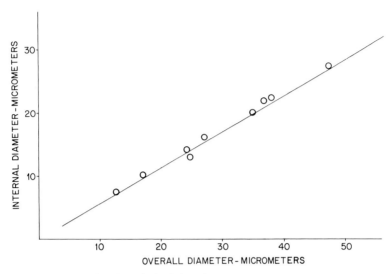

Fig. 7. Graph showing theoretical relationship between overall (o.d.) and internal (i.d.) tip diameter of pipettes pulled from Leitz capillary tubing under ideal conditions. Seventy lengths of unpulled tubing sampled from 8 separate batches of 100 were scored with a diamond and broken perpendicular to the long axis near one end. Each isolated segment was then viewed end-on in a microscope fitted with a calibrated ocular micrometer and its i.d. and o.d. measured. This yielded a mean i.d./o.d. ratio of 0.573 (± 0.029), which was used to construct the graph. Individual data points record the tip dimensions of several pipettes prepared with an electromagnetic puller and De Fonbrune microforge, and bent distally through 90° so that they could be measured end-on.

80 μm or less. The pipette is secured in an instrument tube so that its distal end can be arranged horizontally in the microscope field of the microforge. The tip of the thick filament is then fused by means of a small bulb of molten glass to the lower surface of the capillary at a point between 80 and 100 μm o.d. The aim is to obtain a frim union without bending or locally thickening the capillary wall, by careful adjustment of the filament temperature and air jet controls. The filament heating circuit is then switched off. Contraction of the filament on cooling should break the capillary cleanly perpendicularly to its long axis just proximal to the point of fusion. Finally, the pipette tip is smoothed down to an *apparent* i.d. of 15–20 μm by positioning the reheated filament close to it. An oblique break is usually due to failure to arrange the pipette horizontally or to insufficient rotation in the flame before pulling so that the wall thickness varies circumferentially. When closed down, the aperture of an obliquely broken pipette tends to be sufficiently maloriented to create problems when immobilizing blastocysts. The last stage is to bend the shank of the pipette close to the beginning of the taper in the microburner flame (see Figs. 6 A and B). Holding pipettes are fairly robust, and

can be placed loose in small closed metal boxes for storage and oven sterilization.

Cell injection pipettes are pulled in the electrode puller, which should be set to yield a gradual taper over at least 8 mm to a pointed tip. The o.d. corresponding to the required tip i.d. is determined from the calibration curve (Fig. 7), and the pipette broken in the microforge by the method described above. The only difference is that extra care is needed to avoid thickening its wall during fusion and, though it is advisable to heat polish the tip, this must also be done without reducing the luminal diameter. This is facilitated by having the air jets turned on fully. Finally, the pipette should be bent near the base of the taper until the tip is approximately in line with one side of the shank when held horizontally. This ensures that the distal end of the pipette can be raised into the hanging drops of the manipulation chamber without obstruction due to the shank hitting the under surface of the cover slip. It also aids alignment of the pipette tip between the recurved needles (see below).

The tip i.d. of cell injection pipettes will obviously depend on the size of the donor cells and is rather critical. If the i.d. is less than that of the cells, the latter are liable to be damaged by compression. If, on the other hand, it is much greater, medium may too readily bypass the cell or cells on injection, should their movement be impeded by slight adhesion to the wall of the pipette. Large cells are more of a problem because of the considerable thickness of the wall of Leitz capillary tubing. Thinner walled tubing of 1 mm o.d. does not seem to be available commercially. It can be pulled from larger glass tubing by a competent glass worker but, as discussed earlier, will have greater variation in wall thickness than machine-pulled tubing, so that one cannot construct an accurate calibration curve. The only solution is to determine the i.d./o.d. ratio of samples taken from each end of every length. Providing these do not differ substantially, their average is then used to calculate the o.d. corresponding to the required i.d. Tissue injection pipettes are prepared in the same way as cell injection pipettes except the tip is broken at an o.d. of approximately 25 μm and heat polished down to an *apparent* i.d. of 12–15 μm. Injection pipettes are much more delicate than holding pipettes and should therefore be stored and oven-sterilized in closed containers in which their distal tips stand free from contact with any surface.

B. Microneedles

Pointed needles can be made simply by pulling Leitz capillary tubing in the electrode puller. However, there is a risk that the tips may be open so that fluid is drawn into the lumen by capillarity when such needles are siliconized and sterilized by dipping in Repelcote (Hopkin and Williams) and alcohol, respectively. Hence, both to avoid this problem and in order to produce needles of greater mechanical strength, they are pulled from solid glass as follows. The middle of a length of Leitz capillary is rotated in a hot standard Bunsen flame until its lumen is totally occluded. By pulling the capillary after a brief pause following removal from the flame, one can obtain a straight length without attenuating the solid region. The capillary is then placed in the puller so that the latter region is tapered to a point over a distance of approximately 7 mm.

The front- and back-recurved needles are undoubtedly the most difficult micro-instruments to make, but their careful preparation is crucial for the success of the microsurgical operation. A sharp-tipped solid microneedle is inserted into the forge obliquely (Fig. 8). The thin filament is then used to pull the distal 300 μm through a right angle. For this operation, the apex of the filament should be well flattened and free from adherent glass, so as to achieve a minimal area of slight fusion with one side of the needle. This requires a very careful adjustment of the rheostat and air jet controls. The distal part of the needle is bent by pulling the filament away from it. If the union is too strong, the needle will be broken when the right-angled bend is completed and the heat turned off. It is far better to have too weak a union so that the filament repeatedly detaches during the pull, which is undertaken thus in a series of steps. Next, the instrument tube is rotated about its axis through approximately 35°, so that the tip of the needle points obliquely *toward* the observer. A second right angle is then made roughly 1.0 mm proximal to the first by the same procedure. The filament and air jets are then turned off and the needle repositioned in the microforge with its shank horizontal. The instrument tube is rotated about its long axis until the part of the needle distal to the second bend points directly toward the observer's eye in the microscope field. This is achieved by focusing between the first and second bend during the rotation until both are in line with the same mark in the ocular micrometer. Finally, the microscope is focused on the distal part of the needle, whose point will be directed downwards at approximately 35° from horizontal. The lower surface of the needle is then heated with a low microburner flame close to the base of the taper, causing the distal part to bend downward under its weight. It thus is necessary to raise the needle horizontally at intervals so as to be able to inspect the tip in the microscope. Bending should be continued slowly until the tip is pointing almost horizontally. If it is carried too far, the axis of the needle should be rotated through exactly 180° and the flame applied to the opposite surface. The final result is a front-recurved needle, as illustrated in Fig. 6.

The first step in making a back-recurved needle is the same as for a front one. But, before making the second bend, the long axis should be rotated so that the tip points away from the observer by 35°. Similarly, the part distal to the second right angle must be directed away from the observer before making the final bend. There is one other crucial difference. The distance between the first and second right-angle bends on a back needle needs to

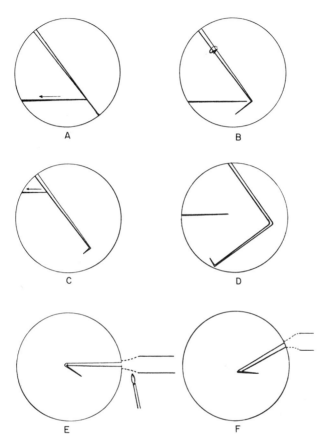

Fig. 8. Stages in the preparation of a front-recurved needle. (The arrangement of the needle and filament is drawn, as it would appear to the naked eye rather than when viewed through the compound microscope of the microforge.) A solid needle is oriented in the microforge obliquely with its pointed tip downwards as indicated in (A). The apex of a flattened fine platinum filament is then brought into contact with the side of the needle at a point roughly 300 μm from the tip. The filament should be just hot enough to enable it to pull the distal segment of the needle through 90°, but detach when the bend is completed and the filament turned off (B). The instrument tube holding the needle is then rotated through approximately 35° so that the tip points obliquely *toward* the observer (C). Next, the needle is pulled through a second right-angle at a point approximately 1 mm proximal to the first one (D). The filament heater and air jets are turned off and the needle repositioned horizontally in the microforge. Its holding tube is rotated until the section distal to the second right-angle points straight *toward* the observer (E). Finally, the needle is heated near the base of its taper with a gas microburner so that the distal region falls until the pointed tip is almost horizontal (F). The procedure for preparing a back recurved needle differs in three respects. First, the tip should be rotated *away* from the observer before making the second right-angled bend. Next, the second right-angled bend should be made at a point between 0.6 and 0.7 mm proximal to the first. Finally, at the stage shown in (E), the needle should be rotated until the segment distal to the second bend points directly away from the observer.

be slightly greater than half the o.d. of the capillary shank (0.6 mm is sufficient) to ensure that the recurved tip can be raised high enough in the
manipulation chamber. However, the length of this region must always be greater
for a front needle than its back partner because the vertical screw control on the
double instrument head only moves the distal end of this needle downwards from
horizontal and cannot be used to raise it. The essential steps in preparing recurved needles are summarized in Fig. 8, and the desired end result is illustrated
in Figs. 1 and 6. The points of a pair of needles should come together at an acute
angle, while their shanks are well separated and approximately parallel for most
of their length, thus enabling the holding pipette to be maneuvered between them.
If the angle between their tips is too acute, the third needle and injection pipette
cannot be positioned inside it; if too large, they will not penetrate the trophectoderm readily. Understanding the rationale of the steps involved in making these
needles is facilitated by going through the sequence of bending and rotation with
lengths of malleable wire.

The third needle is also made from a straight, solid-tipped needle arranged
with its point vertically downwards in the microforge. The apex of the thin
filament is positioned close below the point without touching it, and heated
enough to convert the point into a smooth, rounded end. The distal 300 μm
should then be pulled through an angle of 5–10° so that it can be made parallel
with the injection pipette after insertion into the double instrument head of the
right hand Leitz manipulator unit (Fig. 6).

All needles are dipped in Repelcote immediately after preparation and are
stored in plastic sandwich boxes with their proximal ends firmly embedded in
modeling clay. They are sterilized by dipping in absolute alcohol immediately
prior to use.

VI. SETTING UP THE MICRO-INSTRUMENTS ON THE MANIPULATOR ASSEMBLY

The correct alignment of the five micro-instruments is illustrated in Figs. 1 and
6. Attention to detail in setting them up is vital for the success of subsequent
manipulations. The following points should be noted. All instruments must be
tightly secured in the metal instrument tubes by means of washers and captive
nuts. Slackness is usually attributable to too short a length of rubber washer or to
its being excessively worn or perished. The instrument tubes should, after initial
alignment, be tightly secured in the spring clips on the instrument heads by
means of the appropriate screws. The author proceeds as follows.

The back-recurved needle is inserted into the rear position on the double head
of the left Leitz unit and its distal end brought into the microscope field at the
lower magnification. Its tube is rotated while focusing until the region distal to

the second right-angle bend is vertical. The tube is then secured by the screw clip. The scissor action is then unscrewed so that the tube carrying the front needle can be inserted without risk of contact between the two needles. This needle is also rotated until the section carrying the pointed tip is vertical and then secured. The three knurled screw controls are used to bring the two points together in the same focal plane. Final alignment of the points is done at the higher operating magnification (about × 300). The tip of the back needle should be set a little to the right of the front one when the two are in contact because, on parting them with the scissor action, the latter moves in this direction somewhat. Following exact mutual alignment of the tips, the arm on the scissor screw control is locked while hanging downwards (Fig. 5), so that the needletips are parted on pushing it to the right, and closed on shifting it back to the left.

The next step is to fit the holding pipette into its tube. The captive nut, brass washer, and rubber washer are removed from the tube and slid onto the proximal end of the holding pipette in the same sequence. The injector is operated to bring the continuous column of paraffin oil to the end of the tube. It is advisable, before inserting the pipette, to score it near the base with a diamond and break off the short proximal segment. Otherwise, pieces of rubber, dirt, or even keratinized squamous cells introduced into the lumen during placement of the washers may occlude the tip. The proximal end is then touched against the surface of the oil to introduce a short column of this fluid into the pipette, which is then inserted fully and secured without inclusion of air. The tube is then fitted into the Leitz single instrument head attached to the Prior manipulator and the pipette aligned by means of the universal joint and manipulator controls. The tapering distal end of the pipette is lowered between and parallel to the shanks of the recurved needles and its tip inclined slightly. It must be brought forward into the microscope field very carefully to avoid damaging the delicate needles and the tip set at the same height as the latter. It is then moved to the rear of the field and the needles to the front before all three are withdrawn.

The injection pipette is inserted into its instrument tube, following the same procedure used for the holding pipette, and clamped in the front position on the right double head with its angled tip directed upwards. The tip is centered in the microscope field and the pair of recurved needles reintroduced to check that it will fit into the angle between their points. Rotating the instrument tube will, because of the bend near the base of the taper, facilitate alignment by slightly altering the direction of the distal segment of the pipette. The recurved needles should again be withdrawn while the third needle is fitted in the rear position on the right Leitz head. The latter must be adjusted so that its distal, blunt-tipped segment is parallel with that of the injection pipette and lies just above it. A length of folded aluminum foil placed on the floor of the rear tube insert will ensure that the tip of the third needle can be raised above the pipette. Also, the third needle should be fitted into its instrument tube in such a way that the length of exposed capillary differs from that of the injection pipette by at least 7 mm. Otherwise, contact between the captive nuts of the two tubes will prevent correct alignment of the tips of the instruments by the scissor movement. Finally, the arm on the back-and-forth movement should be locked to the screw control in a downward position when the tip of the third needle projects to the left of the pipette tip by 200–300 μm. Raising this arm will then move the injection pipette to the left, to just beyond the tip of the needle, and lowering should reverse this movement.

The micro-instruments have to be withdrawn from and reintroduced into the microscope field repeatedly, both during the setting up procedure and while carrying out the experimental manipulations. Risk of damage to them during these maneuveres is greatly reduced by making a habit of shifting them to different points within the field before every withdrawal. The author shifts the holding pipette to the rear of the field, the recurved needles to the front, and the injection pipette and third needle to the center. In this way, mutual damage is avoided, even following hasty reintroduction.

VII. BLASTOCYST INJECTION

All manipulations are carried out in hanging drops of medium in Leitz (Puliv) manipulation chambers filled with heavy paraffin oil. Excessive spreading and flattening of the drops is avoided by dipping the cleaned cover slips in Repelcote before oven sterilization. This measure necessitates introduction of the drops on the underside of the cover slip *before* filling the chamber with paraffin oil. Chambers are detergent cleaned, rinsed in distilled water, and wiped with an alcohol-soaked tissue prior to assembly. Oven sterilization tends to cause detachment of the walls from the base of the chambers. Following evaporation of the alcohol, the upper surface of each wall is smeared with a thin layer of vaseline dispensed from a syringe. The cover slip is then pressed on firmly with sterile forceps and a row of six to eight drops of medium is placed on its lower surface with a pulled Pasteur pipette. The two end drops must be located sufficiently far from the respective walls so that the recurved needles can reach them without their shanks contacting the walls. Finally, the chamber is filled with paraffin oil. The medium used for the microdrops, as also for recovery, storage, and postoperative culture of the blastocysts, is essentially the phosphate-buffered medium devised by Whittingham and Wales (1969), differing only in omission of bovine serum albumin and inclusion of 10% (v/v) fetal calf serum.

The drops can be assigned numbers conveniently because one wall of the chamber is much closer to the edge of the base than the other (Fig. 6C). The drop closest to this wall is taken as number one. Disaggregated cells to be transplanted are placed in this drop and host blastocysts in the remainder. If isolated ICMs or other clumps of cells are to be injected, one is placed in each drop, together with a single blastocyst. It is advisable to put only one blastocyst in each drop, at least until one is competent at the injection procedure, because, once the blastocysts have contracted following operation, it is often difficult to distinguish those that have been successfully injected from those that have not.

All five instruments are withdrawn well clear of the center of the microscope stage so that the chamber may be positioned on it with a drop centered in the field of the microscope. If difficulty is experienced in positioning the chamber by hand, it may be aided by applying a little vaseline to its base. However, greater care is then needed when the chamber is eventually removed from the stage, after focusing on a blastocyst on the floor of a drop. The instruments are then reintroduced and adjusted to the focus of the microscope. This obvious but all too readily forgotten step ensures that, following their withdrawal and reintroduction when the chamber is replaced, the micro-instruments will clear the cover slip and floor of the latter.

A cell or cells are drawn carefully into the injection pipette not too close to the medium–paraffin interface, and held stationary by locking the retaining nuts on the De Fonbrune injector. The pipette is withdrawn from the drop and the chamber moved to one containing a blastocyst. All the instruments are brought into this drop at the lower magnification. The height of the tip of the holding pipette is adjusted until its lumen is parfocal with the greatest diameter of the blastocyst. The third needle is then used to maneuver the blastocyst against the tip of the holding pipette, and to orient it so that it can be held over the middle of the ICM. The blastocyst can be rotated by lowering or raising this needle tip against one side. Suction is applied to the embryo only when it is sufficiently close and correctly oriented, in order to avoid drawing more than a minimal volume of medium into the pipette during immobilization. Once the blastocyst is immobilized by firm but gentle suction, the pipette is raised to lift it clear of the floor of the drop. The other instruments are also raised and arranged as shown in Fig. 9A, and the microscope changed to the higher working magnification. The apposed tips of the recurved needles are then pushed well into the blastocoel with the joystick control on the left unit at a point to the rear of the abembryonic pole (see legend to Fig. 9), in the plane of maximum diameter. The needletips are parted by approximately 50 μm by moving the arm locked to the scissor action on the left Leitz head to the right, thereby forming a horizontal slit in the abembryonic polar trophectoderm and overlying zona pellucida (Fib. 9B). The third needle is brought up to this slit by operating the right joystick and very carefully introduced into it, using the fine vertical adjustment to ensure that its rounded tip is parfocal with the regions of the recurved needles at this point. The only way to verify that the tip of this needle is really in the slit is to move it slightly toward the rear and front of the microscope field between the recurved needles. If no resistance to such lateral movement is evident, it can be pushed

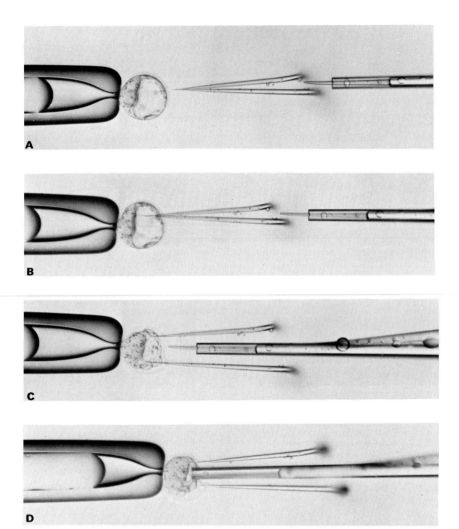

Fig. 9. Stages in the cell injection operation. (A) The blastocyst has been immobilized by applying suction to the ICM pole, and then raised clear of the floor of the hanging drop. The remaining micro-instruments are aligned ready for the operation. (B) The apposed tips of the recurved needles are pushed well into the blastocoel a little to the far side of the abembryonic pole; otherwise, the blastocyst will be pulled sideways when the front needle is parted from the stationary back one by the scissor movement. (C) A fairly wide slit is made in the trophectoderm and overlying zona, into which the third needle has to be maneuvered. Following introduction of the third needle, the slit is converted into a triangular hole by raising the third needle, and lowering the pair of recurved ones. (D) The injection pipette is then moved into the blastocoel relative to the third needle, and the cell injected. The blastocyst has undergone a greater degree of contraction by the stage illustrated in (D) than usual, due to interruptions required for photography.

further into the blastocoel. The fine vertical adjustments near the joysticks of the two Leitz units are then used to raise the third needle and lower the parted recurved needles by an approximately equal distance. It is wise to check by focusing at this juncture that the recurved needles lie below the injection pipette. The tip of this pipette will then be adjacent to a triangular hole in the trophectoderm and zona, through which it can be moved into the blastocoel by raising the arm locked to its back-and-forth screw control. The cells are then ejected slowly against the surface of the ICM, the tips of the recurved needles raised and closed below the pipette, and all the instruments withdrawn. If the recurved needles show a tendency to stick to the damaged trophectoderm, the tip of the pipette or third needle can be used to hold the abembryonic pole while they are pulled out. Finally, the blastocyst is released from the holding pipette and the entire cycle repeated on the next one. The essential steps of the injection procedure are illustrated in Figs. 9A–D. All micro-instruments should be withdrawn clear of the hanging drops each time the chamber is moved from one to another.

It is unnecessary to remove the zona pellucida from host blastocysts prior to injection. There are, in fact, several advantages in using blastocysts whose zonae are intact. First, the polar trophectoderm and underlying ICM are less likely to be damaged during immobilization on the holding pipette. Second, elasticity of the zona aids closure of the wound, trapping of the injected cells, and withdrawal of the instruments. Finally, blastocysts within their zonae are less likely to adhere to the wall of the pipette during removal from the chamber and transplantation into uterine foster mothers.

There are several points of detail to which particular attention must be paid in carrying out the injections. Accurate vertical adjustment of the three needles so that they are coplanar with the maximum diameter of the blastocyst is one. This applies particularly to the apposed tips of the recurved needles because they must penetrate the trophectoderm at the same point. If they fail to do so, a clean slit will not be produced, and strands of cellular debris are liable to traverse the hole formed following introduction of the third needle. Such strands tend to obstruct the aperture of the injection pipette, thereby preventing ejection of the cells into the blastocoel. Similar problems will be encountered if the vertical adjustment of the third needle above the injection pipette is wrong. If it is too close to the upper surface of the pipette, the latter will not clear the edges of the hole, while if it is too high the blastocyst will have to be torn wide open or pulled off the holding pipette in order to get the recurved needles below the level of the injection pipette. It is also important to have the tip of the third needle in view at higher magnification by positioning it close to the right of the apposed recurved needletips in the same plane, since the blastocyst will begin to contract as soon as these needles have penetrated it. Therefore, slitting of the trophectoderm and penetration by the third needle should be carried out as quickly and efficiently as possible. Finally, the injectors must be operated slowly, particularly when applying suction, otherwise medium will bypass the paraffin oil and break it up into a series of small drops. The volume of medium taken into the pipettes should be small enough to ensure that the interface with the paraffin oil is visible in the microscope field at all times when the injectors are handled. It is only by observing this interface that one can tell whether micropipettes are taking in or expelling fluid or in a static condition.

Transplantation of pieces of tissues or mechanically or immunosurgically isolated ICMs (Gardner and Johnson, 1972; Solter and Knowles, 1976) to the blastocoel is carried out in exactly the same way, except that they are held by gentle suction on the tip of the injection pipette, which is closed down for the purpose (see section on making injection pipettes). Operated blastocysts are cultured for 1–4 hours at 37°C to allow repair and integration of the donor cells before transplantation to the uterus. There is some advantage in incubating them in the manipulation chambers after enlarging the drops by adding more medium. Not only does this avoid moving them before repair and integration, but it also enables critical appraisal of the final location of the injected cells by inspection at high magnification while orienting the blastocysts with the third needle. Provided the blastocysts have not been damaged excessively during operation, they should reexpand within 1–3 hours.

Microsurgery is usually carried out at room temperature because the problem of adhesion of cells and cellular debris to the micro-instruments is lessened thereby. However, it is possible to operate at 37°C using a heated microscope stage (Leitz supply such a stage designed to fit the Laborlux microscope). This may be necessary to assist integration of donor cells that do not readily adhere to the surface of the ICM. There are many protocols for dissociating tissues to obtain single cell suspensions (see Kruse and Patterson, 1973, for details), and a number of trials may be necessary to find one that yields a satisfactory rate of integration. Disaggregation of mouse ICMs can be obtained by the method of Cole *et al.* (1966) which gives a cloning efficiency *in vivo* of approximately 25%. A protocol for obtaining suspensions of embryonal carcinoma cells from *in vivo* embryoid bodies is described by Mintz *et al.* (1975).

The author can routinely inject up to 30 blastocysts per hour by the above technique, and has operated on as many as 70 without changing any instruments. However, it is wise to have at least one set of spares ready, and to replace at once any that cease to function properly. Trying to continue with broken needles or partly occluded pipettes leads to a vicious circle of abortive operations and increasing exasperation. Once one is experienced in making instruments, one afternoon every two weeks should be sufficient to prepare enough sets for about 10 days experiments. I make it a rule never to use the same ones on successive days, even if they are still functional after an experiment.

When one has gained proficiency in cell injection, it is possible to dispense with the third needle, providing the dissociated cells to be transplanted are fairly small. The recurved needles are used to make a wide slit in the trophectoderm then brought closer together while the injection pipette is gently maneuvered into the blastocoel. The tip of such a pipette must be carefully polished and have as small an o.d. as is compatible with avoiding damage to the enclosed cells.

So far, the technique has been used only for injecting cells into mouse and rabbit blastocysts (Gardner, 1968; Gardner and Munro, 1974). There are no obvious reasons why it could not be adopted for other species. Attempts to produce chimeras in species like the rabbit, in which the blastocyst undergoes considerable growth and expansion prior to implantation, are more likely to succeed if injection is carried out at the early blastocyst stage. The ratio of donor to host ICM cells will be most favorable, and their integration into the host ICM most probable. Chimerism has been obtained in sheep by injecting cells through the zona at the morula stage (Tucker *et al.*, 1974).

Finally, it is the author's firm belief that the principal quality needed for microsurgical work of the type described in this chapter is patience rather than great manual dexterity. Those who persevere should find themselves competently injecting cells into blastocysts within 3–4 months of assembling the necessary equipment.

ACKNOWLEDGMENTS

I wish to thank Mr. A. J. Copp, Mrs. W. J. Gardner, Dr. C. F. Graham, Dr. J. Rossant, and Dr. P. Thorogood for valuable comments on the manuscript, and Mr. J. Hayward, Mrs. P. Little, and Mrs. M. White for assistance in preparing it. I am also indebted to Professor Joe Daniel, Jr., for providing me with the opportunity to publish the technique in full, and to the Medical Research Council for support.

REFERENCES

Benirschke, K. (1970). *Curr. Top. Pathol.* **51**, 1–61.
Bowman, P., and McLaren, A. (1970). *J. Embryol. Exp. Morphol.* **23**, 693–704.
Buehr, M., and McLaren, A. (1974). *J. Embryol. Exp. Morphol.* **31**, 229–234.
Chambers, R. W., and Kopac, M. J. (1950). *In* "McClung's Handbook of Microscopical Technique" (R. McClung Jones, ed.), 3rd ed., pp. 492–543. Hafner, New York.
Cole, R. J., Edwards, R. G., and Paul, J. (1966). *Dev. Biol.* **13**, 385–407.
Crick, F. H. C., and Lawrence, P. A. (1975). *Science* **189**, 340–347.
De Fonbrune, P. (1949). "Technique de Micromanipulation." Masson, Paris.
Deol, M. S., and Whitten, W. K. (1972). *Nature (London) New Biol.* **240**, 277–279.
Fialkow, P. J. (1973). *Ann. Hum. Genet.* **37**, 39–48.
Ford, C. E. (1969). *Br. Med. Bull.* **25**, 104–109.
Gardner, R. L. (1968). *Nature (London)* **220**, 596–597.
Gardner, R. L. (1971). *Adv. Biosci.* **6**, 279–296.
Gardner, R. L. (1974). *In* "Birth Defects and Fetal Development, Endocrine and Metabolic Factors" (K. S. Moghissi, ed.), pp. 212–233. Thomas, Springfield, Illinois.

Gardner, R. L. (1977). *In* "Genetic Mosaics and Cell Differentiation: Results and Problems in Cell Differentiation" (W. Gehring, ed.). Springer-Verlag, Berlin and New York (in press).

Gardner, R. L., and Johnson, M. H. (1972). *J. Embryol. Exp. Morphol.* **28**, 279–312.

Gardner, R. L., and Johnson, M. H. (1973). *Nature (London), New Biol.* **246**, 86–89.

Gardner, R. L., and Johnson, M. H. (1975). *Cell Patterning, Ciba Found. Symp. 1975 No. 29*, pp. 183–200.

Gardner, R. L., and Lyon, M. F. (1971). *Nature (London)* **231**, 385–386.

Gardner, R. L., and Munro, A. J. (1974). *Nature (London)* **250**, 146–147.

Gardner, R. L., and Papaioannou, V. E. (1975). *In* "The Early Development of Mammals" (M. Balls and A. E. Wild, eds.), pp. 107–132. Cambridge Univ. Press, London and New York.

Gardner, R. L., and Rossant, J. (1976). *Embryogenesis Mammals, Ciba Found. Symp. 1976 No. 40*, pp. 5–18.

Gehring, W., ed. (1977). "Genetic Mosaics and Cell Differentiation: Results and Problems in Cell Differentiation." Springer-Verlag, Berlin and New York (in press).

Hotta, Y., and Benzer, S. (1973). *In* "Genetic Mechanisms of Development." (F. H. Ruddle, ed.). pp. 129–167. Academic Press, New York.

Illmensee, K., and Mintz, B. (1976). *Proc. Natl. Acad. Sci. U.S.A.* **73**, 549–553.

Kopac, M. J. (1964). *Phys. Tech. Biol. Res.* **5**, 191–233.

Kruse, P., Jr., and Patterson, M. K., eds. (1973). "Tissue Culture: Methods and Applications." Academic Press, New York.

Lyon, M. F. (1974). *Proc. R. Soc. London, B Ser.* **187**, 243–268.

McLaren, A. (1976). "Mammalian Chimeras." Cambridge Univ. Press, London and New York.

Melvold, R. W. (1971). *Mutat. Res.* **12**, 171–174.

Mintz, B. (1962). *Am. Zool.* **2**, 432 (Abstr. No. 310).

Mintz, B. (1965). *Preimplantation Stages Pregnancy, Ciba Found. Symp. 1965* pp. 194–207.

Mintz, B. (1971). *In* "Methods in Mammalian Embryology" (J. C. Daniel, Jr., ed), pp. 186–214. Freeman, San Francisco, California.

Mintz, B. (1974). *Annu. Rev. Genet.* **8**, 411–470.

Mintz, B., Illmensee, K., and Gearhart, J. D. (1975). *In* "Teratomas and Differentiation" (M. I. Sherman and D. Solter, eds.), pp. 59–82. Academic Press, New York.

Moustafa, L. A. (1974). *Proc. Soc. Exp. Biol. Med.* **147**, 485–488.

Moustafa, L. A., and Brinster, R. L. (1972a). *J. Exp. Zool.* **181**, 193–201.

Moustafa, L. A., and Brinster, R. L. (1972b). *J. Exp. Zool.* **181**, 181–191.

Mulnard, J. G. (1973). *C. R. Hebd. Seances Acad. Sci., Ser. D* **276**, 379–381.

Mystkowska, E. T. (1975). *J. Embryol. Exp. Morphol.* **33**, 731–744.

Nesbitt, M. N. (1971). *Dev. Biol.* **26**, 252–263.

Nesbitt, M. N., and Gartler, S. M. (1971). *Annu. Rev. Genet.* **5**, 143–162.

Nicholas, J. S., and Hall, B. V. (1942). *J. Exp. Zool.* **90**, 441–460.

Papaioannou, V. E., and Gardner, R. L. (1976). *Embryogenesis Mammals, Ciba Found. Symp. 1976* No. 40, pp. 232–233.

Papaioannou, V. E., McBurney, M. W., Gardner, R. L., and Evans, M. J. (1975). *Nature (London)* **258**, 70–73.

Rossant, J. (1975). *J. Embryol. Exp. Morphol.* **33**, 979–990.

Rossant, J. (1976). *J. Embryol. Exp. Morphol.* **36**, 163–174.

Russell, L. B. (1964). *In* "The Role of Chromosomes in Development" (M. Locke, ed.), pp. 153–181. Academic Press, New York.

Sherman, M. I., and Solter, D., eds. (1975). "Teratomas and Differentiation." Academic Press, New York.

Solter, D., and Knowles, B. B. (1976). *Proc. Natl. Acad. Sci. U.S.A.* **72**, 5099–5102.

Stern, M. S. (1972). *J. Embryol. Exp. Morphol.* **28**, 255–261.

Stern, M. S. (1973). *Nature (London)* **243**, 472–473.

Stern, M. S., and Wilson, I. B. (1972). *J. Embryol. Exp. Morphol.* **28**, 247–254.

Tarkowski, A. K. (1961). *Nature (London)* **190**, 857–860.

Tucker, E. M., Moor, R. M., and Rowson, L. E. A. (1974). *Immunology* **26**, 613–621.

Weissman, I. L., Papaioannou, V. E., and Gardner, R. L. (1977). *Cold Spring Harbor Symp. Quant. Biol.* XLI, 9–21.

Whittingham, D. G., and Wales. R. G. (1969). *Aust. J. Biol. Sci.* **22**, 1065–1068.

Zeilmaker, G. H. (1973). *Nature (London)* **242**, 115–116.

7

Techniques for Separating Early Embryonic Tissues

M. H. L. SNOW

I. INTRODUCTION

The early mammalian embryo is small and relatively inaccessible, and certainly not ideal material for the sort of manipulative experimentation that embryologists used so successfully on amphibian embryos. The comparatively enormous newt and frog embryos, which grow at room temperature and in the simplest of culture media—water, were eminently suited for studies on cell lineage, cell and tissue autonomy, the process of embryogenesis, and cell and tissue movements and interactions. The contributions made by such studies in developing the concepts of determination, differentiation, induction and tissue interaction and, more recently, nuclear–cytoplasmic interactions, are inestimable.

Nevertheless, natural curiosity, if nothing else, demands that other vertebrates, including mammals, should be investigated for similarities and differences in development. An additional impetus to such research on mammalian embryos is provided by the concern about the increasing number of congenital malformations in man, which now survive to birth and, in many instances, for several years thereafter. Such malformations can arise spontaneously or, more insidiously, be induced by the teratogenic action of an outside agent. Whatever the cause, the precise mode and time of their origin is in the majority of cases unknown, but is usually early in embryogenesis.

In recent years, great advances have been made in scaling down many biochemical procedures such that it is now possible to perform sophisticated analyses on samples of only a few hundred cells, and for some specific functions even on single cells (Van Blerkom, this volume; Wales, this volume). There has arisen, therefore, a more widespread interest in the techniques for isolating identified and uncontaminated tissues from the small early mammalian embryo.

The purposes of this chapter are to identify the tissues that can be isolated and to describe in as much detail as space allows the various procedures which can be used. Since these techniques have been developed using rat and mouse embryos, I will confine myself to considering only those two species. Suffice it to say that, with due consideration of embryo size and organization, many of the techniques to be described may well be applicable to other species also, particularly other rodents.

II. THE EMBRYOS

The cell lineages in the rodent embryo have only recently been clarified, and Fig. 1 shows an outline of mouse development from the blastocyst stage (1) to the establishment of the trilaminate embryo immediately propr to the formation of the first somite (3). The derivations of the various tissues are indicated, based upon the work of Gardner and Johnson (1972, 1975) and Gardner and Papaioannou (1975). Various terminologies exist in the literature, but the definitions of the terms used below are those found generally acceptable at the *Ciba Foundation Symposium 40 on Embryogenesis in Mammals* (1976). They are as follows:

Trophectoderm—the single cell thick outer wall of the blastocyst, often called trophoblast.

Inner cell mass (ICM)—all those cells of the blastocyst normally isolated from the external environment by the trophectoderm.

Primary endoderm—the single cell thick layer that forms over the ICM on the surface exposed to the blastocyst cavity. It seems doubtful that this tissue persists into late embryonic development (Gardner and Papaioannou, 1975); other names: hypoblast, endoderm.

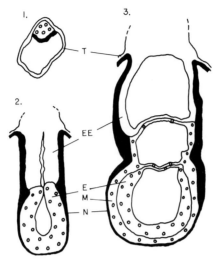

Fig. 1. Developmental stages of mouse and rat embryos. 1, Blastocyst at time of implantation, 4 days p.c. in mouse, 5 days p. c. in rat; 2, pre-primitive streak egg cylinder, 6 ½ days p.c. in mouse, 8 days p.c. in rat; 3, early head fold stage: 7 ½ days p.c. in mouse, 9 ½ days p.c. in rat. T, trophectoderm; EE, extraembryonic ectoderm; E, epiblast, embryonic ectoderm; M, mesoderm; N, primary endoderm. Clear area, trophectoderm derivatives; solid area, primary endoderm derivatives; clear area with circles, epiblast derivatives.

Egg cylinder—the entire, elongated structure which develops projecting into the expanding blastocyst cavity. It consists of:

Extraembryonic ectoderm—a column of cells derived from the trophectoderm to which is attached the

Epiblast—more frequently referred to as embryonic ectoderm. It is currently believed that the entire fetus is derived from this tissue. It represents the nonendodermal portion of the inner cell mass prior to mesoderm formation. The term epiblast is preferred to ectoderm, as it does not prejudge the developmental fate of the tissue, and, hence, gives cognizance to the work of Skreb and his colleagues (1976), who have demonstrated a multipotential role for these cells. Furthermore, the term was used in the first correct description of rodent embryogenesis (Fraser, 1883), and is in keeping with the terminology used in chick embryology.

Proximal endoderm—a derivative of the primary endoderm that covers the outer surface of the epiblast and extraembryonic ectoderm, and completes the early egg cylinder.

After primitive streak formation and the appearance of mesoderm, the inner cell layer of the embryonic portion of the egg cylinder loses its multipotential property and is referred to as embryonic ectoderm.

Development rates of rat and mouse are different, the rat being slower. Table I indicates the approximate ages of comparable developmental stages in the two species. Smaller differences in development rate exist between strains of mice, but in the extreme these do not exceed 6–10 hours at the primitive streak stage.

Methods for obtaining both pre- and postimplantation stage embryos from rat and mouse have been adequately described elsewhere by New (1971) and Kirby (1971), and there are descriptions in the literature of many different culture media which are suitable for the handling of embryos (for references, see Whittingham, 1971; Biggers *et al.*, 1971; New, 1971).

The mouse postimplantation stages are smaller than those of the rat and correspondingly somewhat more difficult to handle, and will yield smaller amounts of tissue. The embryos of both species should only be transferred from dish to dish using flame polished pipettes.

With regard to the *in vitro* culture of embryos, the blastocyst outgrowth system is regarded as postimplantation development *in vitro*. It is clear from a now abundant literature that the optimum culture conditions for trophectoderm and ICM differ and that it is possible to severely restrict ICM development *in vitro* simply by selecting an appropriate medium in which to culture blastocysts (Hsu, this volume; Spindle and Pedersen, 1973; McLaren and Hensleigh, 1975). This fact should be borne in mind when using the blastocyst outgrowth system for isolating trophectoderm (see below).

TABLE I
Comparison of Rates of Development in Mice and Rats[a]

Developmental stage	Age (days p.c.)	
	Mouse	Rat
2-Cell	$1\frac{1}{2}$	$1\frac{1}{2}$
8-Cell	$2\frac{1}{2}$	$3\frac{1}{2}$
Morula	3	4
Blastocyst	$3\frac{1}{2}$	5
Primary endoderm	4	5–6
Implantation	$4–4\frac{1}{2}$	5–6
Extraembryonic ectoderm	$5–6\frac{1}{2}$	$6\frac{1}{2}–9$
Proamniotic cavity	$5\frac{1}{2}–6$	7–8
Primitive streak	$6\frac{1}{2}–7$	$8\frac{1}{2}–9$
Allantois	$7\frac{1}{2}–8$	$9\frac{1}{2}–10$
Head fold	$7\frac{1}{2}–8$	$9\frac{1}{2}–10$
First somite	$8–8\frac{1}{2}$	10

[a]These are average figures, and some variation can be expected according to the strain of animal used.

III. TISSUE SEPARATION

A. Preimplantation Stages

1. Separation of Inner Cell Mass from Trophectoderm

a. Surgical Methods. These are applied to the blastocyst stage embryos. The microsurgical technique was developed by R. L. Gardner, and is described in detail elsewhere in this volume (Chapter 6). It has three advantages over other methods: (1) it is possible to compare trophectoderm and ICM from a single blastocyst; (2) reciprocal reconstructions can be made in circumstances where embryos may be in short supply; and (3) different regions of the trophectoderm can be isolated and compared.

The disadvantages are that it is technically difficult, needs expensive and specialized equipment, and can only be used on comparatively small numbers of embryos at any one time.

b. Nonsurgical Methods. These procedures entail the selective destruction of one cell type but allow the continued development of the other. The advantages are that large numbers of embryos can be processed simultaneously, and the techniques are very simple. They do have the disadvantages that from any one blastocyst only one tissue is available for analysis, and the extent to which that tissue has been changed by the procedures applied are largely unknown.

i. To obtain trophectoderm. It has been found that the mouse ICM is much more susceptible than the trophectoderm to lethal damage by a variety of different agents, and that the ICM can be eliminated using tritium-labeled thymidine (Snow, 1973a,b; Horner and McLaren, 1974), X-irradiation (Goldstein *et al.*, 1975), actinomycin D, cyclohexamide, cordycepin (Rowinski *et al.*, 1975), cytosine arabinoside, Colcemid (Sherman and Atienza, 1975), and bromodeoxyuridine (Sherman and Atienza, 1975; Pederson and Spindle, 1976).

The protocol used for each factor varies, and the stage to which each particular technique is applied ranges from cleavage stages through to cultured blastocyst outgrowths. Fortunately, there appears to be little variation in the reaction shown by different strains of mice, and the following general procedures can be applied. Special culture media are not generally required; where blastocyst outgrowths are needed, one of the techniques described by Hsu (this volume Chapter 10) can be followed, but culture media discouraging ICM development may be preferable.

(a) ³H-thymidine. Mouse embryos should be cultured from the 2- or 8-cell stage in the presence of ^{3}H-thymidine for at least two cleavage divisions. They may be removed from ^{3}H-TdR at the morula stage and allowed to expand in

fresh, unlabeled, medium if required. This maneuver circumvents the possibility that ^{3}H-TdR would accumulate in the blastocyst cavity, which could perhaps affect further development or become a nuisance in subsequent studies of the embryos.

Several factors interact in the production of large ICM-free blastocysts. Thymidine is toxic at concentrations above $10^{-6} M$, but it is the tritium concentration that is critical, so high specific activity ^{3}H-TdR should be used. It should be labeled in the methyl group, and not in carbon 6 of the ring. Thymidine-6-^{3}H is more toxic, and there is a smaller difference in the susceptibility to damage between ICM and trophectoderm (Snow, 1973a).

To obtain ICM-free blastocysts, a concentration of 0.05 μCi/ml methyl ^{3}H-thymidine is used. Concentrations above 0.1 μCi/ml are lethal to trophectoderm also. Between 0.01 and 0.05 μCi/ml, there is only a reduction in the number of ICM cells in the blastocyst, and at concentrations of 0.001 μCi/ml no significant reduction in blastocyst cell numbers occurs. Nevertheless, a 0.005 μCi/ml concentration of tritium is sufficient to impair future development of the ICM *in utero* (Horner and McLaren, 1974).

Trophectoderm vesicles derived in this manner have yet to be shown capable of supporting the development of a donor ICM during pregnancy, but, in other ways, the cells of the vesicles are indistinguishable from trophectoderm isolated surgically or in the intact blastocyst. The cells are invasive, undergo giant cell transformation and polyploidy, do not proliferate unless an ICM is present (Snow, 1973b; Ansell and Snow, 1975), and will enter into an embryonic diapause in the uterus of females in delay of implantation (Snow *et al.*, 1976).

(b) X-irradiation.　Goldstein *et al.* (1975) have shown that irradiation of the mouse morula or blastocyst can effectively prevent development of the ICM in blastocyst outgrowths. At the morula stage, Goldstein *et al.* found that 109 ± 17 rads of X-rays eliminates ICM development in 50% of embryos, whereas 269 ± 21 rads were required to reduce trophectoderm development to a similar extent. At the blastocyst stage, the differences are much greater with an ED_{50} for trophectoderm outgrowth of 1600 rads, but an ED_{50} for ICM development of 180 rads. At the blastocyst stage, fewer than 10% of the ICMs survive 1000 rads, but about 90% of trophectoderm will continue development.

It should be noted that this procedure does not eliminate the ICM from the blastocyst, but only prevents its further growth *in vitro*. ICM cells degenerate in the blastocyst outgrowth, leaving the trophectoderm to continue development as giant cells. It appears that, although lethally irradiated, the ICM is capable of stimulating trophectoderm proliferation before it degenerates, so care should be taken to harvest trophectoderm only from cultures in which all trace of ICM has been lost.

(c) Metabolic inhibitors.　As with X-irradiation, these agents do not eliminate the ICM from the blastocyst but effectively prevent its development in blastocyst outgrowths.

Unfortunately, there is no simple recipe for success with antimetabolites, as there can be interactions between inhibitor and medium that lead to large variations in the concentrations of inhibitor required to prevent ICM growth. With some media, however, clear differences in the lethal dose for ICM and trophectoderm facilitate selection of trophectoderm. The reader is referred to the original papers for greater detail of the culture requirements, using the following antimetabolites: BUdR (Sherman and Atienza, 1975; Garner, 1974; Pedersen and Spindle, 1976), cytosine arabinoside and Colcemid (Sherman and Atienza, 1975), cordycepin, cyclohexamide, and actinomycin D (Rowinski *et al.*, 1975).

ii. To obtain ICM. This operation is carried out on fully expanded blastocysts, and relies upon the fact that the trophectoderm cells form junctions between them, making an effective impermeable seal around the ICM and blastocyst cavity. As a result, it is possible to lyse the trophectoderm cells by a classical immunologic procedure and to harvest the ICM cells undamaged (Solter and Knowles, 1975).

The zona pellucida is generally removed, either mechanically or by the pronase digestion technique of Mintz (1971). This step is not essential, but does remove a barrier of variable efficiency from the blastocyst and, thus, facilitates a more controllable and uniform operation.

Blastocysts are cultured in any standard medium containing complement-free (heat-inactivated) antimouse antiserum, at appropriate concentrations, for 30 minutes or more. Incubations of up to 24 hours have been tested. After washing thoroughly in fresh, serum-free medium, the embryos are incubated in medium with complement for 30 minutes. Trophectoderm cells should lyse, leaving intact ICM's in the cellular debris. There is generally a little membrane and cytoplasm contamination adhering to the ICM, but it is removed by thorough washing. The ICM's are used for further experimentation without additional treatment.

The procedure is simple and applicable on a large scale, but there are certain minimum requirements for success.

Trophectoderm cells have tough membranes and are resistant to rupture, so the antibody titer in the antiserum must be high. In their report, Solter and Knowles (1975) used their own antiserum raised in rabbits injected with mouse spleen cells, and they were able to achieve lysis at a 1 : 3072 dilution of the antiserum. Commercial antisera seldom have that potency, but samples from four different suppliers tested in our laboratory were all effective, although some could not be diluted. Where possible, it is probably advisable to use fresh antiserum, although a 3-year-old stock has been found to be effective.

The source of complement is also important. Rabbit serum, although rich in complement, is usually toxic to mouse embryos (a very few rabbits have non-toxic sera) and should be avoided. Fresh guinea pig serum is very effective and does not damage the embryo. Commercially available complement (except rabbit) is generally satisfactory.

2. Separation of Epiblast from Primary Endoderm

If ICM's are isolated from 4-day-old blastocysts, they may be disaggregated and two populations of cells identified by phase microscopy. The smaller cells, which are smooth surfaced are epiblast and the larger, cells with a rough surface, are primary endoderm (Gardner and Papaioannou, 1975). With the aid of a micromanipulator, cells of the desired type can be collected. There are roughly equal numbers of endoderm and epiblast cells.

B. Postimplantation Stages

The separation of tissues from these embryos involves two processes, one enzymatic, the other surgical. The modern techniques were developed by Levak-Švajger and Škreb (1969) and are described in detail by Švajger and Levak-Švajger (1975). Their work has been with rat embryos, but only minor modifications are needed to adapt to mouse embryos.

1. Pre-Primitive Streak Embryos

Grobstein (1952) demonstrated that mouse proximal endoderm could be separated from epiblast mechanically, but, today, enzymatic digestion of the matrix of the basement membrane between the tissues with trypsin and pancreatin is used prior to and as an aid to surgery. There are two important aspects to the enzymatic digestion that combine to facilitate tissue separation rather than cellular disaggregation.

First, trypsin alone is not sufficient. On its own, trypsin digestion leaves the embryos very sticky and resistant to manipulation. The addition of pancreatin or chymotrypsin to the mixture abolishes this problem. Pancreatin is the more efficient.

Second, the digestions need to be carried out at a low temperature to prevent complete disaggregation of the tissues.

The procedure is as follows: the egg cylinder and ectoplacental cone is dissected from the deciduum and incubated intact in calcium and magnesium-free saline (def-saline) containing 0.5% trypsin and 2.5% pancreatin, at 4°C for 20–30 minutes (for the mouse 10–20 minutes is usually adequate).

Digestion is stopped by either (a) the addition of a few drops of serum to the saline/enzyme solution, or (b) transferring the embryos to fresh def-saline containing 1–2% serum. Any nontoxic serum is suitable.

If procedure (a) is used, then after 5–6 minutes the embryos are washed in fresh pure def-saline and transferred into def-saline/serum mixture for further manipulation. If (b) is used, then further manipulation can commence immediately, provided the volume of enzyme mixture transferred with the embryos was minimal. Ideally, however, it is probably advisable to transfer the embryos after 1–2 minutes into another dish of def-saline/serum mixture for microdissection.

Personal experience indicates that, at least for the mouse, any of the standard buffered salines isotonic with mammalian tissues will suffice, and that the commercial source of enzyme is probably unimportant; trypsin from Worthington, British Drug Houses (BDH), Sigma, and Calbiochem, and pancreatin from Difco and BDH have been used.

The surgery of the embryo is carried out either with glass or tungsten needles and, in the mouse, with the aid of flame-polished micropipettes. Tungsten needles must be sharp and smooth surfaced. They are best sharpened and polished electrolytically in sodium hydroxide, but satisfactory needles can be made in hot molten sodium nitrite. To facilitate observation and also to protect the points of the needles, the surgery can be carried out in plastic petri dishes that contain a thin layer of a dark-colored wax. This is easily achieved by making a suspension of either carmine particles (red) or carbon particles (black) in melted histological wax and pouring a small quantity into each dish. After use, the surface can be smoothed by waving a gas flame over the dish to melt the surface of the wax. These dishes may be used many times.

To remove the primary endoderm, hold the egg cylinder down with one needle pressing on the extraembryonic region, and, with the other needle, make a small nick through the endoderm in the region of the junction between epiblast and

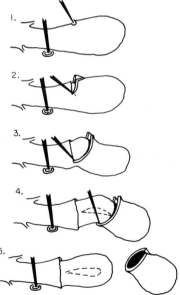

Fig. 2. Stages in the surgical separation of primary endoderm from epiblast in pre-primitive streak stage embryos. See text for explanation.

extraembryonic ectoderm [Fig. 2 (1)]. The initial puncture is then enlarged to cut the endoderm around this junction [Fig. 2 (2 and 3)]. The outer cell layer, the primary endoderm, can then be peeled off the egg cylinder, leaving a denuded epiblast still attached to the extraembryonic region [Fig. 2 (4 and 5)].

This latter tissue is then cut from the egg cylinder, using the needles with a scissorlike action; they represent the perfect dissection. More usually, the endoderm is torn, but it should nevertheless detach as a single sheet of cells. It is not contaminated with epiblast unless that tissue was damaged with a needle.

With mouse embryos, it is probably simpler (because of the small size) to separate the epiblast and primary endoderm with a flame polished glass pipette. The embryonic tissues are cut off the egg cylinder and then pipetted gently in and out of the pipette, whose internal diameter should be marginally less than the cut surface of the embryo. If the tissues are picked up "cut end" first, the two cell layers usually spontaneously separate after a few passages in and out of the pipette.

The pre-primitive streak mouse embryo (about 6 ½ days p.c.) contains, on the average, 100–120 primary endoderm cells and 600–700 epiblast cells. The proportion of those cells in mitosis is approximately 3 and 7%, respectively. These data are not available for the rat, but cell numbers are probably at least double.

2. Post-Primitive Streak Embryos

In this group, I include any embryo with mesoderm. It includes the early primitive streak and headfold stages of Švajger and Levak-Švajger (1975). The presence of mesoderm introduces a complication into the surgery, since, during its early development, it is firmly attached or associated with the epiblast/ embryonic ectoderm at the primitive streak. In order to facilitate the separation of the tissues, part of the surgery is carried out prior to the enzyme treatment (which is the same as for pre-primitive streak stages).

a. Procedure. Using two needles, with a scissorlike action cut the embryonic portion off the egg cylinder. While supporting the embryonic region with one needle, such that the primitive streak is against the petri dish or wax surface, make a single cut along the primitive streak with the second needle. The tissues will thereafter flatten out from their previous cup shape. These flattened embryos are then incubated in the enzyme mixture in the same way as pre-primitive streak embryos, and the reaction halted in the same manner.

Following enzyme digestion, the endoderm often spontaneously detaches from the *lateral* mesoderm and ectoderm. Gentle agitation with a flame-polished glass pipette is usually sufficient to disengage even the most resistant embryonic tissues. If pipetting fails, gentle teasing with needles is required. Manipulation with needles is almost invariably required to separate the mesoderm from ectoderm at its primitive streak attachment. During these manipulations, the endoderm has a marked tendency to shrink and curl up, often around pieces of mesoderm. Needles will be required to unroll it to remove the mesoderm.

In mouse embryos, about 24 hours after the appearance of the primitive streak, i.e., about 7½ days p.c., the embryonic ectoderm contains an average of 8500 cells, the mesoderm 6500 cells, and the primary endoderm covering the embryonic part of the egg cylinder about 650 cells (Snow, 1976).

IV. OTHER POSSIBLE PROCEDURES

A. Restricted Development

When blastomeres of early cleavage stages are separated and cultured individually, they frequently give rise to "false blastocysts" which appear to be composed only of trophectoderm (Tarkowski, 1971).

B. Electrophoresis of Cell Populations

Ave *et al.* (1968) have shown that cells of the presumptive epidermis in amphibian embryos can be separated electrophoretically into three populations whose electrophoretic characteristics correlate well with the properties of ectoderm, mesoderm, and endoderm of later stage embryos. As far as this author is aware, this cell property has not been examined in other embryonic systems.

C. Separation of Cells According to Size

In the early postimplantation mouse embryos (5½ days p.c.), there is about a twofold difference in the volume of epiblast and primary endoderm cells. Such a difference should facilitate their separation by mechanical means, or perhaps by sedimentation characteristics. The size difference does not persist and eventually reverses (Snow, 1976), but this tissue characteristic has not been exploited.

D. Immunosurgery of Egg Cylinder Stages

Theoretically, the techniques described by Solter and Knowles (1975) can be applied to the intact egg cylinder where the primary endoderm acts as an efficient barrier between the embryonic ectoderm and mesoderm, and the external medium. As such, the endoderm should be selectively lysed by the antisera and complement treatments described in Section III,A,b,ii, above. We have investigated this possibility in our laboratories, but so far without success. The reason for failure is obscure, but it seems most probable that our antisera were of insufficient potency to do the job. Possible alternatives are that the primary endoderm is immunologically distinct from the cells (blood, spleen) against which the antisera was raised or that it is deficient in complement-binding sites.

REFERENCES

Ansell, J. D., and Snow, M. H. L. (1975). *J. Embryol. Exp. Morphol.* **33**, 177–185.
Ave, K., Kawakami, I., and Sameshima, M. (1968). *Dev. Biol.* **17**, 617–626.
Biggers, J. D., Whitten, W. K., and Whittingham, D. G. (1971). *In* "Methods in Mammalian Embryology" (J. C. Daniel, Jr., ed.), pp. 86–116. Freeman, San Francisco, California.
Ciba Foundation Symposium. (1976). "Embryogenesis in Mammals," No. 40, Elsevier, Amsterdam.
Fraser, A. (1883). *Proc. R. Soc. London* **34**, 430–437.
Gardner, R. L., and Johnson, M. H. (1972). *J. Embryol. Exp. Morphol.* **28**, 279–312.
Gardner, R. L., and Johnson, M. H. (1975). *Cell Patterning, Ciba Found. Symp. 1975* No. 29, pp. 183–200.
Gardner, R. L., and Papaioannou, V. E. (1975). *In* "The Early Development of Mammals" (M. Balls and A. E. Wild, eds.), pp. 107–132. Cambridge Univ. Press, London and New York.
Garner, W. (1974). *J. Embryol. Exp. Morphol.* **32**, 849–855.
Goldstein, L. S., Spindle, A. I., and Pedersen, R. A. (1975). *Radiat. Res.* **62**, 276–287.
Grobstein, C. (1952). *J. Exp. Zool.* **119**, 355–380.
Horner, D., and McLaren, A. (1974). *Biol. Reprod.* **11**, 553–557.
Kirby, D. R. S. (1971). *In* "Methods in Mammalian Embryology" (J. C. Daniel, Jr., ed.), pp. 146–156. Freeman, San Francisco, California.
Levak-Švajger, B., and Škreb, N. (1969). *Experientia* **25**, 1311–1312.
McLaren, A., and Hensleigh, H. (1975). *In* "The Early Development of Mammals" (M. Balls and A. E. Wild, eds.), pp. 45–60. Cambridge Univ. Press, London and New York.
Mintz, B. (1971). *In* "Methods in Mammalian Embryology" (J. C. Daniel, Jr., ed.), pp. 186–214. Freeman, San Francisco, California.
New, D. A. T. (1971). *In* "Methods in Mammalian Embryology" (J. C. Daniel, Jr., ed.), pp. 305–319. Freeman, San Francisco, California.
O'Connor, M., ed. (1976). *Embryogenesis Mammals, Ciba Found. Symp., 1976* No. 40, Elsevier, Amsterdam.
Pedersen, R. A., and Spindle, A. I. (1976). *Embryogenesis Mammals, Ciba Found Symp., 1976* No. 40, pp. 133–154.
Rowinski, J., Solter, D., and Koprowski, H. (1975). *J. Exp. Zool.* **192**, 133–142.
Sherman, M. I., and Atienza, S. B. (1975). *J. Embryol. Exp. Morphol.* **34,** 467–484.
Škreb, N., Švajger, A., and Levak-Švajger, B. (1976). *Embryogenesis Mammals, Ciba Found. Symp., 1976* No. 40, pp. 27–46.
Snow, M. H. L. (1973a). *J. Embryol. Exp. Morphol.* **29**, 601–615.
Snow, M. H. L. (1973b). *In* "The Cell Cycle in Development and Differentiation" (M. Balls and F. S. Billett, eds.), pp. 311–324. Cambridge Univ. Press, London and New York.
Snow, M. H. L. (1976). *Embryogenesis Mammals, Ciba Found. Symp., 1976* No. 40, pp. 53–70.
Snow, M. H. L., Aitken, J., and Ansell, J. D. (1976). *J. Reprod. Fertil.* **48**, 403–404.
Solter, D., and Knowles, B. B. (1975). *Proc. Natl. Acad. Sci. U.S.A.* **72**, 5099–5102.
Spindle, A. I., and Pedersen, R. A. (1973). *J. Exp. Zool.* **186**, 305–318.
Švajger, A., and Levak-Švajger, B. (1975). *Wilhelm Roux Arch. Entwicklungsmech. Org.* **178**, 303–308.
Tarkowski, A. K. (1971). *In* "Methods in Mammalian Embryology" (J. C. Daniel, Jr., ed.), pp. 172–185. Freeman, San Francisco, California.
Whittingham, D. G. (1971). *J. Reprod. Fertil., Suppl.* **14**, 7–21.

8

Methods for the Preservation of Mammalian Embryos by Freezing

S. P. LEIBO AND PETER MAZUR

I. INTRODUCTION

In 1972, a novel technique was added to the repertoire of procedures available to the embryologist, a technique that permits the storage of viable mammalian preimplantation-stage embryos in the frozen state for at least decades and possibly centuries (Whittingham *et al.*, 1972; Wilmut, 1972). In the ensuing 5 years, more than a dozen different laboratories have successfully used the procedure to freeze embryos of mice, rats, rabbits, sheep, goats, and cattle (Leibo *et al.*,

1974; Maurer *et al.*, 1977; Parkening *et al.*, 1976; Whittingham, 1975, 1977a; Bank and Maurer, 1974; Whittingham and Adams, 1976; Schneider *et al.*, 1974; Maurer and Haseman, 1976; Tsunoda *et al.*, 1976; Wilmut and Rowson, 1973; Moore and Bilton, 1977; Willadsen *et al.*, 1976a,b), and the freezing of embryos has been the subject of one international training course and two international conferences (Mühlbock, 1976; Elliott and Whelan, 1977).

"Successful" freezing not only means that high percentages of frozen-thawed embryos are able to develop *in culture* (where culture techniques are available) but that they are able to develop into normal offspring when the thawed embryos are transferred into the oviducts or uteri of suitably primed foster mothers.

This ability to derive fully functioning normal animals from frozen preimplantation-stage embryos has important potentials in several diverse areas. It means that valuable strains of experimental animals can be protected against possible loss through disease, accident, or genetic drift. Expensive animal facilities that are partially devoted simply to the breeding of infrequently used laboratory strains of animals can be freed for ongoing research. Potentially important mutants, whose value cannot be exploited at the time of isolation, can now be stored at relatively little cost, with the expectation that some at least will eventually become valuable. It is now possible to transport animals, as frozen embryos, around the world (Whittingham and Whitten, 1974). When applied to domestic animals, freezing and transfer of embryos may play a large role in commercial animal husbandry. At a different level, the ability to freeze embryos opens new opportunities for fundamental research. For example, it will permit the testing of hypotheses regarding genetic drift (Bailey, 1977), of hypotheses concerning potential maternal effects on developing fetuses (Uphoff, 1976; Whittingham *et al.*, 1973), and it will permit the stockpiling of viable embryonic material for biochemical analysis, as well as serving as a valuable tool in basic studies of low-temperature biology.

Although the freezing of mammalian embryos can now be performed rather easily and routinely with little need for sophisticated instrumentation, the procedure was derived from an emerging mechanistic understanding of basic cryobiology. The freezing of embryos has even contributed to that understanding by permitting experimental verification of portions of a previously derived theoretical analysis of cell freezing. Some years ago, a quantitative physicochemical model was derived to describe the kinetic response of cells when exposed to subzero temperatures (Mazur, 1963). Briefly, the model is a physicochemical description of the following events.

When a cell suspended in an aqueous medium is cooled to temperatures slightly below 0°C, ice forms first in the extracellular solution. As a consequence, the dissolved solutes become more concentrated as water is removed in the form of ice. As the temperature of the cell suspension is lowered, more ice forms, resulting in a progressively more concentrated extracellular solution. The higher the concentration, the lower the chemical potential of water, and it is known that all cells respond osmotically to equalize the chemical potentials of water across their membranes. Hence, during freezing, they will lose water.

Given a cell's initial water volume, its surface area, its permeability to water, and the temperature coefficient of that permeability, the model permits calculations of cell water volume as a function of subzero temperature when the cell is cooled at specified rates. If a cell is cooled sufficiently slowly, it will progressively lose water as the temperature is lowered so as to remain in osmotic equilibrium with the extracellular solution. But if a cell is cooled at high enough rates, there will be insufficient time for the cell to remain in osmotic equilibrium, and as the temperature is lowered, the cell contents will become increasingly supercooled, until suddenly the cell water freezes within the cell itself. This intracellular ice formation has been shown to be a primary factor responsible for cell death during freezing (Bank and Mazur, 1973; Mazur *et al.*, 1972; Leibo *et al.*, 1977).

The model permits one to estimate quantitatively the extent of supercooling, and, thereby, it permits calculations of the likelihood of intracellular freezing as a function of the rate at which the cell is cooled to low subzero temperatures. The predictions have now been experimentally verified for several cell types, including mouse ova (for review, see Mazur, 1976; Leibo, 1977b). Finally, the model played a significant role in predicting those conditions (especially cooling rate) which would provide the optimum conditions for the freezing of mouse embryos. The procedures, which were developed in the original report (Whittingham *et al.*, 1972) and which are for the most part currently in use, can be summarized as follows.

Fertilized ova or embryos are recovered from the reproductive tracts of female animals that have ovulated naturally or in response to superovulatory hormones. The preimplantation-stage embryos are suspended in $\geq 1\,M$ solutions of a protective compound, namely, glycerol or dimethyl sulfoxide (DMSO) (usually the latter). The suspensions are cooled to temperatures a few degrees below 0°C, and "seeded" with an ice crystal to induce extracellular ice formation—a requisite for successful embryo freezing. The partially frozen suspension is then cooled slowly under controlled conditions to about −100°C, and transferred into liquid nitrogen at −196°C. [Frozen embryos can even be successfully cooled in liquid helium to 4°K (Whittingham *et al.*, 1972).]

To date, the percentage survival has been shown to undergo no diminution when frozen embryos are stored at −196°C. Moreover, theoretical and experimental considerations make it almost certain that the "half-life" of frozen embryos will be certainly decades, if not centuries or millenia (DuFrain, 1976; Mazur, 1976; Ashwood-Smith and Grant, 1977; Lyon *et al.*, 1977). When needed, the frozen embryos are warmed relatively slowly until they thaw, and are then carefully diluted out of the hyperosmotic protective solution. Finally, the thawed embryos are cultured *in vitro* to assess their survival, and are then transferred into foster mothers to develop into living young. Except for the equipment required for the purely embryologic techniques, such as a dissecting microscope and a tissue-culture incubator, the apparatus actually required for embryo freezing can be simple and inexpensive. It is not necessary to use the sophisticated and expensive machines that are marketed for freezing biologic material.

The purpose of this paper is to describe the procedures developed in our laboratory using this simplified apparatus. We recognize that the specific steps and equipment we describe below have been and will continue to be modified by different investigators. Modifications will cause no problems provided that they do not violate the fundamental principles of cell freezing outlined above. Furthermore, these same approaches and equipment can be used with minimal modification for the successful freezing of cell types other than mammalian ova and embryos.

II. EMBRYOLOGIC METHODS

The experimental details of methods for the collection of ova and embryos, for their handling and culture, for media preparation, and for the *in vitro* and *in vivo* assays of viability have all been described in detail (Brinster, 1970, 1972; Whittingham, 1971). An excellent general source of relevant literature is "Methods in Mammalian Embryology" edited by J. C. Daniel, Jr. (1971).

There are, however, a few aspects of the collection and preparation of embryos for freezing that deserve specific mention. The first, while rather trivial, makes the collection of embryos substantially easier than the methods described in most standard texts on the subject. Rather than using 30-gauge needles for flushing mouse oviducts, we have found that substituting blunt-tipped, ½-inch long, 33- or 34-gauge needles (available from Hamilton Co., Reno, Nevada) is much more efficient, especially for the novice embryologist.

The second point is more substantive. When mouse embryos are to be frozen, either for experimental purposes or for preservation, it may be necessary or desirable to freeze as many as 400–500 embryos simultaneously. Since even an experienced worker can collect only about 200 embryos per hour from superovulated mice, the entire collection period may require 2–3 hours. We have found that embryos held in phosphate-buffered saline (PBS) at room temperature for 2 hours or more exhibit a significant delay in further development when placed into culture, and the percentage of embryos, especially of the 2-cell stage, that develop *in vitro* to expanded blastocysts is reduced to an extent that depends roughly on the length of time at room temperature. Both the delay and the lowered percentage development may reflect the fact that embryos held in a nonnutrient solution at 20°C continue to utilize metabolic pools. To avoid these effects when the collection period exceeds ½ hour, we hold the collected embryos in prechilled PBS at about 0°C until the collection is completed. We also find it desirable to avoid the use of bicarbonate-buffered solutions when embryos are to be held for extended times. The reason is simply that the rapid loss of CO_2 from the solutions causes their pH to rise in a matter of minutes to 9 or higher, the exact rate depending on the temperature and volume of the solution.

One item regarding the culture of embryos also warrants mention. Because of the bothersome variability of batches of commercially available mineral or paraffin oils with respect to their use for culturing embryos, we prefer to use a more uniform synthetic oil instead. Furthermore, the physical properties of these oils, such as their permeability to gases and solutes, are known. One oil that serves well for embryo culture is a dimethyl polysiloxane (Dow Corning 200 fluid, 50 centistoke viscosity, available from Dow Corning Corp., Midland, Michigan).

Except for these points, standard embryologic procedures work well for the collection and manipulation of these cells prior to freezing, and for assaying their survival afterwards. Our standard *in vitro* assay of survival of mouse embryos is the percentage of frozen-thawed embryos that develops to expanded blastocysts* relative to the percentage of unfrozen controls undergoing comparable development.

In our hands, there is high correlation between the percentage of frozen-thawed embryos that develop *in vitro* and the percentage that develop *in vivo* in foster mothers (Whittingham *et al.*, 1972).

We have, in addition, recently added a third technique to assay survival, a technique that is invaluable in dealing with forms such as unfertilized ova. It is a fluorescent dye technique first described by Rotman and Papermaster (1966) and first applied to freezing studies by McGrath *et al.* (1975). The principle is the following. Many cell types, including ova and embryos, are impermeable to the fluorescent dye, fluorescein, but are permeable to the nonfluorescent substituted derivative, fluorescein diacetate (FDA). Embryos incubated in a $10^{-6} M$ solution of FDA at room temperature quickly take up the dye. The intracellular esterases of viable cells then cleave the acetate groups, leaving intracellular fluorescein. Hence, a cell that exhibits fluorescence must have a membrane sufficiently intact to prevent the loss of both intracellular fluorescein and the presumably soluble esterases. Recently, Jackowski (1977) has found that the ability of fertilized ova to fluoresce after freezing and thawing shows a high correlation (0.96) with their ability to develop in culture. In use, a stock $1.2 \times 10^{-2} M$ solution of FDA (MW 416) in acetone is prepared and stored in the dark at about -15°C. To assay

---

*The assay for survival of fertilized ova is the percentage that develops to the 2-cell stage. With present procedures, the ova of only a few mouse strains will reproducibly develop *in vitro* to the blastocyst stage.

survival, embryos are placed for about 5 minutes at room temperature in a 10^4 dilution of this stock in PBS. The embryos are then examined for fluorescence, using any microscope fitted with filters appropriate for fluorescein. We use a combination of a Wild No. 313810 interference filter and a No. BG23 blue filter over the light source for excitation and a No. FITC yellow filter between the objective and ocular to observe fluorescence.

III. SAMPLE PREPARATION

A. Suspending Media for Freezing

A variety of compounds, such as glycerol, dimethyl sulfoxide (DMSO), sucrose, polyvinylpyrrolidone (PVP), hydroxyethyl starch, and several proteins, have all been reported to protect various cell types against freezing damage (see Pegg, 1970, for review). Although the mechanisms by which these protective compounds act remain to be determined, they are required in nearly all circumstances if mammalian cells are to survive freezing. Despite the lack of a mechanistic understanding, much is known empirically regarding the influence of glycerol and DMSO on the survival of frozen-thawed cells. Thus far, only these two compounds have been confirmed to protect mammalian embryos against freezing damage; DMSO has been the solute used most often.

The use of protective compounds in freezing studies is a complex subject. At the least, the following variables can affect survival: (1) the concentration of the protective additive; (2) the rate of addition of the compound to embryos; (3) the length and temperature of exposure of embryos to the compound prior to freezing; and (4) the rate and temperature of dilution of the compound after thawing. The influence of each of these variables on cell survival depends to a certain extent on the embryonic stage and also on the species of embryo being treated. We will discuss the role of items (1), (2), and (3) here, deferring item (4) to the discussion below of embryo recovery after freezing (Section V).

1. Concentration of DMSO

All investigators agree that high survivals of embryos after freezing require that the concentrations of DMSO be at least $1 M$. The concentrations reported for maximum survival have ranged from $1.0 M$ (Whittingham et al., 1972; Leibo et al., 1974) to $\sim 1.5 M$ (Wilmut, 1972; Bank and Maurer, 1974; Whittingham and Adams, 1976), to $2.0 M$ (Maurer and Haseman, 1976). Schneider et al. (1974) used 1.0 and 1.6 M solutions of DMSO for freezing of mouse and rabbit embryos, respectively. Cattle, sheep, and rat embryos have been successfully frozen in 1.5 M solutions of DMSO (Moore and Bilton, 1977; Willadsen et al., 1976a,b; Whittingham, 1975). Concentrations some 20–50% above optimum can be quite detrimental. One suggestion has been that the detrimental effect results from the toxic effect of high DMSO concentrations produced during freezing. This conclusion is probably incorrect, however, since the concentration of solutes at subzero temperatures is fixed by temperature alone. This means that cells frozen in different initial concentrations of DMSO are all exposed to approximately the same high concentration of DMSO at a given temperature in partially frozen solutions (Cocks and Brower, 1974).

2. Rate of Addition of DMSO

Some papers on embryo freezing have reported improved results when DMSO is added to embryos in a stepwise fashion (Moore and Bilton, 1977; Parkening *et al.*, 1976; Willadsen *et al.*, 1976b); Wilmut (1972) had emphasized that "direct addition" irreversibly damaged 8-cell and early blastocyst stage mouse embryos. This is not a unanimous view, however, since other workers have obtained equally high survivals of frozen-thawed embryos when DMSO is added in a single step (Whittingham *et al.*, 1972; Leibo *et al.*, 1974; Maurer *et al.*, 1977; Whittingham, 1975).

3. Duration and Temperature of Exposure to DMSO Prior to Freezing

Presumably, the chief effect of the time and temperature of exposure of embryos to the protective compound prior to freezing is on the amount of additive that permeates intracellularly. When a cell is placed into a hyperosmotic solution of a permeating solute, the cell quickly shrinks by water loss to restore osmotic equilibrium across its membrane. Concurrently, the solute begins to permeate the cell, accompanied by water entry. This progressive and coupled entry of solute and water continues until chemical potential equilibrium across the membrane has been restored. The time-dependent permeation of solute into the cell is a function of the initial solute concentration and the temperature of exposure. The greater the concentration and the higher the temperature of exposure, the faster the solute permeates. Mathematical expressions to describe the entry of solutes, at the high concentrations used in cryobiology, have been derived (Mazur *et al.*, 1974) and used to calculate glycerol permeation into ova and embryos (Jackowski, 1977; Jackowski and Leibo, 1976; Mazur *et al.*, 1976). The permeation of glycerol into ova, calculated from these expressions, has been experimentally verified using ^{14}C-glycerol (Jackowski, 1977). The coefficients of permeability for various solutes derived from the mathematical expressions can be used to calculate not only the influx of solutes but their efflux as well.

Using these permeability data, Jackowski (1977) has compared the relation between the survival of frozen-thawed mouse ova and the amount of glycerol present intracellularly prior to freezing. In general, she found that conditions that enhance permeation of glycerol into the cells also increase their survival after freezing. However, other factors including the time after fertilization are involved, since a given concentration of intracellular glycerol did not necessarily produce the same survival in fertilized ova of different ages or in ova of a given age preincubated at different temperatures.

Although glycerol can yield high survivals after freezing, the survival level is rather critically dependent on the time and temperature of incubation prior to freezing and during dilution subsequent to thawing (Leibo, 1976). Some (but not all) of these complexities are explicable in terms of osmotic volume changes associated with the influx and efflux of glycerol.

When DMSO, on the other hand, is used as the protective agent, survivals appear to be not so critically dependent on the exposure time and temperature. This decreased sensitivity is probably a reflection of the higher permeability of embryos to DMSO, which results in a reduced probability of osmotic damage. At any rate, DMSO has been the protective additive used in most studies. Generally, embryos have been preincubated in aqueous solutions of it at 0°C. A few studies have been conducted, however, in which embryos were exposed to DMSO at 20° or 37°C (Whittingham, 1974; Whittingham and Adams, 1976; Willadsen et al., 1976a,b). Most workers have exposed embryos to DMSO for about 15–20 minutes prior to initiating freezing of the samples, although the survival of mouse embryos seems to depend only slightly on the length of exposure (Whittingham et al., 1972; Leibo et al., 1974). The survival of 8-cell rabbit embryos, on the other hand, has been reported to increase from nil to about 55% as the exposure to DMSO at 0°C is lengthened from 1 to 30 minutes (Bank and Maurer, 1974). Yet, in this and a companion study (Maurer and Haseman, 1976), it was found that survival of morula-stage rabbit embryos was only slightly improved by increasing the exposure from 1 to 15 minutes, and that survival decreased slightly with longer exposures.

Clearly, the role of the permeation of additive and of temperature and time of incubation prior to freezing is not yet completely understood. Nevertheless, a general procedure can be suggested. Embryos suspended in a small volume ($\sim$ 0.1 ml) of PBS should be chilled to 0°C. An equal volume of a prechilled solution of $\sim 3\,M$ DMSO prepared in PBS (twice the desired final concentration of $1.5\,M$) is then added to the embryo suspension. The suspension is held at 0°C for about 30 minutes before beginning the actual freezing process.

B. Sample Containers

A variety of containers have been used for embryo freezing. These range from small glass tubes (9 mm o.d. $\times$ 95 mm long), plastic screw-top vials, to glass ampules (1- to 5-ml capacity) that can be sealed to assure sterility for long-term preservation. Recently, Tsunoda and Sugie (1977) have reported the successful freezing of rabbit embryos in the plastic straws frequently used for the preservation of bovine sperm.

Whatever the container used, a small volume (~ 0.1 ml) of PBS is pipetted into an appropriate number of labeled sample tubes. The embryos, numbering from as few as 1 to as many as 50, are pipetted into the PBS in as small a volume as possible, and the sample tubes are chilled to 0°C. When all tubes have been filled, the protective compound is added as described above. It is frequently convenient for handling to secure the sample tubes to a glass or plastic rod using ordinary rubber bands. Alternatively, if glass freezing ampules have been used, once the DMSO has been added and the ampules have been sealed, they can be allowed to float free like miniature buoys in the alcohol baths used for freezing. This approach has the advantage of assuring that the vials have been completely sealed; those with pinhole leaks will become filled with alcohol and sink. (The embryos in such tubes will, of course, be killed. But this step removes the inadequately sealed ampules that might "explode" during thawing. See Section IV.)

C. "Tubal" Freezing

Very recently, a clever alternate method for embryo freezing has been introduced by G. Zeilmaker (Erasmus University, Rotterdam, The Netherlands, personal communication). It has the distinct advantage of avoiding the necessity for embryo collection prior to freezing. Oviducts are removed from day 2 or day 3 pregnant mice, checked briefly for the presence of embryos, and then placed into sample tubes. The rest of the procedure follows the usual pattern, except that the embryos are flushed from the oviducts after they have been frozen and thawed. Zeilmaker reports that the survivals of 2-cell and 8-cell embryos obtained after freezing and thawing approach those obtained with conventional freezing procedures. This procedure will drastically reduce the time required for embryo collection when freezing is being used to preserve mutant stocks. Only those oviducts containing embryos required for initiating new stocks need to be flushed. The balance can be held in the frozen state.

IV. FREEZING AND THAWING PROCEDURES

A. Summary of Steps

If a suspension of mammalian cells is to be successfully frozen, it must be subjected to the following sequence of steps. First, ice must be induced to form in the extracellular milieu by "seeding." Once the cells have equilibrated with the partially frozen external solution, they can be successfully cooled to even lower temperatures. But the rate at which the cells are cooled is critical. It must be sufficiently slow for the cells to remain in approximate osmotic equilibrium until the entire system—cells and solution—has completely solidified.* In practice, complete solidification usually occurs at temperatures of about $-50°$ to $-75°C$. Although some cells in certain solutions will retain viability even at these temperatures, extended storage of mammalian cells for months or years requires that the storage temperatures be below about $-130°C$. Practically, such conditions can be easily achieved by storing the cells in liquified gases, whose boiling points are below $\sim -150°C$, or in the vapor phase above the gases. Liquid nitrogen, because of its availability, relatively low cost, and nonreactivity, is usually the storage fluid of choice. Finally, use of stored cells obviously requires that the frozen suspension be warmed to physiological temperatures. For some cells, the rate of warming is also important. For frozen mammalian embryos, survivals are highest when warming from $-196°$ to $0°C$ is relatively slow.

A detailed discussion of the fundamental basis of all these steps is beyond the primary purpose and scope of this chapter. The fundamentals have been dealt with in several recent reviews (Mazur, 1977a,b,c; Leibo, 1977a,b; see also Mühlbock, 1976; Elliott and Whelan, 1977). But one step of the procedure, seeding to induce ice formation, does deserve special discussion. The reasons are that (1) it is essential if the embryos are to survive freezing; (2) the procedure and rationale may not be familiar even to investigators who routinely preserve other cell types by freezing; and (3) while the technique for seeding a sample is simplicity itself, this step is derived from a firm physicochemical analysis of low-temperature biology.

B. Seeding of Samples

It is increasingly evident that different cell types exhibit characteristic optimum cooling rates for their maximum survival (Mazur et al., 1969). Analytical methods to calculate these optima, rather than to derive them empirically, are also available (Mazur, 1963, 1965, 1966). The discussion to follow will describe practical means to achieve such optimum cooling rates for embryos. In the absence of seeding, however, simply cooling a suspension of embryos from $0°$ to $-100°C$ or below at a previously determined optimum rate will probably yield few if any survivors. The reasons are found in the thermal behavior of a solution that undergoes spontaneous nucleation.

---

*Asahina et al. (1970) and Shimada and Asahina (1972) have found that some types of mammalian cells will survive rapid cooling under conditions in which the cells are not in osmotic equilibrium, and ice apparently forms intracellularly. However, survival requires that the cells be cooled and warmed extremely rapidly.

Figure 1A illustrates the behavior of two samples of a solution with a true freezing point of −2.5°C immersed in a bath cooling at 0.5°C/minute. The samples remain unfrozen below −2.5°C, i.e., they become supercooled. But eventually one of the samples will nucleate spontaneously (a), at which point the released latent heat of fusion causes the sample temperature to "rebound" to close to that of the solution freezing point (b). Ice continues to form at about that temperature (b to c) as the bath temperature continues to fall. Then, the sample temperature decreases relatively rapidly to restore thermal equilibrium (between points c and d). The region e to h in the figure depicts the thermal events that occur if supercooling of a second sample were only to terminate at a considerably lower temperature (e.g., −15°C). The temperature in this second example will also rebound, although to a temperature slightly less than that of the first sample. The ice grows more rapidly in this case (f to g), and this sample exhibits an even

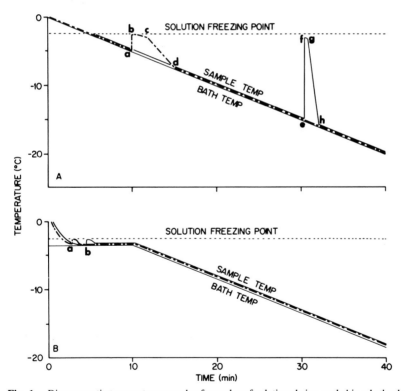

Fig. 1. Diagrammatic temperature records of samples of solutions being cooled in a bath whose temperature decreases at 0.5°C/minute. (A) Samples allowed to supercool before freezing spontaneously at −5°C or −15°C. (B) Samples seeded to induce crystallization at −3.5°C. See text for details.

faster drop in temperature (between points g and h). It is clear, then, that, over a portion of the temperature range, rather than cooling at the optimum rate of 0.5°C/minute, these two samples have cooled at about 1.5°C/minute (first example) and 10°C/minute (second example). Because embryo survival is critically dependent on cooling rate, no embryos in sample 2 would be likely to survive. The reasons for this are relatively straightforward. When cooled below 0°C, the embryos begin to respond osmotically only after ice initially forms (points a or e). In example 1, that osmotic response begins to occur 10 minutes after the bath temperature reaches 0°C. In example 2, the osmotic loss of water only begins 20 minutes later, and, therefore, the time available for the embryos to dehydrate is greatly reduced. As a result, the cells in the second example will contain more intracellular water at any given subzero temperature than the cells in the first example. This, in turn, means that the cells in the second example will have an increased likelihood of intracellular freezing upon reaching their nucleation temperature (Mazur, 1977a; Leibo, 1977a,b).

Various aspects of this deleterious effect of extensive supercooling have been previously discussed (Leibo et al., 1970), and have been experimentally shown to occur in yeast (Mazur and Schmidt, 1968), tissue-culture cells (Bank and Mazur, 1973; Mazur et al., 1972), and embryos (Whittingham, 1977b). The solution to the problem is to make sure that the extracellular medium undergoes little supercooling, as in the first example in Fig. 1A. In practice, this is done as shown in Fig. 1B. The samples of embryos are cooled to a constant temperature only slightly below that of the freezing point of the suspending solution. They generally do not freeze spontaneously and, therefore, are induced to freeze by simply touching the surface with a small ice crystal, i.e., seeding (points a and b). Although the sample temperatures will again rebound, the extent of this rebound will be small. More importantly, since the bath temperature is held constant during this time, the subsequent drop in sample temperature will be much smaller and at a substantially lower rate than when supercooled samples are allowed to freeze spontaneously as the bath temperature falls, as in Fig. 1A. The samples are then held briefly (2–5 minutes) at the seeding temperature, permitting time for the restoration of thermal equilibrium and for the establishment of osmotic equilibrium as well. Then, when the samples are cooled to lower temperatures at the predetermined optimum rate, the embryos can remain in osmotic equilibrium as more ice forms and the solute concentration increases.

A variety of approaches have now been used to seed samples of embryos and other cells. One way is to transfer the sample tubes into a constant temperature bath held about 1–1.5°C below the freezing point of the suspending solution. (The freezing points of 1.0, 1.5, and 2.0 M DMSO solutions prepared in isotonic saline are about $-2.5°$, $-3.5°$, and $-4.5°C$, respectively.) Several different types of equipment can be used as seeding baths, some rather elaborate, others rather simple. One may use ethanol either cooled in a thermoelectric bath (e.g.,

"Minifreezer" Model W 1500, Virtis Co., Gardiner, New York) or cooled in a standard Dewar flask with an immersion cooler ("Cold Finger," Forma Scientific, Marietta, Ohio; Eberbach Thermoelectric Cooler, Arthur H. Thomas Co., Philadelphia, Pennsylvania). If unsealed sample tubes are used, it is inadvisable to cool baths with Dry Ice for the CO_2 vapor will enter the vials and decrease the pH appreciably. If a large number of samples are to be seeded simultaneously, it is possible to use a chilled metal block with holes drilled to accommodate the sample tubes. The holes can be filled with ethanol for good thermal contact and then the block can be cooled to the appropriate subzero temperature in an ordinary freezer. The mass of the block will maintain the temperature sufficiently long for seeding. The samples are then simply cooled to the seeding temperature by placing them into the ethanol-filled holes. Seeding then proceeds as described below.

Seeding the chilled samples is easy. There are several approaches. One is to fill the first few millimeters of the tip of sterile Pasteur pipettes by capillarity with sterile water or media (without DMSO or glycerol), and to freeze the fluid by placing the pipettes into liquid nitrogen or into a freezer. Each sample is then seeded by simply touching its surface with the ice contained in the pipette tip. Another approach is to seed the sample by touching its surface with a sterile wire previously cooled in liquid nitrogen. Or, if the samples have been previously sealed in glass ampules to assure sterility, they may be seeded by touching the outside of the glass with a small piece of Dry Ice or a cold metal rod. The point is simply to induce ice crystal formation under conditions that avoid extreme temperature fluctuations of the sample. Once the samples have been seeded, they can then be cooled to lower temperatures.

C. Cooling of Seeded Samples

If one wishes to preserve cells by freezing, it is necessary to cool them at rates that preclude the formation of intracellular ice. For mammalian embryos, theoretical and experimental analysis demonstrates that appropriate freezing rates are of the order of 0.2°–2°C/minute. Rates above 5°C/minute are lethal because they induce intracellular ice formation. This critical relationship between survival of three stages of mouse embryos and cooling rate is shown in Fig. 2, and a comparison of this response to cooling rate for embryos from three species is shown in Fig. 3.

Fortunately, cooling embryos at an appropriate rate is not difficult. One may use any of a variety of sophisticated, electronically controlled, and expensive machines or one can use simple, reliable, and inexpensive glass assemblies. We will describe only the latter; the former are widely advertised and marketed.

The apparatus is shown diagrammatically in Fig. 4 and photographically in Fig. 5. It consists simply of an inner, double-walled, glass vessel that has been

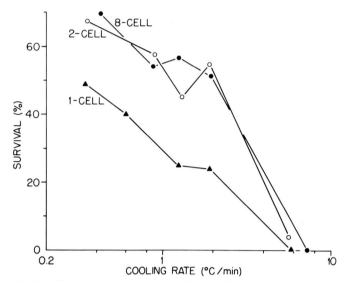

Fig. 2. Survival of mouse ova and embryos as a function of the rate at which they were cooled in solutions of DMSO to −196°C. The data are redrawn from Whittingham *et al.*, 1972, copyright (1972) by the American Association for the Advancement of Science and are used with permission of the publisher.

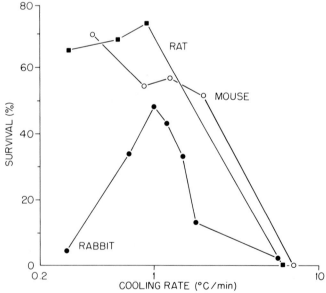

Fig. 3. Survival of 8-cell embryos as a function of cooling rate. The data for mouse, rat, and rabbit embryos are, respectively, those of Whittingham *et al.* (1972), Whittingham (1975), and Bank and Maurer (1974).

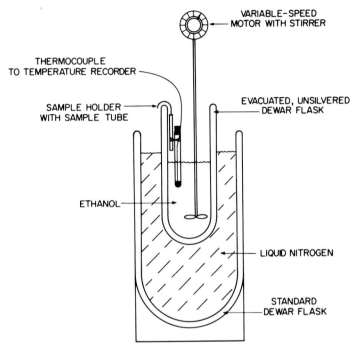

THERMOCOUPLE
TO TEMPERATURE RECORDER

SAMPLE HOLDER
WITH SAMPLE TUBE

VARIABLE-SPEED
MOTOR WITH STIRRER

EVACUATED, UNSILVERED
DEWAR FLASK

ETHANOL

LIQUID NITROGEN

STANDARD
DEWAR FLASK

Fig. 4. Diagram of apparatus used to cool samples at controlled rates. See text for details.

evacuated and contains 95% or 100% ethanol as a coolant. (Any organic solvent with a freezing point of $-90°C$ or below can be substituted. Ethanol or isopropanol are the most convenient and least noxious.) The ethanol is mixed with a variable speed stirrer to prevent the establishment of thermal gradients. After they have been seeded, the samples are placed into the ethanol, which has been prechilled to approximately the seeding bath temperature. Again, the use of Dry Ice should be avoided if the samples are unsealed. For cooling, this entire assembly is simply placed carefully into liquid nitrogen contained in a standard 4-liter wide-mouth Dewar flask. (The liquid nitrogen will "boil" when the warmer inner flask is first transferred into it. Therefore, care and appropriate safety equipment, such as asbestos gloves and goggles or a face shield, should be used at this point.) Once the transfer is complete, the apparatus requires little attention, except to maintain the level of liquid nitrogen in the outer flask as a constant heat sink. The temperature of the samples and/or the bath can be monitored continuously by thermocouples or thermistors attached to appropriate low temperature recorders (e.g., Speedomax Type W, Leeds & Northrop, North Wales, Pennsylvania). Alternatively, the cooling rate achieved with a given inner flask containing a fixed amount of well-stirred ethanol can be measured be-

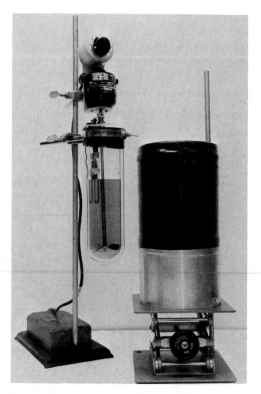

Fig. 5. Photograph of a cooling assembly.

forehand using a low-temperature thermometer. (A wide selection of calibrated thermometers are available from Precision Thermometer and Instrument Co., Southampton, Pennsylvania. Others covering ranges of +50° to −100°C and +30° to −200°C are available from laboratory suppliers such as Curtin Matheson Scientific Co., International Division, Houston, Texas, and VWR Scientific, International Dept., San Francisco, California.) As long as the ambient temperature is approximately constant, and the volume of ethanol is also held constant, a given flask cooled in liquid nitrogen will repeatedly yield the same nearly constant cooling rate.

The approach of using this type of lagged vessel for cooling cell suspensions at various rates was developed empirically in our laboratory over a period of several years. It has been used to study fundamental aspects of low temperature biology of yeast (Mazur and Schmidt, 1968), mammalian cells (Mazur *et al.*, 1969; Leibo *et al.*, 1970), as well as embryos (Whittingham *et al.*, 1972; Leibo *et al.*, 1974). The principle of the approach is to use a constant heat sink of liquid nitrogen at −196°C. The samples are cooled in ethanol so as to provide good thermal conduction. The cooling vessel itself is made from an unsilvered Dewar flask blank. (These are available in a variety of sizes from Ace Glass, Vineland, New Jersey, and from Kontes/Martin and Co., Evanston, Illinois.) These blanks can be sealed without a vacuum, providing less insulation, or sealed after having been evacuated to various pressures, providing greater insulation. We have used such Dewar flasks ranging in size from 50 mm o.d. × 210 mm long, 65 × 265 mm, 85 × 285 mm, up to 150 mm o.d. × 380 mm long. Normally, the flask is filled to about one-half its capacity with ethanol, i.e., about 100 ml of ethanol in the smallest and about 2000 ml in the largest. Obviously, the larger the flask and the more ethanol it contains, the slower will be its cooling rate. However, cooling rate is more affected by whether the flask is unevacuated or evacuated. For example, a flask with a capacity of about 900 ml (85 mm o.d. × 285 mm long) containing about 500 ml ethanol will yield a cooling rate of about 0.5°C/minute if it is evacuated, and about 1.8°C/minute if it is unevacuated. Some control over the cooling rate can also be exercised by varying the depth to which the inner flask is immersed in the liquid nitrogen. In fact, by placing the liquid nitrogen flask onto an adjustable laboratory stand, one can gradually immerse more and more of the inner flask into the nitrogen. In this fashion, it is possible (but by no means necessary) to obtain an almost constant cooling rate over a very broad temperature range. If, however, the inner flask is immersed in liquid nitrogen to a constant depth during the entire process, the resultant cooling will be slightly curvilinear with time. In practical terms, the gradual reduction in cooling rate with falling temperature may actually be desirable, since it provides a longer time for the cells to achieve osmotic equilibrium at lower temperatures.

An essential aspect of any study in low temperature biology is knowing the numerical value of the rates at which the cell suspensions are cooled or warmed. As mentioned above, the temperature changes are most easily monitored using thermistors or thermocouples. When samples are small, the low heat capacity of thermocouples is a distinct advantage; the temperature measured is that of the sample, rather than the measuring device. However, in the case of embryo freezing for which low rates are used, no significant error is introduced by measuring the bath temperature with a thermometer. There will be less than 1°C difference between the sample and the bath.

The numerical value of the rate depends on the temperature range over which it is calculated. Therefore, we recommend the use of the following convention, which has been followed in most published studies on embryo freezing. Express the rate in terms of the time required for a given bath or set of samples to decrease from −10° to −65°C. The cooling profiles obtained with the cooling vessels described above are essentially constant over that temperature range.

The cooling of samples in the fashion just described can be continued to about −117°C, the freezing point of pure ethanol although in practice, it is generally sufficient to cool embryos in DMSO solutions at a controlled rate to about −80°C (Leibo *et al.*, 1974; Whittingham *et al.*, 1972). (However, Whittingham and Adams (1976) and Maurer and Haseman (1976) have reported somewhat better survivals of rabbit embryos when slow cooling was continued down to −110° and −100°C, respectively.) Once the samples have reached about −80° to −100°C, they can be simply transferred directly into liquid nitrogen at −196°C.

All available evidence indicates that survival of frozen embryos is unaffected by the length of storage; to date, information is available for storage times up to 2½ years at −196°C (Whittingham *et al.*, 1972; Leibo *et al.*, 1974; Maurer, 1976; Lyon *et al.*, 1977). No thermally driven chemical reactions can occur at −196°C, and estimates based on calculations of cumulative damage from background radiation of frozen embryos suggest that little damage would occur even after a century or more (Mazur, 1976; DuFrain, 1976; Lyon *et al.*, 1977).

A variety of liquid nitrogen refrigerators for storage of biologic materials are available. One caveat to their use is that appropriate arrangements must be made to maintain the level of liquid nitrogen. Sophisticated commercial devices and alarm systems are available for this purpose. The occasional reports of apparent loss of biologic activity of cells stored at −196°C are likely due to the transient evaporation of all the liquid nitrogen in the refrigerator. Another practical aspect of embryo storage is that, as this procedure becomes more widespread, the problem of the proper nomenclature for stocks of animals derived from frozen-thawed embryos will become significant. It is a problem that is already receiving attention (see discussions in Mühlbock, 1976; Elliott and Whelan, 1977).

D. Warming of Frozen Samples

The next step in embryo freezing is the return of the frozen cells to physiological temperatures. The rate at which many types of frozen cells are warmed is frequently not critical, but this is much less true for frozen embryos. Their survival can depend as much on the rate at which they are warmed as on the rate at which they were initially cooled (Whittingham *et al.*, 1972; Leibo *et al.*, 1974; Maurer and Haseman, 1976). Generally, the more slowly the embryos are cooled, the more slowly they need to be warmed for maximum survival (Fig. 6). The damage from warming too rapidly seems to be related to osmotic phenomena occurring at subzero temperatures.

The appropriate warming rates (between −65° and −10°C) lie between 2° and 30°C/minute, the exact value in this range being of relatively little consequence. Simple methods exist for achieving these rates. The simplest is to suspend the frozen samples in room temperature air.* Tubes containing 0.2 ml of sample will

---

*If sealed vials have been used, care must be taken that liquid nitrogen has not entered through a pinhole leak. If it has, the vial will explode violently during warming. Because of this potential danger, some prefer to store sealed vials in the vapor phase above liquid nitrogen. However, the entry of liquid nitrogen into unsealed vials or tubes causes no problems.

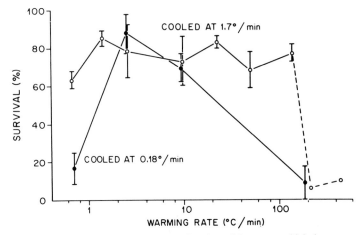

Fig. 6. Survival of 8-cell mouse embryos as a function of the rate at which they were warmed following cooling in 1 *M* DMSO to −196°C at each of the indicated rates. The figure is from Leibo *et al*. (1974) and is used with permission of the publisher.

warm at 20° to 30°C/minute. Lower warming rates can be achieved simply by transferring the frozen samples into small volumes of ethanol previously cooled to about −100°C in liquid nitrogen. The prechilled ethanol containing the frozen samples is allowed to warm in air. The resulting warming rates will depend on the volumes of ethanol used as "warming baths." For example, two to four samples (each of 0.2 ml volume) placed in 30 ml of ethanol in a 35 × 200 mm glass tube will warm at about 5°C/minute. Samples placed in 200 ml of cold ethanol in a 500-ml tall-form beaker will warm at about 2°C/minute.

Regardless of the specific rate used, samples of frozen embryos are normally warmed just until the last ice in the sample melts, at which point the average temperature of the sample is close to 0°C. The thawed samples are then transferred into an ice bath in preparation for the critical step of the dilution of the concentrated suspending medium.

V. SAMPLE RECOVERY

A. Dilution of Suspending Media

An important yet often neglected step in the use of freezing to preserve cells is the final one of returning the frozen-thawed cells to physiological conditions. In this step, the osmolality of the solution in which the embryos were frozen, 1.5 Osm or higher, is reduced to that of standard growth medium, about 0.3 Osm.

The response of ova and embryos to the decreased solute concentration in the external medium depends on how much protective additive permeated them prior to or during freezing, and on their relative permeabilities to solutes and water. Since the latter usually greatly exceeds the former, cells respond osmotically to dilution by rapidly taking up water. The rate and extent of the osmotic response depends on the concentration difference and on temperature. To avoid damage, the rate of dilution must be low enough to prevent damage from osmotic shock.

Two practical solutions to prevent shock have been used. The first is simply to dilute the external DMSO in a number of small steps at a constant temperature, with short intervening holding periods to permit equilibration. Because of the temperature dependence of the permeability coefficients for both DMSO and H_2O, the higher the temperature the more rapidly the cell will reach osmotic equilibrium at each step of the dilution. The following stepwise procedure has been demonstrated to work successfully to dilute various preimplantation stages of mouse embryos out of concentrated DMSO solutions. To each 0.2 ml of sample volume containing embryos at 0°C is successively added 0.2, 0.2, 0.4, and 1 ml of PBS at 0°C. After each addition, the samples are mixed gently and held for 1 minute before the next addition. The net effect is to reduce the external DMSO concentration tenfold. We have more recent unpublished evidence that survivals are slightly improved by using more and smaller dilution steps, or by carrying out the dilution at 37°C.

A second approach is based on that commonly used to recover frozen-thawed erythrocytes from hypertonic glycerol solutions for clinical transfusions (see Valeri et al., 1969, for review). It involves the initial transfer of thawed embryos into media containing a hypertonic concentration of a nonpermeating solute such as sucrose. The rationale is that the nonpermeant solute maintains a constant external osmolality and has sufficient osmotic pressure to prevent injurious cell swelling during the efflux of intracellular DMSO. Bank and Maurer (1974) found that a variant of this procedure was required to obtain high survival of frozen-thawed 8-cell rabbit embryos. They found that the DMSO had to be diluted rapidly while the total osmolarity was diluted slowly. To accomplish this, they added PBS at a concentration four times that of isotonic in a volume equal to that of the original sample, and immediately warmed the sample to 37°C. They then added increasing volumes of twice concentrated PBS, and finally relatively large volumes of single-strength PBS.

We have used a somewhat different procedure employing sucrose as the non-permeant species. A 0.2-ml sample of embryos in 1 M DMSO in PBS is diluted in one step with 2 ml of 0.75 M sucrose in PBS, but containing no DMSO. The embryos are held in this solution at room temperature for about 20–30 minutes to permit time for the intracellular DMSO to diffuse out of the embryos. Finally, the sucrose solution is diluted relatively rapidly in three steps with PBS. The embryos can then be safely washed by isotonic PBS to prepare them for the assay.

B. Embryo Recovery

A variety of procedures have been successfully used to recover frozen-thawed embryos from the tubes in which they were frozen. Since the actual manipulations are largely a matter of preference of the individual investigator, we present only the barest outline of our approach. Once the thawed suspension of embryos has been diluted out of the concentrated solution of DMSO, the embryos are recovered by gently mixing the tube contents and pouring them into a sterile watchglass or a disposable 33-mm diameter petri dish. (The latter has the advantage of avoiding the necessity for the careful washing of glassware required for routine embryologic manipulations. Its disadvantage is that the bottom of the dish is flat, so that the embryos are more dispersed than in a concave watchglass.) Alternatively, the diluted contents of the tube are gently aspirated into a sterile Pasteur pipette and then transferred into a sterile recovery dish. In either case, the frozen-thawed and diluted embryos are recovered using a low-power microscope, washed two or three times with fresh PBS, and finally assayed for survival by the standard *in vitro* and *in vivo* methods already cited.

VI. CONCLUSIONS

The procedures described in this chapter are being used in more than a dozen laboratories around the world to freeze preimplantation-stage embryos of several mammalian species. Exploitation of this approach for the conservation of the genetic information of mammals is only beginning. It is being applied as insurance against potential, irrevocable loss by disease or catastrophe of specific valuable strains of laboratory animals used in a variety of biomedical investigations. It is being applied as an approach to the preservation of unusual mutants, the preservation of which by standard breeding methods would be prohibitively expensive. It is being applied as a method of preventing genetic drift and as a method of assessing the magnitude of genetic drift. Although it is premature to draw definitive conclusions, the procedure appears to offer potential economic benefits in the husbandry of both laboratory and domestic animals. Furthermore, the ability to freeze mammalian embryos provides an approach to explore certain fundamental aspects of mammalian reproductive biology (Whittingham *et al.*, 1973). For example, it has been suggested that the maternal environment alters the developing fetus in some fashion (Uphoff, 1976). The use of frozen embryos would permit the simultaneous comparison of an original strain, a substrain established by embryo transfer, and a substrain obtained from the original strain many generations previously but preserved in the frozen state. Other advantages of this procedure for investigations in immunology, genetics, and radiation biology have also recently been suggested (Elliott and Whelan, 1977). Finally, the procedure itself is providing basic information both with respect to fundamental low temperature biology and to the fundamental physiology of mammalian embryos.

REFERENCES

Asahina, E., Shimada, K., and Hisada, Y. (1970). *Exp. Cell Res.* **59**, 349–358.
Ashwood-Smith, M. J., and Grant, E. (1977). *In* "The Freezing of Mammalian Embryos" (K. Elliott and J. Whelan, eds.), Ciba Found. Symp. No. 52. Elsevier, Amsterdam, pp. 251–267.
Bailey, D. W. (1977). *In* "The Freezing of Mammalian Embryos" (K. Elliott and J. Whelan, eds.), Ciba Found. Symp. No. 52. Elsevier, Amsterdam, pp. 291–299.
Bank, H., and Maurer, R. R. (1974). *Exp. Cell Res.* **89**, 188–196.
Bank, H., and Mazur, P. (1973). *J. Cell Biol.* **57**, 729–742.
Brinster, R. L. (1970). *Adv. Biosci.* **4**, 199–233.
Brinster, R. L. (1972). *In* "Growth, Nutrition, and Metabolism of Cells in Culture" (G. H. Rothblat and V. J. Cristofalo, eds.), Vol. II pp. 251–286. Academic Press, New York.
Cocks, F. H., and Brower, W. E. (1974). *Cryobiology* **11**, 340–358.
Daniel, J. C., Jr., ed. (1971). "Methods in Mammalian Embryology." Freeman, San Francisco, California.
DuFrain, R. J. (1976). *In* "Basic Aspects of Freeze Preservation of Mouse Strains" (O. Mühlbock, ed.), pp. 73–84. Fischer, Stuttgart.
Elliott, K., and Whelan, J., eds. (1977). "The Freezing of Mammalian Embryos," Ciba Found. Symp. No. 52. Elsevier, Amsterdam.
Jackowski, S. C. (1977). Ph.D. Dissertation, University of Tennessee, Knoxville.
Jackowski, S. C., and Leibo, S. P. (1976). *Cryobiology* **13**, 646.
Leibo, S. P. (1976). *In* "Basic Aspects of Freeze Preservation of Mouse Strains" (O. Mühlbock, ed.), pp. 13–33. Fischer, Stuttgart.
Leibo, S. P. (1977a). *In* "Cryoimmunologie" (D. Simatos, D. M. Strong, and J.-M. Turc, eds.), pp. 311–334. INSERM, Paris.
Leibo, S. P. (1977b). *In* "The Freezing of Mammalian Embryos" (K. Elliott and J. Whelan, eds.), Ciba Found. Symp. No. 52. Elsevier, Amsterdam, pp. 69–92.
Leibo, S. P., Farrant, J., Mazur, P., Hanna, M. G., Jr., and Smith, L. H. (1970). *Cryobiology* **6**, 315–332.
Leibo, S. P., Mazur, P., and Jackowski, S. C. (1974). *Exp. Cell Res.* **89**, 79–88.
Leibo, S. P., McGrath, J. J., and Cravalho, E. G. (1977). *Cryobiology* (in press).
Lyon, M. F., Whittingham, D. G., and Glenister, P. (1977). *In* "The Freezing of Mammalian Embryos" (K. Elliott and J. Whelan, eds.), *Ciba Found. Symp.* No. 52. Elsevier, Amsterdam, pp. 273–282.
McGrath, J. J., Cravalho, E. G., and Huggins, C. E. (1975). *Cryobiology* **12**, 540–550.
Maurer, R. R. (1976). *Can. J. Anim. Sci.* **56**, 131–145.
Maurer, R. R., and Haseman, J. K. (1976). *Biol. Reprod.* **14**, 256–263.
Maurer, R. R., Bank, H., and Staples, R. E. (1977). *Biol. Reprod.* **16**, 139–146.
Mazur, P. (1963). *J. Gen. Physiol.* **47**, 347–369.
Mazur, P. (1965). *Ann. N. Y. Acad. Sci.* **125**, 658–676.
Mazur, P. (1966). *In* "Cryobiology" (H. T. Meryman, ed.), pp. 213–315. Academic Press, New York.
Mazur, P. (1976). *In* "Basic Aspects of Freeze Preservation of Mouse Strains" (O. Mühlbock, ed.), pp. 1–12. Fischer, Stuttgart.

Mazur, P. (1977a). *Cryobiology* **14**, 251–272.

Mazur, P. (1977b). *In* "Cryoimmumologie" (D. Simatos, D. M. Strong, and J.-M. Turc, eds.), pp. 37–60. INSERM, Paris.

Mazur, P. (1977c). *In* "The Freezing of Mammalian Embryos" (K. Elliott and J. Whelan, eds.), *Ciba Found. Symp.* No. 52. Elsevier, Amsterdam, pp. 19–40.

Mazur, P., and Schmidt, J. J. (1968). *Cryobiology* **5,** 1–17.

Mazur, P., Farrant, J., Leibo, S. P., and Chu, E. H. Y. (1969). *Cryobiology* **6**, 1–9.

Mazur, P., Leibo, S. P., and Chu, E. H. Y. (1972). *Exp. Cell Res.* **71**, 345–355.

Mazur, P., Leibo, S. P., and Miller, R. H. (1974). *J. Membr. Biol.* **15**, 107–136.

Mazur, P., Rigopoulos. N., Jackowski, S. C., and Leibo, S. P. (1976). *Biophys. J.* **16**, 232a.

Moore, N. W., and Bilton, R. J. (1977). *In* "The Freezing of Mammalian Embryos" (K. Elliott and J. Whelan, eds.), *Ciba Found. Symp.* No. 52. Elsevier, Amsterdam, pp. 203–219.

Mühlbock, O., ed. (1976). "Basic Aspects of Freeze Preservation of Mouse Strains." Fischer, Stuttgart.

Parkening, T. A., Tsunoda, Y., and Chang, M. C. (1976). *J. Exp. Zool.* **197**, 369–374.

Pegg, D. E. (1970). *In* "Current Trends in Cryobiology" (A. U. Smith, ed.), pp. 153–180. Plenum, New York.

Rotman, B., and Papermaster, B. (1966). *Proc. Natl. Acad. Sci. U.S.A.* **55**, 134–141.

Schneider, U., Hahn, J., and Sulzer, H. (1974). *Dtsch. Tiererztl. Wochenschr.* **81**, 445–476.

Shimada, K., and Asahina, E. (1972). *Low Temp. Sci., Ser. B* **30**, 65–75.

Tsunoda, Y., and Sugie, T. (1977). *J. Reprod. Fertil.* **49**, 173–174.

Tsunoda, Y., Parkening, T. A., and Chang, M. C. (1976). *Experientia* **32**, 223–224.

Uphoff, D. E. (1976). *In* "Basic Aspects of Freeze Preservation of Mouse Strains" (O. Mühlbock, ed.), pp. 85–102. Fischer, Stuttgart.

Valeri, C. R., Runck, A. H., and Brodine, C. E. (1969). *J. Am. Med. Assoc.* **208**, 489–492.

Whittingham, D. G. (1971). *J. Reprod. Fertil., Suppl.* **14**, 7–21.

Whittingham, D. G. (1974). *J. Reprod. Fertil.* **37**, 159–162.

Whittingham, D. G. (1975). *J. Reprod. Fertil.* **43**, 575–578.

Whittingham, D. G. (1977a). *J. Reprod. Fertil.* **49**, 89–94.

Whittingham, D. G. (1977b). *In* "The Freezing of Mammalian Embryos" (K. Elliott and J. Whelan, eds.), *Ciba Found. Symp.* No. 52. Elsevier, Amsterdam, pp. 97–108.

Whittingham, D. G., and Adams, C. E. (1976). *J. Reprod. Fertil.* **47**, 269–274.

Whittingham, D. G., and Whitten, W. K. (1974). *J. Reprod. Fertil.* **36**, 433–435.

Whittingham, D. G., Leibo, S. P., and Mazur, P. (1972). *Science* **178**, 411–414.

Whittingham, D. G., Leibo, S. P., and Mazur, P. (1973). *Science* **181**, 288.

Willadsen, S. M., Polge, C., Rowson, L. E. A., and Moor, R. M. (1976a). *J. Reprod. Fertil.* **46**, 151–154.

Willadsen, S. M., Trounson, A. O., Polge, C., Rowson, L. E. A., and Newcomb, R. (1976b). *In* "Egg Transfer in Cattle" (L. E. A. Rowson, ed.), pp. 117–124. Comm. Eur. Commun. Publ., Luxembourg.

Wilmut, I. (1972). *Life Sci.* **11**, 1071–1079.

Wilmut, I., and Rowson, L. E. A. (1973). *Vet. Rec.* **92**, 686–690.

9

Immunologic Inhibition of Development

ANTHONY G. SACCO AND C. ALEX SHIVERS

I. INTRODUCTION

Much interest has recently been shown in the concept of immuno-contraception—the inhibition of fertilization and development by immunologic means. The feasibility of this approach to contraception is dependent upon the existence of an antigen or antigens specific to a particular reproductive tissue (i.e., not present in other reproductive or nonreproductive tissues). Presumably due to this specificity, this antigen would also possess a unique reproductive role. Such an antigen would serve as the target against which to direct an immunologic attack in the form of specific antibodies that would neutralize the reproductive function of this antigen and subsequently prevent fertilization or development.

The search for antigens specific to either male or female reproductive tissues has occurred for numerous years and many claims for the existence of such antigens have been made (see Mancini, 1971; Diczfalusy, 1974; World Health Organization, 1976). Most recently, specific antigens associated with the mammalian ovary and, particularly, the zona pellucida have gained much attention (for reviews, see Fox and Shivers, 1972; Dunbar and Shivers, 1976). While the emphasis of this chapter will be on descriptions of the approaches and procedures used to detect antigens specific to the ovary and zona, such techniques should also apply for initial attempts to detect antigens specific to other tissues as well.

II. ANTISERUM PRODUCTION AND COLLECTION

A. Preparation of Antigen

Two approaches can be taken in attempting to demonstrate and to produce heteroantibodies against reproductive tissue specific antigens. Both have their obvious advantages and disadvantages. One can initially produce an antiserum against a biochemically purified protein or glycoprotein which nonimmunologic data suggest may be specific to a reproductive tissue. Examples of such specific antigens for the male would be sperm hyaluronidase, LDH-X, and acrosin; for the female, β-HCG and the placental protein SP_1. Following the production of a monospecific iso- or heteroantiserum, immunologic testing designed to establish the tissue specificity of this antigen can then be performed. The major disadvantage of this approach is that the presence of a substance in a reproductive tissue, which perhaps on a functional level appears specific, does not guarantee its antigenic specificity.

The second approach, which is most commonly used to date, involves the production of heteroantiserum against an entire reproductive tissue (e.g., ovary, uterus, testes, etc.). The resulting antiserum is then absorbed with various nonreproductive tissues to remove all antibodies directed against antigens shared by the reproductive tissue and those tissues used for absorption. Following appropriate immunologic testing for tissue cross-reactivity, such an absorbed antiserum should contain only antibodies directed against antigens specific to the reproductive tissue, if such antigens exist.

Antiserum has been produced against the ovaries from at least seven mammalian species—hamster, rabbit, mouse, guinea pig, rat, pig, and human—for the explicit purpose of detecting antigens specific to either the ovary or zona pellucida. For the smaller species, several ovaries (approximately 6–10) obtained from animals in various stages of the estrous cycle are used per injection. For the larger species (e.g., pig and human), a single ovary or portion of ovary per injection is sufficient. We attempt to inject as much and as concentrated a sample as is feasible, since we are attempting to produce an immune response to as many different ovarian antigens as possible. The ovaries are minced with scissors and then homogenized in a tissue grinder (4°C) in 1–2 ml of either 0.15 M NaCl, a phosphate-buffered saline (PBS;0.1 M PO$_4$,0.85% NaCl, pH 7.3) or appropriate buffer. We prefer injecting the total homogenate (i.e., without any centrifugation), since by this procedure the immunized animal will be exposed to both soluble and insoluble antigens. If centrifugation to remove tissue debris is preferred, the homogenate should be exposed to sonication and/or multiple freeze-thawing prior to the centrifugation to allow for adequate membrane disruption. If centrifugation is performed, the resulting supernatant is then used as the antigenic preparation for the immunization. The total protein content of the antigenic preparation is determined by the method of Lowry *et al.* (1951).

B. Immunization Format

Rabbits have been used most frequently for the production of anti-ovary sera. A notable exception would be the report describing specific antigens in the rabbit ovary (Sacco and Shivers, 1973a) where sheep were used for antiserum production. We prefer using young animals of opposite sex to the material being injected, since if the immunizing material does contain a reproductive tissue specific antigen, then an animal of opposite sex should have a greater chance of recognizing that antigen as being foreign. Therefore, male rabbits approximately 3–4 months of age are used for antiserum production against female tissues.

Each investigator has a favorite injection and bleeding format, and descriptions of the various techniques are readily available (Weir, 1973; Vaitukaitis *et al.*, 1971). We use the following. For the first injection, the ovarian homogenate (or supernatant), volume approximately 1–2 ml, is emulsified with an equal volume of Freund's complete adjuvant and injected subscapularly on each side (total volume injected approximately 2–4 ml). Two booster injections follow at weekly intervals, and the first antiserum bleeding (a bleeding to obtain preimmune serum is taken prior to the first immunization) is taken 3 days following the second booster (third injection). Booster injections are identical except that Freund's incomplete adjuvant is used. Blood is collected via the marginal ear vein and bleedings are continued on a weekly basis. Additional booster injections may be given depending upon the initial response of the rabbit, how long weekly bleedings are continued, or if any drop in titer is observed. If the rabbit is bled on a weekly schedule, booster injections usually are given every 6–8 weeks. Blood is allowed to coagulate for 1 hour at 25° or 37°C, and then left at 4°C overnight. It is then centrifuged and the antiserum stored at −20°C until used.

If enough antigen is available, we recommend immunizing a minimum of two rabbits to allow for variances in response and possible loss of a rabbit due to illness. If several rabbits are injected with the same antigen, then either antiserum from the best responding rabbit or a pooled preparation consisting of equal quantities from each of the rabbits can be used.

The antiserum is eventually used as three different preparations: "whole" antiserum, a crude γ globulin preparation obtained by salt fractionation, and a pure γ globulin preparation obtained by chromatographic techniques (see Weir, 1973). Initial testing for antibody activity and specificity is performed with the whole antiserum, and all tests are later reconfirmed using the more purified preparations.

III. DETERMINATION OF ANTISERUM ACTIVITY AND SPECIFICITY

Antiserum activity and specificity is initially tested by agar gel double diffusion. Macroimmunodiffusion is preferred over microimmunodiffusion because of the better resolution obtained. However, if the quantity of reagents is a limiting factor, the microtechnique should be used to conserve material.

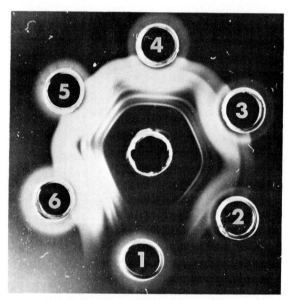

Fig. 1. Immunodiffusion plate testing initial bleedings from a rabbit immunized with pig ovary. Center well, pig ovary; well 1, preimmune serum; wells 2–6, rabbit anti-pig ovary, first to fifth bleedings, respectively.

For macroimmunodiffusion, 5 ml of 1% agarose (SeaKem) dissolved (by autoclaving for 15 minutes) in 0.1 M PO$_4$ buffer, pH 7.0–7.1, is poured onto 2 × 2 inch glass plates (Kodak slide cover glass), and the gel cut with a template to produce a pattern of one central well and six peripheral wells. The buffer used for preparing plates will vary, depending upon the nature of the antigens being tested, but we try to use the same buffer for preparing the plates and for homogenizing tissues to be reacted in the plates. Tissues are homogenized to a final concentration of either 25% or 50% (w/v) and following centrifugation, the supernatants are used as the antigenic preparations in double diffusion.

TABLE I

Precipitin Bands Produced against Different Tissues in Immunodiffusion Using Anti-Ovary Sera[a]

	Antisera		
Tissue	Anti-hamster ovary	Anti-rabbit ovary	Anti-human ovary
Adrenal gland	NT	9	7
Brain	3	4	6
Duodenum	NT	14	9
Fat	NT	7	6
Follicular fluid	NT	NT	4
Heart	5	10	8
Ileum	5	11	5
Kidney	5	14	10
Liver	5	11	9
Lung	5	13	7
Ovary	7	15	9
Oviduct	4	12	NT
Pancreas	NT	8	9
Plasma	5	15	8
Red blood cells	NT	3	6
Seminal plasma	NT	NT	7
Serum	5	14	6
Skeletal muscle	NT	7	7
Spleen	NT	10	9
Stomach	NT	6	7
Testis	3	13	9
Thyroid gland	NT	6	8
Uterus	5	12	9

[a] Each numeral represents maximum number of precipitin bands produced in agar-gel double diffusion when unabsorbed anti-ovary sera were allowed to react against various tissues. Each antiserum was reacted against tissues obtained only from the same species. NT, not tested. From Ownby and Shivers (1972), Sacco and Shivers (1973a), and Sacco (1977a).

The first reactions carried out are those designed to test the initial bleedings to determine how the rabbit(s) is responding to the immunization regime (see Fig. 1). Once an antiserum of good titer is obtained (i.e., successive bleedings produce no additional precipitin bands), then the cross-reactivity of the antiserum with other reproductive and nonreproductive tissues can be tested. The largest possible number of different tissues is tested, since the greater the number of tissues involved the more convincing will be the data for the existence of a specific antigen. Table I demonstrates the number of precipitin bands observed when various anti-ovary sera are reacted against different tissues. As seen, antiserum produced against ovary cross-reacts with a large number of different tissues, thus demonstrating that the ovary shares a large number of antigens. Similar findings have also been shown for antiserum produced against other female reproductive tissues as well (Sacco and Shivers, 1973a; Fox and Shivers, 1975).

A. Antiserum Absorption

Because of this large number of antigens shared among various tissues an antiserum produced against one tissue will quite likely produce a significant number of precipitin bands when tested against other tissues by immunodiffusion (see Table I). Rendering such an antiserum specific to the tissue against which it was produced requires the removal of these cross-reacting antibodies (i.e., the antibodies which react with the shared antigens). This is accomplished by absorbing the antiserum with the cross-reacting tissue(s). The type of tissue or number of tissues required for absorption will obviously vary depending upon the antisera. Plasma (or serum) is commonly used as the first absorbing material, although it may not be necessary for all antisera since other absorbing tissues may contain enough plasma components to successfully remove all antibody activity directed against the plasma proteins. This is apparently true for anti-hamster ovary serum, where absorption with only small intestine is sufficient to render the antiserum specific to hamster ovary (Shivers et al., 1972). However, anti-human ovary serum must be absorbed with plasma, since initial absorption with liver alone does not remove all antibody activity directed against the plasma components (Sacco, 1977a). Plasma is preferred over serum, since it still contains all the components of the blood coagulation system, and these are obviously antigenic and will induce an immune response.

The actual amount of a tissue required to completely absorb a particular antiserum can be determined only by trial and error testing. We normally begin with a small volume of antiserum (1–5 ml) and absorb initially with plasma. Usually, an equal volume of lyophilized plasma is added to the antiserum. For example, if 2 ml of an anti-human ovary serum are to be absorbed, 2 ml of human plasma are lyophilized and then added to the antiserum. After thorough mixing, the antiserum is left at 25° or 37° for 60 minutes with occasional shaking, placed at 4°C overnight, and then centrifuged (12,000 g) the following morning. The supernatant, which is now referred to as plasma-absorbed antiserum, is reacted against plasma in double diffusion analyses to test the effectiveness of the absorption. The failure of any precipitin bands to form between the plasma-absorbed antiserum and the plasma is interpreted that the absorption was successful and that the absorbed antiserum no longer contains antibody activity directed against plasma components. If precipitin bands are produced in this reaction, then additional lyophilized plasma must be added to the antiserum to accomplish complete absorption. This procedure of absorption followed by testing of the absorbed antiserum by immunodiffusion against the absorbing tissue is continued until no precipitin bands are observed. An absorbed antiserum is always reacted against the tissue used for absorption to verify the complete removal of all antibody activity against the tissue.

Following successful absorption with plasma, the absorbed antiserum is next reacted by immunodiffusion against as many reproductive and non-reproductive tissues as is feasible, including the homologous tissue (i.e., the tissue against which it was produced). The formation of a precipitin band(s) against any other tissue except the homologous tissue indicates that antigens other than plasma proteins are shared and that absorption with additional tissue(s) is necessary. The

TABLE II
Antigens of Hamster Ovary[a]

Antigens	Antisera to hamster ovary			
	A	B	C	D
Ovary	7	4	2	1
Oviduct	4	2	1	0
Uterus	5	3	1	0
Kidney	5	3	1	0
Serum	5	0	2	0
Plasma	5	0	2	0
Small intestine	5	4	0	0
Testis	3	3	1	0
Brain	3	2	0	0
Heart	5	3	2	0
Lung	5	3	2	0
Liver	5	4	2	0

[a] Numbers represent precipitin bands formed when the antigen was reacted with the antisera in agar-gel diffusion plates. A, unabsorbed antisera; B, antisera absorbed with plasma; C, antisera absorbed with small intestine; D, antisera absorbed with small intestine and lung. From Ownby and Shivers (1972).

somatic tissue finally selected for the next absorption procedure is usually the tissue against which the largest number of precipitin bands are produced, but, in some cases, availability of a tissue may be a deciding factor.

When absorbing with a somatic tissue, two procedures can be used. The tissue can be homogenized, lyophilized, and then added to the antiserum, or the minced tissue can be homogenized directly in the antiserum. Both procedures work well, but the major advantage of the latter procedure is that it is more rapid since the lyophilization step is eliminated.

The amount of somatic tissue required for successful absorption, as with absorption by plasma, is determined by trial and error. Once all antibody activity against the absorbing tissue is removed, the absorbed antiserum is checked again by immunodiffusion against the test series of reproductive and nonreproductive tissues. This procedure of absorption, followed by checking against the test

TABLE III

Antigens of Rabbit Tissues Detected by Sheep Anti-Rabbit Ovary Serum[a]

Antigen	(A) Unabsorbed antiserum	(B) Absorbed with rabbit plasma	(C) Absorbed with rabbit plasma and kidney	(D) Absorbed with rabbit plasma, kidney, and spleen
Ovary	15	7	4	2
Oviduct	12	6	2	0
Uterus	12	7	2	0
Adrenal gland	9	7	1	0
Brain	4	0	0	0
Duodenum	14	5	2	0
Fat	7	0	0	0
Heart	10	3	0	0
Ileum	11	5	2	0
Kidney	14	6	0	0
Liver	11	7	2	0
Lung	13	4	1	0
Pancreas	8	2	0	0
Plasma	15	0	0	0
Red blood cells	3	1	0	0
Serum	14	0	0	0
Skeletal muscle	7	2	0	0
Spleen	10	6	2	0
Stomach	6	3	0	0
Testis	13	5	1	0
Thyroid gland	6	1	0	0

[a] Each numeral indicates the maximum number of precipitin bands observed in Ouchterlony plates when the antiserum was allowed to react against a particular rabbit tissue and represents 10 separate tests involving different preparations of the reactants. From Sacco and Shivers (1973a).

series of tissues, is continued until the absorbed antiserum fails to produce precipitin bands against any tissue except the homologous tissue. These bands are then interpreted as indicating the presence of reproductive tissue specific antigens. Following completion of the absorption procedure, the antiserum is heat inactivated at 56°C for 30 minutes, centrifuged (12,000 g), and the supernatant stored frozen (-20°C or -70°C) until used. Tables II–IV present the results obtained for three different anti-ovary sera absorbed following the above procedures.

All initial testing of antiserum for tissue specificity, due to the large number of tissues involved, is usually performed by immunodiffusion analyses using whole

TABLE IV
Antigens in Human Tissues Detected by Rabbit Anti-Human Ovary Serum Using Agar Gel Double Diffusion[a]

Human tissues	(A) Unabsorbed antiserum	(B) Human liver absorbed antiserum	(C) Human liver and plasma absorbed antiserum
Adrenal gland	7	—	0
Brain	6	—	0
Duodenum	9	—	0
Fat	6	—	0
Follicular fluid	4	—	0
Heart	8	—	0
Ileum	5	—	0
Kidney	10	—	0
Liver	9	1	0
Lung	7	—	0
Ovary	9	2	1
Pancreas	9	—	0
Plasma	8	2	0
Red blood cells	6	—	0
Seminal plasma	7	—	0
Serum	6	—	0
Skeletal muscle	7	—	0
Spleen	9	—	0
Stomach	7	—	0
Testis	9	—	0
Thyroid gland	8	—	0
Uterus	9	—	0

[a] Each numeral represents the maximum number of precipitin bands observed in agar gel double diffusion plates when the antiserum was allowed to react against a particular human tissue and represents five separate tests involving different preparations of the reactants. (—), Not tested. From Sacco (1977a).

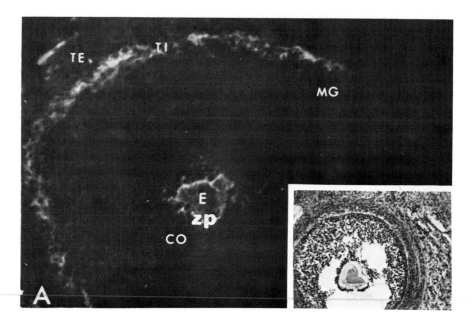

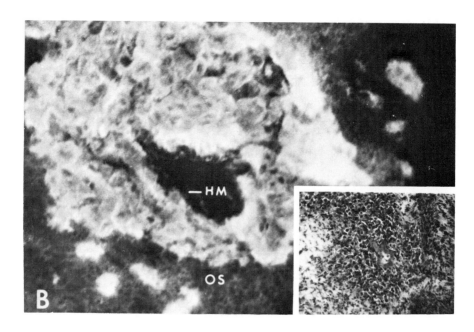

antiserum. The investigator must be aware that these immunodiffusion procedures demonstrate only soluble antigens, and that once specific antigens are indicated, these results must be reconfirmed both by using more sensitive techniques and by using a purified preparation of the absorbed antiserum. Testing the various tissues involved by the indirect fluorescent antibody technique using a chomatographically pure preparation of the absorbed antiserum is the most convenient method to confirm the immunodiffusion data. Procedures describing the fluorescent antibody technique and the isolation of the immunoglobulin fraction from serum are readily available (Goldman, 1968; Glass, 1971; Weir, 1973). *In vivo* tissue clearance of radiolabeled specific antiserum as described by Yanagimachi *et al.* (1976) can also be used to verify tissue specificity, or if a purified preparation of the antigen is available, a radioimmune assay can be developed for this purpose.

B. Antigen Localization

The availability of a monospecific antiserum directed against a reproductive tissue specific antigen allows for the localization of that antigen within its respective reproductive tissue. The indirect fluorescent antibody technique can be used to localize the specific antigen (see Fig. 2).

IV. EVALUATION OF ANTIBODY ACTIVITY

Once a reproductive tissue has been found to contain a specific antigen and a monospecific antiserum directed against this antigen is available, then the effect of this antiserum on the reproductive function of the antigen can be evaluated. How this is determined will depend upon the nature and reproductive role of the specific antigen involved. For example, if the specific antigen is known to be an enzyme, then antibody-produced inhibition of enzymatic activity may result from exposing the antigen to its specific antibody. This in turn may result in impairment or inhibition of fertility.

In regard to ovarian specific antigens, only the effects of antibodies directed against the antigen(s) localized in the zona pellucida have been evaluated to any

---

Fig. 2. Cryostat sections of rabbit ovary treated with sheep anti-ovary serum and FITC-labeled anti-sheep serum. The anti-ovary serum was rendered specific to ovary by absorption with rabbit plasma, kidney, and spleen. (A) Section through follicle showing localization of fluorescence in the zona pellucida and theca interna, × 250. Inset: hematoxylin and eosin stained section of a comparable region, × 90. (B) Section through an atretic follicle showing localization of fluorescence. Hyaline material does not fluoresce, × 445. Inset: hematoxylin-and-eosin-stained section of a comparable region. × 128. From Sacco and Shivers (1973c). CO, cumulus oophorus; E, egg; HM, hyaline material; MG, membrana granulosa; OS, ovarian stroma; TE, theca externa; TI, theca interna; ZP, zona pellucida.

great extent. The procedures by which anti-zona pellucida activity can be demonstrated are described below.

A. Obtaining Eggs and Isolated Zonae Pellucidae

1. Egg Collection Procedures

Two procedures are used to collect eggs for obtaining zonae. For the smaller species, such as mouse, hamster, rat, guinea pig, and rabbit, superovulation techniques followed by killing the animal and flushing the reproductive tracts to obtain the eggs is the most convenient and productive method. The hormonal regimes necessary to produce superovulation vary among species, and are available in the literature (see Daniel, 1971).

For the larger species such as pig and cow, collection of eggs directly from the ovary is more convenient than the superovulation technique (see Sacco and Palm, 1977). Ovaries are collected at a commercial packing house, brought back to the laboratory, and the follicular fluid aspirated from the follicles with a tuberculin syringe and 26-gauge needle. The follicular fluid should be kept on ice during the collection procedure to retard coagulation which will interfer with egg collection. The ovarian eggs are then collected from the pooled follicular fluid under a stereomicroscope using a micropipette (see Fig. 3).

2. Cumulus Cell Removal

To obtain eggs having an exposed zona pellucida requires the removal of the cumulus cell layer. This can be effectively accomplished either by incubating the eggs in hyaluronidase (usually 0.1% for 5–30 minutes at either 22°C or 37°C), or

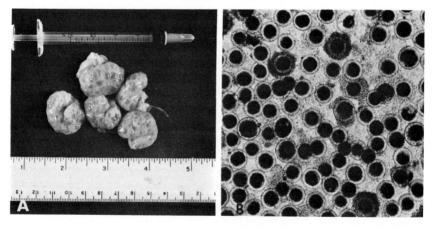

Fig. 3. Ovarian pig eggs collected from follicular fluid. (A) Pig ovaries demonstrating follicles which are aspirated with tuberculin syringe and 26 gauge needle. (B) Pig eggs in cumulus cells isolated from follicular fluid, × 75. From Sacco and Palm (1977).

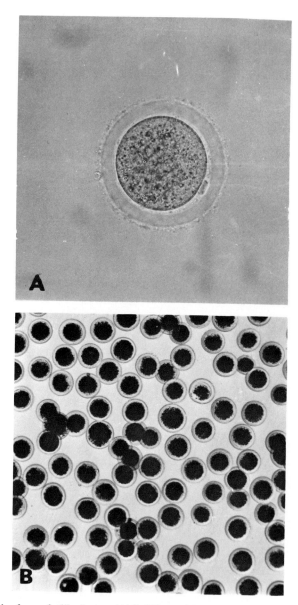

Fig. 4. Cumulus-free unfertilized eggs. (A) Rabbit egg following hyaluronidase treatment, ×
540. (B) Pig eggs following sodium citrate treatment, × 75.

by agitating the eggs in 0.01% sodium citrate solution in 0.15 M NaCl or PBS for 30 seconds (see Fig. 4). Following either treatment, the cumulus-free eggs are thoroughly washed in the appropriate buffer medium (usually PBS or 0.15 M NaCl). The major advantages of the latter treatment are that it is rapid and does not result in contamination of the eggs by extraneous proteins (i.e., hyaluronidase or the contaminants present in commercial preparations of the enzyme). Drawbacks, however, are that the procedure usually results in a greater egg loss than the enzyme treatment, and, to date, the fertilizability and viability of such treated eggs has not been tested. However, the procedure works well for purposes of acquiring isolated zonae (see below), and no observable differences in zona pellucida antigenicity following cumulus cell removal by either procedure have been reported (see Sacco, 1977a,b; Shivers and Dunbar, 1977).

3. Isolation of Zona Pellucida

Isolated zonae are obtained by mechanical means. Groups of eggs devoid of cumulus cells (50–100) are drawn into a micropipette with an internal-bore diameter slightly less than that of the egg plus its zona. Drawing the eggs once into the pipette followed by expulsion back into the medium is in most cases sufficient to break the zonae. A repeated passage into the pipette is usually successful in removing any egg contents which may be adhering to the interior

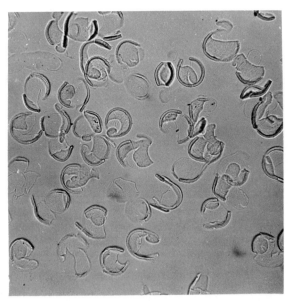

Fig. 5.   Isolated pig zonae obtained following procedures described in text, × 75. From Sacco and Palm (1977).

portion of the zona. The micropipettes are made in the laboratory from Pyrex glass tubing. The procedure works best if the suction and expulsion is done by mouth by means of latex tubing connected to the pipette. Once the isolated zonae are obtained, they are washed in several changes of buffer using the standard size micropipette for handling eggs (see Fig. 5).

B. Testing Effect of Antiserum on Antigen (Zona Pellucida)

Treatment of zonae with either antisera containing antibody activity directed against zona pellucida (e.g., unabsorbed anti-ovary sera) or with antisera rendered specific to zona pellucida by absorption (anti-zona sera) has been found to produce several different effects regarding the zona. Several of these procedures are now routinely used to assay antisera for antizona activity. These antibody produced effects on the zona include:

1. Agglutination of cumulus-free eggs.
2. Formation of a precipitation layer on the outer surface of the zona (also referred to as an alteration in the light-scattering properties of the zona).
3. Inhibition of zona lysis by proteolytic enzymes or reducing agents.
4. Inhibition of sperm attachment to and penetration of the zona.
5. Inhibition of zona "hatching" by embryos.

In all cases, similar treatment of zonae with preimmune serum or control preparations (buffer medium alone or anti-ovary serum absorbed with ovary) does not produce the observed effect.

1. Agglutination of Cumulus-Free Eggs

Eggs devoid of cumulus cells are placed in a small volume of serum (0.1–0.5 ml) at room temperature and pushed together with a finely drawn glass rod so that the eggs (and zonae) remain in contact with each other. After approximately 10 minutes, medium is gently flushed over the eggs with the micropipette. Eggs incubated in antiserum will remain adhered together in groups even after relatively forceful flushing, whereas those incubated in preimmune serum or the control preparations will separate (see Fig. 6).

2. Formation of Precipitation Layer

Eggs incubated in antisera as described in Section IV,B,1 when viewed by light microscopy are found to possess a dark layer on the outer surface of the zona under bright-field illumination or a white layer similarly located when viewed under dark-field illumination. This phenomena has been described as either the formation of an antibody-produced precipitation layer on the surface of the zona or a modification in the light-scattering properties of the zona pellucida. Eggs treated with preimmune serum or the control preparations have never been observed to undergo this change (see Fig. 7).

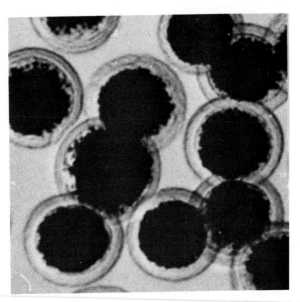

Fig. 6. Small group of cumulus-free pig eggs agglutinated by a rabbit anti-pig zona serum, ×
380.

The indirect fluorescent antibody technique has also been used to visualize
antibody activity directed against zona. For this procedure, once eggs (or isolated
zonae) have been pretreated with antisera, as described above, they are
thoroughly washed in several changes of medium and then incubated for 15–30
minutes at 25°C in a fluorescein isothiocyanate-labeled antiserum. The labeled
antiserum is usually an anti-rabbit IgG, but this will vary depending upon the
species used for the initial production of the anti-ovary or anti-zona serum. Such
labeled antisera are available commercially, and, in most instances, must be
diluted 1:10 or 1:100 before use. Following incubation in the labeled antiserum,
the eggs are thoroughly washed by repeated pipetting in several changes of
medium, transferred to glass depression slides, and viewed by fluorescent microscopic techniques. Zonae treated with antiserum fluoresce a bright green, while
very little fluorescence is associated with the control-treated zonae (see Fig. 7).

3. Inhibition of Zona Lysis

As described in the literature (Bowman and McLaren, 1970; Krzanowska,
1972; Sacco and Shivers, 1973b; Inoue and Wolf, 1974), certain proteolytic
enzymes, such as trypsin and pronase, or reducing agents, such as mercaptoethanol, have been used to dissolve the zonae of certain species. It has been
found that when zonae are first treated with antiserum containing antibody activity against zona and possess the precipitation layer, the zonae become resistant to

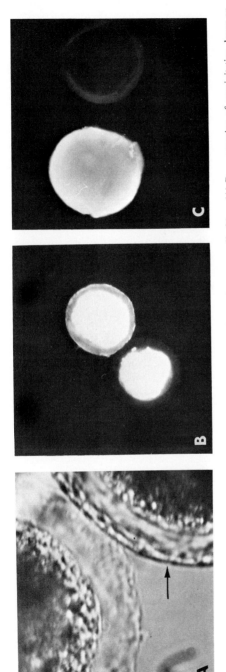

Fig. 7. Eggs or isolated zonae treated with antisera possessing antibody activity against zona pellucida. (A) Demonstration of precipitation layer on outer surface of pig zona. Egg at upper left treated with preimmune serum and no precipitation layer is observed, × 1480. (B) Appearance of precipitation layer under dark-field illumination. Preimmune serum treated pig egg is at left, × 340. (C) Fluorescing isolated human zona following antiserum treatment and testing by the indirect fluorescent antibody technique. Preimmune serum treated zona is on right, × 330.

dissolution by these reagents (Ownby and Shivers, 1972; Sacco and Shivers, 1973b; Oikawa and Yanagimachi, 1975).

Cumulus-free eggs are pretreated in 0.1–0.5 ml of anti-ovary or anti-zona sera at 25°C for 5–15 minutes. During this incubation period, the precipitation layer forms on the zona. They are then washed in several changes of medium to remove the serum components and transferred to the medium containing the enzyme or reducing agent. The concentration of these reagents and the incubation time required to effectively dissolve the zona varies depending upon the particular reagent and the species being used. The most common procedures are: trypsin (0.1–3.0%, 25°C for 5–20 minutes for rabbit or hamster zonae); pronase (0.5%, 37°C, for 5 minutes for mouse zonae); mercaptoethanol (0.1–0.75 M, 37°C for 30–60 minutes for mouse and hamster zonae). Zonae possessing the antibody-produced precipitation layer do not dissolve, whereas zonae treated with control preparations, which do not possess the precipitation layer, will dissolve within the normal period of time for those conditions being used (see Table V).

TABLE V

Effect of Anti-Ovary Sera on Zona Pellucida Dissolution by Trypsin[a]

	Effect of Trypsin on zona removal[d]	
Pretreatment	Hamster	Rabbit
Anti-ovary serum[b]	−	−
Specific immune serum[c]	−	−
Preimmune serum	+	+
Medium alone	+	+
Anti-ovary serum absorbed with ovary	+	NT

[a] Cumulus-free hamster or rabbit eggs were treated as described in text. Trypsin concentrations used were 0.2% for hamster eggs and 3.0% for rabbit eggs. Hamster and rabbit eggs pretreated only with the homologous sera preparations.

[b] Anti-hamster ovary serum; anti-rabbit ovary serum.

[c] Anti-hamster ovary absorbed with hamster small intestines and lung; anti-rabbit ovary absorbed with rabbit plasma, kidney, and spleen.

[d] −, Zona pellucida not removed; +, zona pellucida removed; NT, not tested. Modified from Ownby and Shivers (1972) and Sacco and Shivers (1973b).

4. Inhibition of Sperm Attachment and Penetration

The presence of the precipitation layer on the outer surface of the zona has been found to inhibit both sperm attachment to and penetration of the zona (Shivers *et al.*, 1972; Oikawa and Yanagimachi, 1975). For the hamster system, either eggs in cumulus or cumulus-free eggs are incubated in antiserum, preimmune serum, and/or the control preparations at 37°C for 20–30 minutes. The eggs can be incubated directly in 0.1 ml of the serum sample or in Tyrode's solution containing 20–50 mg/ml of the appropriate serum sample or control preparation. Following incubation, the eggs are washed in several changes of Tyrode's solution to remove unreacted serum components, placed in 0.1 ml Tyrode's solution under mineral oil, inseminated with 0.05 ml of an epididymal sperm suspension in Tyrode's solution ($12–57 \times 10^6$ sperm/ml), and incubated at 37°C for 5–6 hours. Insemination procedures can vary depending upon the investigator. Following this incubation, the eggs are placed on microscope depression slides and viewed by light microscopy. Eggs pretreated with the control preparations are found to have numerous sperm firmly attached to the zona pellucida, which cannot be removed by washing. Such treated zonae have also been penetrated as evidenced either by the presence of sperm in the perivitelline space or by pronuclear development (see Table VI; Fig. 8). In contrast, very few sperm are attached to the precipitated zona surface of eggs pretreated with antiserum, and these sperm can easily be removed by washing. Also, antiserum-treated eggs show no evidence of penetration (see Table VI; Fig. 8).

TABLE VI
Sperm Attachment and Penetration in Hamster Ova Treated with Antiserums[a]

Absorbing agent	Zona precipitation	Ova examined	No. of sperm attached per ovum		Ova penetrated		
			Range	Average	No. observed	No. penetrated	Percent penetrated
Saline							
None	−	22	17–54	31.9			
Normal serum							
None	−	66	17–58	38.9	58	28	48.3
Antiserum to ovary							
Ovary	−	15	11–54	31.0	80	61	76.3
None	+	57	0–21	6.5	64	0	0
Small intestine	+	82	0–15	2.7	106	0	0

[a] From Shivers *et al.* (1972). Copyright 1972 by the American Association for the Advancement of Science.

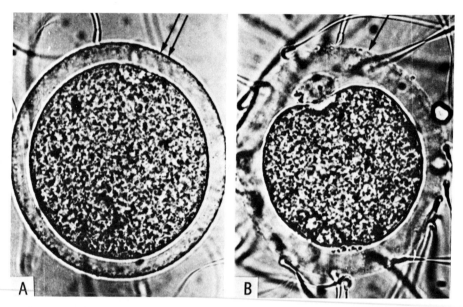

Fig. 8. Inhibition of sperm attachment to and penetration of the hamster egg by zona-precipitating antibody. (A) Hamster egg treated with zona precipitating antibody and then inseminated. Very few sperm can be seen attached to the densely precipitated zona (double arrows). (B) Hamster egg treated with preimmune serum and then inseminated *in vitro*. Numerous sperm can be seen attached to the zona pellucida. The zona is not precipitated (single arrow). From Shivers *et al*. (1972). Copyright 1972 by the American Association for the Advancement of Science.

5. Inhibition of Hatching

Evidence suggests that at least two mechanisms are available whereby the zona pellucida is removed from the embryo prior to implantation (for review, see Dickmann, 1969; McLaren, 1970). One of these includes a "hatching" or shedding mechanism where the embryo, by means of pulsating contractions, is capable of splitting and emerging from the zona. It has been demonstrated, using the mouse (Shivers, 1974), that the presence of the antibody produced precipitation layer on the zona greatly inhibits this hatching mechanism.

Female mice are superovulated and mated. Females demonstrating vaginal plugs are killed 36 hours after mating and the reproductive tracts flushed with culture medium (Brinster, 1971) to obtain the embryos which are at the 2- to 4-cell stage of development. The embryos are placed in either 0.1–0.5 ml of antiserum or the control preparations for 20 minutes at 37°C, washed in culture medium, and allowed to develop *in vitro* for approximately 74 hours (for culture procedures, see Brinster, 1965; Hoppe and Pitts, 1973). Examination of the embryos following the culture period shows that the hatching mechanism in

TABLE VII
Inhibition of Zona Shedding in the Mouse by Zona Precipitating Antibody[a]

Treatment	Total	Number of blastocysts			
		Without zona	Zona shedding	With zona	Shed or shedding (%)
Brinster's medium	90	58	18	13	84.5
Control serum	48	19	15	14	71.0
Antibody absorbed with ovary	28	23	2	3	92.0
Unabsorbed antibody	88	1	2	85	3.3

[a] Embryos at the 2 to 4-cell stage were exposed to the appropriate solutions and cultured *in vitro* for 74 hours. Antibody was prepared in the rabbit against mouse ovary. From Shivers (1974).

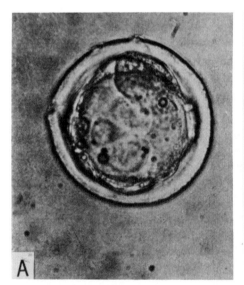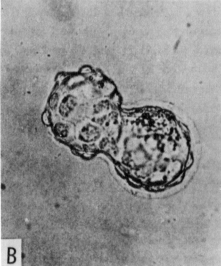

Fig. 9. Inhibition of zona hatching or shedding in the mouse by zona precipitating antibody. (A) Mouse embryo treated at 2-cell stage with a zona precipitating antiserum and then cultured *in vitro* for 74 hours. Note the precipitate is still on the zona surface; the embryo was unable to escape from the zona. (B) Embryo treated at 2-cell stage with preimmune serum and cultured as in (A). No precipitate is present and the embryo is in the process of escaping from the zona. From Shivers (1974).

TABLE VIII
Effect of ZPA on Implantation

Treatment[a]	Pregnant uterine horns[b]	No. of embryos transferred[c]	No. of implantation sites[d]	Percentage implantation[e]
CM	7/11 (63.6)	84	18(1)	19/84 (22.6)
PRS	9/12 (75.0)	111	10(5)	15/111(13.5)
ZPA	2/10 (20.0)	110	0(5)	5/110 (4.5)

[a] CM, control medium (Tyrode's, Brinster's, Ham's F–10); PRS, preimmune rabbit serum; ZPA, zona-precipitating antibody. From Dudkiewicz et al. (1975).

[b] Number of uterine horns showing implantation sites/total number of horns. The percentage is shown in parentheses.

[c] Most of the embryos transferred were cavitated blastocysts; however, some preblastocyst stages were also transferred.

[d] The number of resorptions is shown in parentheses.

[e] Comparison of percentage implantation; CM versus ZPA, $p < 0.001$; PRS versus ZPA $p < 0.02$; PRS versus CM, not significant.

embryos treated with antibody to zona has been greatly inhibited (see Fig. 9; Table VII).

Both inhibition of zona lysis and the hatching mechanism have been shown to occur *in vivo* by the reduced ability of hamster embryos pretreated with antibodies against zona to undergo normal implantation when transferred to pseudopregnant hosts (Dudkiewicz et al., 1975). Embryo donors were killed approximately 5–13 hours prior to implantation on day 3 p.c., the reproductive tracts flushed with Brinster's medium (Brinster, 1971), and the embryos (most were cavitated blastocysts) immediately treated for 10–15 minutes at 37°C with anti-zona serum, preimmune serum, or control medium. The treated embryos were then transferred surgically into the uterine lumen of synchronous pseudopregnant hosts on day 3 of a second pseudopregnant cycle. The uterine horns of these embryo recipients are then examined on days 6 and 9 of the pseudopregnancy for the presence of implantation sites (see Table VIII).

C. Testing Effect of Antiserum on Fertility

The ultimate test of any immunocontraceptive approach to fertility regulation is the inhibition of fertility by antiserum without the production of adverse side effects. This fertility inhibition may be achieved following either active or passive immunization procedures (for reviews, see Celada, 1974; Tung, 1976). Both *in vitro* and *in vivo* fertilization have been inhibited in at least three species (hamster, mouse, and rat) by antibodies directed against zona pellucida antigen(s) (Jilek and Pavlok, 1975; Oikawa and Yanagimachi, 1975; Tsunoda and

Chang, 1976a–d). The methods used to demonstrate this inhibition by anti-zona serum are described below.

1. Inhibition of in Vitro Fertilization

Procedures describing the various methods to accomplish *in vitro* fertilization for different species are available in the literature (for reviews, see Seitz *et al.*, 1973; Gould, 1973; Brackett *et al.*, 1972). To demonstrate the inhibition of fertilization by specific antibody against zona requires the exposure of the unfertilized eggs to the antiserum either prior to or during the fertilization process. The former approach seems more popular. Unfertilized eggs, either with or without cumulus cells, are incubated at 35–37°C for 30–40 minutes in culture medium containing either antiserum with antibodies against zona, preimmune serum, or the control preparations. The concentration of serum in the culture medium has varied from 1.25 to 50% or 20 to 50 mg protein/ml, depending upon the investigator. Following this incubation step, the sperm suspension is added to the culture medium. In some instances, the sera to be tested are preabsorbed with sperm to remove any natural sperm agglutinins if present. A modification of this

TABLE IX
Effect of Anti-Ovarian Rabbit Heteroimmune Serum on Fertilization in Mice[a]

Treatment	Concentration of sera (%)	In Vitro			Time after PMSG (hours) in vivo	
		Intact ova (Exp. 1)	Zona-free ova	Intact ova (Exp. 2)	7	31
Specific	10	0 (21)	100(21)		0.6(158)	0 (48)
immune	5	0 (57)	100(53)	0 (73)		
serum	2.5	—	—	1.7(60)		
	1.25	—	—	7.2(69)		
Ovary-	5	—	—	57.9(57)	—	—
absorbed	2.5	—	—	60 (75)		
immune	1.25	—	—	77.8(63)		
serum						
Control	10	94.4(18)	100(20)	—	97.1(139)	91.4(35)
serum	5	93 (57)	96.4(55)	—		
Untreated	—	89 (82)	97.3(76)	70.9(55)	—	—
medium						

[a] The values show the percentage of eggs fertilized. The number of eggs examined is given in parentheses. Specific immune serum, rabbit anti-mouse ovary serum absorbed with mouse serum, liver, spleen, and kidney. From Jilek and Pavlok (1975).

approach is the addition of the sera to be tested in the sperm suspension which is made up of culture medium. Thirty minutes later, the unfertilized eggs are added to the sperm suspension. Table IX shows the inhibition of *in vitro* fertilization in the mouse by anti-ovary serum rendered specific to the mouse zona by absorption.

2. Inhibition of in Vivo Fertilization

The majority of investigations to date have concerned the effect of passive immunization with antibodies against zona antigen(s) on fertilization. Animals (mouse, hamster, rat) subjected to procedures to induce superovulation are passively immunized (either intraperitoneally or subcutaneously) with antiserum, control serum, or the control preparations. Either 0.3 ml of the antiserum (whole serum or crude γ globulin fraction obtained by salt fractionation) or preparations containing > 40 mg protein/ml have been found to inhibit effectively fertilization. Animals can be immunized either prior to or immediately following natural or artificial insemination (see Oikawa and Yanagimachi, 1975, for artificial insemination procedure). The animals are killed approximately 24 hours following insemination, the oviducts flushed, and the eggs examined for evidence of fertilization. Tables IX and X summarize the results obtained using these procedures in the mouse and hamster, respectively.

TABLE X
Block to Fertilization of Hamster Eggs *In Vivo*[a] by Anti-Hamster Ovary Serum Fraction

Fraction injected	Amount of fraction injected (mg protein)	No. of animals	Eggs		Light scattering of outer region of zona[c]
			No. examined	Percentage fertilized[b]	
Anti-ovary	4	4	74	100.0	± to +
serum	20	3	47	55.3	+ +
fraction	30	3	52	28.8	+ +
(AOSF)	40	3	49	0	+ + +
	50	4	61	0	+ + +
Control	4	3	38	100.0	−
serum frac-	20	3	41	100.0	−
tion (CSF)	50	3	47	100.0	−

[a] Estrous females were naturally or artificially inseminated and injected with serum fraction, then killed the next morning.

[b] All fertilized eggs were in the pronuclear stage with well-developed pronuclei, and all were monospermic. Unfertilized eggs showed no sign of sperm passage through the zona pellucida.

[c] Examined under dark-field illumination: very strong ($+ + +$), moderate ($+ +$), weak ($+$), faint ($\pm$), and no ($-$) light scattering. From Oikawa and Yanagimachi (1975).

V. SUMMARY

The inhibition of fertility and development by immunologic means is a broad and continuously expanding area of research. It is beyond the scope of the present chapter to describe in intimate detail the myriad procedures involved for the preparation of different antigens, production and collection of antisera, testing antisera specificity, absorbing antisera, and testing antisera effect both on the target antigen and on fertilization and development. The major purpose of this chapter was to familiarize the reader with the concepts of immunocontraception, and to present a description of the procedures one should take to explore this approach to fertility regulation. The antigens associated with the ovary and zona pellucida were used as the model system.

For those interested in working in the area of immunocontraception, two topics discussed in this chapter warrant reemphasis due to their critical importance to this approach of reproduction control. These include (1) the absolute necessity for establishing the tissue specificity of the antigen involved by the examination of numerous tissues by several different techniques such as immunodiffusion, immunofluorescence, RIA, etc.; (2) the need to reconfirm *all* findings using purified [IgG or F(ab')₂ fractions] antiserum preparations. By this critical examination of specific antigens that may be present in reproductive tissues, there exists the potential for a new and effective means of fertility regulation.

REFERENCES

Bowman, P., and McLaren, A. (1970). *J. Embryol. Exp. Morphol.* **24**, 331–334.
Brackett, B. G., Seitz, H. M., Rocha, G., and Mastroianni, L. (1972). *In* "Biology of Mammalian Fertilization and Implantation" (K. S. Moghissi and E. S. E. Hafez, eds.), p. 165. Thomas, Springfield, Illinois.
Brinster, R. L. (1965). *J. Reprod. Fertil.* **10**, 227–240.
Brinster, R. L. (1971). *In* "Methods in Mammalian Embryology" (J. C. Daniel, Jr., ed.), p. 215. Freeman, San Francisco, California.
Celada, F. (1974). *In* "Immunological Approaches to Fertility Control" (E. Diczfalusy, ed.), Karolinska Symp. No. 7, p. 419. Karolinska Inst., Stockholm.
Daniel, J. C., Jr., ed. (1971). "Methods in Mammalian Embryology." Freeman, San Francisco, California.
Dickmann, Z. (1969). *Adv. Reprod. Physiol.* **4**, 187.
Diczfalusy, E., ed. (1974). "Immunological Approaches to Fertility Control," Karolinska Symp. No. 7. Karolinska Inst., Stockholm.
Dudkiewicz, A. B., Noske, I. G., and Shivers, C. A. (1975). *Fertil. Steril.* **26**, 686–694.
Dunbar, B. S., and Shivers, C. A. (1976). *Immunol. Commun.* **5**, 375–385.
Fox, L. L., and Shivers, C. A. (1972). *In* "Embryonic and Fetal Antigens in Cancer" (N. G. Anderson *et al.*, eds.), Vol. 2, p. 35. Natl. Tech. Inf. Serv., U.S. Dept. of Commerce, Springfield, Virginia.
Fox, L. L., and Shivers, C. A. (1975). *Fertil. Steril.* **26**, 579–608.

Glass, L. E. (1971). *In* "Methods in Mammalian Embryology" (J. C. Daniel, Jr., ed.), p. 355. Freeman, San Francisco, California.

Goldman, M. (1968). "Fluorescent Antibody Methods." Academic Press, New York.

Gould, K. G. (1973). *Fed. Proc., Fed. Am. Soc. Exp. Biol.* **32**, 2069–2074.

Hoppe, P. C., and Pitts, S. (1973). *Biol. Reprod.* **8**, 420–426.

Inoue, M., and Wolf, D. P. (1974). *Biol. Reprod.* **10**, 512–518.

Jilek, F., and Pavlok, A. (1975). *J. Reprod. Fertil.* **42**, 377–380.

Krzanowska, H. (1972). *J. Reprod. Fertil.* **31**, 7–14.

Lowry, O. H., Rosebrough, N. J., Farr, A. L., and Randall, R. J. (1951). *J. Biol. Chem.* **193**, 265–275.

McLaren, A. (1970). *J. Embryol. Exp. Morphol.* **23**, 1–19.

Mancini, R. E. (1971). *In* "Control of Human Fertility" (E. Diczfalusy and U. Borell, eds.), p. 157. Wiley (Interscience), New York.

Oikawa, T., and Yanagimachi, R. (1975). *J. Reprod. Fertil.* **45**, 487–494.

Ownby, C. L., and Shivers, C. A. (1972). *Biol. Reprod.* **6**, 310–318.

Sacco, A. G. (1977a). *Biol. Reprod.* **16**, 158–163.

Sacco, A. G. (1977b). *Biol. Reprod.* **16**, 164–173.

Sacco, A. G., and Palm, V. S. (1977). *J. Reprod. Fertil.* **51**, 165–168.

Sacco, A. G., and Shivers, C. A. (1973a). *J. Reprod. Fertil.* **32**, 403–414.

Sacco, A. G., and Shivers, C. A. (1973b). *Biol. Reprod.* **8**, 481–490.

Sacco, A. G., and Shivers, C. A. (1973c). *J. Reprod. Fertil.* **32**, 415–420.

Seitz, H. M., Brackett, B. G., and Mastroianni, L. (1973). *In* "Human Reproduction: Conception and Contraception" (E. S. E. Hafez and T. N. Evans, eds.), p. 119. Harper, Hagerstown, Maryland.

Shivers, C. A. (1974). *In* "Immunological Approaches to Fertility Control" (E. Diczfalusy, ed.), Karolinska Symp. No. 7, p. 223. Karolinska Inst., Stockholm.

Shivers, C. A., and Dunbar, B. S. (1977). *Science* **197**, 1082–1084.

Shivers, C. A., Dudkiewicz, A. B., Franklin, L. E., and Russell, E. N. (1972). *Science* **178**, 1211–1213.

Tsunoda, Y., and Chang, M. C. (1976a). *J. Reprod. Fertil.* **46**, 379–382.

Tsunoda, Y., and Chang, M. C. (1976b). *Biol. Reprod.* **14**, 354–361.

Tsunoda, Y., and Chang, M. C. (1976c). *Biol. Reprod.* **15**, 361–365.

Tsunoda, Y., and Chang, M. C. (1976d). *J. Exp. Zool.* **195**, 409–416.

Tung, K. S. K. (1976). *In* "Development of Vaccines for Fertility Regulation," World Health Organ. Symp., 1975, p. 127. Scriptor, Copenhagen.

Vaitukaitis, J., Robbins, J. B., Nieschlag, E., and Ross, G. T. (1971). *J. Clin. Endocrinol. Metab.* **33**, 988–991.

Weir, D. M., ed. (1973). "Handbook of Experimental Immunology," 2nd ed. Blackwell, Oxford.

World Health Organization. (1976). "Development of Vaccines for Fertility Regulation." Scriptor, Copenhagen.

Yanagimachi, R., Winkelhake, J. L., and Nicolson, G. L. (1976). *Proc. Natl. Acad. Sci. U.S.A.* **73**, 2405–2408.

10

In Vitro Development of Whole Mouse Embryos beyond the Implantation Stage

Y-C. HSU

I. INTRODUCTION

In vivo, the trophoblast invades the uterine stroma during implantation, forming a three-dimensional structure which interlocks with the inner cell mass. On a glass or plastic surface, however, the trophoblast spreads out in a two-dimensional monolayer. Jenkinson and Wilson (1970) attempted to injected mouse blastocysts into a network of bovine lens fibers to provide a three-

229

dimensional support *in vitro* for blastocysts. They obtained a relatively high ratio of development up to an early egg cylinder stage (stage 9 of Fig. 1). Further development *in vitro*, however, was never achieved. Cole and Paul (1965) were first to have used reconstituted rat tail collagen for blastocyst attachment to mimic *in vivo* implantation. They have developed a small percentage of "cysts" which morphologically resembled yolk sacs. It has also been reported that an egg cylinder of mouse embryos of 7 days' gestation (stage 12) has been developed to the early somite (stage 15) stage (Tamarin and Jones, 1968; Moore and Metcalf, 1970). Although rat embryos have been developed *in vitro* for about 2 days at any stage between day 8 and day 14 of gestation, it is not possible yet to continuously develop rat embryos *in vitro* from days 8 to 14 (New, 1971; Robkin

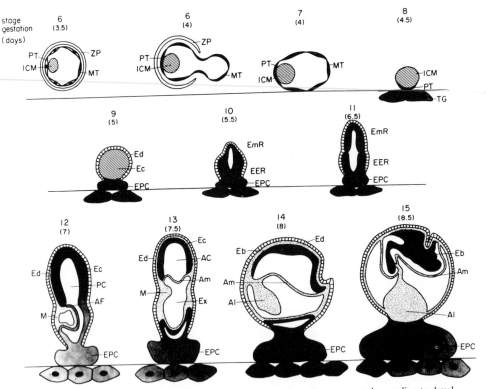

Fig. 1. Mouse embryos developed *in vitro* from blastocysts are represented according to developmental stages (upper) in relation to gestational days (in parentheses). AC, Amniotic cavity; AF, amniotic fold; Al, allantois; Am, amnion; Eb, embryo; Ec, ectoderm; Ed, endoderm; EER, extraembryonic region; EmR, embryonic region; EPC, ectoplacental cone; Ex, exocoelum; ICM, inner cell mass; M, mesoderm; MT, mural trophoblast; Pc, proamniotic cavity; PT, polar trophoblast; TG, trophoblastic giant cell; ZP, zona pellucida.

et al., 1972). This paper will deal exclusively with the *in vitro* development of mouse embryos beyond the implantation stage.

After using many experimental methods during the last 8 years (Hsu, 1971; Hsu, 1972), our laboratory has developed a successful procedure. Although many modifications on developing mouse embryos *in vitro* beyond the implantation stage have been reported (Spindle and Pedersen, 1973; Wilson and Jenkinson, 1974; Pienkowski *et al.*, 1974; Sherman, 1975a,b; McLaren and Hensleigh, 1975; Juurlink and Fedoroff, 1977), to develop mouse embryos *in vitro* is to reconstruct the delicate and precise *in vivo* processes in an artificial environment. The slightest deviation from this procedure may cause complete arrest of differentiation, although many modifications or alternatives are possible. However, an effort was made to make the procedure as simple as possible without using elaborate equipment. Two excellent descriptions of methodology on cultivating preimplantation mouse embryos by Biggers *et al.* (1971) and Mintz (1971) should be referred to. Mouse embryos developed *in vitro* are schematically depicted in Fig. 1, which is based on the classification of Witschi (1972) and Theiler (1972). It is now possible to develop mouse embryos from the 2-cell stage (stage 2) to the early somite stage with well-organized ectoplacental cones (stage 15) (Hsu *et al.*, 1974). Figure 1 shows development of the mouse embryo only from the stage of the blastocyst (3.5 days' gestation) to early somite (8.5 days' gestation). With the current method, it takes 7 to 8 days to develop mouse embryos *in vitro* (from stage 6 to 15), compared to 5 days' gestation *in utero*. The developmental delay of 2 days occurs from stages 7 to 9. Part of the delay *in vitro* at this stage may be caused by adaptation of the blastocyst to the new environment of culture medium. Another reason for delay may be the difficulty in inducing differentiation of endoderm and ectoderm from inner cell mass. The remainder of the *in vitro* development is comparable to *in vivo* development from stages 10 to 15.

II. COLLAGEN

It has been reported that mouse blastocysts attach and differentiate on plastic culture dishes (Spindle and Pedersen, 1973; Pienkowski *et al.*, 1974; McLaren and Hensleigh, 1975; Sherman, 1975a,b). However, the egg cylinders that develop beyond stage 12 on the surface of plastic tend to be more abnormal than those developed on collagen. Therefore, it is recommended that plastic surfaces be coated with collagen. It has been demonstrated that collagen has the function of maintaining tissue architecture. This extracellular structural material maintains cellular arrangement by fixing relative positions and distances between cells and tissues and also supplies adhesive sites. Collagen is in this way essential for cell polarity and may produce sieving effects and diffusion gradients. All these functions of collagen may have some relevance in tissue interactions *in vitro* for the control of cell differentiation.

Our method of collagen preparation is a slight modification of that used by Ehrmann and Gey (1956). Collagen is prepared in a horizontal laminar flow hood (Edgegard, Baker Co., Sanford, Maine) under strict sterilization precautions. After anesthetizing the rats, the tails are amputated, scrubbed thoroughly with soap, then 70% alcohol and soaked for 15 minutes in a large petri dish containing 70% alcohol. Tendons are recovered by successively fracturing the tail (beginning at the tip) with large Kelly clamps (Fig. 2). By using a shearing and pulling motion, the tendons are freed from the long tail segment. The long tendons from each tail segment were cut and placed in a 90-mm diameter petri dish two-thirds full of distilled water. The tendons from one rat tail were teased into finer filaments with two pairs of fine forceps, transferred to two 100-ml centrifuge bottles containing 80 ml each of a 1:1000 dilution of glacial acetic acid, and stored for 24 hours at 4°C. The bottle of collagen suspension is swirled occasionally. Collagen is extracted from the swollen fibers after centrifugation for about 1 hour at 1500 rpm in a Sorvall refrigerated centrifuge (RC-5). The clear supernatant contains the collagen. The extraction is repeated two to three times at 24-hour intervals. The supernatant is replaced each time with only one-half its original volume of the acetic acid solution. The pooled collagen solution is centrifuged once more at 1500 rpm for 1 hour at 4°C with a Sorvall refrigerated centrifuge. Clarified collagen extracts may be frozen at −20°C in 50-ml aliquots. When

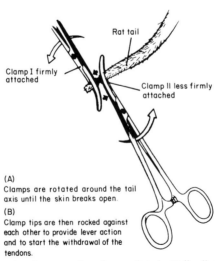

Fig. 2.   Isolation of tendons for preparation of reconstituted rat tail collagen (see text for details).

aliquots are needed, they are thawed and dialyzed in cellulose dialysis tubing (A. H. Thomas Co., inflated diameter ⅝ inch) against 2 liters of sterilized distilled water with two to three changes for 10- to 24-hour intervals. The viscosity of the collagen was tested with each water change. Dialysis is terminated before the collagen becomes too thick to pipette. One milliliter of collagen solution is used to coat a 35-mm plastic culture dish (Falcon Cat. No. 3001). Sterilized filter paper (23 mm in diameter) (Whatman 3MM) is placed on the cover of a 35-mm plastic culture dish. Three to four drops of NH_4OH is put on the filter paper in the cover of the culture dish in a vertical laminar flow hood for 15 minutes so that the ammonium vapor will neutralize the collagen. The blower motor of the laminar flow hood is stopped during this period. Residual NH_4OH is removed by soaking the dishes in sterile water. The collagen-coated dishes are incubated at 37°C in a humidified CO_2 incubator overnight. The sterile water for soaking plates is warmed previously at 37°C to prevent shrinkage and detachment of collagen from the culture dishes. The sterile water was changed two more times at intervals of 9–24 hours. A few hours before use, culture medium is introduced into the dishes to equilibrate them.

III. SERA

Three kinds of sera are used; calf serum (CS), fetal calf serum (FCS), and human cord serum (HCS). The most important part in developing mouse embryos *in vitro* is proper preparation of sera. The optimal concentration of sera in Eagle's minimal essential medium (MEM) is 10–20%, and all serum is heat inactivated at 56°C for 30 minutes before use.

A. Calf Serum (CS)

Commercial calf serum is divided in small glass vials, 4 ml each, and frozen at −20°C. It should be used within 3 months. Calf serum is used to culture blastocysts from stages 6 to 8.

B. Fetal Calf Serum (FCS)

Before purchasing a large stock, we obtained samples of fetal calf serum from the Grand Island Biological Company, New York to confirm the biologic activity of developing egg cylinders from blastocyst (from stages 8 to 10). FCS is also divided into 4 ml each in small glass vials and stored at −20°C.

The FCS can be used to develop mouse embryos only up to the stage of early egg cylinder (stage 11). Most mouse embryos developed in FCS became abnormal as the embryo develops to the later stages. We have never succeeded in developing mouse embryos to the early somite stage by cultivating in FCS. The embryonic region of the egg cylinder grown in FCS becomes atrophic after stage 12 and eventually disappears, leaving a yolk sac without an embryo proper. (This may correspond to the blighted ova in human pregnancy.) Mouse embryos are cultured in human cord serum after stage 12.

C. Human Cord Serum (HCS)

Blood is withdrawn from the umbilical cord while the placenta is still in the uterus. Usually, 30–50 ml of blood can be obtained from one delivery by an experienced obstetrician. The glass tube containing cord blood is placed on the bench top at room temperature until the blood coagulates. The coagulated blood is then stored overnight in a refrigerator at 4°C. The next morning, serum is separated from the blood clot by centrifuging twice at 3000 rpm. Two to four milliliters of nonhemolyzed serum is placed in small vials, and heat-inactivated at 56°C for 30 minutes. The yellowish serum is stored in a −40°C refrigerator.

Hemolyzed serum cannot be used in the early implantation stages. The hemolyzed serum does not affect shedding of the zona pellucida or attachment of blastocysts, but growth of the inner cell mass at stage 8 (usual implantation stage) will be inhibited and disorganized.

IV. CULTURE MEDIA

Levels of circulating ovarian steroid hormones increase immediately prior to and at the time of implantation. When mouse blastocysts are cultured in a physiological concentration of progesterone and estradiol, the steroids do not seem to directly induce differentiation of endoderm and ectoderm from the inner cell mass (from stages 8 to 9) (Y-C. Hsu, unpublished results). It has been shown that steroid hormones stimulate the biosynthesis of many proteins and lipoproteins in distant organs such as liver and oviduct in birds and amphibia. Although the chemical nature of the active component(s) in fetal calf serum and human cord serum which is essential for embryo development is not known, to mimic the in vivo conditions, mouse blastocysts were initially cultured in calf serum for 48 hours, during which shedding of the zona pellucida and attachment and outgrowth of the mural trophoblast took place. Calf serum was then replaced by fetal calf serum or human cord serum, which presumably act as gene activators on stage 8 to induce the differentiation of endoderm and ectoderm (stage 9).

Eagle's minimum essential medium (MEM) with Earle's base (Gibco Cat. No.

109 or Microbiological Associates Cat. No. 12-125) is used. The MEM is supplemented with 1 mM l-glutamine and 1 mM sodium pyruvate. Antibiotics are not added because it is not yet clear whether they interfere with embryo development. Three kinds of heat-inactivated serum are added at a final concentration of 10–20%. The medium is changed every day after the blastocysts attach to the collagen.

The heat inactivated serum in MEM may be as shown in the following tabulation:

Schedule of changing serum	
Day 0 of culture	10% CS
Day 2 (after 48 hours of incubation)	10% FCS
Day 3	20% FCS
Day 4	10% FCS + 10% HCS
Day 5 and thereafter	20% HCS

For culture of trophoblasts, medium CMRL-1066 was used beyond stage 15 (see tabulation below).

CMRL-1066	78ml
Heat-inactivated human cord serum	20 ml
100 mM l-glutamine	1 ml
100 mM sodium-pyruvate	1 ml
Total medium	100 ml

V. OBTAINING BLASTOCYSTS FROM MICE

Both inbred and random bred mice can be used. For economical reasons, we usually use random bred CF No. 1 from Charles River Co., Massachusetts. We consistently obtain a large yield of blastocysts from 8- to 11-week-old female mice. Six-week-old female mice are purchased from a commercial farm and placed five to a box in a light-controlled room for at least 1 week before hormone treatment. Male mice should be between 3 and 9 months old. The mating rate decreases abruptly when male mice reach the age of 10 months. All outdoor light is excluded from the animal colony. In our colony, the light is automatically controlled to maintain 11 hours of darkness and 13 hours of light, that is a light period from 5:30 A.M. to 6:30 P.M. in winter and from 6:30 A.M. to 7:30 P.M. in summer. The animal room temperature is kept at 23°C. Our central animal room is fully accredited by the American Association for Accreditation of Laboratory Animal Care. Pregnant mare serum gonadotropin (PMSG) is given to stimulate follicular growth, then human chorionicgonadotropin (HCG) is injected 48 hours later to stimulate ovulation (Runner and Gates, 1954). Ovulation generally follows HCG injection by 11–14 hours, and mating usually precedes ovulation by 1–5 hours. Optimal dose response to hormone treatment varies, depending on the mouse strain.

Hormones

1. Pregnant Mare's Serum Gonadotropin (PMSG)

Gestyl (Organon, Inc., West Orange, New Jersey), or gonadotropin (Sigma Co., Cat. No. G4877), is dissolved with phosphate buffered saline (PBS) to a concentration of 400 IU/ml. The PMSG solution is divided into small aliquots and stored at −20°C as the stock solution. Stock solution (0.1 ml) was diluted on the day of injection with 1.5 ml of PBS (25 IU/ml). Each 0.2 ml of diluted PMS at the concentration of 25 IU/ml was injected ip.

2. Human Chorionic Gonadotropin (HCG)

APL (chorionic gonadotropin for injection, USP, Ayerst Laboratories, 685 Third Avenue, New York, New York), chorionic gonadotropin (Sigma Co., Cat. No. CG-2, CG-5, or CG-10), or Pregnyl (Organon, Inc., West Orange, New Jersey) were used to stimulate ovulation. HCG is dissolved to a concentration of 500 IU/ml with PBS, divided into 1-ml aliquots, and stored at −20°C as a stock solution. The stock solution, which should be used within 3 months, is thawed on the day of injection and diluted to the final concentration of 25 IU/ml with PBS. Each 0.2-ml aliquot is injected ip into the mice.

All 8- to 11-week-old female mice are injected at 4:00 P.M. with 5 IU of PMSG; 48 hours later the same mice are injected with 5 IU of HCG. They are placed with males, one pair to a freshly cleaned cage. The next morning, the females are checked for the presence of a vaginal sperm plug (day 0 of pregnancy).

VI. PREPARATION OF BLASTOCYSTS

1. On the 3rd day of pregnancy, mice are killed by cervical dislocation. The uteri are removed from their mesometrium and placed in a 100-mm plastic

culture dish. All operations under this section are performed under a horizontal laminar flow hood (Edgegard, Baker Co., Sanford, Maine).

2. The dish is placed under a dissecting microscope (Bausch and Lomb, Zoom 7), with reflected light.

3. Under the dissecting microscope with $10-70 \times$ magnification, the filed syringe needle (25 gauge) is inserted into the vaginal end of each uterine horn, which is then flushed with 1 ml of culture medium.

4. Blastocysts are located by scanning the flushing medium under the dissecting microscope. They are sucked up into a capillary pipette, operated by a 1-ml Hamilton microsyringe (No. 0010). Preparation of capillary pipettes is described by Rafferty (1970).

5. Blastocysts are pooled in a 35-mm diameter plastic culture dish containing 2 ml of culture medium which is constantly flushed with 5% CO_2 and 95% air (Mintz, 1971).

6. Blastocysts are drawn up into a capillary pipette and distributed into plastic culture dishes.

7. The culture dishes are incubated at 37°C in a humidified CO_2 incubator with 5% CO_2 and 95% air.

VII. THE WATER-JACKETED, AUTOMATIC CO_2 CONTROL INCUBATORS

Since the mammalian embryo is highly adapted to the mother's environment, the pH should be kept at an optimal 7.4 ± 0.5 by equilibration with $5 \pm 0.5\%$ CO_2 and 95% air at 37°C. The CO_2 concentration in the incubator should be standardized by a Fyrite test kit (Bacharach Instrument Co., Pittsburgh, Pennsylvania). To avoid CO_2 stratification, an incubator equipped with a small fan to circulate the chamber atmosphere continuously is recommended (Forma Scientific, Marietta, Ohio, Model 3156 or 3171). The distilled water in the bottom of the CO_2 incubator is changed every 2 weeks to avoid mold contamination.

VIII. MOUSE DEVELOPMENT *IN VITRO*

In some blastocysts, part of the trophoblast or inner cell mass may herniate through a hole in the zona pellucida immediately after being placed in the incubator (Fig. 3D). This shedding of the zona pellucida may continue for the next 24 hours by slow contraction and relaxation of the trophoblast (Fig. 3E). In other blastocysts, the zona pellucida becomes thinner without a noticeable hole and eventually disappear from the blastocysts. It appears that blastocysts release some enzyme(s) upon response to some serum components and dissolve the zona

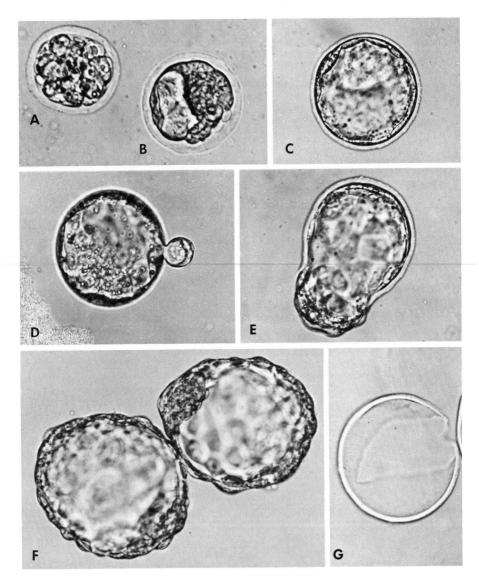

Fig. 3.   Mouse blastocysts hatching from zona pellucida equivalent to 4 days' gestation, × 200. Morula (A), early (B) and late (C) blastocyst stages. Blastocysts escaping from the zona pellucida (D and E). Denuded and expanded blastocysts (F) and empty zona pellucida shell (G).

pellucida. The denuded blastocysts (stage 7 in Fig. 1 and Fig. 3F) expand their diameter by about 1.5 times during the next 12 hours. The mural trophoblasts of expanded blastocysts sink on the collagen's surface. Many such trophoblasts have their inner-cell mass downward and extend many pseudopods from their cell surfaces. The pseudopods of a mural trophoblast anchor on the collagen and

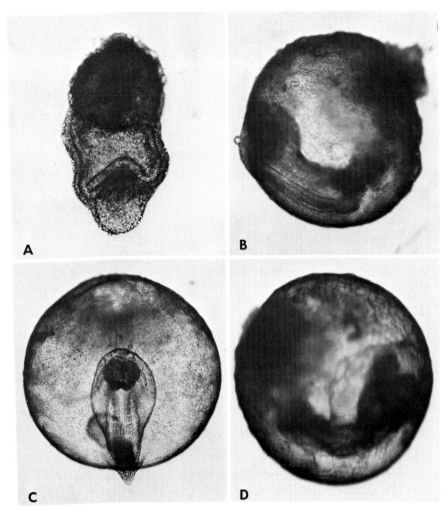

Fig. 5. Mouse embryo development *in vitro* from late egg cylinder stage to early somite stage. (From Hsu, 1973 by permission from Academic Press). (A), × 100; (B), × 60; (C), × 40; (D), × 30.

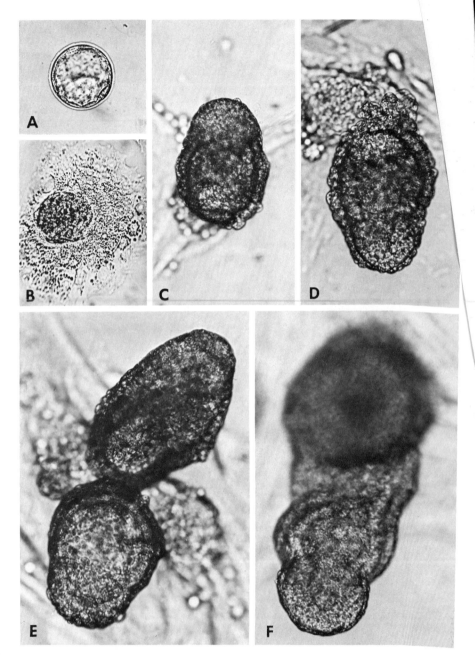

Fig. 4. Stages seen as mouse blastocysts developed in culture to late egg cylinder stage, × 200. From Hsu, 1973, by permission from Academic Press.

begin to spread out on the surface to form primary giant cells within 48 hours of incubation. Thus, the three-dimensional structure of the trophoblast wall collapses as the mural trophoblast spreads out and migrates outwards, leaving the inner cell mass on the center of the trophoblast sheet (stage 8 in Fig. 1 and Fig. 4B). On the collagen surface, the inner cell mass remains round, and mounds of three-dimensional structures with a smooth edge surround the trophoblasts (Fig. 4B). While on the plastic surface, the inner cell mass becomes completely flat and spreads out with irregularly shaped edges and proliferates rapidly. Therefore, the inner cell mass loses its three-dimensional structure by spreading on the surface of the plastic dish which is coated with unknown chemicals by the manufacturer, presumably for supporting growing cells in monolayers. In fetal calf serum, the inner cell mass grows away from the collagen surface with a perfect spherical shape as the polar trophoblast proliferates instead of spreading on the plastic surface. Apparently, some component of the fetal serum causes the cell surfaces in the inner cell mass to stick together so that cells can grow as a spherical mass in the culture medium without external physical support to maintain a three-dimensional structure. Preserving the three-dimensional structure by

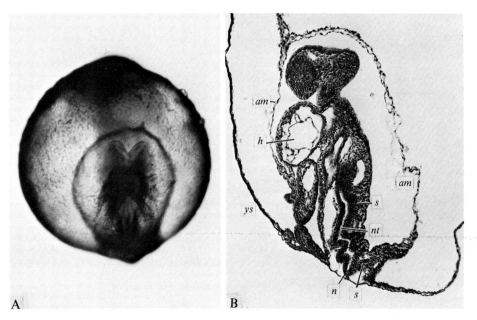

Fig. 6. (A) Live embryo developed *in vitro* which shows vitelline vessels (× 56) and (B) its histological section, × 140. am, Amnion; h, heart; ys, yolk sac; s, somite; nt, neural tube; and n, notochord. (From Hsu *et al.*, 1974 by permission from Cambridge University Press).

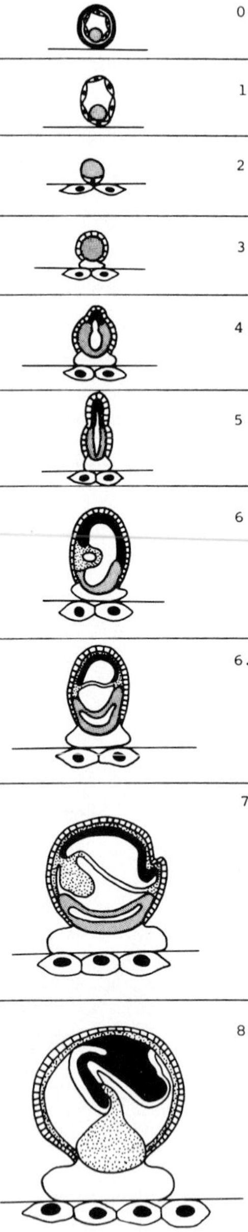

Stages Witschi	Theiler	Gestation Age		Culture in Days	Characteristics
6	5	(3.5)		0	Blastocyst with zona pellucida
7	5	(4)		1	Free blastocyst
8	6	(4.5)		2	Implanting blastocyst
9 (Gastrula)	7	(5)		3	Inner cell mass covered with endoderm (doughnut shape)
10	8	(5.5)		4	Inner cell mass begins differentiation into embryonic and extra-embryonic part
11	9	(6.5)		5	Proamniotic cavity, ecto-placental cone (snowman shape)
12 (Primitive streak)	10	(7)		6	Connecting ectochorionic and amniotic cavities; rudiments of amniotic folds; primitive streak
13 (Neurula)	11	(7.5)		6.5	Presomite neurula, fusion of chorioamniotic folds; amniotic stalk; bud of allanotic stalk
14	12	(7.75)		7	Somites 1-4 (occipital). neurula plus 3 cavities: ecto-chorionic cyst, exocoelom and amniotic cavity; ectochorionic cavity collapsing; allantoic stalk projects into exocoelom embryo bent dorsally
15	13	(8-8.5)		8	Somites 5-12 (cervical); 1st visceral arch; ectochorionic cyst fused with ectoplacenta and allantoic stalk.

Fig. 7. Developmental stages, gestation days, days *in vitro* development, and characteristics of mouse embryos.

cultivating blastocysts on the collagen surface and stimulating the rapid proliferation of the inner cell mass by some components of the fetal calf serum and human cord serum are two keys to developing mouse embryos at stage 15. The polar trophoblast proliferates at the abembryonal pole to form a conical shape partly enclosing the inner cell mass, which forms an ectoplacental cone at a later stage. The ectoplacental cone becomes a chorioallantoic placenta which is the main nutritional and gas exchange organ of embryos after 8.5 days' gestation. Within 72 hours of incubation, the inner cell mass (embryoblast) differentiates into epiblast (ectoderm) and hypoblast (endoderm) to form a doughnut-shaped structure (stage 9 of Fig. 1, Fig. 4C, and Fig. 7). The part of the epiblast opposite the ectoplacental cone proliferates rapidly and grows away from the embryoblast. Therefore, the whole embryoblast becomes elongated and forms an elipsoid shape (stage 10 of Fig. 1, Fig. 4D, and Fig. 7). The elongated egg cylinder soon divides into embryonic and extraembryonic regions (stage 11 of Fig. 1, Fig. 4F, and Fig. 7). The ectoderm of the extraembryonic region is depicted as the derivative of the trophoblast (Gardner and Papaioannou, 1975). The embryonic region develops into the embryo proper, while the extraembryonic region gives rise to the visceral yolk sac at stage 15. As the tip of the embryonic region proliferates and grows away from the ectoplacental cone, a primitive streak develops in between the endoderm and ectoderm to generate the mesoderm (stage 12 of Fig. 1 and Fig. 7). At stage 13 (neurula stage), a notochord can be observed under a dissecting microscope (Fig. 5B). At stage 14 (Fig. 1 and Fig. 5C), a neural fold and about five somites enclosed by amnion develop within the yolk sac. Allantois is extended from the caudal part of the embryo to the exocoelom. At stage 15 (Fig. 1 and Fig. 5D), the heart begins to beat. Blood islands are formed in the mesoderm of the yolk sac and soon communicate with each other to complete the blood circulatory system as the heart chambers contract. The primary erythroblasts within the vitelline vessels circulate in a pulsatory way as the heart contracts. Apparently normal development can occur *in vitro*, as judged by light and electron microscopic examination (Fig. 6; Hsu *et al.*, 1974).

IX. PROLIFERATION OF TROPHOBLAST

Soon after the inner cell mass attaches on the collagen, after 48 hours of incubation, the polar trophoblast proliferates to form an ectoplacental cone on top of the mural trophoblast which formed the primary giant cells (stage 9 in Fig. 1). The nuclear diameter of the primary giant cell gradually increases without cell division (Fig. 8C). As the cytotrophoblasts, from the polar trophoblast, divide rapidly and push the primary giant cell outward, the distal end of the cytotrophoblast mass transforms into secondary giant cells. The nuclear size of the trophoblast is variable. Numerous multinucleated syncytia (Fig. 8D) can be

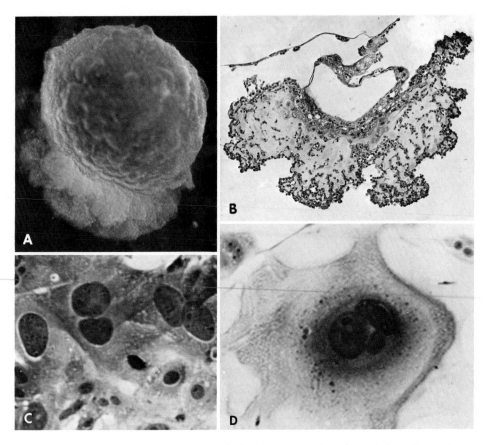

Fig. 8. Proliferation of placental labyrinth. In this example, after polar trophoblasts formed the ectoplacental cone in MEM plus 20% human cord serum for 7 days' cultivation, the medium was changed to CMRL-1066 plus 20% human cord serum. (A) The explacental cone continued to proliferate on the top of the collagen surface at the abembryonal pole of yolk sac. (B) A histological section of placental labyrinth in (A), which shows the cell islands composed of cytotrophoblasts. (C) The giant nuclei on the collagen surface among the smaller nuclei of cytotrophoblasts, and (D) syncytia formation of polykaryon formed on the collagen surface.

observed among the cytotrophoblasts. A three-dimensional discoid form of a well-organized placental labyrinth consisting of many lobuli may form on top of the giant cells (Fig. 8A). A histological section of this labyrinth shows many cytotrophoblast islands within the lobuli (Fig. 8B). However, the vascularization and other two cell layers of the giant cell which are normal components of placental labyrinth (Enders, 1965) do not develop. Differentiation *in vitro* of the chorionic placenta from of a 7-day stage mouse embryo has been reported (Hernandex-Verdin, 1975). Many clusters, each composed of various members of cytotrophoblasts, float free in the medium and resemble trophoblastic deportation *in vivo*. These clusters attach to the collagen and eventually degenerate.

ACKNOWLEDGMENT

This investigator was supported by Grant CA12336, awarded by the National Cancer Institute and in part by the Biomedical Research Support Branch, Grant FR05445, Division of Research Facilities and Resources, National Institute of Health, DHEW.

REFERENCES

Biggers, J. D., Whitten, W. K., and Whittingham, D. G. (1971). *In* "Methods in Mammalian Embryology" (J. C. Daniel, Jr., ed.), pp. 86–116. Freeman, San Francisco, California.

Cole, R. J., and Paul, J. (1965). *Preimplantation Stages Pregnancy, Ciba Found. Symp., 1965* pp. 82–122.

Ehrmann, R. L., and Gey, G. O. (1956). *J. Natl. Cancer Inst.* **16**, 1375–1390.

Enders, A. (1965). *Am. J. Anat.* **116**, 29–68.

Gardner, R. L., and Papaioannou, V. E. (1975). *In* "The Early Development of Mammals" (M. Balls and A. E. Wild, eds.), pp. 107–132. Cambridge Univ. Press, London and New York.

Hernandex-Verdin, D. (1975). *J. Embryol. Exp. Morphol.* **33**, 633–642.

Hsu, Y-C. (1971). *Nature (London)* **231**, 100–102.

Hsu, Y-C. (1972). *Nature (London)* **239**, 200–202.

Hsu, Y-C. (1973). *Dev. Biol.* **33**, 403–411.

Hsu, Y-C., Baskar, J., Stevens, L., and Rash, J. (1974). *J. Embryol. Exp. Morphol.* **31**, 235–245.

Jenkinson, E. J., and Wilson, I. B. (1970). *Nature (London)* **228**, 776–778.

Juurlink, B. H. G., and Fedoroff, S. (1977). *In Vitro* **13**, 790–798.

McLaren, A., and Hensleigh, H. C. (1975). *In* "The Early Development of Mammals" (M. Balls and A. E. Wild, eds.), pp. 45–60. Cambridge Univ. Press, London and New York.

Mintz, B. (1971). *In* "Methods in Mammalian Embryology" (J. C. Daniel, Jr., ed.), pp. 186–214. Freeman, San Francisco, California.

Moore, M. A. S., and Metcalf, D. (1970). *Br. J. Haematol.* **18**, 279–296.

New, D. A. T. (1971). *In* "Methods in Mammalian Embryology" (J. C. Daniel, Jr., ed.), pp. 305–319. Freeman, San Francisco, California.

Pienkowski, M., Solter, D., and Koprowski, H. (1974). *Exp. Cell Res.* **85**, 424–428.

Rafferty, K. A., Jr. (1970). "Methods in Experimental Embryology of the Mouse." Johns Hopkins Press, Baltimore, Maryland.

Robkin, M. A., Shepard, T. H., and Tanimura, T. (1972). *Teratology* **5**, 367–376.

Runner, M. N., and Gates, A. (1954). *Nature (London)* **174**, 222–223.

Sherman, M. I. (1975a). *Cell* **5**, 343–349.

Sherman, M. I. (1975b). *Differentiation* **3**, 51–67.

Spindle, A., and Pedersen, R. A. (1973). *J. Exp. Zool.* **186**, 305–318.

Tamarin, A., and Jones, K. W. (1968). *Acta. Embryol. Morphol. Exp.* **10**, 288–301.

Theiler, K. (1972). "The House Mouse." Springer-Verlag, Berlin and New York.

Wilson, I. B., and Jenkinson, E. J. (1974). *J. Reprod. Fertil.* **39**, 243–249.

Witschi, E. (1972). *In* "Biology Data Book," 2nd ed., Vol. 1, pp. 178–180. Fed. Am. Soc. Exp. Biol., Washington, D.C.

11

Implantation of Mouse Blastocysts *in Vitro*

MICHAEL I. SHERMAN

I. INTRODUCTION

Although implantation has been studied extensively by reproductive biologists, physiologists, and endocrinologists, some gaps still exist in our understanding of the event. For example, we are ignorant of the nature of changes taking place at the molecular level which result in the adhesion of the blastocyst to the uterine epithelium. Recently, approaches have been developed which may allow us to address this and other remaining questions more easily. For instance, with some available *in vitro* techniques, blastocysts behave in many respects as they do during implantation in the uterus (see Sherman and Wudl, 1976, for a review). Large numbers of blastocysts can thus be studied at characteristic pre- or peri-implantation stages (i.e., nonadhesive, adhesive but noninva-

247

sive, invasive, postinvasive) based upon their behavior in these *in vitro* systems (Sherman and Wudl, 1976). It is also possible to monitor blastocysts continuously during these stages, not feasible *in utero* where the tissue must be fixed, sectioned, and stained for observation.

All the *in vitro* techniques used in this laboratory have been geared to following the transformation of the blastocyst during implantation; at present, the systems are not at all optimized for studying changes in uterine cells. It is probably due to this lack of attention to the state of uterine cells that our *in vitro* systems have been unresponsive to hormones [since the bulk of available evidence supports the view that hormones act primarily on the uterus and only indirectly upon the blastocyst during implantation *in vivo* (Sherman and Wudl, 1976)]. With pure cultures of uterine epithelial cells now available (Section III,B), it may be possible to develop an *in vitro* implantation system subject to hormonal control.

II. PREPARATION AND HANDLING OF BLASTOCYSTS

Blastocysts are obtained from previously superovulated females as described in detail elsewhere (Sherman, 1976). They are washed in calcium- and magnesium-free phosphate-buffered saline (PBS; solution A of Dulbecco and Vogt, 1954), and can be kept in this buffer at room temperature with no apparent damage for an hour or more.

In some cases, it is necessary to remove the zona pellucida. This is done with pronase (Mintz, 1971). We have found that naked (pronase-treated or spontaneously hatched) blastocysts are very sticky, particularly in PBS. Consequently, necessary transfers are carried out with capillary pipettes that have been drawn out, flame-polished, siliconized with 1% Siliclad (Clay Adams, Parsippany, New Jersey) and washed extensively with distilled water. We reuse these micropipettes several times, cleaning them with distilled water after each use, and storing them in a sterile hood under germicidal lamps.

Naked blastocysts tend to adhere tenaciously to plastic culture dishes in PBS. This can be overcome either by adding bovine serum albumin (final concentration of 1–2%) to the buffer, or by using culture dishes coated with a pad of agarose (see Section V).

We routinely culture blastocysts through the implantation period in NCTC-109 (Microbiological Associates, Bethesda, Maryland) or Dulbecco-modified Eagle's medium (Gibco, Grand Island, New York), supplemented with heat-inactivated fetal calf serum and antibiotics (Sherman, 1975, 1976). However, other serum-supplemented media, including Eagle's medium and the amino acid-enriched medium of Spindle and Pedersen (1973), may be used.

III. PREPARATION OF UTERINE MONOLAYERS

Others have studied the behavior of blastocysts *in vitro* on strips of uterine tissue (e.g., Glenister, 1965) or even enclosed in intact uteri (e.g., Grant, 1973). We have investigated "implantation" *in vitro* on monolayers of uterine cells (Salomon and Sherman, 1975; Sherman and Salomon, 1975), and we have provided a rationale for doing so by detailing the similarities in blastocyst behavior *in utero* and on these monolayers (Sherman and Wudl, 1976). One decided shortcoming of the system we have used in the past is that the primary cultures were generated from a mixture of uterine epithelial and stromal cells, and the monolayers so formed were assumed to consist mainly of the latter. Thus, while a stromal cell monolayer might be useful for a study of invasiveness of trophoblast cells, it offers less value in investigations on blastocyst attachment, since contacts *in utero* are initially made with the uterine epithelium. We have now utilized a technique suggested to us by Dr. Richard Gardner of the Zoology Department, University of Oxford (originally devised for separating embryonic germ layers by Levak-Švajger *et al.*, 1969) for generating relatively pure monolayers of uterine epithelial cells for attachment studies. At the same time, equally pure cultures of uterine stromal cells can be obtained. Descriptions of our techniques for making mixed and pure cultures are described below.

A. Mixed Monolayers from Whole Uteri

This procedure has been described previously by Salomon and Sherman (1975). Briefly, uteri are removed from mice (pregnant, nonpregnant, or ovariectomized), placed in PBS, and cleared as thoroughly as possible of fat, mesentery, and blood vessels. Oviducts are removed by cutting with scissors a few millimeters distal to the uterotubal junction. The uteri are then cut up at short intervals (about 3 mm), picked up with forceps, and placed in 25-ml flasks containing 2.5 ml 0.05% trypsin–0.02% EDTA solution (Gibco), 1 ml collagenase (0.5 mg/ml; *Clostridium*, type III, Sigma Chemicals, St. Louis, Missouri), and 0.5 ml DNase (200 units; bovine pancreatic, Sigma). The flasks are shaken in a 37°C water bath for 30 minutes, the incubation being interrupted periodically to force the pieces of tissue through a Pasteur pipette (it may be necessary to break the pipette off farther up along the tapered part of the stem so that the pieces of tissue can pass through the aperture). After incubation, 0.3 ml fetal calf serum is added, and the suspension is filtered through sterile cheesecloth. Cells are sedimented at low speed, resuspended in medium, and plated at moderate-to-high density (one uterus per 35 mm culture dish) in supplemented NCTC-109 medium. The next day, the cultures are washed, and new medium is added. The cells should be confluent over most of the dish prior to the addition of blastocysts.

B. Monolayers of Uterine Epithelial Cells

Uteri are cleaned and trimmed in PBS as described above and slit along their lengths with fine dissecting scissors. They are then placed in an ice-cold solution made by adding powdered trypsin (final concentration 0.5%; bovine pancreatic, type III, Sigma) to a 2.5% solution of pancreatin in Hank's balanced salt solution, calcium- and magnesium-free (Microbiological Associates). After 2 hours at 4°C, the uteri are incubated for 30 minutes to 1 hour at room temperature, still in the proteolytic solution. The uteri are then transferred to PBS. When inspected under a dissecting microscope, it may be seen that the uterine epithelial layer has begun to lift off the stromal surface in transparent sheets. These can be freed from the stroma in relatively large pieces with the use of watchmakers' forceps (Fig. 1).

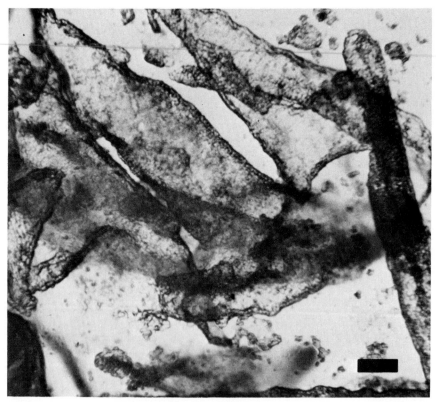

Fig. 1.   Sheets of epithelial cells obtained by trypsin–pancreatin treatment of uteri. Scale marker = 100 μm.

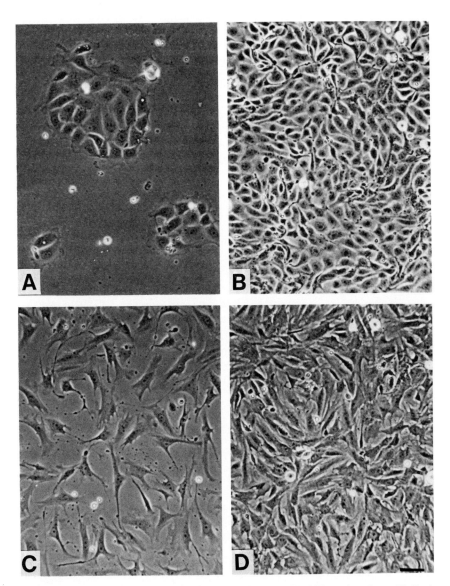

Fig. 2. Primary cultures of uterine epithelium and stroma after 24 hours in culture. (A) Uterine epithelial cells plated at low density. The epithelial layer has been reduced to small aggregates by the proteolytic treatment. (B) Monolayer of uterine epithelial cells plated at moderate density. (C) Uterine stroma cells plated at low density. The preparation consists primarily of individual fibroblastlike cells. (D) Monolayer of uterine stroma cells plated at moderate density. Note that the morphology of the epithelial and stromal cells are quite different, both at low and high density. All photographs taken with phase optics. Magnification bar (in D) = 50 μm.

The uterine epithelium is then placed in a trypsin-EDTA-DNase solution (the same as in Section II,A, except that collagenase is omitted) and incubated in a shaking water bath at 37°C for 5 minutes. (The uterine stroma may be processed simultaneously as described in the next section.) The reaction is stopped by adding 1/10 volume of cold fetal calf serum, and the epithelium is sedimented by low-speed centrifugation. The supernate is decanted, the cells resuspended in supplemented NCTC-109 medium, and plated at moderate density (epithelial cells from two uteri will give a confluent monolayer in a 60-mm culture dish 24 hours later). The epithelial cells, present mainly in small sheets (e.g., Fig. 2a), attach to the culture dish with high frequency. At high density, a confluent mosaiclike monolayer characteristic of epithelioid cells is observed (Fig. 2b).

C. Monolayers of Stromal Cells

After the sheets of epithelium have been removed from the uteri, the remaining tissue is cut into small pieces and placed in trypsin-EDTA-DNase solution (as in Section II,A, except that collagenase is omitted). After 5 minutes of shaking at 37°C, the pieces are pipetted up and down and returned to the water bath for a further 10 minutes incubation. Fetal calf serum (1/10 volume) is added to stop the reaction. The tissue is vigorously pipetted up and down. While the mucosal layers of the uterus are resistant to this treatment, the stromal cells are disaggregated and are displaced from the intact mucosae. The total suspension is placed in a conical centrifuge tube, and the intact mucosae are allowed to sediment by gravity. The turbid suspension of stromal cells, which consists largely of single cells (Fig. 2c), is then drawn off, sedimented by low-speed centrifugation, and plated at medium-to-high density. One to two uteri per 60-mm dish gives a confluent culture of fibroblastlike cells (Fig. 2d) within 24 hours.

IV. *IN VITRO* BLASTOCYST IMPLANTATION STUDIES

We have shown elsewhere that the surface of the blastocyst undergoes a programmed conversion from nonadhesive to adhesive *in vitro* at the time that implantation would take place *in utero* (Sherman and Atienza, 1978). Since we feel it likely that this phenomenon signals the capacity of the blastocyst to implant, we have used attachment to a culture dish surface or a cellular monolayer as an *in vitro* criterion of the "implantability" of the blastocyst. A cellular monolayer is used when it is desirable to study morphology, certain aspects of cell–cell interactions, or extents of invasiveness under a variety of conditions. It may be preferable to use the simpler system of blastocyst attachment to the surface of a culture dish for biochemical or immunologic experiments and for studies involvings drugs or antimetabolites. We have also carried out comparative studies between implantation of blastocysts on a culture dish or a cellular surface in the same medium by forming a cellular monolayer on a culture dish and then scraping the cells off half the surface. A capillary pipette is cut to the inside diameter of the dish, wedged so as to separate the two surfaces, and the dish is filled with medium. Blastocysts then placed on either side of the capillary pipette will be exposed to the same medium but to different substrata (Sherman and Salomon, 1975).

For studying the effects of hormones on *in vitro* implantation, we have removed endogenous steroid hormones from the serum by treatment with a dextran–Norit A mixture (Salomon and Sherman, 1975). Implantation of blastocysts can occur on washed uterine monolayers in the absence of added serum or serum factors, but serum is necessary for blastocyst attachment to, and outgrowth along, a tissue culture dish surface (Sherman and Salomon, 1975).

In scoring the attachment of blastocysts, we have routinely used 35-mm tissue culture dishes with or without a cellular monolayer. We add 15–30 blastocysts to each dish, and we use duplicate dishes for each set of conditions under study. Adhesiveness is scored by counting under a dissecting microscope the number of blastocysts which remain attached to the substratum when the contents of the dish are swirled in a circular motion.

We obtain kinetics of blastocyst attachment by scoring the dishes three or four times per day. A typical experiment is plotted in Fig. 3. Duplicate dishes usually give results in close agreement with each other, as is the case here. From one day to another, however, the curves can be displaced by as much as 5–10 hours in either direction. Under our conditions of culture (Sherman, 1976), often all blastocysts hatch from their zonae pellucida and attach, whether to a culture dish

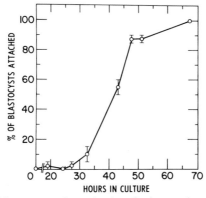

Fig. 3. Kinetics of blastocyst attachment *in vitro*. In the experiment shown here, blastocysts were removed from uteri on the afternoon of the 4th day of pregnancy. Twenty blastocysts were placed in each of two tissue culture dishes and monitored for attachment as indicated in the text. The bars indicate the variation between the two dishes, the circles represent the average values.

surface or a cellular monolayer. In some cases, however, one or a few blastocysts will fail to hatch or show extensive delay (greater than 72 hours when culture is begun on the middle of the 4th day) in attachment after hatching. In order to avoid giving undue emphasis to the behavior of the few blastocysts which do not attach or which attach abnormally late or even prematurely (e.g., in the experiment shown in Fig. 3, one blastocyst had attached to the culture dish after 19 hours but had become detached 5 hours later), we have put most weight on the time at which 50% of the blastocysts have attached to the culture dish (T_{50}). Furthermore, when studying agents that may alter the T_{50}, results from one experiment to the next can be compared in terms of ΔT_{50} (i.e., the increased number of hours required for blastocysts to reach T_{50} in the presence of a perturbant compared to control blastocysts). In this way, variability in the T_{50} of control blastocysts on different days does not complicate interpretation of the data.

V. PREVENTION OF BLASTOCYST IMPLANTATION *IN VITRO*

As mentioned earlier, a satisfactory *in vitro* system for demonstrating hormonal control of blastocyst implantation has not been developed. Consequently, although it might be desirable in some experiments to prevent blastocysts from attaching to a cellular or culture dish surface until hormone is added to the medium, such experiments cannot yet be carried out. Nevertheless, it is possible to "delay" blastocyst attachment *in vitro* in two different ways. The first method, developed by Gwatkin (1966), involves omitting two amino acids, arginine and leucine, from the medium. According to Gwatkin, blastocysts can be maintained in this medium, supplemented with dialyzed serum, for up to 7 days, and will resume development when the missing amino acids are added to the culture. We reported that blastocysts delayed in this medium for 4 days developed normally when transplanted to uteri of foster mothers (C. F. Graham and M. I. Sherman, unpublished results, cited in Sherman and Barlow, 1972). However, we noted some degenerative changes in the blastocysts after 7 days in arginine- and leucine-free medium.

A technique that we have used to advantage in our *in vitro* studies is to prevent blastocyst implantation by culturing embryos on a nonadhesive surface, most commonly agarose. Unlike the previous procedure, blastocysts do become competent to implant but are physically prevented from doing so (see Fig. 4).

Agarose-coated dishes are prepared by boiling a 2% solution of agarose in water, pouring some in a tissue culture dish, and then quickly pouring it off again. This procedure leaves a thin film across the bottom of the dish. After the agarose has cooled, the dishes are soaked with at least five changes of PBS over a period of 4 hours or more in order to remove toxic products which leach out from

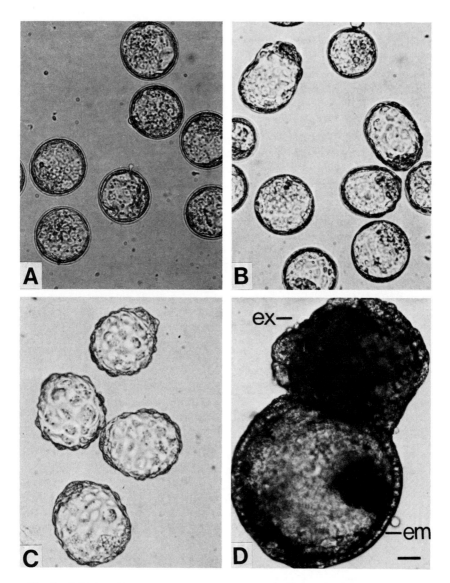

Fig. 4. Behavior of blastocysts prevented from attachment *in vitro*. (A) Blastocysts on the 4th "equivalent gestation day" (their age had they been left *in utero*). (B) Blastocysts on the 5th equivalent gestation day. Most have expanded and are hatching but are not adhesive. (C) Blastocysts on the 6th equivalent gestation day, now in the adhesive phase, are prevented from attaching by being placed on an agarose pad. Note that they have expanded markedly and have maintained their rounded shape. (D) Blastocyst on the 11th equivalent gestation day, cultured on an agarose pad. Substantial growth has taken place (compare with a) and the structure has a bilobed appearance, presumably representing embryonic (em) and extraembryonic (ex) moieties. Magnification is the same in all photos. Scale bar (in d) = 50 μm.

the gel. PBS is again added, and the dish is sterilized under a germicidal lamp for 30 minutes. The dish is then filled with medium. After this medium has been discarded 30 minutes later, the agarose-coated dishes can be safely used for blastocyst culture. The dishes, filled with PBS, may also be stored in a sterile hood for 2 or 3 days. They should then be washed as described above just before being used.

We have tested a number of different brands of agarose and have found that although all are refractory to blastocyst attachment, some seem to cause the blastocysts to agglutinate. In our experience, SeaKem agarose (MCI Biomedical, Rockland, Maine) minimizes the tendency of blastocysts to stick to each other and appears to be nontoxic after washing.

In some cases, agarose-coated dishes may not be suitable for use. In these instances, Nucleopore filters can be used (Nucleopore Corporation, Pleasanton, California). These polycarbonate filters generally do not permit blastocyst attachment, presumably because they are nonwettable. We normally use large pore (8μm) Nucleopore filters because they are translucent and, therefore, allow inspection of the blastocysts through the filter with an inverted phase optics microscope.

Nucleopore filters initially float when placed in medium. It is necessary to force the filters to the bottom of the culture dish with a forceps several times before they will remain there. Blastocysts tend to agglutinate when cultured on Nucleopore filters, so each culture dish should contain only small numbers of embryos. Furthermore, after several days, some of the blastocysts will begin to adhere to the filter. Finally, the available filter diameters do not coincide very closely with tissue culture dish diameters so that if the dishes are jostled, the blastocysts can roll off the filter and attach to the surface of the culture dish. This problem can be circumvented by cutting down larger (47 mm) filters so that they will fit snugly in small (35 mm) culture dishes. Because of these inconveniences, we prefer to use agarose-coated dishes where possible.

We have also attempted to use siliconized culture dishes or bacteriological dishes for preventing blastocyst attachment. Although these are suitable for short-term use, a few hours at most, blastocysts which have acquired their adhesive properties seem eventually to find sticky patches on the surface of these dishes and, after having done so, quickly attach and outgrow.

Blastocysts cultured on agarose-coated dishes or Nucleopore filters show substantial growth (Fig. 4), acquire enzyme levels characteristic of normal development *in vitro* (M. I. Sherman, S. B. Atienza, L. Wudl and D. S. Salomon, unpublished observations) and, when transferred to regular tissue culture dishes, adhere almost immediately (Fig. 5). Thus, blastocysts can be treated with agents that might be expected to reverse their adhesiveness and tested to see whether they will attach when offered a compatible surface (see, e.g., Sherman and Atienza, 1978). This procedure is ideal as well for studying blastocysts in the

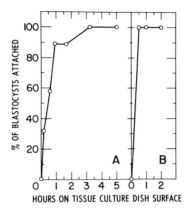

Fig. 5. Kinetics of attachment of blastocysts after culture on agarose pads. Blastocysts, removed from the uterus on the 4th day, were placed in agarose-coated dishes for 48 (A) or 72 (B) hours and were then transferred to regular tissue culture dishes. The figures illustrate that blastocyst attachment occurs very quickly following transfer.

early postimplantation phase, a time at which it is very difficult to obtain them from the uterus. It also obviates the need to scrape the developing embryos off a culture dish surface.

REFERENCES

Dulbecco, R., and Vogt, M. (1954). *J. Exp. Med.* **99**, 167–182.

Glenister, T. W. (1965). *In* "The Early Conceptus Normal and Abnormal" (W. W. Park, ed.), pp. 24–26. University St. Andrews Press, Edinburgh.

Grant, P. S. (1973). *J. Embryol. Exp. Morphol.* **29**, 617–638.

Gwatkin, R. B. L. (1966). *J. Cell. Physiol.* **68**, 335–344.

Levak-Švajger, B., Švajger, A., and Škreb, N. (1969). *Experientia* **25**, 1311–1312.

Mintz, B. (1971). *In* "Methods in Mammalian Embryology" (J. C. Daniel, Jr., ed.), pp. 186–214. Freeman, San Francisco, California.

Salomon, D. S., and Sherman, M. I. (1975). *Exp. Cell Res.* **90**, 261–268.

Sherman, M. I. (1975). *Differentiation* **3**, 51–67.

Sherman, M. I. (1976). *In* "Tissue Culture Association Manual" (V. J. Evans, V. P. Perry, and M. M. Vincent, eds.), pp. 199–201. TCA, Inc., Rockville, Maryland.

Sherman, M. I., and Atienza, S. B. (1978). *In* "Human Fertilization" (H. Ludwig and P. F. Tauber, eds.). Thieme, Stuttgart (in press).

Sherman, M. I., and Barlow, P. W. (1972). *J. Reprod. Fertil.* **29**, 123–126.

Sherman, M. I., and Salomon, D. S. (1975). *In* "The Developmental Biology of Reproduction" (C. L. Markert and J. Papaconstantinou, eds.), pp. 277–309. Academic Press, New York.

Sherman, M. I., and Wudl, L. R. (1976). *In* "The Cell Surface in Animal Development" (G. Poste and G. R. Nicolson, eds.), pp. 81–125. North Holland Publ., Amsterdam.

Spindle, A. I., and Pedersen, R. A. (1973). *J. Exp. Zool.* **186**, 305–318.

12

Advances in Rabbit Embryo Culture

RALPH R. MAURER

I. INTRODUCTION

The rabbit zygote and/or embryo has been one of the most responsive to development *in vitro*. All the preimplantation stages have undergone development in culture. Fertilization *in vitro* and subsequent early cleavages were observed by Chang (1959). Development from early cleavage stages to morulae were reported by Lewis and Gregory (1929), Pincus and Enzmann (1936), Adams (1956), and Purshottam and Pincus (1961); development of blastocyst stages have been reported by Brachet (1913), Pincus and Werthessen (1938),

259

Huff (1962), Daniel (1965), Staples (1967), and Ogawa and Imagawa (1969). Using heat-treated rabbit and bovine serum and 5% CO_2 in air, Onuma et al. (1968) cultured 2- and 4-cell rabbit embryos to the hatching blastocyst stage; 80–90% of the embryos developed a blastocoel. Maurer et al. (1969) were the first to demonstrate the development of zygotes to the blastocyst stage; using heat-treated bovine serum plus glucose, they reported 40% of the zygotes developed into blastocysts. Forty-eight percent of Dutch-Belted zygotes developed into blastocysts in a defined medium (Kane and Foote, 1971), while 81% of New Zealand White zygotes cultured in a defined medium without glucose grew to the blastocyst stage (Kane, 1972).

Rabbit embryos developed in vitro have shown a requirement for amino acids and vitamins and are affected by changes in osmotic and atmospheric pressure. Zygotes, 2-, and 4-cell embryos do not develop to the blastocyst stage without methionine and have a reduced development when tyrosine, cysteine, serine, and threonine are absent (Kane and Foote, 1970). Removal of vitamins from defined medium results in a decreased percentage of zygotes and early cleavage stage embryos developing during culture (Kane and Foote, 1970). The addition of thymidine inhibited the development of 2- and 4-cell embryos into expanding blastocysts, while the addition of 1.5% bovine serum albumin (BSA) has been shown to have a beneficial effect (Kane and Foote, 1971). The development of zygotes did not require glucose or pyruvate. The optimal osmolarity for the culture of rabbit embryos was 270 mOsM (Naglee et al., 1969), while maximum growth in vitro occurred at an atmospheric pressure of 3 cm Hg (4052 Newton/ m^2; Elliott et al., 1974).

The test for viability of embryos maintained in vitro is their subsequent development into fetuses upon transfer to suitable recipients. In early studies, 2- to 16-cell embryos maintained in vitro for 24–48 hours did develop into viable fetuses upon transfer to foster mothers (Pincus and Enzmann, 1934; Chang, 1948; Adams, 1956). However, as the length of time the embryos are maintained in vitro is increased beyond 48 hours, fewer embryos retain the ability to develop into fetuses (Maurer et al., 1970; Adams, 1970). Two- and four-cell embryos were cultured for 72 (Adams, 1970) and 88 hours (Maurer et al., 1970) and upon transfer to recipients some embryos developed into fetuses. Increased atmospheric pressure during culture improved the viability of rabbit embryos (Elliott et al., 1974). After transfer to suitable recipients, viable fetuses were obtained from embryos maintained in vitro for 96 hours (Maurer, Elliott and Staples, in preparation).

Viability of rabbit embryos can be maintained in vitro for an extended period of time (at least 4 days) if care is used in mating the females producing the embryos and in the subsequent embryo manipulations. Embryos are more likely to continue development in vitro if they are obtained from a healthy nonstressed doe that was mated to a fertile buck. The factors which have been identified as important for development *in vitro* are described below.

II. PREPARATION OF EMBRYO DONORS

Mature 5-(small breed) or 6-(large breed) month-old does, which have been caged individually for 18–21 days, should be used to obtain the embryos. The does should be housed in an area with controlled lighting (12/12 or 14/10 hours light/dark cycle), temperature (18°–20°C), and humidity (50–55%). Animals should have free access to water, and they should receive daily 200 (small breed) to 250 (large breed) gm of a 17–18% protein rabbit ration.

A. Natural Mating

The rabbit is an induced ovulator and will ovulate approximately 12 hours after a coital stimulus (Harper, 1963) or an injection of pituitary luteinizing hormone (PLH, Burns-Biotec, Oakland, California; Foote *et al.*, 1963). To mate animals naturally, place the doe in a cage with a fertile buck and observe if the female will accept the male. Does readily receive the buck every 4–5 days, which is the estimated length of the rabbit estrous cycle (Stranzinger, 1970; Myers and Poole, 1962; Hamilton, 1951). Most active bucks will mate a receptive doe immediately. Allowing the doe to be mated twice either by the same male or by two different males increases the percentage of secondary oocytes which will be fertilized. Exhaustive use of one male is not recommended because sperm number and quality decrease, reducing the number of secondary oocytes that will be fertilized, as well as subsequent embryo viability.

B. Induced Ovulation and Artificial Insemination

Does caged individually for 18 days (this protects against using pseudopregnant does) can be induced to ovulate by an iv injection of 25 international units (IU) human chorionic gonadotropin (HCG) or 0.5 mg/kg PLH. Shortly after the ovulating hormone injection, each doe is artificially inseminated with motile spermatozoa obtained from a fertile male with an artificial vagina (Foote *et al.*, 1963; Varian *et al.*, 1967). The collected semen can be extended with a fructose–citrate or a Tris–egg yolk extender (Roche *et al.*, 1968; Stranzinger *et al.*, 1971). The composition of each extender is listed in Table I. Each female should be inseminated with 20×10^6 motile spermatozoa (1×10^6 motile spermatozoa minimum) in a volume of 0.4–0.6 ml. Proper iv injections, using the correct dosage of PLH, will result in 100% of the does ovulating. The use of

TABLE I
Extenders for Rabbit Semen

Extender	Amount (gm/100 ml twice-distilled water)
Fructose–citrate extender[a,b]	
D-Fructose ($C_6H_{12}O_6$)	0.5
Sodium citrate ($Na_3C_6H_5O_7 \cdot 2\ H_2O$)	2.9
Tris–egg yolk extender[a,c]	
Tris (hydroxymethyl)amino methane ($C_4H_{11}NO_3$)	3.028
Citric acid ($C_6H_8O_7 \cdot H_2O$)	1.675
D-glucose ($C_6H_{12}O_6$)	1.250
To the 100 ml are added 20 ml of egg yolk	

[a] To each milliliter of extender, 1000 units each of penicillin and streptomycin can be added.
[b] Roche et al. (1968).
[c] Stranzinger et al. (1971).

induced ovulation allows maximum utilization of animals and permits exact timing of experiments. If many embryos are needed, the doe can be superovulated by injecting sc once daily for 4 days 0.4 mg follicle-stimulating hormone (FSH-P Burns-Biotec, Oakland, California) in 1% aqueous methyl cellulose (Maurer and Haseman, 1976; Maurer et al., 1968; Kennelly and Foote, 1965). On the 4th day, each doe is induced to ovulate with PLH and is artificially inseminated.

III. EMBRYO COLLECTION

Zygotes and/or embryos can be collected in vitro by removing and flushing the reproductive tract or by anesthetizing the doe and flushing the reproductive tract in situ (Maurer et al., 1968; Hafez, 1971). The supplies and equipment needed are listed in Table II. To remove the reproductive tract the female is killed by cervical dislocation and then, via an incision in the linea alba, the oviducts and uterine horns are dissected from the broad ligament (ligamentum latum uteri). Maintaining the identity of each horn (left or right), the reproductive tract is placed in a sterile 100 × 15 mm petri dish. The ovaries are removed, and ovulation points (corpora hemorrhagica) are counted to determine the percentage of embryos recovered. Remnants of fatty tissue are then trimmed from the tract. The oviducts and uterine horns are separated at the tubouterine junction and the appropriate organ flushed with 3–5 ml of flushing medium (culture medium with 0.1% BSA). The oviduct or uterine horn is attached to a blunted 20-gauge needle with a hemostat and mounted to a ringstand or a blunted 20-gauge needle is

TABLE II

Equipment and Supplies Needed to Collect Rabbit Embryos

Equipment for collections *in vitro*
 1. Surgical scissors (5½ inches)
 2. Hemostat (6 inches)
 3. Blunted 20-gauge needle (1½ inches long)
 4. Sterile syringe (3 or 5 ml)
 5. Watchglasses or 10 × 60 mm Falcon tissue culture dishes
 6. Gauzettes (2 × 2 inches)
 7. Stereomicroscope or low power microscope
 8. Flushing medium
Equipment for collections *in situ*
 1. Same equipment as listed above plus
   a. Polyethylene tubing (Intramedic PE 160, 1.14 mm i.d. × 1.57 mm o.d.)—30-cm length
      flanged slightly at one end
   b. Serrefine, straight 1½ inches, lined with rubber or miniature plastic clothespin lined with
      rubber
   c. Pasteur pipette, bent at a 45°–90° angle, with one end having a 2–3 mm diameter

---

placed in the lumen of the oviduct or uterine horn and held firmly with the thumb and index finger. The organ should be dried with a gauzette to prevent any blood from entering the collection container. For collection of embryos *in vivo*, the doe in anesthetized with pentobarbital sodium and the oviducts and/or uteri are exteriorized through a midventral incision. Surgical anesthesia is produced by injecting 1 ml of a pentobarbital sodium solution (50 mg/ml) rapidly and, thereafter, 0.2 ml/min until surgical anesthesia is achieved. To collect embryos from the oviduct, a 30-cm length of polyethylene tubing flanged slightly at the end is inserted into the fimbriated end of the oviduct and held in place with a miniature plastic clothespin or a rubber-lined 4-cm serrefine hemostat (bulldog clamp). A blunted 20-gauge needle is inserted through the wall of the uterus and passed beyond the tubouterine junction into the isthmus of the oviduct. The zygotes and/or embryos are flushed toward the fimbriated end of the oviduct into a 15 × 60 mm sterile petri dish or sterile watchglass (50-mm diameter) with 3 ml of culture medium containing 0.1% BSA. To flush the uterus, a small incision is made in the cranial portion of the vagina and the small end of a Pasteur pipette (bent 45°–90° and drawn out at one end) is inserted into the incision and threaded through the cervix. The pipette is held in place with the thumb and index finger. At the cranial end of the uterine horn, a blunted 20-gauge needle is inserted through the wall, and the uterine horn is flushed with 5 or more ml of medium.

 All secondary oocytes and/or embryos are examined under a stereomicroscope for evidence of fertilization, cleavage stage, and morphological appearance (uniformity of blastomeres, homogeneity of blastomere texture, thickness of zona pellucida, and presence of mucin covering). The unfertilized (no male and

TABLE III

Stage of Rabbit Embryo Development and Location within the Reproductive Tract after the Time of Mating or the Ovulating Hormone Injection

Stage of embryo development	Time (hours) after mating or PLH injection	Location
Zygote	14–22	Oviduct
2-Cell	20–28	Oviduct
4-Cell	26–32	Oviduct
8-Cell	32–44	Oviduct
Morula	60–72	Oviduct (mainly) uterus
Blastocyst	70–144	Uterus

female pronuclei) secondary oocytes and the embryos having fragmented blastomeres or other morphological aberrations are removed. The remaining embryos are washed at least once in culture medium and pooled according to cleavage stage. The stage of embryo development and the location within the reproductive tract after mating or the ovulating hormone injection are listed in Table III.

IV. CULTURE METHODS

The culture of mammalian embryos has been reviewed by Mintz (1967) and Brinster (1968; 1970), and only techniques that differ or have been modified will be discussed.

A. Work Area

A tissue culture room with positive pressure and equipped with ultraviolet and fluorescent lamps should be used for large-scale culture work. For most research laboratories a sterile work area within the laboratory can be produced by a transparent plastic hood equipped with an ultraviolet and fluorescent light or with a laminar or vertical flow hood. The ultraviolet light is used only for sterilizing the air and surface area and embryos or medium should not be exposed to it. Within the sterile work area, room for a stereomicroscope should be provided.

B. Culture Medium

Rabbit embryos have been grown *in vitro* in various media—heat-treated serum, Brinster's BMOC-3, McCoy's 5a, Medium 199, Ham's F10 and F12 for various periods of time. The medium which has given the most consistent results has been described by Kane and Foote (1970) and Naglee *et al.* (1969). The current composition (Table IV) has been modified slightly as the NaCl content has been decreased to 6.019 gm/liter, and the nucleic acid precursors have been deleted. The medium is prepared in 1- or 5-liter quantities according to Table IV, with all ingredients except glucose, BSA, and sodium bicarbonate being added. The medium is filtered through a 0.22-μm filter (Millex) into a sterile 100-ml serum bottle and stoppered with a sterile rubber stopper. The medium without glucose, BSA, and sodium bicarbonate can be stored at 5°C for as long as 6 months. To make up the complete medium, the appropriate amounts of glucose, BSA, and sodium bicarbonate are added, and the medium is again filtered (0.22-μm Millex filter) into a sterile serum bottle and stoppered with a sterile

TABLE IV
Composition of Synthetic Medium for Rabbit Embryo Culture[a]

Component		Component	
Basic salt solution	(gm/liter)	Amino acids	(mg/liter)
NaCl	6.019	L-Alanine	8.90
KCl	0.356	L-Arginine-HCl	211.00
$CaCl_2 \cdot 2H_2O$	0.251	L-Aspartic acid	13.30
KH_2PO_4	0.162	L-Asparagine·H_2O	15.00
$MgSO_4 \cdot 7H_2O$	0.294	L-Cysteine-HCl	31.50
$NaHCO_3$[b]	2.106	L-Glutamine	146.20
Glucose[b]	1.800	L-Glutamic acid	14.70
BSA[b]	15.000	Glycine	7.50
		L-Histidine-HCl	23.00
Vitamins	(mg/liter)	L-Isoleucine	2.60
		L-Leucine	13.10
Biotin, cystalline	0.024	L-Lysine-HCl	29.30
DL-Calcium pantothenate	0.72	L-Methionine	4.50
Choline choride	0.70	L-Phenylalanine	5.00
Folic acid	1.30	L-Proline	11.50
i-Inositol	0.54	L-Serine	10.50
Niacinamide	0.62	L-Threonine	3.60
Pyridoxine-HCl	0.21	L-Tryptophan	0.60
Riboflavin	0.38	L-Tyrosine	1.80
Thiamine-HCl	1.04	L-Valine	3.50
DL-Thioctic acid (α-lipoic acid)	0.20		
Vitamin B_{12}, crystalline	1.40	Trace elements	(μg/liter)
		$CuSO_4 \cdot 5H_2O$	2.50
		$FeSO_4 \cdot 7H_2O$	834.00
		$ZnSO_4 \cdot 7H_2O$	28.80

[a]From Kane and Foote (1971) and Naglee et al. (1969).

[b]These ingredients are not added until the medium is needed for culture. The completed medium is stable for 14 days when stored at 5°C. The medium should be gassed with 5% CO_2:air after the sodium bicarbonate has been added, and, after each time medium is withdrawn from the bottle.

rubber stopper. The medium is gassed for 30 seconds with 5% CO_2 in air. The gassing is done via a sterile 20-gauge needle attached to a 5% CO_2 in air source and inserted through the rubber stopper. A second sterile 20-gauge needle (vent) is inserted through the rubber stopper and the CO_2 in air passed over the medium (gas is not bubbled through the medium) for 20 seconds. The vent needle is removed first, and the medium is gassed an additional 10 seconds before the needle attached to the 5% CO_2 in air is removed. The medium is shaken gently and allowed to stand at least 15 minutes before the pH and osmolarity are measured. The completed medium should have a pH of 7.4 ± 0.1 and an osmolarity of 270 ± 5 mOsM. Antibiotics have been excluded from the composition of the medium because they are not necessary if the culture work is done under sterile conditions. However, if conditions are such that antibiotics are needed, 100 IU of penicillin G (potassium salt) and 50 μg streptomycin sulfate should be added per milliliter of medium. The medium used for culture contains 15 mg/ml BSA, whereas the medium used to flush the reproductive tract contains 1.0 mg/ml BSA. Crystallized BSA (Pentax, Miles Laboratories, Inc.) with greater than 99% purity is used as the albumin source.

C. Incubators

The physical conditions necessary for rabbit embryo culture are a temperature of 37°C, relative humidity of 99%, an atmosphere of 5% CO_2 in air, and atmospheric pressure of 16 inches of water (3 cm mercury or 4052 Newton/m^2 at 352 ft above sea level; Elliott et al., 1974). The actual atmospheric pressure needed will fluctuate from laboratory to laboratory depending upon the elevation above sea level of the specific laboratory.

A simple incubator, which maintains a temperature of 37° ± 1°C, will suffice. Three systems may be used to maintain the desired gaseous atmosphere, as well as the optimal atmospheric pressure. The continuous flow system as illustrated in Fig. 1A has a continuous gas flow through the incubation chambers (see Biggers et al., 1971, for a further description). The desired atmospheric pressure is attained by adjusting the depth of the water above the outlet tube and/or by restricting the gas flow through the vent tube. Using air supplied from a compressor, a gas proportioner, and 99.9% bone dry CO_2, the 5% (or other concentrations) CO_2 in air mixture is produced. The CO_2 concentration can be monitored quickly and accurately by using a Fyrite CO_2 Gas Analyzer (Fisher Scientific Co.). The high relative humidity is produced by bubbling the gas through distilled water and by placing a tray of distilled water on the bottom of the culture chamber. The advantages of the continuous flow system are that many embryos can be cultured, culture chambers can be hooked in series and that a homogeneous composition of the gaseous atmosphere is maintained (provided

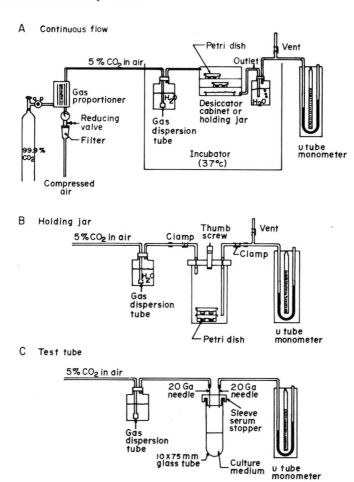

Fig. 1. Three systems used to maintain the desired gas composition and atmospheric pressure. (A) The continuous flow system has an uninterrupted flow of 5% CO_2 in air, and the desired atmospheric pressure is regulated by adjusting the depth of the water above the outlet tube and/or by restricting the gas flow through the vent tube. (B) The holding jar system flushes out the existing air and replaces it with 5% CO_2 in air. The desired atmospheric pressure is produced by restricting the flow of gas through the vent valve. Upon reaching the desired pressure, the gas source is clamped first, and then the exhaust vent is closed. Care must be taken to prevent loss of pressure. The unit is then placed in an incubator. (C) The test tube system uses the same principles as the holding jar to produce the desired gas composition and atmospheric pressure. Upon reaching the desired atmospheric pressure, the inlet needle is removed, and then the vent needle is removed. The test tube is then placed in a rack in an incubator.

the chambers are not opened frequently). Disadvantages are the expensive equipment and the continuous air and CO_2 supply.

An inexpensive method is the closed system (Fig. 1B) in which the air in a holding or anaerobic jar is displaced with 5% CO_2 in air. Humidified 5% CO_2 in air is flushed through the jar for at least 3 minutes after the embryos have been placed in the container. The outlet tube is connected to a U-tube manometer, and, after the desired atmospheric pressure is reached, the inlet tube is clamped first and then the outlet tube. The jar is then placed in an incubator at 37°C. The main disadvantage of the closed system is that the chamber has to be gassed each time the jar is opened.

The third system (Fig. 1C) described by Whitten (1971) uses a stoppered 12 × 75 mm test tube in which the atmospheric gas composition and pressure can be adjusted to the desired level. Using a sleeved rubber stopper instead of a cork, the desired atmospheric pressure can be attained in the same manner as described for the holding jar. The gas source is removed and the tubes placed in an incubator at 37°C. An alternative to the test tube is a screw-cap reaction vial (5 ml volume) with a Mininert valve (Applied Science Laboratories, Inc.). The later system is especially useful where potential harmful substances are added to the culture medium or may be produced during culture. Embryos in both the test tube and reaction vials can be observed under a stereomicroscope in the closed vessels; however, for a close examination, the embryos must be removed and placed in a watch glass or a glass slide with a concavity.

D. Culture Vessels

The many different vessels used to culture mammalian embryos will not be discussed since these were reviewed by Brinster (1968, 1970). Rabbit zygotes and/or embryos readily develop in open plastic wells. Linbro Disposotrays containing 100 wells (Model 96CV "old style" or equivalent models) are cut into smaller trays containing six wells each. The smaller trays are washed with 7X Cleaner (Linbro Chemical Co., Inc.) and rinsed seven times each with tap, single- and triple-distilled water (Whittingham, 1971). The cleaned trays are stored in a 70% ethyl alcohol solution until needed. Thirty to forty-five minutes before the wells are to be filled with medium, the trays are removed from the 70% alcohol and allowed to air dry in a sterile area (laminar flow hood under ultraviolet lighting). The tray is then placed into a sterile petri dish (100 × 15 mm) that contains 2 ml of sterile distilled water (filtered through a 0.22-μm filter) to ensure adequate humidity. One milliliter of culture medium is added to each well, using a 10-ml syringe and filter unit (Millex, 0.22-μm pore size). The dishes containing the medium are placed either in a culture chamber or under a 5% CO_2 in air atmosphere at room temperature (usually an inverted 150-mm funnel with the gas supply attached to the stem) until needed.

E. Embryo Manipulation

The embryos are collected from the flushing medium using a sterile capillary tube (0.5–0.9 mm i.d.) attached to a suction apparatus (Clay Adams No. 4555) and placed in culture medium. All embryos are washed at least once and pooled according to cleavage stages. From the pooled embryos, five are drawn into a sterile capillary tube and placed in a culture well. This procedure is repeated until all six wells have five embryos each. Depending upon the experiment, six different treatments (one treatment/well) can be placed in one petri dish. A sterile capillary tube is used for each treatment to avoid any intratreatment contamination. If any of the substances added to the medium volatilize or react with the culture medium to produce a gas, then all six wells must contain the same treatment. Usually one well per dish serves as the culture control (no treatment). The treatments can be replicated numerous times using a new petri dish each time. With the well method and without a covering of mineral oil or medical fluid, many substances (including those lipid soluble) can be added to the culture medium. The test substance(s) can be added to individual wells, or several different media can be prepared and placed in different wells.

F. Embryo Observation

The embryos can be observed within the petri dish using a stereo, inverted, or regular microscope with low-power objectives. The petri dish cover is removed when using the stereo or regular microscope, but can be left on if using an inverted microscope. Photomicrographs can be taken with the embryos in the wells, but the petri dish cover should be removed because light aberration may be produced. Embryos should not be exposed to light for a prolonged period of time as visible light retards growth of the embryo (Daniel, 1964).

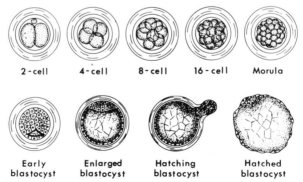

| 2-cell | 4-cell | 8-cell | 16-cell | Morula |

| Early blastocyst | Enlarged blastocyst | Hatching blastocyst | Hatched blastocyst |

Fig. 2. Developmental stages of rabbit preimplantation embryos as occur *in vitro*. Stages through the enlarged or expanding blastocyst stage occur *in vivo*, while the hatching and hatched blastocyst occur only *in vitro*.

Observations are usually taken every 24 hours but can be taken with any frequency. The embryos develop *in vitro* as depicted in Fig. 2. The hatching and hatched blastocyst stages occur *in vitro* but do not occur *in vivo* (Enders and Schlafke, 1971). The uterine milieu contains substances which allowed the zona pellucida to expand *in vivo*. If uterine proteins replace the BSA in the culture medium, then the zona pellucida of cultured embryos will also expand (Maurer and Beier, 1976). The embryos can be placed in fresh medium daily, however, 2- and 4-cell embryos develop normally up to 72 hours in the same medium.

G. Culture Results

Two- and four-cell embryos placed in synthetic medium under 16 or 32 inches atmospheric pressure developed into embryos with diameters up to 4 mm after 6–10 days in culture. This expansion occurred only if the embryos completely

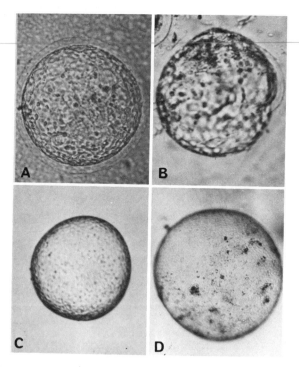

Fig. 3. Blastocysts developed *in vitro* and *in vivo*. (A) Blastocyst with a diameter of 150 μm developed from a 4-cell embryo after 72 hours in culture, $\times$ 217. (B) Hatching blastocyst with diameters of 300 $\times$ 320 μm developed from a 2-cell embryo after 120 hours in culture. $\times$ 103. (C) Day 5 blastocyst (*in vivo*) with a diameter of 1210 μm. $\times$ 22. (D) Hatched blastocyst with a diameter of 1444 μm developed from a 2- to 4-cell embryo after 168 hours in culture, $\times$ 24.

TABLE V

**Summary Development *in Vivo* of 2- and 4-Cell Rabbit Embryos Cultured for
72 or 96 Hours[a]**

	72-Hour cultured	Transfer control	96-Hour cultured	Transfer control
No. pregnant/(No. females) (%)	46/66 (70)		22/42 (52)	
No. embryos transferred	329	279	211	159
No. implanted (%)	71 (22)	154 (55)	29 (14)	74 (47)
No. viable fetuses (%)	47 (14)	126 (45)	13 (6)	63 (40)

[a] Cultured embryos were transferred to one horn, while the contralateral horn received control embryos. The does were killed on day 28 of gestation.

escaped (hatched) from the zona pellucida and if the atmospheric pressure was maintained at 16 or 32 inches of water. Figure 3 displays typical blastocysts that developed *in vitro* from 2- and 4-cell embryos.

Embryos maintained under conditions described in this chapter have developed into fetuses after 96 hours *in vitro*. Summarized in Table V are data of subsequent *in vivo* development of 2- and 4-cell rabbit embryos which were cultured for 72 or 96 hours. Although the viability is low (6%) after 96 hours *in vitro*, it is remarkable that any survived, as the rabbit embryo appears to have a requirement for uterine secretions to maintain viability (Kendle and Telford, 1970; Beier *et al.* 1972).

REFERENCES

Adams, C. E. (1956). *Proc. Int. Congr. Anim. Reprod. Artif. Insem., 3rd.* Vol. 3, pp. 5–6.

Adams, C. E. (1970). *J. Embryol. Exp. Morphol.* **23**, 21–34.

Beier, H. M., Mootz, U., and Kühnel, W. (1972). *Proc. Int. Congr. Anim. Reprod. Artif. Insem., 7th.* Vol. 3, pp. 1891–1896.

Biggers, J. D., Whitten, W. K., and Whittingham, D. G. (1971). *In* "Methods in Mammalian Embryology" (J. C. Daniel, Jr., ed.), pp. 86–116. Freeman, San Francisco, California.

Brachet, A. (1913). *Arch. Biol.* **28**, 447–503.

Brinster, R. L. (1968). *J. Anim. Sci.* **27**, Suppl. I, 1–14.

Brinster, R. L. (1970). *Adv. Biosci.* **4**, 199–232.

Chang, M. C. (1948). *Nature (London)* **161**, 978–979.

Chang, M. C. (1959). *Nature (London)* **184**, 466–467.

Daniel, J. C., Jr. (1964). *Nature (London)* **201**, 316–317.

Daniel, J. C., Jr. (1965). *J. Embryol. Exp. Morphol.* **13**, 83–95.

Elliott, D. S., Maurer, R. R., and Staples, R. E. (1974). *Biol. Reprod.* **11**, 162–167.

Enders, A. C., and Schlafke, S. (1971). *Am. J. Anat.* **132**, 219–240.

Foote, R. H., Hafs, H. D., Staples, R. E., Grégoire, A. T., and Bratton, R. W. (1963). *J. Reprod. Fertil.* **5**, 59–66.

Hafez, E. S. E. (1971). In "Methods in Mammalian Embryology" (J. C. Daniel, Jr., ed.), pp. 177–132. Freeman, San Francisco, California.

Hamilton, C. E. (1951). Anat. Rec. 110, 557–568.

Harper, M. J. K. (1963). J. Endocrinol. 26, 307–316.

Huff, R. L. (1962). Am. Zool. 2, 416.

Kane, M. T. (1972). Nature (London) 238, 468–469.

Kane, M. T., and Foote, R. H. (1970). Proc. Soc. Exp. Biol. Med. 133, 921–925.

Kane, M. T., and Foote, R. H. (1971). Biol. Reprod. 4, 41–47.

Kendle, K. E., and Telford, J. M. (1970). Br. J. Pharmacol. 40, 759–774.

Kennelly, J. J., and Foote, R. H. (1965). J. Reprod. Fertil. 9, 177–188.

Lewis, W. H., and Gregory, P. W. (1929). Science 69, 226–229.

Maurer, R. R., and Beier, H. M. (1976). J. Reprod. Fertil. 48, 33–41.

Maurer, R. R., and Haseman, J. K. (1976). Biol. Reprod. 14, 256–263.

Maurer, R. R., Hunt, W. L., and Foote, R. H. (1968). J. Reprod. Fertil. 15, 93–102.

Maurer, R. R., Whitener, R. H., and Foote, R. H. (1969). Proc. Soc. Exp. Biol. Med. 131, 882–885.

Maurer, R. R., Onuma, H., and Foote, R. H. (1970). J. Reprod. Fertil. 21, 417–422.

Maurer, R. R., Elliott, D. S., and Staples, R. E. In preparation.

Mintz, B. (1967). In "Methods in Developmental Biology" (F. H. Wilt and N. K. Wessells, eds.), pp. 379–400. Crowell-Collier, New York.

Myers, K., and Poole, W. E. (1962). Nature (London) 195, 358–359.

Naglee, D., Maurer, R. R., and Foote, R. H. (1969). Exp. Cell Res. 58, 331–333.

Ogawa, S., and Imagawa, D. T. (1969). Nature (London) 223, 409–410.

Onuma, H., Maurer, R. R., and Foote, R. H. (1968). J. Reprod. Fertil. 16, 491–493.

Pincus, G., and Enzmann, E. V. (1934). Proc. Natl. Acad. Sci. U.S.A. 20, 121–122.

Pincus, G., and Enzmann, E. V. (1936). J. Exp. Zool. 73, 195–208.

Pincus, G., and Werthessen, N. T. (1938). J. Exp. Zool. 78, 1–18.

Purshottam, N., and Pincus, G. (1961). Anat. Rec. 140, 51–55.

Roche, J. F., Dziuk, P. J., and Lodge, J. R. (1968). J. Reprod. Fertil. 6, 155–157.

Staples, R. E. (1967). J. Reprod. Fertil. 13, 369–372.

Stranzinger, G. F. (1970). Tierzuechter 8, 219.

Stranzinger, G. F., Maurer, R. R., and Paufler, S. K. (1971). J. Reprod. Fertil. 24, 111–113.

Varian, N. B., Maurer, R. R., and Foote, R. H. (1967). J. Reprod. Fertil. 13, 67–73.

Whitten, W. K. (1971). Adv. Biosci. 6, 129–139.

Whittingham, D. G. (1971). J. Reprod. Fertil., Suppl. 14, 7–21.

13

Advances in Large Mammal Embryo Culture

GARY B. ANDERSON

I. INTRODUCTION

Most of what is known about culturing mammalian embryos has been learned from research carried out with embryos of the laboratory species. Culture systems that are used for sheep and cattle embryos are based largely upon techniques and procedures developed for mouse and rabbit embryos. However, while chemically defined media have been developed and are widely used for the culture of mouse (Brinster, 1965; Whitten and Biggers, 1968) and rabbit (Kane and Foote, 1970) embryos, progress with development of chemically defined media for the culture of embryos from domestic livestock has been much slower. Reports in the scientific literature of ''successful'' attempts to culture sheep and cattle embryos have usually described poorer survival *in vitro* than is achieved with embryos of the laboratory species.

Recently, a great deal of interest has developed for *in vitro* culture systems for embryos of the livestock species, especially the cow. This interest has been stimulated by the application of embryo transfer techniques to livestock improvement. Successful application of embryo transfer techniques to practical livestock production requires that the embryo be maintained in a viable state outside the maternal environment for variable periods of time. In many cases this period is short, a matter of hours. But for maximum flexibility, it is desirable that procedures are available whereby embryo viability can be maintained for longer periods. In addition, the development of culture systems for embryos of the domestic livestock is necessary if we are to study early embryonic development in these species.

There have been several recent reports of the successful culture at 37°C of embryos of the ewe (Moore, 1970; Moor and Cragle, 1971; Tervit *et al.*, 1972; Tervit and Rowson, 1974; Wright *et al.*, 1976b; Christenson and Lunstra, 1976; Peters *et al.*, 1977; Boone *et al.*, 1976b) and cow (Tervit *et al.*, 1972; McKenzie and Kenney, 1973; Seidel, 1974; Shea *et al.*, 1974; Kanagawa *et al.*, 1975; Boone *et al.*, 1976a; Wright *et al.*, 1976a,c). Procedures have also been described for successful storage of bovine and ovine embryos at temperatures below body temperature. These reports have included storage at −196°C in liquid nitrogen (cow: Wilmut and Rowson, 1973a,b; Wilmut *et al.*, 1975; Willadsen *et al.*, 1976b; Bilton and Moore, 1976; sheep: Willadsen *et al.*, 1976a). Shorter term storage systems at 0°–20°C have also been described (Sreenan *et al.*, 1970; Kardymowicz, 1972; Moore and Bilton, 1973; Wilmut *et al.*, 1975; Trounson *et al.*, 1976).

It is worth noting that systems designed for storing embryos, even if storage is at room temperature or body temperature, may be quite different from those designed to support cleavage *in vitro*. Requirements for holding bovine embryos *in vitro* for several hours prior to transfer to a recipient female may be different than for continued *in vitro* development for several days. For example, tissue culture medium 199, containing 25 m*M* Hepes buffer (GIBCO) and supplemented with 5% heat-treated bovine serum, is an excellent medium for storing bovine embryos for several hours either at 37°C (Drost *et al.*, 1975) or at room temperature (Seidel, 1974). This medium, however, will not support continued development *in vitro* for long periods.

Different criteria for assessing embryo viability and the adequacy of a culture system have been used by various authors. Some have used continued cleavage *in vitro* and "normal embryo morphology" as criteria for successful culture. Others have used growth *in vitro* to a particular stage of embryonic development, such as the morula or blastocyst stage, to define successful culture. Others have transferred cultured embryos to recipient females and counted fetuses at slaughter or young at birth.

Culture techniques and conditions used by authors also vary considerably. One of the most common and conspicuous differences in techniques reported is the type of culture medium used. Some authors have described systems using simple media, while others have used complex media; some have used media that are chemically defined, while others have included natural media such as homologous or fetal calf serum. However, differences in culture systems other than culture media may be equally important to evaluating the success of the various workers. Some workers have cultured embryos in test tubes; others have cultured embryos in small (0.01 ml) drops of medium under oil, or relatively large amounts of medium (1.0 ml) in tissue culture wells. Bovine and ovine embryos have been collected and cultured at different stages of embryonic development and in different gas atmospheres. Tervit *et al*. (1972) used an atmosphere of 5% oxygen, 5% carbon dioxide, and 90% nitrogen for their culture systems for cattle and sheep embryos, rather than the 5% carbon dioxide–95% air atmosphere used by many workers. Wright *et al*., using a different culture system, found this low oxygen atmosphere beneficial for the culture of cattle embryos (1976a), but not for sheep embryos (1976b).

It is important to remember that each of these variables, as well as the number of embryos cultured per drop of medium, the temperature at which embryos are held, and possibly the female from which the embryos are collected can affect the success of a culture system. Since all the variables that affect the viability of bovine and ovine embryos *in vitro* have not yet been established, slight modifications in culture systems may affect rates of development. Furthermore, since, in many of the reports previously mentioned, there were a number of factors that differed among the various culture systems, combinations of factors described in different reports may or may not provide a system that supports *in vitro* development.

In this chapter, the culture systems used in this laboratory for the culture at 37°C of bovine and ovine embryos are described. No attempt has been made to compare these procedures with those used and reported by other workers. Specific techniques adapted from systems utilized for embryos of laboratory species and described elsewhere have been referenced, but not outlined in detail. Since the conditions under which sheep and cattle embryos have been cultured have differed in various reports, the reader is cautioned against adopting portions of these or other procedures without consideration of other differences in the culture systems.

II. CULTURE OF OVINE EMBRYOS

A. Superovulation and Embryo Collection

The breeds of sheep most commonly used in embryo culture studies in this laboratory are Targhee, Finnish Landrace, Suffolk, and their crossbreds. Embryos are generally collected from cycling ewes that have been superovulated. Estrus synchronization and superovulation are accomplished by the insertion of progestagen-impregnated vaginal pessaries for 12 days and injection of 1200–1500 IU pregnant mare serum gonadotropin (PMSG) at the time of pessary removal. Ewes are exposed to fertile rams and estrus is observed approximately 24–72 hours after sponge removal. An alternate means of estrus synchronization involves daily sc injections of 5 mg progesterone in corn oil for 12 consecutive days. PMSG is administered at the time of the last progesterone injection, and, again, estrus is observed approximately 24–72 hours later.

Four-cell and eight-cell embryos can be collected 48 and 72 hours, respectively, after the onset of estrus. Comparable intervals for breeds with long estrus periods are 72 and 96 hours, respectively. It is not unusual to collect some embryos with fewer blastomeres than otherwise expected. It is not known whether these embryos result from late ovulations or from oocytes whose development is abnormally slow. The developmental potential of these earlier stage embryos is not known, but in some cases, they have developed into blastocysts when placed in culture at 37°C. Embryos are flushed from the donor's uterine horns and oviducts with tissue culture medium 199 (TCM199) at surgery or slaughter. With the aid of a dissecting microscope, they are counted and their morphology is examined. If embryos are not to be immediately observed after collection, they are held in the flushing medium in an incubator at 37°C in an atmosphere of 5% CO_2–95% air.

B. Culture Techniques

In an experiment which compared various culture media for the maintenance of viability of sheep embryos *in vitro* (Wright *et al.*, 1976b), Whitten's mouse ova culture medium (Whitten and Biggers, 1968), supplemented with 0.1% or 0.2% bovine serum albumin (BSA), was shown to be superior to several more complex tissue culture media. We have subsequently increased the level of BSA in the medium to 0.5% and improved the development observed *in vitro* (Peters *et al.*, 1977). Embryos are cultured by the microdrop technique described by Brinster (1963) for mouse embryos. A gas mixture of 5% CO_2–95% air is gently bubbled through the culture medium for approximately 5 minutes. The medium is then sterilized by filtering through a Millipore filter (0.22-μm pore size). Eight individual drops of medium (approximately 0.01 ml each) are placed in a plastic 60 × 15 mm petri dish (Falcon Plastics) and covered with 10 ml light-weight paraffin oil (Saybolt viscosity, 125/135; Fischer Products) that has been previously equilibrated with the medium and gas atmosphere. Culture plates are generally made 1 day prior to embryo collection and are stored in an incubator at 37°C in a 5% CO_2–95% air atmosphere until needed.

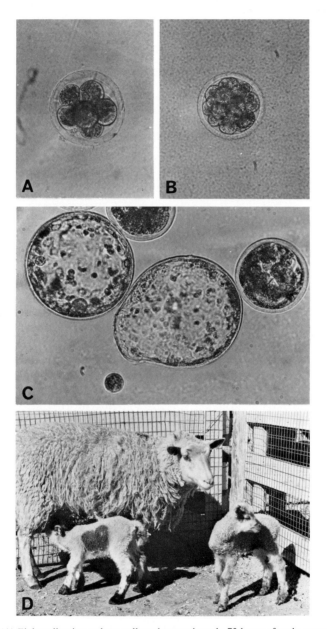

Fig. 1. (A) Eight-cell ovine embryo collected approximately 72 hours after the onset of estrus. (B) Ovine morula collected at the 8-cell stage and cultured at 37°C for 24 hours in Whitten's mouse ova culture medium supplemented with 0.5% bovine serum albumin. (C) Ovine embryos cultured at 37°C for 129 hours from the 8-cell to the expanded and hatching blastocyst stages in supplemented Whitten's medium. [(A, B, and C) photographed at × 40]. (D) Twin lambs born following transfer of ovine embryos cultured at 37°C for 24 hours in supplemented Whitten's medium.

To equilibrate the oil with the medium and gas atmosphere, approximately 500 ml oil is heated to 160°C for 60 minutes. After it has cooled, approximately 50 ml culture medium without BSA is added and 5% CO_2–95% air is bubbled slowly (3 liters/min) through the mixture for 15 minutes. After thorough shaking, the medium and oil mixture is allowed to sit and separate for 48 hours. When oil is needed for culturing embryos, it is carefully pipetted from this equilibrated oil, taking care not to disturb the medium phase under the oil.

After the embryos are removed from the TCM199 flushing medium, they are moved sequentially through three washes of culture medium and placed into culture. They are photographed, and culture plates are immediately returned to the incubator, where they are maintained at 37°C in an atmosphere of 5% CO_2–95% air for the culture period. The culture plates are removed from the incubator at daily intervals, and embryos are photographed at 80 × with an inverted stage phase-contrast microscope. With this culture system, ovine embryos have been cultured from the 1-cell to the blastocyst stage and from the 8-cell to the hatching blastocyst stage (Fig. 1). In contrast to the results of Tervit *et al.* (1972), we have found no advantage to culturing sheep embryos in an atmosphere containing 5% oxygen, rather than the approximately 20% level found in air (Wright *et al.*, 1976b). Tervit cultured his embryos in glass test tubes (Biggers *et al.*, 1971), however, rather than in small drops of medium under paraffin oil.

C. Viability of Cultured Embryos

This culture system which has supported *in vitro* development of sheep embryos to the expanded and hatching blastocyst stage has also been tested on a limited basis in terms of the viability of cultured embryos. Eighteen embryos that were cultured from the 8-cell stage for 24 hours were transferred two each to nine synchronized recipient females. Seven lambs were subsequently born from five recipients. It is worth noting that the estrous cycles of all recipients were not exactly synchronized with the stage of development of the cultured embryos, and viability may have been adversely affected. All recipients that lambed (five of nine) showed estrus within 12 hours of the time estrus was first observed in the donors. The remaining recipients showed estrus at a period of greater than 12 hours from the time estrus was observed in the donors.

D. Staining of Ovine Embryos

Upon removal from culture, sheep embryos can be stained with either acetoorcein or hematoxylin. With these staining procedures, it is possible to estimate the number of nuclei in each embryo. The presence of nuclei indicates that cleavage has occurred *in vitro* rather than simply fragmentation of the cytoplasm. To stain with acetoorcein, four drops of a 9:1 mixture of Vaseline and paraffin are placed on a clean glass slide. The drops should be placed so that when a 22 × 22 mm cover slip is placed over them, one drop is located at each corner of the cover slip. The embryo to be stained is placed in a minimum amount of medium in the center of the field among the drops of Vaseline/paraffin mixture. A clean cover slip is placed over the embryo. With the aid of a dissecting microscope, the embryo can be observed while light pressure is exerted with the fingers at each corner of the cover slip. The embryo is held in place when the cover slip contacts it and slightly distorts its shape. The slide is carefully moved to a staining jar containing Carnoy's fixative (1:3 glacial acetic acid and ethanol) and left for 24 hours. Upon removal from the fixative, embryos are stained by slowly and repeatedly passing a 1% acetoorcein stain under the cover slip. The stain is drawn off by touching the opposite edge of the cover slip with a piece of paper tissue. The stain is filtered immediately before using to reduce the number of crystals that can make visual observations difficult. The method used in this laboratory involves filtering the stain directly onto the slide from a 1.0 cc disposable syringe attached to a Millipore Swinnex filter holder containing a 0.22-μm pore size filter. Staining generally takes 10–20 minutes. The degree of staining can be continuously monitored. Final counting of nuclei is best accomplished at 100 × or 200 × magnification. This technique produces a temporary preparation that should be observed and photographed as soon as the embryo has reached the desired degree of staining.

An alternative means that we have used for staining sheep embryos uses hematoxylin stain and different procedures than described for acetoorcein. The advantage of this second technique is that a permanent specimen is prepared. Embryos to be stained are moved in a minimum amount of medium to a clean glass slide that has been thinly coated with Mayer's albumin fixative. The slides are air-dried and carefully moved to a staining jar containing Carnoy's fixative for 30 minutes. Slides are again air-dried and then moved to a staining jar containing hematoxylin stain. The period of time required for staining depends upon the stage of development of the embryo. Morulae and blastocysts are stained for 15 minutes at room temperature. Earlier stage embryos tend to require a longer staining period and/or slightly higher temperatures. Slides are rinsed briefly in water and dehydrated with a series of ethanol rinses. A permanent specimen is made by mounting the cover slip with any compound used for that purpose.

III. CULTURE OF BOVINE EMBRYOS

A. Superovulation and Embryo Collection

Most of the embryos used in our studies are collected from superovulated Hereford, Angus, and crossbred heifers. Females are observed for signs of estrus to establish estrous cycles. Normally cycling females are given an im injection of 2000 IU PMSG, followed 48 hours later with 30 mg prostaglandin $F_{2\alpha}$ (Upjohn Co.). Estrus is observed 48–60 hours later. $PGF_{2\alpha}$ is effective in inducing luteolysis between days 5–17 of the bovine estrous cycle, but we generally arrange our injection schedule so the $PGF_{2\alpha}$ is administered between days 10 and 16 of the estrous cycle. An alternate method of synchronizing estrus in donor animals is with daily im injections of 50 mg progesterone for 13 days. On the fifth day of progesterone administration, a luteolytic dose of 6 mg estradiol valerate is injected im. PMSG is given at the time of the last progesterone injection, and estrus is observed approximately 72 hours later. Regardless of the method used for synchronization, donors are mated or inseminated at estrus. Embryos are collected at surgery by midventral laparotomy or at slaughter by flushing the uterine horns and oviducts with TCM199 (GIBCO) according to procedures described by Rowson *et al.* (1969). The interval between estrus and embryo collection varies, depending upon the stage of embryonic development desired. Generally, 1- and 2-cell embryos are collected 2 days after estrus, 4- and 8-cell embryos are collected 3–4 days after estrus, and early morulae are collected 5 days after estrus. Embryos are counted, and morphological examination for normality is made with a dissecting microscope.

B. Culture Techniques

Embryos are removed from the flushing medium and transferred sequentially through three washes of culture medium. They are examined and photographed at 80 × with a phase-contrast microscope and then placed into culture. The system for culturing embryos is the microdrop technique described for culturing sheep embryos. A number of culture media, including modified Eagle's medium, TCM199, synthetic oviduct fluid, Brinster's mouse ova culture medium (BMOC-3), and Whitten's mouse ova culture medium, have been tested in this laboratory for maintenance of viability of bovine embryos *in vitro* (Wright *et al.*, 1976a). The best medium tested so far under the conditions used in this laboratory is Ham's F-10 medium supplemented with 10% heat-treated fetal calf serum.

The Ham's F-10 medium is purchased and stored at 4°C in dry form (GIBCO). The day before the embryos are to be cultured, the medium is made with twice deionized and three times distilled water, and sodium bicarbonate and fetal calf serum (GIBCO) are added. A gas mixture of 5% CO_2–5% oxygen and 90% nitrogen is bubbled through the medium for approximately 5 minutes. The medium is sterilized by filtering through a sterile Millipore filter (0.22-μm pore size). Equilibration of paraffin oil with the medium is carried out with Ham's F-10 without serum and with the 5% oxygen gas mixture.

Culture plates are held in an anaerobic chamber flushed with the low oxygen gas mixture and held at 37°C. A beaker of water is placed in the bottom of the

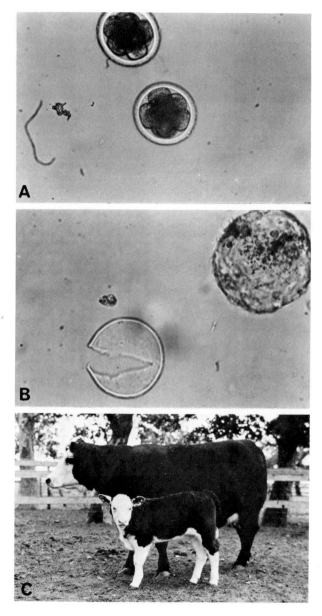

Fig. 2.   (A) Eight-cell bovine embryos collected approximately 96 hours after the onset of estrus. (B) Bovine embryo cultured at 37°C for 165 hours from the 8-cell to the hatched blastocyst stage in Ham's F-10 medium supplemented with 10% heat-treated fetal calf serum [(A and B) photographed at × 40]. (C) Calf born following transfer of bovine embryo cultured at 37°C for 24 hours in supplemented Ham's F-10 medium.

chamber to provide a humidified atmosphere. The culture plates are removed daily from the chamber to evaluate embryonic development. The anaerobic chamber is reflushed with the gas mixture after each time it is opened. Using this relatively simple system, bovine embryos have been cultured from the 1-cell to the early blastocyst stage, from the 2-cell to the expanded blastocyst stage (after 155–165 hours *in vitro*), and from the 8-cell to the hatched blastocyst stage (after 165 hours *in vitro*) (Fig. 2).

C. Viability of Cultured Embryos

The viability of embryos cultured with this system has been tested. Ten embryos collected 5 days after estrus and cultured for 24 hours were transferred to the uteri of six heifers. Four recipients each received two cultured embryos, and two each received one cultured and one noncultured embryo. In these latter two recipients, coat color markers were used to differentiate calves born from cultured and noncultured embryos. Recipients were selected that showed estrus 1 day after the donors to allow for any retardation of development that may occur *in vitro*. Five normal calves were born from cultured embryos in four recipients (Fig. 2).

D. Staining of Bovine Embryos

Bovine embryos can be fixed and stained with acetoorcein, as described for staining of ovine embryos. Because of the granular nature of the cytoplasm in bovine embryos, we have found that this procedure produces specimens that can be studied more easily than those produced with the hematoxylin staining procedure.

REFERENCES

Biggers, J. D., Whitten, W. K., and Whittingham, D. G. (1971). *In* "Methods in Mammalian Embryology," (J. C. Daniel, Jr., ed.), pp. 86–116. Freeman, San Francisco, California.
Bilton, R. J., and Moore, N. W. (1976). *J. Reprod. Fertil.* **46**, 537–538.
Boone, W. R., Dantzler, J. R., Luszcz, L. J., Dickey, J. F., and Kennedy, S. W. (1976a). *J. Anim. Sci.* **43**, 276 (abstr.).
Boone, W. R., Luszcz, L. J., Dantzler, J. R., Dickey, J. F., and Kennedy, S. W. (1976b). *J. Anim. Sci.* **43**, 276 (abstr.).
Brinster, R. L. (1963). *Exp. Cell Res.* **32**, 205–208.
Brinster, R. L. (1965). *J. Reprod. Fertil.* **10**, 227–240.
Christenson, R. K., and Lunstra, D. D. (1976). *9th Annu. Meet Soc. Study Reprod.* Abstr. No. 120.
Drost, M., Anderson, G. B., Cupps, P. T., Horton, M. B., Warner, P. V., and Wright, R. W. Jr. (1975). *J. Am. Vet. Med. Assoc.* **166**, 1176–1179.

Kanagawa, H., Bedirian, K., Ringelberg, C., and Basrur, P. K. (1975). *8th Annu. Meet. Soc. Study Reprod.* Abstr. No. 74.

Kane, M. T., and Foote, R. H. (1970). *Proc. Soc. Exp. Biol. Med.* **133**, 921–925.

Kardymowicz, O. (1972). *Proc. Int. Congr. Anim. Reprod. Artif. Insem., 7th,* 1972 pp. 500–503.

McKenzie, B. E., and Kenney, R. M. (1973). *Am. J. Vet. Res.* **34**, 1271–1275.

Moor, R. M., and Cragle, R. G. (1971). *J. Reprod. Fertil.* **27**, 401–409.

Moore, N. W. (1970). *Aust. J. Biol. Sci.* **23**, 721–724.

Moore, N. W., and Bilton, R. J. (1973). *Aust. J. Biol. Sci.* **26**, 1421–1427.

Peters, D. F., Anderson, G. B., and Cupps, P. T. (1977). *J. Anim. Sci.* **45**, 350–354.

Rowson, L. E. A., Moor, R. M., and Lawson, R. A. S. (1969). *J. Reprod. Fertil.* **18**, 517–523.

Seidel, G. E., Jr. (1974). *Proc. Soc. Study Breed. Soundness,* p. 9.

Shea, B. F., Church, R. B., and Tervit, H. R. (1974). *7th Annu. Meet. Soc. Study Reprod.* Abstr. No. 147.

Sreenan, S. J., Scanlon, P., and Gordon, I. (1970). *J. Agric. Sci.* **74**, 593–594.

Tervit, H. R., and Rowson, L. E. A. (1974). *J. Reprod. Fertil.* **38**, 177–179.

Tervit, H. R., Whittingham, D. G., and Rowson, L. E. A. (1972). *J. Reprod. Fertil.* **30**, 493–497.

Trounson, A. O., Willadsen, S. M., Rowson, L. E. A., and Newcomb, R. (1976). *J. Reprod. Fertil.* **46,** 173–178.

Whitten, W. K., and Biggers, J. D. (1968). *J. Reprod. Fertil.* **17**, 399–401.

Willadsen, S. M., Polge, C., Rowson, L. E. A., and Moor, R. M. (1976a). *J. Reprod. Fertil.* **46**, 151–154.

Willadsen, S. M., Trounson, A. O., Polge, C., Rowson, L. E. A., and Newcomb, R. (1976b). *In* "Egg Transfer in Cattle" (L. E. A. Rowson, ed.), pp. 117–124. Commission of the European Communities, Luxembourg.

Wilmut, I., and Rowson, L. E. A. (1973a). *J. Reprod. Fertil.* **33**, 352–353.

Wilmut, I., and Rowson, L. E. A. (1973b). *Vet. Rec.* **92**, 686–690.

Wilmut, I., Polge, C., and Rowson, L. E. A. (1975). *J. Reprod. Fertil.* **45**, 209–211.

Wright, R. W., Jr., Anderson, G. B., Cupps, P. T., and Drost, M. (1976a). *Biol. Reprod.* **14**, 157–162.

Wright, R. W., Jr., Anderson, G. B., Cupps, P. T., Drost, M., and Bradford, G. E. (1976b). *J. Anim. Sci.* **42**, 912–917.

Wright, R. W., Jr., Anderson, G. B., Cupps, P. T., and Drost, M. (1976c). *J. Anim. Sci.* **43**, 170–174.

14

Embryo Transfer in Large Domestic Mammals

FINNIE A. MURRAY

I. INTRODUCTION

Transfer of embryos in large farm animals is currently a widely applied technology, both as a research tool and as a commercial enterprise. The technology has evolved through the efforts of many scientists, but originated with Heape (1890). No attempt will be made in this chapter to review the literature on embryo transfer; rather, the chapter will deal with methodology that reflects the current state of the procedure.

Embryo transfer in large animals involves a number of steps, each of which is essential for the overall success of the transfer. These include herd management, superovulation, estrus synchronization and detection, insemination, embryo collection, evaluation, and transfer, pregnancy diagnosis, and proof of parentage of the offspring. All embryo transfer programs require attention to these points to a greater or lesser degree; however, transfer operations necessarily vary somewhat with different species of animals. Therefore, it is necessary to discuss specific methods for each of the four major species of farm mammals (cattle, horses, sheep, and swine).

II. FACILITIES AND EQUIPMENT

Work with large animals necessitates adequate housing and handling facilities for each species used. It is essential to have sorting pens and chutes for separating animals for treatment, surgery, and pregnancy diagnosis. These facilities are important, but can be varied to meet the needs of a specific program. It is suggested, however, that if new facilities are to be constructed, the expertise of an agricultural engineer be employed with specific attention to space, convenience of operation, and waste disposal to meet local codes.

A. Surgery

A spacious and clean area is essential for surgery. It is recommended that space for at least two simultaneous operations be provided in the surgery area. For example, a space of approximately 40 m^2 should be available for cattle surgery, 30 m^2 for swine, and 25 m^2 for sheep. The surgery room for cattle, horses, or pigs should be equipped with convenient oxygen outlets and mobile machines for halothane anesthesia. Two adjustable overhead surgical lamps for each surgical location are recommended. Electrocautery is also very helpful, especially on cattle. A scrub area for the surgeons in or near the surgery room is essential, as are spark-retardant electrical outlets and wall switches. Wide, tightly closing swinging doors with windows are also helpful. It is also recommended that fresh, filtered air be used to create a positive pressure for maintaining a clean surgical field.

A scrub room in which animals can be prepared for surgery should be provided adjacent to, but not in, the surgery room. An anesthesia induction area should be near the surgical preparation area, and a spacious recovery area near the surgery room is also necessary. To prevent congestion, it is advantageous to have animals enter and leave each area in opposite directions. Oxygen outlets conveniently located at each area are also very helpful.

B. Embryologic Laboratory

The embryologic laboratory should be located adjacent to the surgery room, but it should be completely separate. A fresh, filtered air supply to the embryo lab should provide positive pressure to this area to minimize influx of the atmosphere from the surgery room. In the experience of the author, the surgery room atmosphere can be extremely detrimental to embryo survival and should not be allowed to contaminate the atmosphere for the embryos. The embryo lab should be equipped with sufficient germicidal ultraviolet lamps to minimize microbial contamination of the area. An embryo manipulation hood should be provided with fresh filtered air, germicidal lamps, warming capacity, and a stero dissection microscope. Several models of embryologic hoods have been described for use with laboratory animals (e.g., Staples, 1971), and one can construct a suitable hood from such a pattern. The embryologic laboratory should provide an incubator for temporary storage or culture of embryos. As most media currently in use employ bicarbonate buffering, it is necessary to provide a mechanism to supply humidified 5% CO_2 in air, unless one plans exclusively to use media buffered without bicarbonate. It is wise to provide a convenient desk area near the embryologic hood for record keeping.

III. PROCEDURES

A. Herd Management

Herd management must be considered the first priority for any embryo transfer program to be successful. The best animals may yield poor results if attention is not given to the welfare, health, and nutrition of both donors and recipients. In fact, problems can occur in this regard under ''good'' management, due to subtle factors not normally encountered or expected. For example, Segerson et al. (1977) recently observed fertilization failure in cattle due to what appeared to be lack of selenium in the diet and poor quality of hay fed the animals. In spite of the great importance of good herd management, it would be inappropriate to use space in this chapter to include this topic, since it is described in a variety of texts on the husbandry of domestic animals. Furthermore, it is suggested that professional consultation be used for each aspect of herd management.

B. Estrus Synchronization

Survival of transferred embryos requires a hospitable intrauterine environment in all species. This is most satisfactorily accomplished by transferring embryos to recipients that are in the same endocrinologic condition as the donor. In practice, this is achieved by use of recipients that are naturally or artificially synchronized at estrus with the donor female. Synchronization within 24 hours of the donor is considered adequate to achieve excellent results from transfer (Newcomb and Rowson, 1975).

1. Natural Synchronization

Natural synchronization is the simpler approach to estrus synchronization, and it is necessary in certain situations at the present time due to drug restrictions and lack of effective alternatives. Large numbers of recipient females are required, so that on any day there are enough in the right stage to receive all available embryos from synchronous donors. The large herd size required for this type of synchronization creates very large costs for herd maintenance, estrus detection, and acquisition of animals. For the smallest embryo transfer operation in cattle, for example, the natural estrus synchronization method requires 250–300 cycling females in the recipient herd in order to provide 10–15 recipients in estrus on any 1 day during a 21-day estrous cycle. Obviously, with this degree of expense and labor, other methods of estrus synchronization are preferable, if available.

2. Artificial Synchronization

Presently, there are several products that are effective in achieving satisfactory estrus synchronization without creating fertility problems; however, most of these are not yet commercially available. These products have been and are being used effectively in research programs involving embryo transfer. Use of artificial synchronization reduces the number of recipient females required and, therefore, improves the economy of the transfer procedure. Procedures for artificial synchronization are outlined below.

a. Prostaglandins. Prostaglandin $F_2\alpha$, its THAM salt or synthetic analogues, have been demonstrated to provide good estrus synchronization with no impairment of fertility. Intramuscular administration of prostaglandins works well with cattle (Lauderdale, 1972), horses (Douglas and Ginther, 1975), and sheep (Douglas and Ginther, 1973). Prostaglandins are effective in producing luteal regression only between days 5 and 16 in cattle (Lauderdale, 1972; Rowson et al., 1972; Tervit et al., 1973); therefore, either it must be administered to females with well-established corpora lutea or administered twice at intervals sufficient in length to allow regression of corpora lutea formed after the first treatment. The two-injection sequence is recommended for the recipient herds. The literature is voluminous on this subject. Therefore, only representative reports are cited in Table I, which summarizes treatment schedules for the various products.

b. Progestogens. Progestogens have long been used for estrus synchronization; however, poor fertility following their use has limited their value until

TABLE I
Treatment Schedule to Achieve Estrus Synchronization with Prostaglandins

Agent	Species	Dose	Site	Estrus dates unknown (two injections)	Estrus dates known (one injection)	Reference
Prostaglandin $F_{2\alpha}$-THAM salt[a]	Cattle	25 mg	im	12-Day interval		Manns et al. (1976)
	Horse	10 mg	im		Day 6 after ovulation	Miller et al. (1976)
	Sheep	6 mg	im		Day 8 of cycle	Douglas and Ginther (1973)
Prostaglandin $F_{2\alpha}$-THAM salt[a]	Cattle	33.5 mg	im		After day 4	Lambert et al. (1976); Cupps et al. (1976)
Analogues ICI 80,996[b]	Cattle	500 μg	im		Day 5–15	Sreenan et al. (1975)
Equimate[b]	Horse	250 μg	im	14-Day interval[c]	Between 5th and 13th day of diestrus[c]	Allen et al. (1976)

[a] Upjohn Company, Kalamazoo, Michigan.
[b] I.C.I. Pharmaceuticals, Ltd., Macclesfield, Cheshire, U.K.
[c] Follow each Equimate injection with 2500–3000 IU HCG at 6 days.

recently. The progestogen method relies on the suppression of follicular development by the agent until the entire group of animals so treated no longer possess luteal function. Therefore, when the progestogen is withdrawn, follicular development occurs synchronously in the whole group. This method requires constant release of the agent throughout the treatment period. Table II summarizes typical protocols for use of progestogens.

There are a number of ways to achieve estrus synchronization, all of which can yield a high degree of synchronization without producing fertility problems. The method of choice will depend upon the cost of the products, the program, and the facilities available.

TABLE II
Treatment Schedules to Achieve Estrus Synchronization with Progestogens

| Agent | Species | Treatment | | | Reference |
		Dose	Site	Duration (days)	
Progesterone	Cattle	10% Progesterone in silicone rubber over stainless steel coils for cows, 6.6% for heifers[a]	Intravaginal	12	Roche (1976)
Norgestamet[b]	Cattle	6 mg	Subcutaneous implant	8	Stauffer et al. (1976)
Cronolone[c]	Sheep	Prepared pessary	Intravaginal	12	Wright et al. (1976)
Progesterone	Sheep	5 mg/day	Subcutaneous	12	Wright et al. (1976)
A-35957[d]	Swine	12.5 mg/day	Feed	18–19	Webel (1976); Davis et al. (1976); Knight et al. (1976)

[a] All cattle receive 5 mg estradiol benzoate and 50 mg progesterone, im, in corn oil at the time of insertion of the coil.

[b] SC 21009, Searle Laboratories.

[c] 9-Fluoro-11β, 17-dehydroxypregn-4-ene-3,20-dione, 17-acetate, Searle Laboratories.

[d] 17-α-allyl-estrateine-4-9-11, 17-β-ol-3-one, Abbott Laboratories, North Chicago, Illinois.

TABLE III
Effect of Superovulation on Number of Usable Ova on Days 3–5 p.c. in Swine[a]

Treatment	No. of gilts	No. of corpora lutea	No. of ova recovered	No. of fertilized ova	No. of embryos developing normally
PMSG	18[b]	15.56±3.01	9.44±1.94	8.78±1.79	8.22±1.78
No PMSG	23	11.35±0.75	8.74±0.73	8.65±0.74	8.04±0.81

[a] Data are means ± SEM.

[b] Includes two gilts that failed to ovulate after treatment.

TABLE IV

Superovulation Schedules

Gonadotropin	Species	Dose	Time (estrus = day 0)	Secondary treatment Site	Agent	Dose	Time	Site	Reference
PMSG	Cattle	2200 IU	Days 15–16	im	None				Segerson et al. (1976)
	Cattle	2000 IU	Mid-late luteal	sc	ICI-80,996	100 μg	48 hrs after	im	Trounson et al. (1976)
	Horse	Not recommended							
	Sheep	1000 IU	Day 12	sc	None				Willadsen et al. (1976)
	Swine	1200 IU	Day 15	sc	None				Curnock et al. (1976)
FSH	Cattle	FSH:LH, 5:1 total dose: 32 mg FSH, 5.3 mg LH divided into multiple injections	Two injections per day, mg of FSH given: Day 10 5,5 Day 11 4,4 Day 12 3,3 Day 13 2,2 Day 14 2,2	sc	PG $F_{2\alpha}$-THAM salt	45 mg in two doses: 30 mg in AM. 15 mg in P.M.	Day 12, A.M. and PM	im	Elsden et al. (1976)

C. Superovulation

For many embryo transfer situations superovulation is essential to provide enough embryos for efficient operation. This may not apply to mares and sows, or for certain nonsurgical transfer procedures in cattle. In my laboratory, superovulation of pigs for embryo work is no longer practiced because 8–10 embryos per gilt are routinely obtained, and superovulation introduces a great deal of variation. This variation stems from widely ranging ovulation rates, and greater frequency of fertilization failure (Table III). Thus superovulation of the gilt for embryo transfer is not advised in most instances.

The materials used to achieve superovulation are pregnant mare serum gonadotropin (PMSG) and follicle-stimulating hormone (FSH). Both of these products are available in forms which are of high purity and which cause relatively few problems of side effects. PMSG is convenient to use, since only one injection is required; however, due to rapid turnover (Catchpole, 1963), FSH must be administered in a series of injections.

With the possible exception of donor females, which are to be superovulated repeatedly, there is little reason to use FSH, since its use is more complex than that for PMSG (Moore, 1975). If the donor is to be superovulated repeatedly, FSH and PSMG may be alternated to reduce the possibility of decreased response to the gonadotropin treatment. Regardless of the gonadotropin employed, it is desirable to determine the dose response to each lot placed in use. The optimum dose level is that which produces the greatest ovulation rate with minimum numbers of unruptured follicles. Once the optimal dose is determined, it is best to use that as a standard level in the group of animals for which it was determined. Ovulation rates after superovulation are highly variable in all cases; therefore, the information in Table IV provides general dose levels only. Prostaglandins are often used in the superovulation protocol to achieve estrus synchronization and to decrease the variation in time of ovulation in cattle (Moore, 1975).

D. Estrus Detection

Whether natural or artificial synchronization is used, detection of estrus is crucial. Animals exhibiting estrus at the same heat check as the donor are the best candidates for recipients in cattle (Newcomb and Rowson, 1975), pigs (Webel et al., 1970), and sheep (Hancock and Hovell, 1961). Regardless of the methods employed, human judgment is the key to estrus detection. The procedures briefly described below are well established and are more fully presented elsewhere (e.g., Hafez, 1962; Anderson, 1969).

1. Cattle

In cattle, the strongest criterion for behavioral estrus is standing rigidly for mounting by other cattle (males or females), although other criteria are at times useful (Anderson, 1969). With standing for mounting as the primary criterion, visual detection is performed in the early morning and late afternoon. Several worthwhile estrus detection aids are available to capitalize on the standing behavior. These aids include pressure-sensitive dye patches worn on the cow's back, chin ball markers worn on teaser bulls, and various types of surgically altered marker bulls.

2. Horses

Teaser stallions are employed to aid in estrus detection. Estrous mares also exhibit several external signs: frequent urination, squatting, "winking" of the vulvar labia, and tail raise. Sullivan *et al.* (1973) considered mares to have entered estrus when three of the four external signs were observed. Mares have extended estrous periods (Anderson, 1969), and ovulation time is variable within this interval. Even when artificial control of luteal life is exercised, the interval from treatment to ovulation is 7–12 days and variable (Allen and Rowson, 1973; Douglas and Ginther, 1975; Allen *et al.*, 1976). For this reason, rectal palpation of the mare throughout estrus at 12-hour intervals to detect ovulation is essential.

3. Sheep

Estrus detection in ewes depends upon the use of a ram, since ewes exhibit no clear external signs of estrus except in association with a male. Cryptorchid, vasectomized, or aproned rams fitted with a marking crayon are used for estrus detection.

4. Swine

Sows and gilts exhibit several external signs which can be exploited in estrus detection. Swelling and reddening of the vulva, restlessness, and frequent attempts to urinate indicate approaching estrus. At the onset of estrus, females stand rigidly for mounting by other females, as well as males, and become immobile when hand pressure is applied to the back. This immobilization reflex is considered the onset of estrus.

E. Insemination

Whether donors are bred naturally or artificially, several inseminations at 12-hour intervals, beginning approximately 12 hours prior to expected ovulation and continuing until at least 12 hours after ovulation, are highly recommended. Many workers use multiple ampules or straws at each artificial insemination.

F. Embryo Collection

The collection of embryos for transfer involves essentially the same thing, regardless of the species. The exact manner by which collection of embryos from the uterus is performed varies with species. Procedures successful in the author's experience and/or in the literature are described below.

1. Cattle

a. Surgical. The basic approach to embryo transfer in cattle was developed by Rowson *et al.* (1969). These methods have been modified by many researchers to meet needs of their own programs, and the procedures described here are those used by my colleagues and myself. In addition, a review of this subject was recently published elsewhere (Newcomb, 1976).

The donor and a group of synchronized recipients are subjected to rectal palpation to verify that ovulation occurred in the recipients, as well as to estimate the number of ova shed by the donor. Surgery is performed 5–7 days after estrus in the donor. The donor is anesthetized with thiamylal sodium iv, and is allowed to fall onto a mobile surgical table on which she is situated in a supine position and to which her legs are secured by ropes. An endotrachial tube is installed and connected to a gas anesthesia apparatus dispensing halothane, nitrous oxide, and oxygen. The animal is shaved, scrubbed, and draped in a preparation room, from which she is moved to the surgery room. Surgery is performed under sterile conditions. A 15-cm midline incision is made just anterior to the udder. Hemostasis is maintained with electrocautery. The reproductive tract is exposed with firm but gentle force to allow manipulation of the oviducts and ovaries. The number of corpora lutea on each ovary is determined and recorded. A sterile polyvinyl tube, approximately 40 cm in length, is selected from a stock ranging from 1.5 to 4.0 mm in diameter, so that its outside diameter can be forced (without tissue damage) 2–3 cm into the infundibular end of the oviduct (Fig. 1). Two cross-acting tissue forceps are clamped on the oviduct and cannula to retard slippage of the cannula within the oviduct. One pair of forceps is placed on the oviduct near the end of the cannula and the other about 1 cm behind the first (Fig. 1). A large pair of compression forceps protected with rubber tubing is placed on the uterine horn near the external bifurcation. The uterine horn is now ready to flush.

A syringe containing 50–60 ml of bicarbonate-buffered tissue culture medium 199 (TCM 199) with Earle's salts is used to flush the uterine contents into the oviduct and cannula. The syringe is equipped with a blunt 18-gauge hypodermic needle. (The blunt needle aids in locating the uterine lumen, without lacerating the uterine wall, which can result in hemorrhaging.) The needle is introduced through the uterine wall at a point near the compression forceps, and about 10 ml of medium is injected to test the location of the tip of the needle. If it is in the lumen, another 15–20 ml is injected, and gentle pressure is applied to the uterus to aid in forcing fluid through the tubouterine junction. The flushing is collected into a series of culture tubes, which are immediately capped and taken to the

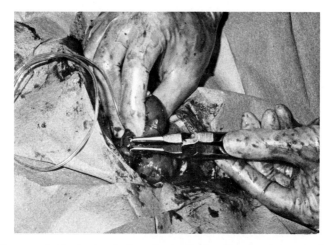

Fig. 1.   Cow reproductive tract ready for embryo collection. The cannula is secured within the infundibular end of the oviduct with cross-action forceps.

embryologic laboratory. The process is repeated with the second oviduct and uterine horn.

Once it is established that most or all embryos have been recovered from the donor, the peritoneum and linea alba are simultaneously closed with discontinuous suturing with No. 3 chromic catgut. Antibiotic powder is applied, and the skin is closed with discontinuous suturing of synthetic suture. The animal receives penicillin–streptomycin (im) and close supervision following surgery.

b.   Nonsurgical Embryo Collection.   Elsden *et al.* (1976) recently developed a procedure for nonsurgical recovery of bovine embryos which was highly successful with substantial numbers of cattle in a total of 115 attempts. Success rates for unsuperovulated and superovulated cattle were 71% and 92%, respectively. Such a consistently successful nonsurgical recovery method marks a significant breakthrough in the field of embryo transfer in cattle. Essentially similar techniques have recently been reported by Drost *et al.* (1976) and Rowe *et al.* (1976). An outline of the method of Elsden *et al.* (1976) is presented below.

Elsden and collegues recover embryos between days 5 and 8, but mainly on days 6 or 7 (estrus = day 0). The donors receive no feed or water for 24 hours prior to the collection, which is performed in a squeeze chute. An epidural block is achieved with 8–10 ml of 2% procaine–HCl. The collection apparatus is a slightly modified three-way Foley catheter (Fig. 2). Insertion of the catheter follows cervical dilation with a long rod, having a maximum diameter of 1 cm. The dilator is then removed to allow insertion of the Foley catheter. A stiff rod

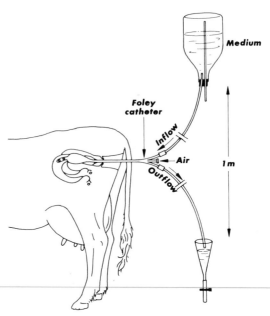

Fig. 2. Diagrammatic representation of the Elsden *et al.* procedure for nonsurgical collection of cow embryos. Adapted with permission from Elsden *et al.* (1976), Figures 2 and 3.

inside the Foley catheter aids in its placement in the horn, at a point just beyond the external bifurcation. The air cuff is inflated and the rod removed. The influx tube of the Foley catheter is connected to a flask containing about 800 ml of warm (37°C) Dulbecco's phosphate-buffered saline with 1% heat-inactivated bovine serum and antibiotics added. The outlet of the Foley catheter is extended to a 250-ml sedimentation funnel. The tubouterine junction is held closed by rectal manipulation, and, with the outlet to the catheter closed, the uterine horn is distended with fluid. The outlet is then opened, and, with the inlet to the Foley catheter closed, the uterine contents are allowed to flow into the funnel while the uterus is being gently massaged. The process is repeated until the flushing medium is used up. When full, the funnels are placed in an incubator (37°C) until the fluids can be drawn off the bottom in the search for embryos. At the end of the uterine flush, all donors receive an intrauterine infusion of antibiotics.

As mentioned above, this nonsurgical collection procedure allows reliable collection of bovine embryos from as many as 92% of females attempted. This level of success makes nonsurgical embryo recovery the method of choice except for certain research purposes. Nevertheless, Elsden and co-workers caution that the procedure requires correct placement of the collection catheter (therefore, skill and practice) and reliable embryo searching technique, since large volumes of fluid containing cervical mucus and cellular debris are involved.

2. Horses

The number of experiments investigating embryo transfer in horses is relatively small. The methods (both surgical and nonsurgical) employed have been modifications of the procedures developed in cattle and are described fully in the literature. Surgical methods are presented by Allen and Rowson (1975), and nonsurgical methods are described by Oguri and Tsutsumi (1972, 1974) and Allen and Rowson (1975). Interestingly, the success rate for nonsurgical embryo recovery in horses is moderately to highly acceptable (39%, Allen and Rowson, 1975; 90%, Oguri and Tsutsumi, 1972, 1974). Although attempts have been made on only small numbers of horses, nonsurgical collection may be the method of choice for most applications. Flushing media employed have been TCM199 (Allen and Rowson, 1975) or physiological saline with 2% gelatin (Oguri and Tsutsumi, 1974).

3. Sheep

In sheep, embryos are obtained during midventral laparotomy under barbiturate or gas anesthesia. We use iv (jugular) injection of pentobarbital sodium to achieve the surgical level of anesthesia. For most large ewes, this requires about 1 gm. The ewe is placed into a laparotomy cradle, described by Hulet and Foote (1968). Once secured, the cradle is tilted, bringing the abdomen of the ewe to a convenient position for surgery. The abdomen is shorn, shaved, washed, and disinfected with povidone–iodine. A midventral incision is made just anterior to the udder, and the uterus and ovaries are exposed to allow embryo recovery.

Collection of sheep embryos was described by Hunter et al. (1955), and several others in subsequent reports used their collection method (e.g., Moore et al., 1960; Hancock and Hovell, 1961; Hancock and McGovern, 1968). Hunter et al. (1955) described methods for collection of both tubal and uterine embryos. Tubal embryos were obtained by putting a 15-gauge hypodermic needle into the oviduct at the tubouterine junction, and cannulating the infundibular end with a bent 2-mm bore glass tube. About 2 ml of flushing medium was infused into the oviduct and collected through the glass tube into a graduated centrifuge tube.

More recently, Wright et al. (1976) adapted the bovine procedure of Rowson et al. (1969) for sheep embryo collection. In this technique, the infundibulum is cannulated, and flushing medium is injected into the ipsilateral uterine horn and forced through the tubouterine junction. This procedure allows simultaneous collection from oviduct and uterus with high recovery rates. Wright and co-workers used TCM199 as the flushing medium.

4. Swine

Swine embryos are obtained surgically. The gilts are initially anesthetized with 1 gm of thiamylal sodium or thiopental sodium via ear venipuncture. The gilt is placed on her back into a surgical cradle, to which her legs are secured with rope (Fig. 3). Cuffed endotrachial tubes are inserted into each nostril and are connected to a closed-circuit anesthesia apparatus dispensing oxygen and halothane or methoxyflurane. The surgical cradle is secured to a surgical table with the head tilted downward approximately 30°. The abdomen is clipped, washed, and disinfected with povidone–iodine. A sterile drape and towels are secured with towel clamps and a 10-cm long incision is made in the midline between the second last and third last sets of teats. The subcutaneous fat and fascia are separated with blunt dissection, and an incision is made in the linea alba. If the incision is on midline, no muscle tissue will be cut and little or no bleeding will occur during the surgery. In this laboratory, we perforate the peritoneum by tearing it with the fore and middle fingers (we have found it unnecessary to suture the peritoneum when closing). The uterus is exposed, one horn and ovary at a time.

Collection of oviducal embryos is achieved by modification of the procedure of Vincent *et al.* (1964). A 3–4 mm diameter polyvinyl cannula is inserted into the infundibulum and clamped in position with cross-acting forceps. The free end of the cannula is placed into a sterile culture tube and flushing medium (bicarbonate-buffered TCM199 with Earle's salts and antibiotics) is injected into the oviduct at the tubouterine junction, using enough force to achieve a moderate velocity of flow within the oviduct.

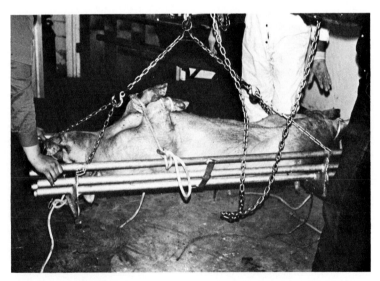

Fig. 3. Anesthetized sow in surgery cradle. The cradle is lifted with a manual hoist on a monorail track leading to the surgery room.

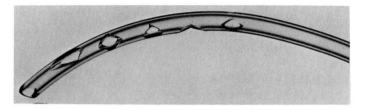

Fig. 4.   Notched end of cannula used for collection of uterine embryos in swine. The notches minimize cannula blockage and, therefore, facilitate embryo recovery. Cannula diameter is 1.2 mm (o.d.).

Uterine embryos are more commonly used for embryo transfer, and these are collected by a modification of the method of Fenton *et al.* (1972). For this procedure, a polyvinyl cannula about 40 cm in length and 1.2–1.7 mm (o.d.) is used. One end of the cannula is notched with several 0.5 mm holes 1–2 cm from the tip, which is cut at a slight angle (Fig. 4). (The purpose of the holes in the side of the cannula is to promote continuous flow of fluid into the cannula during the uterine flush.) Taking care to avoid blood vessels, a small incision is made in the oviduct, with the tip and edge of a cutting suture needle approximately 1 cm from the tubouterine junction. The end of the cannula with the holes is pushed into the oviduct lumen (Fig. 5) and through the tubouterine junction until it is 3–5 cm into the uterine lumen. The tubouterine junction is clamped with two cross-acting forceps. The surgical assistant grasps the uterine horn at the external

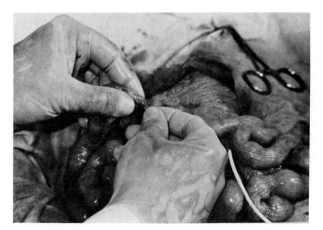

Fig. 5.   Introduction of a cannula into the oviduct and through the tubouterine junction in a sow to allow collection of uterine embryos.

bifurcation to prevent fluid passage, and 20 ml of medium (as described above) is infused into the uterus via the cannula. As soon as the fluid is in the uterine lumen, the free end of the cannula is placed into a culture tube to receive the embryos. The fluid in the uterine horn is moved through the uterus by squeezing the horn and sliding the fingers to the constriction imposed by the assistant. The direction of stripping is then reversed, and fluid is forced out of the uterus through the cannula into the culture tube. The procedure is repeated with the remaining uterine horn.

G. Embryo Isolation and Evaluation

Sterile surgical procedures are highly recommended to avoid infection of the animals as well as the embryos. Clean procedures, sterile instruments, and flushing solutions are equally important for nonsurgical collection. Residue-free and sterile vessels are essential to the success of the transfer operation. Where possible the use of disposable, nontoxic tubes, dishes, pipettes, syringes, and cannulae is advised. This eliminates the risk of residual contamination and is labor saving. The quality of water used in preparation of media and rinsing glassware is equally important (Whittingham, 1971). Therefore, triple glass-distilled water must be considered essential. In this laboratory, we utilize water with conductivity from 0.5 to 1.0 μSiemens/cm with good results. All glassware is washed in a tissue culture grade detergent such as 7X (Linbro Scientific, Inc., Hamden, Connecticut) or chromic acid and is thoroughly rinsed prior to use.

The flushings are inspected for embryos under dissection microscopy. Since embryos are quite dense and settle to the bottom of the tube, 23–cm sterile Pasteur pipettes are used to transfer 3–5 ml of medium from the bottom of each culture tube into 6.5-cm diameter watchglasses housed in 10-cm diameter plastic petri dishes. Each watch glass is covered by the petri dish cover, which remains in place during embryo evaluation. The embryos are located at low magnification (10–15 ×) and transferred to fresh medium, where they are pooled. If the anticipated number of embryos is not located, the uterus may be flushed a second time. If the flushing is bloody, smaller aliquots are diluted with clean fresh medium, to improve visibility.

Embryo evaluation is performed under dissection microscopy at 135 × and is based upon criteria that are quickly determined and are not harmful to the embryos. The criteria used for this purpose are (1) uniformity of blastomere size and appearance, (2) stage of development of embryo in relation to presumed ovulation time, and (3) compactness and symmetry of the blastomeric mass. The embryos which fail to satisfy any of these criteria are considered unfit for transplantation. The acceptable cattle embryos are ranked according to quality and placed into individual watchglasses, each with 1 ml of fresh flushing medium containing 1% heat-inactivated fetal calf serum. For swine and sheep embryos, the same procedure is used except all embryos constituting a single prospective litter are pooled into a single dish. The watchglasses in petri dishes are transferred to a 37.5°C incubator supplied with 5% CO_2–95% humidified air until needed for transfer.

H. Embryo Transfer to Recipients

1. Surgical Methods

Aside from different surgical techniques, with different species as outlined above in Section III,F, the actual method of transfer of embryos to recipient females is similar for all species. For very early embryos (less than four blastomeres), a small incision is made in the ampulla of the oviduct, and a Pasteur pipette containing the embryo(s) in a small volume (0.5 ml or less) of transfer medium are deposited into the isthmus. (A 1-ml syringe fitted with a 2-cm section of rubber tubing, such that Pasteur pipettes can be quickly connected and removed, is a very satisfactory volume control device.) Older embryos are transferred to the uterus, usually in the anterior end. To achieve this, the uterus is punctured with the blunt end of a suturing needle and the pipette containing the embryo(s) is inserted into the uterine lumen via the puncture wound.

In cattle, horses and sometimes sheep, there is only one corpus luteum in the recipient animal. If only one embryo is to be transplanted, it is better to transfer it into the uterine horn ipsilateral to the corpus luteum (Sreenan et al., 1975). However, when two embryos are transferred in cattle, the survival rate can be very good (Sreenan et al., 1975; Anderson et al., 1976; Sreenan and Beehan, 1976).

2. Nonsurgical Transfer

At the present time, nonsurgical transfer of cow and mare embryos has been achieved, but, in the case of cattle, the embryo survival rates are not nearly equal to that achieved by surgical methods (Sugie et al., 1972; Boland et al., 1975; Lawson et al., 1975; G. E. Seidel, personal communication, 1976). On the other hand, nonsurgical transfer in the horse, while involving very small numbers of embryos, seems to be more promising (Oguri and Tsutsumi, 1974; Allen and Rowson, 1975).

There have been two basic approaches to nonsurgical transfer of embryos: (1) passage of a tube through the cervix to deposit into the uterus (e.g., Allen and Rowson, 1975), or (2) cervical bypass, puncturing both the vaginal and uterine walls with a large needle (Sugie, 1965; Oguri and Tsutsumi, 1974). The earlier attempts with both methods also involved inflation of the uterus with CO_2; however, Boland et al. (1975) and Allen and Rowson (1975) did not follow this practice, since it proved deleterious (Lawson et al., 1975).

It has been postulated (supported by unpublished evidence as cited by Allen and Rowson, 1975) that manipulation of the cervix during transcervical transfer causes expulsion of the embryo in cattle. The work of Boland *et al.* (1975), while involving only 24 recipient cattle, suggests that the lower success rates with nonsurgical methods is not always due to embryo expulsion. Boland *et al.* achieved 25% survival of transferred embryos at 1 month, while the native embryo survival rate was 62.5%, indicating that they were neither killed by intrauterine infection nor expelled by the uterus. Similarly Seidel *et al.* (1975) and Elsden *et al.* (1976) found no evidence of intrauterine infection after nonsurgical collection or sham nonsurgical transfers.

I. Pregnancy Diagnosis

It is normally desirable to know the success of the transfer as soon as possible after transplantation. Observation of return(s) to estrus following transfer is not a reliable indication of pregnancy, since it tends to be quite variable (e.g., Rowson *et al.,* 1969). Cattle and horses can be diagnosed pregnant by rectal palpation of the uterus and ovaries at 35–40 days after breeding. These methods are described elsewhere (e.g., Ulberg, 1962; Nishikawa and Hafez, 1962) and are well established. Sheep and swine require other methods to diagnose pregnancy.

In sheep, pregnancy can be detected by use of ultrasonic equipment. Lindahl (1971) described the method presently used in sheep. This involves turning the ewe on her back and inserting a lubricated probe bearing a Doppler transducer into the rectum. Fetal heart beat, fetal pulse, or fetal movements, when detected, are the parameters used in diagnosis. Accuracy of diagnosis was greater than 90% with 2111 ewes checked. This method can be successfully used from about 50 days of pregnancy. It is anticipated that an immunologic test for pregnancy in the sheep will be available shortly. Cerini *et al.* (1976) reported the basis for such a test and indicated that pregnancy can be detected as early as day 6 after breeding. The test is based upon detection of pregnancy specific antigens, and it encourages the hope that similar tests might be developed for cattle, horses, and swine.

The current pregnancy diagnosis method in swine was reported by Lindahl *et al.* (1975). This method detects acoustical impedance in the abdomen of the sow. Due to the presence of large amounts of fluid the pregnant uterus possesses different acoustical properties than do other abdominal tissues and the nonpregnant uterus. Linddahl *et al.* reported accuracy approaching 100% with 801 sows. The method is accurate from 30 days of pregnancy.

J. Proof of Parentage

For research purposes, proof of parentage is often not necessary since the investigator will be aware of the breeding or insemination status of each donor and each recipient. When identification of two or more possible parentages is necessary, as in transfers to recipients already pregnant to achieve twinning, etc., the investigator can utilize easily distinguishable breeds for the donors and recipients.

In situations in which the offspring resulting from embryo transfer are to be registered as purebred animals, more exacting proofs of parentage are required. This involves blood typing of the sire, the donor, and the offspring. The criteria are established by the breed associations which permit registry of animals resulting from embryo transfer, and, thus, the breed association must be consulted when registry is anticipated.

K. Rate of Success

Success rates vary considerably, even within the same organization and same species, but the embryo survival rate after transfer in some cases can reach 80% or greater (e.g., Newcomb and Rowson, 1975; Sreenan and Beehan, 1976). However, survival rates of 40–60% are more common for established programs and can be poorer for beginners. As a ''rule-of-thumb,'' a transferred embryo survival rate of 50% may be considered about average, regardless of species. Pregnancy rates may be considerable higher in transfers involving two or more embryos per recipient.

IV. FUTURE DIRECTIONS

There have been, and undoubtedly will be, many applications of embryo transfer for research purposes. Recently, this technology has been put to use commercially in the cattle and swine industries. It is not difficult to understand how embryo transfer, when combined with other procedures, such as prolonged embryo storage, will be as standard an agricultural technology as is artificial insemination in cattle at the present time. The combination of nonsurgical collection, embryo culture, sexing, storing (e.g., freezing), and nonsurgical transfer will enable a producer of cattle, for example, to order an embryo or a set of embryos for which he knows the parentage, the sex, and the probability of survival. It also seems certain that greater use for embryo transfer will be made by nonembryologists. since the technique provides the possibility of delineating between genetic and prenatal environmental effects. It is expected that developments and improvements in this field of science will occur at even greater rates in the future than have occurred in the past 10 years.

ACKNOWLEDGMENT

The original observations used in this chapter were aided by Edward C. Segerson, Anthony P. Grifo, and Donald R. Redman and by a grant from Erwin J. Nutter, KBJ Ranch, Xenia, Ohio.

REFERENCES

Allen, W. R., and Rowson, L. E. A. (1973). *J. Reprod. Fertil.* **33,** 539–543.

Allen, W. R., and Rowson, L. E. A. (1975). *J. Reprod. Fertil., Suppl.* **23,** 525–530.

Allen, W. R., Stewart, F., Trounson, A. O., Tischner, M., and Bielanski, W. (1976). *J. Reprod. Fertil.* **47,** 387–390.

Anderson, G. B., Baldwin, J. N., Cupps, P. T., Drost, M., Horton, M. B., and Wright, R. W. (1976). *J. Anim. Sci.* **43,** 272.

Anderson, L. L. (1969). *In* "Reproduction in Domestic Animals" (H. H. Cole and P. T. Cupps, eds.), 2nd ed., pp. 541–568. Academic Press, New York.

Boland, M. P., Crosby, T. F., and Gordon, I. (1975). *Br. Vet. J.* **131,** 738–740.

Catchpole, H. R. (1963). *In* "Gonadotropins" (H. H. Cole, ed.), pp. 40–70. Freeman, San Francisco, California.

Cerini, M., Findley, J. K., and Lawson, R. A. S. (1976). *J. Reprod. Fertil.* **46,** 65–69.

Cupps, P. T., Anderson, G. B., Drost, M., Darien, B., and Horton, M. B. (1976). *J. Anim. Sci.* **43,** 280–281.

Curnock, R. M., Day, B. N., and Dziuk, P. J. (1976). *Am. J. Vet. Res.* **37,** 97–98.

Davis, D. L., Killian, D. B., and Day, B. N. (1976). *J. Anim. Sci.* **42,** 1358.

Douglas, R. H., and Ginther, O. J. (1973). *J. Anim. Sci.* **37,** 990–993.

Douglas, R. H., and Ginther, O. J. (1975). *J. Anim. Sci.* **40,** 518–522.

Drost, M., Brand, A., and Carts, M. H. (1976). *Theriogenology* **6,** 503–507.

Elsden, R. P., Hasler, J. F., and Seidel, G. E. (1976). *Theriogenology* **6,** 523–532.

Fenton, F. R., Schwartz, F. L., Bazer, F. W., Robinson, O. W., and Ulberg, L. C. (1972). *J. Anim. Sci.* **35,** 383–388.

Hafez, E. S. E., ed. (1962). "The Behavior of Domestic Animals." Baillière, London.

Hancock, J. L., and Hovell, G. J. R. (1961). *J. Reprod. Fertil.* **2,** 295–306.

Hancock, J. L., and McGovern, P. T. (1968). *Res. Vet. Sci.* **9,** 411–415.

Heape, W. (1890). *Proc. R. Soc. London* **48,** 457–458.

Hulet, C. V., and Foote, W. C. (1968). *J. Anim. Sci.* **27,** 142–145.

Hunter, G. L., Adams, C. E., and Rowson, L. E. (1955). *J. Agric. Sci.* **46,** 143–149.

Knight, J. W., Davis, D. L., and Day, B. N (1976). *J. Anim. Sci.* **42,** 1358–1359.

Lambert, P. W., Greene, W. M., Strickland, J. D., Han, D. K., and Moody, E. L. (1976). *J. Anim. Sci.* **42,** 1565.

Lauderdale, J. W. (1972). *J. Anim. Sci.* **35,** 246.

Lawson, R. A. S., Rowson, L. E. A., Moore, R. M., and Tervit, H. R. (1975). *J. Reprod. Fertil.* **45,** 101–107.

Lindahl, I. L. (1971). *J. Anim. Sci.* **32,** 922–925.

Lindahl, I. L., Totsch, J. P., Martin, P. S., and Dziuk, P. J. (1975). *J. Anim. Sci.* **40,** 220–222.

Manns, J. G., Wenkoff, M. S., and Adams, W. M. (1976). *J. Anim. Sci.* **43,** 295.

Miller, P. A., Lauderdale, J. W., and Gengy, S. (1976). *J. Anim. Sci.* **42,** 901–911.

Moore, N. W. (1975). *Aust. J. Agric. Res.* **26,** 295–304.

Moore, N. W., Rowson, L. E. A., and Short, R. V. (1960). *J. Reprod. Fertil.* **1,** 332–349.

Newcomb, R. (1976). *Vet. Rec.* **99,** 40–44.

Newcomb, R., and Rowson, L. E. A. (1975). *J. Reprod. Fertil.* **43,** 539–541.

Nishikawa, Y., and Hafez, E. S. E. (1962). *In* "Reproduction in Farm Animals" (E. S. E. Hafez, ed.), pp. 266–276. Lea & Febiger, Philadelphia, Pennsylvania.

Oguri, N., and Tsutsumi, Y. (1972). *J. Reprod. Fertil.* **31,** 187–195.

Oguri, N., and Tsutsumi, Y. (1974). *J. Reprod. Fertil.* **41,** 313–320.

Roche, J. F. (1976). *J. Anim. Sci.* **43,** 164–169.

Rowe, R. F., Dellampo, M. R., Eilts, C. L., French, L. R., Winch, R. P., and Ginther, O. J. (1976). *Theriogenology* **6**, 471–483.

Rowson, L. E. A., Moor, R. M., and Lawson, R. A. S. (1969). *J. Reprod. Fertil.* **18**, 517–523.

Rowson, L. E. A., Lawson, R. A. S., Moor, R. M., and Baker, A. A. (1972). *J. Reprod. Fertil.* **28**, 427–431.

Segerson, E. C., Redman, D. R., and Murray, F. A. (1976). *Ohio Rep.* **61**, 57–59.

Segerson, E. C., Murray, F. A., Moxon, A. L., Redman, D. R., and Conrad, H. R. (1977). *J. Dairy Sci.* **60**, 1001–1005.

Seidel, G. E., Bowen, J. M., Homan, N. R., and Okun, N. E. (1975). *Vet. Rec.* **97**, 307–308.

Sreenan, J. M., and Beehan, D. (1976). *J. Reprod. Fertil.* **47**, 127–128.

Sreenan, J. M., Beehan, D., and Mulvehill, P. (1975). *J. Reprod. Fertil.* **44**, 77–85.

Staples, R. E. (1971). *In* "Methods in Mammalian Embryology" (J. C. Daniel, Jr., ed.), Vol. 1, pp. 290–304. Freeman, San Francisco, California.

Stauffer, G. D., Ellington, E. F., and Nielsen, M. K. (1976). *J. Anim. Sci.* **42**, 1564.

Sugie, T. (1965). *J. Reprod. Fertil.* **10**, 197–201.

Sugie, T., Soma, T., Fukumitse, S., and Otsuki, K. (1972). *Bull. Natl. Inst. Anim. Ind. Chiba, Jpn.* **25**, 35–40.

Sullivan, J. J., Parker, W. G., and Larson, L. L. (1973). *J. Am. Vet. Med. Assoc.* **162**, 895–898.

Tervit, H. R., Rowson, L. E. A., and Brand, A. (1973). *J. Reprod. Fertil.* **34**, 179–181.

Trounson, A. O., Willadsen, S. M., Rowson, L. E. A., and Newcomb, R. (1976). *J. Reprod. Fertil.* **46**, 173–178.

Ulberg, L. C. (1962). *In* "Reproduction in Farm Animals" (E. S. E. Hafez, ed.), pp. 229–239. Lea & Febiger, Philadelphia, Pennsylvania.

Vincent, C. K., Robinson, O. W., and Ulberg, L. C. (1964). *J. Anim. Sci.* **23**, 1084–1088.

Webel, S. K. (1976). *J. Anim. Sci.* **42**, 1358.

Webel, S. K., Peters, J. B., and Anderson, L. L. (1970). *J. Anim. Sci.* **30**, 565–568.

Whittingham, D. G. (1971). *J. Reprod. Fertil., Suppl.* **14**, 7–21.

Willadsen, S. M., Polge, C., Rowson, L. E. A., and Moor, R. M. (1976). *J. Reprod. Fertil.* **46**, 151–154.

Wright, R. W., Anderson, G. B., Cupps, P. T., Drost, M., and Bradford, G. E. (1976). *J. Anim. Sci.* **42**, 912–917.

15

Manipulation of Marsupial Embryos and Pouch Young

MARILYN B. RENFREE AND C. H. TYNDALE-BISCOE

I. INTRODUCTION

Marsupials offer unique opportunities for studies of mammalian development, yet the potential has hardly been realized. This has been because of the difficulty of establishing and maintaining colonies of breeding animals of any species in captivity, and the lack of success so far in attempts to induce superovulation in the monovular species of choice. It may also have been due to a lack of awareness of the particular opportunities that marsupials afford. The difficulties of husbandry have now been largely overcome for several species, and awareness of their value for developmental biology is increasing (Jurgelski, 1974).

There are three features of marsupial reproduction that are pertinent to experimental embryology. The chromosomes of marsupials are large and the karyotype low ($2n = 10$–28) (see Hayman and Martin, 1974, for review), which make marsupial embryos potentially excellent material for studies correlating gene activation with early differentiation. The discovery that, in females of some species, the paternally derived X chromosome is predominantly inactivated in somatic cells has stimulated much current work in this field (see Sharman, 1973b, for review). The relatively long period during intrauterine development when the embryo is not attached to the uterus and is surrounded by the maternally derived shell membrane offers great potential for *in vitro* culture. This has been demonstrated by the successful culture of vesicles of *Didelphis virginiana* by New and Mizell (1972). Finally, the undeveloped state of several organ systems at birth and the long period of pouch life afford special opportunities to study the differentiation of biochemical and endocrine processes and physiological functions (Sharman, 1973a; Tyndale-Biscoe, 1973).

Intrauterine development has been reviewed by Tyndale-Biscoe (1973) and Gomot (in press), and only a brief summary will be given here.

With a few exceptions in the Dasyuridae (Woolley, 1973), all marsupials are polyestrous, and ovulation is spontaneous. The number of eggs shed varies from very large numbers in some Didelphidae and Dasyuridae, to less than 10 in the Peramelidae, Caenolestidae, and Phalangeridae, and to 1 in the Macropodidae. The egg at ovulation is larger than that of Eutheria (Table I) and is invested by a zona pellucida (Fig. 1A). Passage through the oviduct is rapid and takes about 1 day in *Didelphis virginiana, Trichosurus vulpecula, Setonix brachyurus,* and *Macropus eugenii.* During this time, a second glycoprotein membrane is provided from secretions of oviductal glands (Fig. 1B), while a keratinous shell membrane is overlaid on this by glands at the uterotubal junction (Fig. 1C). The properties of the egg membranes have been reviewed by Hughes and Shorey (1973) and Hughes (1974). Some cleavages may take place during passage through the oviduct, but 1-cell or 4-cell eggs have been recovered from the uteri of several species.

TABLE I
Dimensions (μm) of Eggs and Egg Membranes of Marsupials Used for Experiment

Species	Vitellus diameter	Zona pellucida	Muco-lemma	Shell membrane	Total diameter
Didelphis virginiana[a]	135–165	1	140	1.2	500–700
Trichosurus vulpecula[b]	245	3.9	39–69	3.2–6.7	
Macropus eugenii (n = 9)	126.4 ± 13.3[c]	6.3 ± 1.4	24.3 ± 7.8	5.9 ± 1.8	200.3 ± 18.57

[a] Hartman (1916).
[b] Hughes and Shorey (1973).
[c] Mean ± SD.

Cleavage and blastocyst formation differ markedly from eutherian patterns. At the first cleavage, a noncellular yolk body is extruded. Subsequent cleavage of the blastomeres results in 60–80 similar cells that surround the yolk body. Junctional complexes are established between adjacent cells so that a unilaminar blastocyst is formed (Fig. 1D). There is no inner cell mass and, at this stage, no indication of differentiation of a presumptive embryonic region; all cells appear to be totipotent, though no experiments have been performed to test this. For this reason, this layer of cells is termed "protoderm," rather than trophectoderm or trophoblast (McCrady, 1938).

Differentiation and polarity are established at endoderm formation. Some cells of the protoderm layer migrate inward and form an incomplete layer beneath it. The overlying cells increase in height and become cuboidal, and the area so formed is the medullary plate. As the blastocyst expands, the protoderm cells become attenuated, but the cells of the medullary plate do not, so that this area becomes clearly visible in living vesicles (Fig. 2A). By the time the endoderm layer is complete in the abembryonal pole, the zona pellucida and mucoid layer have disappeared, and the attenuated shell membrane alone surrounds the vesicle. The shell membrane persists for two-thirds or more of gestation, during which time the embryo is formed and the vascularized yolk sac and vitelline circulation is established (Table II). Up to the end of this period, the fetal trophoblast is wholly separated from the maternal uterine epithelium by the enveloping shell membrane, and the whole conceptus can be rolled out of the opened uterus undamaged. In the remaining relatively brief period of gestation, after rupture of the shell, embryogenesis and organogenesis are completed, the fetal compartments are differentiated, and the fetus is brought to a state sufficient

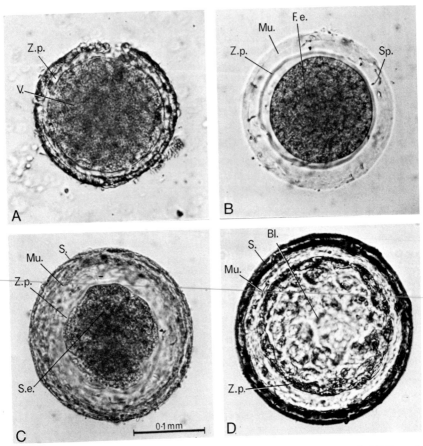

Fig. 1. Living stages in the early development of the tammar, *Macropus eugenii*. (A) Preovulatory follicular oocyte at estrus, to show vitellus, V., and zona pellucida, Z.p. (B) Fertilized egg, F.e., recovered from the oviduct less than 1 day p.c. It is surrounded by the mucolemma, Mu., and entrapped spermatozoa, Sp. (C) Segmenting egg, S.e., recovered from the uterus 30 hours p.c. The shell membrane, S., covers the mucolemma. (D) Unilaminar blastocyst, Bl., in diapause surrounded by a thicker shell membrane.

Fig. 2. Later stages of intrauterine development of the tammar, *Macropus eugenii*. (A) Vesicle, 16-mm diameter, with somitic embryo recovered from the uterus on day 17, still enclosed by the shell membrane. (B) Fetus at day 21–22 during organogenesis, when the allantois, al, is growing and the vascular yolk sac membrane, ysm, is well developed. (C) Fetus at day 25. 1–2 day before term. The yolk sac and allantois have collapsed after fluid collection, but the amnion and the vitelline veins are still intact. Note the well-developed forelimbs with claws and the subcutaneous vasculature, adaptations for perinatal life. (From Renfree, 1973b, by permission.)

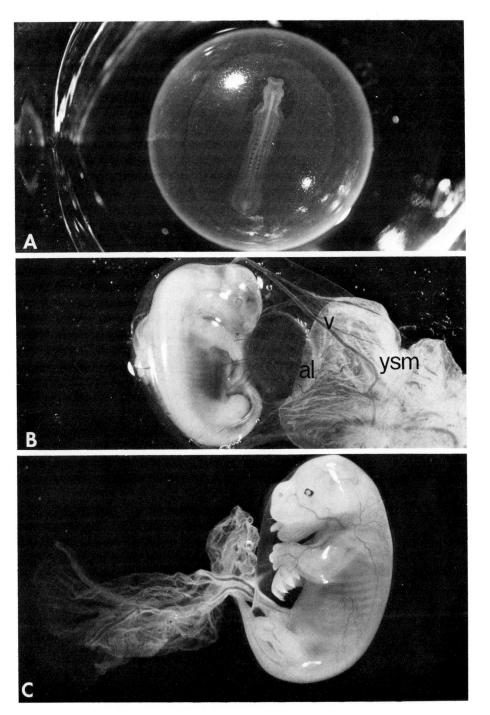

TABLE II
Stages in Intrauterine Development of Marsupials Used for Experiment[a]

Species	Tubal ova	Uterine cleavage stages	Unilaminar blastocyst	Bilaminar blastocyst	Presomite embryo	Vascular circulation	Shell ruptures	Yolk sac fluid yellow	Allantois fluid-filled	Birth
Didelphis virginiana[b]	1	2	3	5–6	7–8		9	11	11	13
Trichosurus vulpecula[c]	1–2	—	—	—	12	14	12	14	14	17
Macropus eugenii[d]	2	2–4	5–250[e]	9	12–14	18	20	21	22	27

[a] Days p.c. for *D. virginiana* and *T. vulpecula*, and *M. eugenii* to unilaminar blastocyst; days after removing pouch young for *M. eugenii* from bilaminar blastocyst.
[b] Hartman (1928), McCrady (1938), Renfree (1974).
[c] Sharman (1961); C. H. Tyndale-Biscoe and N. J. Cother (unpublished).
[d] Renfree (1973b); C. H. Tyndale-Biscoe (unpublished).
[e] If diapause intervenes.

for independent life. The disruption of the shell allows a close apposition of fetal and maternal tissues to take place, and a more or less intimate connection is established. In the majority of species, the connection consists of no more than an interdigitation of fetal and maternal microvilli (Tyndale-Biscoe, 1973; Hughes, 1974), but, in a few species, the fetal trophoblast may invade the uterine epithelium or form a symplasma with it (Enders and Enders, 1969; Padykula and Taylor, 1977).

All the fetal compartments are fluid-filled, but the yolk sac is by far the largest. The allantois increases in volume at the end of gestation, and small amounts of fluid can be aspirated from both the allantois and the amnion at these stages (Renfree, 1973b).

The small size and fetal appearance of the newborn marsupial has led to the view that it is equivalent to an "exteriorized" fetus and may be used as a convenient experimental model for fetal physiology. This is valid only in some respects. Differentiation of small lymphocytes and their migration to the thymus takes place in the first few days after birth (Block, 1964; Ashman et al., 1975a); thus, experimental thymectomy can be achieved at an earlier developmental stage than in any eutherian. Similarly, the gonads are indifferent at birth, and this has been exploited for study of differentiation of the gonads and genital ducts (review by Burns, 1961; Alcorn, 1976).

However, in other respects, the physiological state of the neonatal marsupial is well differentiated and resembles that of the neonatal rat (Janssens et al., 1977), so caution must be exercised before attempting to use them in lieu of fetuses.

For convenience in describing experimental procedures, we recognize four phases of development.

1. Ovum transport to the uterus and development to the blastocyst stage.
2. The preattachment phase while the shell membrane remains intact. In the Macropodidae, this phase may be greatly extended by interpolation of a period of embryonic diapause.
3. The attachment phase and organogenesis.
4. The pouch young.

II. ANIMAL HUSBANDRY TO OBTAIN TIMED STAGES OF GESTATION

A. The American Opossums, *Didelphis virginiana* and *Marmosa mitis*

The Virginia opossum, *Didelphis virginiana,* has a widespread distribution over North America up to the –7.0°C isotherm and westward as far as the Rocky Mountains. This ubiquitous animal has, like the Australian brush possum, exploited human habitations. Female opossums weigh about 2 kg, although males may be much heavier. They are polyovular, polyestrous marsupials with a gestation period of 13 days, which is the same duration as the luteal phase of the cycle (Hartman, 1923, 1925). The next proestrous phase and ovulation are suppressed by the presence of suckling young in the pouch. During the breeding season (which extends from January to July), females carrying pouch young can be stimulated to resume follicular growth and estrous activity by removal of the pouch young (RPY). After RPY, daily vaginal smears are taken from days 3–10, following the method described by Pilton and Sharman (1962), and illustrated by Jurgelski and Porter (1974). The usual time of estrus and mating is between days 5 and 7; the day of mating as determined by the presence of spermatozoa in the smear is commonly designated by 0. Only a few animals show obvious vaginal plugs, and sperm counts are always very low.

Most workers have had difficulty in breeding opossums, but this was probably due to too much confinement in small, inside cages. On a small scale, good success is achieved by accommodating animals in large open cages of about 5 × 12 m, divided into two sections, where animals are provided with individual nest boxes and housed in the ratio of four to five females : two males (Renfree, 1974). As McCrady (1938) emphasized, nutrition (especially bone meal) is critical, and the diet of Purina Dog Chow should be supplemented daily with fruit or vegetables, chicken bones, and meat. Opossums are clean animals and will habitually defecate in one place; several large litter boxes are adequate for this area.

A much more elaborate and very successful breeding compound has been developed by Jurgelski et al. (1974). The facility design has allowed dependable large scale production of opossum young under controlled conditions. Again, success has been attributed to the semioutdoor breeding pens. Jurgelski's papers provide a comprehensive description of husbandry and laboratory techniques used for this species.

The embryology of the opossum as described by Hartman (1928) and McCrady (1938) still remains the most complete description of the embryology of any marsupial. Between 15 and 30 eggs may be produced, but not all are fertilized or survive the first days of gestation. Development is slow at first, although 8 to 16-cell eggs are in the uterus by day 2, and the blastocysts are formed by day 3 (Table II). The shell membrane is not lost until about day 9, after which development is extremely rapid, with birth occurring on day 13. The newborn young weigh 150 mg, and between 8 and 15 young are usually produced. Of those born, some may die before weaning and independence.

Of the South American species, the murine opossum *Marmosa mitis* seemed ideal for laboratory establishment because of its karyogram ($2n = 14$), lack of pouch, large litters, and small size (Barnes and Barthold, 1969). Different species of *Marmosa* range from central Mexico to Central Chile, and animals have been available from dealers. Detailed descriptions of the husbandry of *Marmosa* suggest that although diet, bedding, and caging have been carefully controlled, reproductive efficiency in colonies declines, with F_1 matings being particularly unsuccessful (Barnes and Wolf, 1971). The estrous cycle in *Marmosa* is 28 days and may be detected by vaginal smears using the method described by Barnes and Wolf (1971). Gestation is 14 days, and newborn young each weigh 100 mg (Barnes and Barthold, 1969). They are permanently attached to the mothers' nipples for 21 days and remain with the mother for 35–60 days. At 60–70 days, antagonistic behavior of the young necessitates their weaning and separation if they are held in captivity.

B. The Brush Possum, *Trichosurus vulpecula*

The brush possum is an arboreal marsupial that weighs 1–3 kg. It is widespread in Australia and New Zealand and has adapted to city gardens. Because it is readily available near all the main Australian cities, little attempt has been made to establish breeding colonies, but it has been used for a variety of investigations in endocrinology and neurophysiology, and its reproduction is well known.

Females will breed in captivity if held in large cages or rooms, but they do not respond well to close confinement. They are strictly nocturnal, so that handling in the daytime is disturbing to them. Possums kept in a room on reversed photoperiod give more satisfactory results (Dr. J. C. Rodger, personal communication). Females isolated from males undergo regular estrous cycles of 25.69 (22–32) days from early February to October (Pilton and Sharman, 1962). Estrus can be detected by vaginal smears, and ovulation occurs 1–2 days later (Shorey and Hughes, 1975). If copulation has taken place, it can be detected by the presence of a large copulatory plug composed of coagulated semen and vaginal secretions or by the presence of sperm and prostatic bodies in the vaginal smear. A lactating female will return to estrus about 8 days after removing the pouch young and, as with *Didelphis,* this provides a convenient means of synchronizing the cycles of females or of obtaining timed stages of gestation.

The species is monovular, and attempts to induce superovulation have so far not given consistent results. Segmenting eggs (16 blastomeres) have been obtained (Hughes, 1974) from the oviduct and from the uterus (4 blastomeres) (Sharman, 1961). The presomite embryo has formed by day 12, when the shell membrane breaks down (Table II). Birth occurs 16–17 days after copulation, and the neonatal young weighs 210 mg (Pilton and Sharman, 1962). Nonpregnant and even virgin females at day 17 of the estrous cycle can receive a neonatus (Sharman, 1962), which can then be suckled through pouch life.

C. The Tammar Wallaby, *Macropus eugenii*

In recent years, the tammar wallaby has become the most thoroughly studied macropod marsupial in Australia, and the species of choice for reproduction studies. It breeds readily in captivity, is docile, and withstands surgery very well.

Females weigh 3-6 kg and males may reach 8 kg. In its natural distribution, it is now restricted to several offshore islands around the coast of south and western Australia, and the mainland of south west Australia. The largest population lives on Kangaroo Island, South Australia, and most breeding colonies are derived from this population. The several island populations have been isolated for at least 9000 years since the last glacial period, and this has resulted in genetic differences, which can be exploited for experiments. The species has a very well-defined annual breeding pattern. The large majority of females give birth during late January and February and undergo a postpartum estrus at which conception usually occurs. The estrous cycle is 29 days, and gestation is 27.5 days. The first offspring occupies the pouch for 8 months and associates with its mother for the remainder of the year. Young females come into estrus and conceive at 9 months of age, soon after weaning. The embryo conceived postpartum and its associated corpus luteum remain quiescent until the end of December (at the summer solstice), when they both reactivate. It is this highly synchronized reactivation that results in the peak of births in January–February (Renfree and Tyndale-Biscoe, 1973a).

Reactivation of the blastocyst can be achieved throughout the year by several means. Up to the end of May, reactivation is most easily achieved by removing the pouch young, since suckling is the proximate inhibitory factor. However, after May this maneuver is no longer reliable, as the females progressively enter seasonal quiescence. Three treatments have been found to be effective during this period. The simplest is to inject 10 mg progesterone in oil im for 10 days. This bypasses the corpus luteum (CL), which remains quiescent, and stimulates the uterus and directly or indirectly the blastocyst. However, parturition is inhibited. A second method is to alter the photoperiod. Six animals exposed in winter to summer photoperiod for 6 weeks followed by a drop to equinoctial photoperiod gave birth 30-33 days after the second change (Sadleir and Tyndale-Biscoe, 1977).

The third method is to abolish the pituitary inhibition of the CL exerted by prolactin (Tyndale-Biscoe and Hawkins, 1977), which was achieved by either adenohypophysectomy or less drastically by an im injection of bromocriptine (CB 154) at a dose of 1 or 5 mg/kg. (C. H. Tyndale-Biscoe and L. Hinds, unpublished results).

III. SURGERY

A. Anesthesia

For simple laparotomy required to obtain embryos, barbiturate (Nembutal, Surital, sodium amytal or Dial) injection without premedication or analgesic is sufficient. However, for hypophysectomy or skin transplantation, which require analgesia, we use themalon (diethylthiambutene) in conjunction with thia-mylal sodium (Surital), or halothane anesthesia. While we have no evidence that barbituates adversely affect fetal development *in utero,* the anesthetic does appear to pass into the milk of suckling females. It is advisable, therefore, to remove young from the pouch during anesthesia of the mother and return them later. Alternatively, where no surgery is planned Brietal sodium (Eli Lilly & Co.) can be used to control the female without affecting the pouch young. Themalon may affect hypothalamic centers and the secretion of pituitary hormones, so that its use may have unexpected and unwanted effects on embryo development.

The commercial preparation of veterinary Nembutal contains propylene glycol as preservative, and this appears to cause irritation during injection and subsequent necrosis at the site of injection. We prefer to prepare solutions in sterile saline of Surital and store under refrigeration. Three routes for anesthesia are available for the opossum, brush possum, and tammar. The route of first choice is one of the lateral tail veins. The animal will remain quiet in a sack while a tourniquet is applied to the base of the tail. A No. 19 to 21 gauge needle with catheter tubing and disposable syringe are used to deliver the anesthetic. When the animal is relaxed, the catheter is taped to the tail with the needle still in the vein. This allows the level of anesthesia to be maintained by supplementary injections later, without risk of dislodging the needle.

If the tail is not available, a second route is via a marginal ear vein using a No. 26 needle. It is more difficult to retain the syringe in place, and, after induction, the needle may be withdrawn and a fine polythene catheter filled with saline inserted into the vein, and subsequent injection can be made through it.

For longer term experiments where serial samples of blood are required, the most satisfactory method is to insert a catheter into the jugular vein and bring it to the exterior on the dorsal surface of the neck (see McDonald and Than, 1976). In our experience with tammars and McDonald's with brush possums, the catheter remains patent for up to 8 weeks, provided it is cleared once a day with sterile heparinized saline. If this method is used for serial plasma sampling, the red blood cells stored in RBC preservative can be replaced daily by the same route to prevent anemia.

B. Laparotomy

The most satisfactory access to the ovaries and genital tract is by a midline incision in the anterior part of the pouch (Fig. 3). After light anesthesia has been induced, the animal is laid on its back. Small sand bags help to keep a tammar in this position without strain to the hind limbs. However, it is advisable to have loose ties around the limbs. The fur around the pouch and the sparse hair in the anterior part of the pouch are clipped. The inside of the pouch is washed with

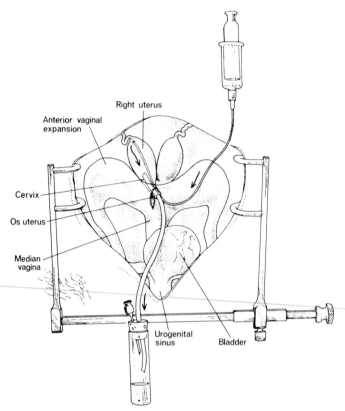

Fig. 3. Surgical approach by midline laparotomy through pouch, illustrating procedure for reverse flushing the uterus to recover blastocysts *in vivo*.

alcoholic Cetavlon solution and the pouch held open with a retractor. A sterile cloth with a central hole is laid over the exposed pouch area and an incision made in the thin pouch skin through the hole, anterior to and avoiding the teats and mammary glands. This exposes the linea alba along which an opening is made with round-tipped scissors. If the animal was denied food and water during the night before surgery, the intestine and bladder are small and the large flat loops of the lateral vaginae come into view clearly. By moving these aside, the paired uteri are seen. The ovaries can be examined by drawing the adjacent uterus toward the midline.

To remove the corpus luteum, the ovary is held at the hilus with a curved hemostat closed sufficiently to reduce the blood flow to it, and the corpus is dissected free with fine, sharp-pointed scissors. The cut surface of the ovary is fulgurated by coagulation, and it is then released. To remove the entire ovary, the hemostat is fully closed, a suture tied, and the ovary severed with the cutting mode.

Ovarian tissue can be transplanted to a site between the body wall and the pouch skin, where it becomes vascularized and functional. The progress of the graft can be easily gauged through the thin, translucent skin.

To obtain expanded vesicles or advanced embryos, it is usually necessary first to remove the gravid uterus. This is done by suturing and dividing the oviduct, mesometrium, and associated branches of the ovarian artery and vein. The uterus can then be separated from its pair and the rest of the mesometrium as far as its junction with the vaginal wall. Because of the enlarged vasculature in this region of the gravid uterus, it is best to tie two sutures of silk around the cervical canal and divide between using the cutting mode of the diathermy knife.

It is possible to obtain early embryos, especially blastocysts in diapause, from living donors by cannulating the cervical canal (Fig. 3). The vaginal loops are drawn anteriorly by retractors and the midventral surface blanched with a diathermy knife. A 5 mm incision is made in the vaginal wall, and the uterus to be flushed is grasped at the cervical region and pushed toward the incision. When the os uterus appears through the incision, a small, blunt-nosed forcep is eased into the canal and allowed to open. This procedure relaxes the canal and allows a fine polythene catheter (1.0 mm o.d.) to be passed into the uterus as far as the uterotubal junction. The catheter is attached to a syringe and is filled with warm sterile Krebs–Ringer solution (for preparation see Section IV,A). A second larger catheter (1.2 mm i.d., 2.0 mm o.d.) with a beveled end is now eased into the cervix alongside the first until it has just entered the uterine lumen, but no further. It is connected at the other end to a small collecting tube. A soft-jaw arterial clamp is placed around the cannulated cervix. Tension is applied to the tubal end of the uterus, while the Ringer solution is driven in through the fine cannula. Saline should appear immediately in the wide cannula and pass into the collecting tube. If this does not happen, the uterus is moved slightly each way until the flow starts. After about 2 ml of saline has been discharged from the syringe, the collecting tube is replaced by a second tube, and the initial sample is searched under a binocular microscope for the blastocyst. If it is not found, successive aliquots of 2 ml are run through until it is found. The most common cause of failure is that the wide cannula has passed into the uterus, and so it should be drawn out of the cervix a few millimeters before the second flushing. The second uterus can be flushed later through the same incision in the vaginal wall.

After the blastocyst is recovered, the two catheters are withdrawn from the cervix, and it is drawn back into the vagina. The vaginal incision is closed with two or three interrupted fine sutures using an eyeless needle (J. Pfrimmer, Erlangen, No. 120 and braided silk BPC 5/0).

The body wall is closed with silk sutures (Mersilk No. 2). It is very important to use a strong grade of silk to close the abdomen because the animal exerts strain on the wound as soon as it recovers from anesthesia and stands up. Fine silk or catgut are liable to break or unravel, leading to hernia, which can be fatal. Sulfanilamide powder is dusted in the skin incision which is closed with 9-mm skin clips (Clay Adams, No. 7631) or with silk sutures.

IV. MANIPULATION OF EARLY EMBRYOS

A. Medium for Handling Embryos

The most satisfactory medium with which to flush the genital tract and in which to store embryos before transfer is Krebs–Ringer bicarbonate equilibrated with Carbogen to pH 7.4 (see Umbreit et al., 1972). The addition of 5% by volume of isologous serum helps to prevent small blastocysts from adhering to glass, but is not essential. The stock solutions for the Ringer can be held under refrigeration and the solution and serum prepared fresh each day and sterilized through a Millipore filter.

B. Flushing

The oviduct of the tammar wallaby is about 6-cm long when dissected from the mesometrium, and it has a much-folded fimbria. To flush the oviduct, it is placed on a cavity slide under a dissecting microscope and is cut at the uterotubal junction. A fine hypodermic needle (No. 26) is inserted into the ampullary region and about 1 ml Krebs–Ringer solution driven through it into the cavity slide. It is then searched by transmitted light for ova, which are about 200 μm diameter.

To recover early embryos from the uterus, the oviduct is removed and fine-pointed scissors inserted at the uterotubal junction so as to enlarge the passage. A blunt No. 18 hypodermic needle is inserted through the cervix and the uterus flushed with 2×2 ml of Krebs-Ringer solution into two solid watchglasses. These are searched for embryos by transmitted light under a binocular microscope. Alternatively, the technique for in vivo collection may be used, and this has the advantage that, since no tissue is cut, there is no contamination of the flushings with extravasated blood. If neither technique proves successful, the uterus is cut longitudinally, everted, and irrigated with more solution into a solid watchglass.

Expanded vesicles cannot be recovered by either method of flushing, so to recover those that still contain a shell membrane, the myometrium is cut longitudinally and the underlying endometrium gently torn apart with fine-toothed forceps in a dish of Krebs–Ringer solution. As this is done, the vesicle eases out of the enclosing folds into the dish.

The shell membrane is refractive and easily seen, and, in fresh blastocysts or vesicles, the yolk sac membrane is closely applied to it (Fig. 2A). If the solution is hypertonic, the yolk sac rapidly collapses and separates from the shell membrane, but will recover if transferred to isotonic conditions.

C. Blastocyst Transfer

Blastocysts in diapause and those up to 8 days after reactivation are less than 0.33 mm diameter and can be readily transferred to uteri of foster mothers. No success has been achieved in attempts to transfer vesicles of 1.0 mm or more, probably because of the mechanical difficulties of putting them into the uterus.

For transfer, both donor and recipient are prepared for laparotomy. When the blastocyst has been obtained, it is held in Krebs–Ringer in an incubator at 31°C, while the recipient's uteri are exposed. It is essential to maintain very precise control over the blastocyst during the actual transfer; we use a micrometer screw-controlled bulb pipette (Fig. 4). With the screw out, a fine pipette (*i.d.* = 0.5 mm) is immersed in saline, which rises about 2 cm by capillary force. This is then opposed by the micrometer screw so that the fluid can then be moved very precisely. The main danger is due to fluctuation in temperature of the contents of the system; this is reduced if the majority of the space is filled with liquid paraffin. The blastocyst is taken up in about 3 μl of saline in a sterile pipette tip and is conveyed in this to the recipient. A stab incision is made in the anterior pole of the uterus with a triangular needle, and the pipette is inserted through this

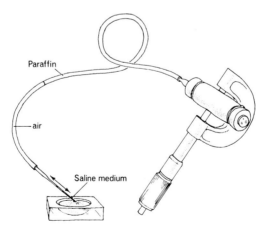

Paraffin

air

Saline medium

Fig. 4.   Fine pipette with micrometer control for transferring small blastocysts to recipient uteri.

into the uterine lumen. The upper meniscus of the saline should still be visible outside the uterus; this is watched as pressure is applied with the micrometer screw until the meniscus disappears. The incision is held for half a minute with fine-toothed forceps as the pipette is withdrawn. The pipette is returned to the binocular microscope and flushed a few times to ensure that the blastocyst has left it before the recipient is stitched up.

Recipients should be females that are undergoing a nonpregnant cycle, so that there are two uteri available to receive blastocysts. Thus, two experimental conditions can be tested in one individual, and each act as the other's control. At autopsy, the transferred blastocysts or the fetuses developed from them are recovered, as well as the native unfertilized egg.

By this technique, the relationship of the blastocyst to the uterus and corpus luteum have been explored (Tyndale-Biscoe, 1963, 1970), and the identity of proteins in the yolk sac fluid identified as of fetal origin, using as a genetic marker the transferrin polymorphism between the two races of tammar wallaby (Renfree and Tyndale-Biscoe, 1973b). This experimental design has also been used successfully with mice (Renfree and McLaren, 1974), and it could have wider application in genetic studies using identifiable embryos.

D. *In Vitro* Culture

Marsupial embryos remain free in the uterus for up to two-thirds of gestation, and, even after attachment, little erosion of maternal tissue occurs. It might be expected, therefore, that *in vitro* culture of marsupial embryos would be easier than with eutherian embryos, whose fetal membranes erode the uterine epithelium. A common problem in growing larger eutherian fetuses in culture is the failure of the allantoic placenta to develop while the yolk sac grows very well (New, 1975). However, at present, the only successful culture of marsupial embryos *in vitro* has been by New and Mizell (1972), grown after the embryos had reached the free vesicle, or early limb bud stages. Opossum embryos, explanted at 11 days gestation, were cultured in TC199 or Ham's F10 in 20% serum, with antibiotics and under 5% CO_2 in 95% O_2 or air (New and Mizell, 1972), using the rotating culture tube apparatus described by New *et al.* (1973). Blood circulation was maintained, and organogenesis continued at about the same rate as *in vivo* for up to 20 hours. The yolk sac presumably mediates most of the respiratory and nutritional requirements of the embryo (New, 1975). The most advanced stage reached in culture was the size of a day 12 embryo of normal gestation (McCrady stage 33), and it is conceivable that cultured opossum fetuses could be subsequently reared in the pouch (New and Mizell, 1972). It is possible that use of uterine fluid instead of serum might enhance survival, but the numbers of embryos are still too small to confirm this trend. However, the success of New and colleagues shows great promise for the possibility of culturing mammalian embryos throughout an entire gestation period.

So far, no early marsupial embryos have been cultured successfully, and the following comments are derived from numerous unsuccessful attempts to culture early blastocysts of red kangaroo, tammar, and opossum (C. H. Tyndale-Biscoe, M. B. Renfree, and J. C. Daniel, unpublished results).

The flushing medium must be isotonic or the protoderm shrinks away from the shell membrane, giving the blastocyst a shriveled appearance. In our experience, the simplest medium works best—either 0.9% sterile saline or Krebs–Ringer gassed with 95% O_2–5% CO_2. Other common media (e.g., TC199, Brinsters, Ham's F10 supplemented with 10 or 20% serum) caused more shrinkage. In opossum, wallaby, and red kangaroo cultures, the blastocysts remained apparently unchanged in Krebs–Ringer for up to a week before collapsing. Opossum embryos maintained their "normal" appearance for longer periods if galactose, but not glucose, and if endometrial fluids, but not serum, was added. In the tammar and red kangaroo, the blastocyst is in diapause when flushed from the uterus, but freeing the blastocyst from the uterine environment did not cause reactivation; this may be an added complication when using these species.

V. COLLECTION OF FETAL AND UTERINE FLUIDS AND TISSUES

A. Uterine Fluids and Tissues

Collection of flushings has already been described (Section IV,B), but, in any flushing method for the purposes of analysis of uterine fluid, there is always the possibility of contamination with blood. The reverse flushing method (Fig. 3) gives least contamination, but a better source of uterine glandular secretion is derived from the endometrium itself.

Endometrium samples can be collected throughout pregnancy from both the pregnant and the nonpregnant uterus of each animal. The uterus is removed from the body at surgery or immediately after killing and is blotted free of blood. It is then moistened in saline and cut longitudinally. After removal of embryonic tissue, the endometrium can be carefully stripped from the myometrium with curved forceps and stored frozen. After thawing, a fluid exudes from the thawed tissue, which has a high protein content and varies in volume and composition according to the stage of gestation (Renfree, 1972, 1973a, 1975). When compared with isologous serum, many unique proteins are observed in the exudate, which can be collected by this means in fair quantity. The exudate does not differ significantly in its protein composition from an endometrial homogenate.

B. Embryo Measurements

All embryos should be measured fresh, either on removal from the uterus or after the collection of fetal fluids. In early pregnancy, vesicle diameters and somite numbers are easily recorded (Fig. 2A), while at later stages crown-rump length (C.R.L.) and head length (H.L.) can be taken (Fig. 2B). The diameter of the allantois can also be taken when it is present in the later stages of gestation (Fig. 2C).

Greatest length (G.L.), H.L., and C.R.L. are usually measured according to the following definitions. G.L. is measured from the crown to the tail fold. H.L. is measured from the occiput to the anterior limit of the nose. C.R.L. is measured from the crown to the rump. The growth curves so obtained are given for the tammar, *M. eugenii* (Fig. 5).

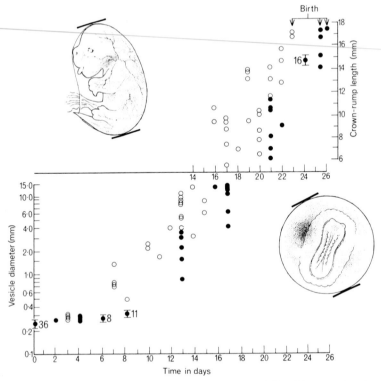

Fig. 5.   Growth curve of tammar embryos during pregnancy initiated by removing the pouch young (●) and initiated by progesterone treatment (○). Redrawn from Renfree and Tyndale-Biscoe (1973a).

C. Fetal Fluids

Methods of sampling the fluids in early, mid, and late pregnancy are outlined below, and are shown diagrammatically in Figs. 6A and B.

The earliest stage sampled to obtain sufficient quantities of fluid occurs at day 17 in the tammar after the blastocyst has developed into a vesicle of about 14 mm diameter, and the embryo has formed about 12 somites (Fig. 2A). The pregnant uterus is swollen, distinguishing it from the nonpregnant uterus. The uterus, once removed from the mother, is opened by carefully blotting away all blood, washing the uterus with sterile saline and then cutting the myometrium and tearing the endometrium so that the blastocyst rolls out into a small dish. It should be washed in sterile saline several times before transferring to a small, sterile vial when the membrane is punctured with a sterile needle. Up to 1.0 ml of yolk sac fluid can be collected from the largest vesicles. The collapsed yolk sac and embryonic disc can be withdrawn from the fluid with forceps.

Collection of middle and late stage pregnancy samples is shown in Fig. 6B. The pregnant uterus in each case is large and conspicuously vascularized. Yolk sac fluid is collected by inserting a 26 gauge hypodermic needle directly into the

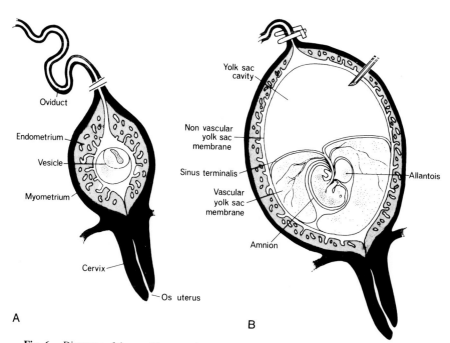

Fig. 6. Diagrams of the gravid uterus of tammar during (A) early and (B) late pregnancy to show the tissues and fluids that can be sampled. Redrawn from Renfree (1973b).

yolk sac through the wall of the uterus. The point of insertion is determined by holding the pregnant uterus up to the light to discover where the embryo is resting. The uterus is then clamped at both the cervical and tubal end, and placed on a moist gauze swab so that the embryo rests on the lower surface. The index finger and thumb gently squeeze the uterus so that the yolk sac membrane pushes up tight against the endometrium. The needle (attached to a sterile 2 ml syringe) should be jabbed, bevel upwards, through the uterine wall at the tubal end about 1 cm from the uterotubal junction to a depth of about 5 mm and then tilted so that the needle rests at about 45° to the plane of the uterus and laboratory bench. A second person is usually required to pull the plunger of the syringe, as the uterus has to be squeezed and the needle carefully held so that the maximum amount of fluid can be collected without sucking the yolk sac membrane onto the bevel of the needle and occluding it. Late in pregnancy, especially near to term, up to 3 ml of yolk sac fluid can be obtained in this way.

The uterus can then be gently torn open as described in Section IV,B, and the embryo, with intact amnion and allantois, tipped into a dish. A maximum of 0.6 ml of allantoic fluid and 0.1 ml of amniotic fluid can be collected from tammars by careful insertion of a syringe with a 26 gauge needle directly into the still fluid-filled sacs. Fetal serum is collected by clamping the vitelline veins between the embryo and point of attachment to the uterus (Fig. 2C), cutting the veins on the uterine side, removing the clamps, and allowing the blood to drip into a small vial or capillary tube directly from the umbilicus. A less satisfactory method is to sever the jugular veins and collect directly into capillary tubes.

All samples should be placed on ice immediately and deep frozen at −15°C within 30 minutes to prevent any change in components. Stored in this way, they appear to be stable for at least 1 year.

D. Fetal Organs

Since organogensis occurs relatively late in gestation, specified fetal organs may only be obtained within a few days of birth. However, with careful dissection under a binocular dissecting microscope, fetal gonads (undifferentiated), liver, heart, adrenals, and kidney can be obtained for assay of hormones, enzymes, etc. (e.g., Renfree and Fox, 1975; Catling and Vinson, 1976). Standard incubation methods for mammalian tissues work effectively for marsupial embryonic tissue.

E. Yolk Sac Placenta

After fluids have been sampled, yolk sac membrane can be carefully pulled from the opened uterus with fine forceps. If the pulling is very gentle, the entire placenta (vascular and nonvascular) can be recovered, and yields about 150 mg of tissue. The placenta is easily minced with fine scissors if a small volume of the incubating medium is added before mincing. The vascular and nonvascular parts of the yolk sac may be easily distinguished by the pinkish color and obvious vessels of the vascular part. Allantoic and amniotic membrane are also easily teased away from the embryo with fine forceps after the yolk sac has been removed. In polyovular species, such as the opossum, yolk sac is not so easily identified, as parts of it are common to more than one embryo (see Enders and Enders, 1969).

VI. POSTNATAL DEVELOPMENT

A. Milk

Milk may be readily obtained from the mammary gland of lactating females carrying pouch young of different ages. A single iv or im injection of 10 IU oxytocin (with or without anesthesia) induces lactation very rapidly, and, with gentle massaging, samples can be obtained direct from the nipple to a tube. Milk whey is obtained by spinning the milk at 20,000 rpm for 20 minutes at 5°C. The supernatant containing the milk proteins when removed from the pellet containing fats, etc., can be satisfactorily stored at $-15°C$ until used for analysis.

B. Pouch Young as Experimental Material

The neonatal marsupial reaches the pouch by its own effort, and within a few minutes attaches firmly to a teat. This attachment is not relinquished for several weeks or months. The end of the teat enlarges within the buccal cavity of the young, so that artificial removal can damage the lips, and, in any event, the young has difficulty reattaching. For this reason, some experimental procedures are done on young attached to the teat and with the mother anesthetized. Jurgelski (1974) has described a technique for introducing fluid to the stomach of the young by inserting a fine catheter (0.024 mm o.d.) into the mouth along the side of the teat. There is a risk in this procedure from the transfer to the young of the anesthetic used to control the mother which may outweigh the risk of detaching the young. For delicate surgery also, the abdominal movements of the mother, being transmitted to the young, make this an unsatisfactory procedure.

In our experience and that of Ashman *et al.* (1975b), very small young, 1–10 days old, will reattach to the teat without assistance, provided the mother is kept quiet in a sack for a few hours.

No attempts to rear small pouch young in an artificial pouch on an artificial milk diet have been successful. More needs to be known about the precise composition of milk as it changes through lactation, and the suckling behavior of the young needs to be examined. Nothing is known about the daily pattern of suckling by the young, nor how much milk is consumed.

During the first half of pouch life, while the young is ectothermic it can be immobilized for surgery by cooling. The heart rate slows down to 25 beats/min^{-1}, and breathing may cease. Apnea is not serious in very small pouch young, as cutaneous exchange is evidently sufficient to maintain respiration, provided the skin is kept moist with saline. A satisfactory device to hold such pouch young designed by K. Hogarth is illustrated in Fig. 7. It is a stainless steel plate with a molded depression in the center to accommodate the young animal on its back. A pattern of pegs radiating away from the depression provide anchorage for rubber bands held at appropriate tension across the head, trunk, and limbs. The plate rests on a bed of crushed ice or other cooling device, and surgery can be performed under a dissecting microscope. Cold light can be brought to the site of work by attaching a tapered glass or Lucite rod to a flexible light source. The taper can be shaped to double as a retractor as well as an illuminator.

The most serious problem in surgery of very small pouch young (< 2.0 gm) is loss of blood. Hemorrhage cannot be controlled by thrombin because the blood coagulates very slowly. It is necessary, therefore, to use a fine cautery or dia-

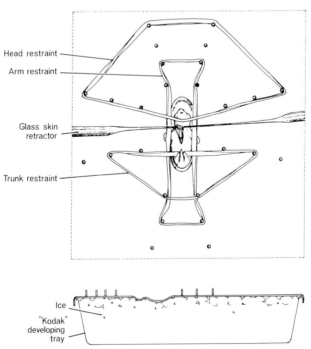

Fig. 7. Restraining and cooling plate used for surgery on neonatal and very small pouch young.

thermy for cutting tissue. With this technique on tammar pouch young less than 3 days after birth, the cervical and thoracic thymus lobes have been removed (K. Hogarth, personal communication). Six out of 13 young aged 2½–3 days recovered and reattached to a teat in the pouch.

After surgery, iridectomy sutures on eyeless needles (Ethicon Micropoint needle 9–7, silk 8/0) are used, and healing is very rapid.

The following experiments have been performed on very small pouch young. Total thymectomy in *M. eugenii* and *Setonix brachyurus* has been achieved on day 3, before small lymphocytes have reached the cervical thymus (Ashman *et al.*, 1975a). Partial thymectomy of the superficial cervical thymus is, of course, much easier to perform and does lead to immunologic deficiency in *Setonix,* but it does not remove the immunologic responses altogether. Kidney grafts and introduction of pathogens to young *Didelphis* during the first week of life have been performed (Mizell and Isaacs, 1970). Gonadectomy and gonad transfer has been undertaken on *M. eugenii* (Alcorn, 1976) and *D. virginiana* (see Burns, 1961) during the first 2 weeks of life when differentiation of the gonad is taking place.

For older pouch young that have developed homeothermy, normal anesthesia can be employed, and the techniques are similar to those used on adults, but the instruments must be scaled down. In *M. eugenii,* thyroidectomy has been performed on young of 140–180 days (Setchell, 1974), and hypophysectomy by a parapharyngeal route on young weighing 200–400 gm, about 8 months old (Hearn, 1975). The young survived for only a few days after the latter procedure, although adults can survive for up to 4 months after hypophysectomy (Hearn, 1975).

Studies published before 1972 on various aspects of the ontogeny of physiological functions in pouch young marsupials have been reviewed by Sharman (1973a) and Tyndale-Biscoe (1973). Since then, Setchell (1974) has described the development of thyroid function in the tammar and Catling and Vinson (1976) steroid secretion by the developing adrenal cortex from birth to pouch exit in the same species. Janssens *et al.* (1977) have examined the regulation of gluconeogenesis in the liver of fed and fasted tammar pouch young, and they conclude that the ability to regulate this pathway precedes the ability to maintain homeothermy reported by Setchell (1974). Renfree and Fox (1975) have examined the ontogeny of some lactate and malate dehydrogenases in opossums from before birth until adult.

VII. CONCLUSIONS

The marsupial embryo and pouch young can yield much unexpected information on the mechanisms and control of mammalian development, and yet the methods described in this chapter have only been tried on a very few marsupial species and can provide a preliminary insight into a potentially vast field. We hope that it will encourage further studies on these fascinating mammals.

REFERENCES

Alcorn, G. (1976). "Ovarian Development in the Tammar Wallaby." Ph.D. Thesis, Macquarie University, Sydney.
Ashman, R., Keast, D., Stanley, N. F., and Waring, H. (1975a). *Am. Zool.* **15,** 155–166.
Ashman, R., Shield, J., and Waring, H. (1975b). *J. Reprod. Fertil.* **42,** 179–181.
Barnes, R. D., and Barthold, S. W. (1969). *J. Reprod. Fertil., Suppl.* **6,** 477–482.
Barnes, R. D., and Wolf, H. G. (1971). *Int. Zoo Yearb.* **11,** 50–54.
Block, M. (1964). *Ergeb. Anat. Entwicklungsgesch.* **37,** 237–366.
Burns, R. K. (1961). *In* "Sex and Internal Secretions" (W. C. Young, ed.), 3rd ed., Vol. 1, pp. 76–160. Williams & Wilkins, Baltimore, Maryland.
Catling, P. C., and Vinson, G. P. (1976). *J. Endocrinol.* **69,** 447–448.
Enders, A. C., and Enders, R. K. (1969). *Anat. Rec.* **165,** 431–450.
Gomot, L. (in press). *In* "Traité de Zoologie" (P.-P. Grassé, ed.), Vol. 16, Part 8. Masson, Paris.
Hartman, C. G. (1916). *J. Morphol.* **27,** 1–84.
Hartman, C. G. (1923). *Am. J. Anat.* **32,** 353–421.
Hartman, C. G. (1925). *Am. J. Physiol.* **71,** 436–454.
Hartman, C. G. (1928). *J. Morphol.* **46,** 143–200.
Hayman, D. L., and Martin, P. G. (1974). *Anim. Cytogenet.* **4,** 1–110.
Hearn, J. P. (1975). *J. Endocrinol.* **64,** 403–416.
Hughes, R. L. (1974). *J. Reprod. Fertil.* **39,** 173–186.
Hughes, R. L., and Shorey, C. D. (1973). *J. Reprod. Fertil.* **32,** 25–32.
Janssens, P. A., Jenkinson, L. A., Paton, B. C., and Whitelaw, E. (1977). *Aust. J. Biol. Sci.* **30,** 183–196.
Jurgelski, W. (1974). *Lab. Anim. Sci.* **24,** 376–403.
Jurgelski, W., and Porter, M. E. (1974). *Lab. Anim. Sci.* **24,** 412–425.
Jurgelski, W., Forsythe, W., Dahl, D., Thomas, L. D., Moore, J. A., Kotin, P., Falk, H. L., and Vogel, F. S. (1974). *Lab. Anim. Sci.* **24,** 404–411.
McCrady, E. (1938). *Am. Anat. Mem.* **16,** 1–233.
McDonald, I. R., and Than, K. A. (1976). *J. Endocrinol.* **68,** 257–264.
Mizell, M., and Isaacs, J. J. (1970). *Am. Zool.* **10,** 141–155.
New, D. A. T. (1975). *In* "Environmental Agents and Congenital Defects: Methods for Detection" (T. H. Shepard, J. R. Miller, and M. Marois, eds.), pp. 145–160. North-Holland Publ., Amsterdam.
New, D. A. T., and Mizell, M. (1972). *Science* **175,** 533–535.
New, D. A. T., Coppola, P. T., and Terry, S. (1973). *J. Reprod. Fertil.* **35,** 135–138.
Padykula, H., and Taylor, M. (1977). *In* "Reproduction and Evolution" (J. H. Calaby and C. H. Tyndale-Biscoe, eds.), pp. 303–323. Aust. Acad. Sci., Canberra.
Pilton, P. E., and Sharman, G. B. (1962). *J. Endocrinol.* **25,** 119–136.
Renfree, M. B. (1972). *Nature (London)* **240,** 475–477.
Renfree, M. B. (1973a). *Dev. Biol.* **32,** 41–49.
Renfree, M. B. (1973b). *Dev. Biol.* **33,** 62–79.
Renfree, M. B. (1974). *J. Reprod. Fertil.* **39,** 127–130.
Renfree, M. B. (1975). *J. Reprod. Fertil.* **42,** 163–166.

Renfree, M. B., and Fox, D. J. (1975). *Comp. Biochem. Physiol. B* **52**, 347–350.

Renfree, M. B., and McLaren, A. (1974). *Nature (London)* **252**, 159–161.

Renfree, M. B., and Tyndale-Biscoe, C. H. (1973a). *Dev. Biol.* **32**, 28–40.

Renfree, M. B., and Tyndale-Biscoe, C. H. (1973b). *J. Reprod. Fertil.* **32**, 113–115.

Sadleir, R. M. F. S., and Tyndale-Biscoe, C. H. (1977). *Biol. Reprod.* **16**, 605–608.

Setchell, P. J. (1974). *Comp. Biochem. Physiol. A* **47**, 1115–1121.

Sharman, G. B. (1961). *Proc. Zool. Soc. Lond.* **137**, 197–220.

Sharman, G. B. (1962). *J. Endocrinol.* **25**, 375–385.

Sharman, G. B. (1973a). *In* "The Mammalian Fetus *in vitro*" (C. R. Austin, ed.), pp. 67–90. Chapman & Hall, London.

Sharman, G. B. (1973b). *In* "Cytotaxonomy and Vertebrate Evolution" (A. B. Chiarelli and E. Capanna, eds.), pp. 485–527. Academic Press, New York.

Shorey, C. D., and Hughes, R. L. (1975). *J. Reprod. Fertil.* **42**, 221–228.

Tyndale-Biscoe, C. H. (1963). *J. Reprod. Fertil.* **6**, 41–48.

Tyndale-Biscoe, C. H. (1970). *J. Reprod. Fertil.* **23**, 25–32.

Tyndale-Biscoe, H. (1973). "Life of Marsupials." Arnold, London.

Tyndale-Biscoe, C. H., and Hawkins, J. H. (1977). *In* "Reproduction and Evolution" (J. H. Calaby and C. H. Tyndale-Biscoe, eds.), pp. 245–252. Aust. Acad. Sci., Canberra.

Umbreit, W. W., Burris, R. H., and Stauffer, J. F. (1972). "Manometric and Biochemical Techniques." Burgess, Minneapolis, Minnesota.

Woolley, P. A. (1973). *Exp. Anim.* **22**, 161–172.

16

Experimentation Involving
Primate Embryos

BENJAMIN G. BRACKETT

I. INTRODUCTION

The processes of fertilization and early embryonic development have intrigued biologists during the last century. During the last three decades, along with renewed awareness of the exponential increase in human population, much progress has been made toward understanding these critical steps in ontogeny. Progress in efforts to better understand human gamete interaction, fertilization, and early development was given impetus in this country by the Department of Health, Education and Welfare (D.H.E.W.), National Institute for Child Health and Human Development Center for Population Research, which, in 1969, initiated a program for contract funding administered through its Contraceptive Development Branch. At about the same time, small groups of scientists in Australia, Germany, Great Britain, Japan, South America, and elsewhere around the world began experimentation with human gametes and embryos, and these relatively recent studies account for much of our present knowledge of fertilization and early development in our own species.

Although they are somewhat neglected as experimental laboratory animals, progress has been made using nonhuman primates. Research in primate reproduction has received impetus by a commitment in the United States to seven Regional Primate Research Centers, administered by the Division of Research Resources of the National Institutes of Health (N.I.H.) since 1962, and additional support by N.I.H. for primate research resources in several major medical centers.

Unfortunately, progress in experimentation on the primate front—both human and nonhuman—has been somewhat hindered during recent years. Ethical concerns in the United States led to a moratorium on human *in vitro* fertilization and fetal studies. At the time of this writing, "certain types of activities involving human subjects may not be supported or conducted with the aid of N.I. H. or P.H.S. or D. H. E. W. funds regardless of the type of grant, contract, or other support mechanism involved." Such prohibited or restricted research applies to "any research whatsoever involving *in vitro* fertilization of human ova, unless previously approved by the D.H.E.W. Ethical Advisory Board, N.I.H., Bethesda, Maryland 20014. [Authority: 45 CFR 46.204(3)]" (N.I.H. Guide for Grants and Contracts 5(18), Oct. 8, 1976.) The National Research Act requires The Institutional Review Board of each site to review all proposed human experimentation, non-D.H.E.W.-supported as well as D.H.E.W.-supported research.

Hindrance of nonhuman primate experimentation has resulted from export restrictions rather arbitrarily imposed by countries of origin. These restrictions have made many important nonhuman primate species in short supply. As a result, nonhuman primate research is increasingly expensive. The Interagency Primate Steering Committee, composed of representatives of seven components of the United States government, was established in 1974, by the Assistant Secretary for H.E.W., and charged with coordinating and representing the combined interests of the government in the supply, use, and conservation of nonhuman primates. The Committee has recommended criteria to be used by all government agencies that conduct or support research using nonhuman primates, recognizing that these animals are essential in biomedical research, biologics production, and testing compounds for toxicity. The criteria are that (1) the research proposed can be done best with primates; i.e., that no other known system or other kind of animal could produce comparable results; (2) the species of primate proposed is the most appropriate, and that some other more plentiful species would not be adequate; (3) the number of primates proposed is the minimum that will produce acceptable scientific results; (4) the primates will not be sacrificed during or at the end of the study, except in those cases requiring termination as part of the investigation; (5) if sacrifice is deemed necessary, positive action will be taken to share body material when feasible.

The situation regarding availability of nonhuman primates for biomedical research will undoubtedly be, at least temporarily, worsened by recent actions of the Convention of International Trade in Endangered Species of Wild Fauna and Flora, which added all chimpanzees, lemurs, and five species of marmosets to Appendix I: Endangered Species, with all remaining species of the entire order of primates being placed on Appendix II: Threatened Species. The United States delegation from the Department of the Interior supported the Swiss proposal to add all primates to Appendix II. With the addition of the family Pongidae, all great apes now have Appendix I status.

The purpose of this chapter is to summarize progress in human and nonhuman primate embryology with specific emphasis on methods that have enabled the attainment of the present state of the art. Although specimens falling within Streeter's "Horizons" (Streeter, 1942, 1945, 1948, 1951) of less than 34-mm crown–rump length or about 54 gestational days are accurately classified as embryos (Shepard et al., 1971), usage here equates fertilized ovum or egg, or various cleavage stages of the ovum with "embryo," and attention is focused primarily on early aspects of embryology within this context. Included in this survey are references to studies involving recovery of ova and embryos from female reproductive tracts, in vitro fertilization and embryo culture, and initial efforts to transfer primate embryos.

II. RECOVERY OF OVA AND EMBRYOS FROM THE FEMALE REPRODUCTIVE TRACT

A. Human Studies

Surgical recovery of unfertilized human tubal ova from women on cycle days 14–16 was reported around 50 years ago (Allen et al., 1928, 1930; Newell et al., 1930). The appropriate oviduct was flushed by clamping off the cervix and the contralateral fallopian tube and forcing saline through a hypodermic needle into the uterine lumen. In women, fluid passes readily through the fallopian tube to the fimbriated end, at which a watchglass was placed to catch the ovum. Unfertilized tubal ova were also recovered by Lewis (1931) and Pincus and Saunders (1937). These early studies established the size of the unfertilized human tubal ovum as varying in diameter from 115 to 151 μm. Five additional unfertilized tubal ova were recovered from 24 oviducts by Miller et al. (1938).

Human ova undergoing fertilization have been recovered from oviducts removed in the course of surgically indicated procedures. Hamilton (1949) reported the first penetrated tubal ovum, a single-celled, pronuclear specimen. Khvatov (1959) found a pronuclear egg in a serially sectioned oviduct. Dickmann et al. (1965) studied, by means of phase contrast microscopy, a pronuclear egg found following flushing the oviducts of a woman who had an intrauterine contraceptive device. Zamboni et al. (1966) recovered a pronuclear ovum from an oviduct of a 33-year-old patient 26 hours after coitus. Their report marked the first ultrastructural study of a sperm-penetrated human ovum. Remnants of the penetrating sperm cell were found close to one of the pronuclei. The similarities in structure among mammalian species at this stage of development are striking.

The first cleaved oviductal specimen was recovered in the systematic studies of Hertig and associates (1954). This 2-cell ovum was recovered within an estimated 1½–2½ days after ovulation. A 3-cell stage tubal ovum was reported by Doyle and her colleagues (1966). There are several other reports involving human ova and early embryos recovered from oviducts and uteri of patients undergoing surgery during the luteal phase of their menstrual cycle (Rock and Hertig, 1944; Hertig et al., 1956; Noyes et al., 1966; Clewe et al., 1971). From these reports, one concludes that ova are not normally found in the fallopian tubes after the 4th postovulatory day. Hertig et al. (1956) described seven ova that were found free in the uterine cavity. Four of these were abnormal morulae of about 3–5 days, one was a normal morula of 3 days, and two normal blastocysts were of about 4½ days of age.

Difficulties associated with human ovum recovery studies were discussed by Noyes and colleagues (1966). Collection of human embryos (and fetuses) for teaching, research, and monitoring embryonic (and fetal) losses requires well-organized coordination and cooperation between hospital and laboratory personnel (Shepard et al., 1971).

In recent experiments carried out by Croxatto and colleagues (1972a,b), efforts were made to use more appropriate criteria for estimation of ovulation time. The previous studies had estimated probable time of ovulation retrospectively according to the length of the menstrual cycle, the temperature record, ovum cytology, stage of development of endometrium, and ovarian histology. Since ovulation dating by most of those criteria is based on the assumption that the interval between ovulation and the next expected menstruation is about 14 days, on the average, errors can be expected because individual cycles vary and the luteal phase can be as short as 8 days. Noteworthy features of Croxatto's studies were that the women were normal, a rise in the luteinizing hormone (LH) concentration in urine was used as an additional criterion to date ovulation, and a nonsurgical technique was developed to recover the ovum lying free in the uterine cavity.

Croxatto and his colleagues (1972a,b) studied 42 healthy women between 20 and 35 years of age, each with 1 or more children and without contraceptive treatment other than spermicides or the rhythm method used during the 2 cycles preceding the cycle studied. In the cycle of the study, several determinations were made: (1) LH concentration of the first morning urine beginning on the 10th day after the onset of menstruation was assayed by the hemagglutination inhibition assay (Luteonosticon, Oss, Holland); (2) physical characteristics of cervical mucus (Davajan and Nakamura, 1975) every 2 or 3 days; (3) daily record of basal body temperature (BBT); (4) endometrial dating of a biopsy taken in the luteal phase (Noyes *et al.*, 1950); and (5) total urinary excretion of pregnanediol determined once during the luteal phase (Chattoraj and Wottiz, 1967). Interpretation of these parameters for dating ovulation were based on the assumption that follicular rupture would occur: (1) on the day in which LH attained a concentration of 50 IU/liter or more; (2) on the day following maximal estrogenic features, i.e., maximal viscoelastic property (*spinnbarkeit*) and microscopically observable "ferning pattern," of the cervical mucus; (3) on the day preceding a sustained rise in BBT; or (4) on the day corresponding with endometrial development characteristic of day 14. If an LH peak was observed on a single day, this was taken as the leading criterion, whereas in the absence of an LH peak or when high levels were present in more than 1 day, ovulation dating was based upon coincidence of compatibility among the various criteria available in each case. The uterine cavity was flushed with saline through the cervical canal at intervals after presumed ovulation, and the flushings were examined with low-power magnification to determine presence or absence of an egg (Croxatto *et al.*, 1972b). Ova were photographed in a drop of saline or in tissue culture medium 199 (Difco Lab., Detroit, Michigan) on a depression slide under bright field and phase contrast microscopy. Diameters of eggs were measured from negative film using a stage micrometer for reference. Volumes of eggs recovered were calculated. In 8 of the 42 cases, ova were recovered. Although patients in all cases were requested to avoid intercourse from the last menstrual period until after the uterine cavity had been flushed, these instructions were not adhered to in four of the eight patients from whom ova were obtained. In three of these cases, fertilization had taken place, resulting in recovery of two morula-stage embryos estimated to be 4–6 days after ovulation and one blastocyst containing 186 cells which was 5 or more days after ovulation. The latter embryo was recovered 10 days after reported coitus.

The best uterine ovum recovery technique developed by these investigators employed a stainless steel cannula. The end of the cannula, which was inserted into the cervix, was 5-cm long and slightly curved with a 3-mm diameter bore. It had three rows of small holes near the tip to ensure free flow of fluid from the uterine cavity into the collection cannula. A side arm near the extrauterine end allowed the introduction of a polyethylene tube (PE 160) through the cannula up to the uterine fundus. Fluid for flushing the uterine cavity was introduced through this tubing, and washings collected through the stainless steel catheter into test tubes. All washings were done with 10–20 ml of sterile 0.9% NaCl with 5 IU/ml of heparin added to avoid formation of clots in case of endometrial bleeding during the procedure. Washings collected in 10-ml conical tubes were left undisturbed a few minutes before small aliquots were aspirated from the bottom of each tube and examined for eggs in embryologic watchglasses under a dissecting microscope. The entire procedure from arrival of the patient until an egg was found usually required no more than 30 minutes.

The peak of LH as determined by radioimmunoassay of serum at 8-hour intervals was reported to occur 16 hours prior to ovulation as dated by corpus luteum biopsies (Yussman and Taymor, 1970), and it appears that LH in urine peaks about the same time as in serum (Stevens, 1969; Thomas and Ferin, 1970). However, in the present studies, ovulation timing based on LH peak of first morning urine proved inadequate as a general procedure. Arrival of the egg into the uterus was most accurately determined following serial flushings in which the ovum was recovered at an interval of several hours after an earlier unsuccessful uterine flushing. Loss of the zona pellucida and disintegration of unfertilized eggs probably occurred within 24 hours after reaching the uterine cavity, based on failure to find unfertilized eggs beyond day 3 after ovulation (Croxatto *et al.*, 1972a,b). In an extension of these studies, 22 ova were recovered between 48 and 168 hours following the estrogen peak (as detected by daily serum assays) from flushings obtained from various segments of the oviduct and endometrial cavity of 39 women undergoing surgical sterilization (Croxatto *et al.*, 1977). Human ova were found to spend nearly 72 hours in the fallopian tubes, reaching the proximal end of the ampulla within a few hours where they remain 2–3 days before transport during a short period of time through the isthmus and into the uterus.

A human blastocyst reported by Hertig and colleagues (1956) had 107 cells and was about the same size as less developed or unfertilized eggs. The human blastocyst described by Croxatto and colleages (1972a) had 186 cells discernible by counting nuclei following lacmoid staining (Yanagimachi and Chang, 1961), and was at least twice as big as any unimplanted human egg described (7.76 × 10^{-3} mm^3 versus around 2.70 × 10^{-3} mm^3 volume). From available data regarding the human blastocyst, then, it would appear that expansion begins between 107- and 186-cell stages, that shedding of the zona pellucida and implantation occur after the egg has attained the stage of 186 cells, and, at the 186-cell stage, two and perhaps three types of cells are recognizable in the human blastocyst (Croxatto *et al.*, 1972a).

B. Nonhuman Primate Studies

Much progress has been made in embryologic studies involving the baboon, *Papio cynocephalus* (Hendrickx, 1971). Mature female baboons offer an advantage in the accuracy with which the time of ovulation can be estimated by observations of their sex skin deturgescence. The estimated ovulation day (day 0) is the 3rd day preceding initiation of sex skin deturgescence, and mating can be scheduled according to timing anticipated from observations of the previous cycle (Hendrickx and Kraemer, 1968). This feature has facilitated the examination of cleavage and morula stage baboon embryos by presently available morphological technology, including histological (Hendrickx and Kraemer, 1968; Kraemer and Hendrickx, 1971), ultrastructural (Panigel *et al.,* 1975), and surface ultrastructural approaches (Flechon *et al.,* 1976).

In addition to irrigation of excised oviducts and uteri, baboon embryos were collected using an *in situ* flushing procedure which was a combination of the one mentioned above for collection of human embryos (Allen *et al.,* 1928), and that of Alliston and Ulberg (1961) for recovery of sheep embryos. This involved insertion of fluted plastic catheters (Intramedic, PE160 or PE100, Clay Adams, New York) approximately 3 mm into the infundibular ostia of oviducts, where they were secured by a ligature or by a Hagenbarth wound clip applicator (Hendrickx and Kraemer, 1968). An 18-gauge intravenous catheter approximately 5 cm in length was inserted through the uterine wall with the tip in the uterine lumen and secured by a purse-string suture. If oviductal washings were of major interest, the cervix was clamped, and lactated Ringer's solution was introduced, using a 30-ml syringe for flushing the fluid through the uterus, oviducts, and plastic catheters into embryologic watchglasses. For recovery of embryos from the uterus, the cervix was not clamped, and a glass speculum, 17–24 mm in diameter, was inserted into the vagina and held firmly against the external cervical os. Approximately 90 ml of fluid was forced through the uterine lumen, cervix, and speculum into petri dishes. The cervix was then clamped, and additional fluid was forced through the oviducts. Two, 3, and 24 blastomeres were found in 2-, 3-, and 4-day-old baboon embryos, respectively; 30–40 cells were present at 5 days and more than 60 cells in latter stages (Panigel *et al.,* 1975).

Preimplantation development of the fertilized rhesus monkey ovum was documented in detail for the first time by Lewis and Hartman (1933, 1941). Descriptions of tubal ova ranging from two to eight cells were provided. In addition, a 16-cell uterine specimen was recovered; the time after ovulation was estimated to be 96 hours. More recent ovum recovery experiments in the rhesus monkey provide additional evidence for a 3- to 4-day residence of the ovum within the oviduct (Marston *et al.,* 1969a,b; Eddy *et al.,* 1975).

Awareness of the value of and possibilities of exhausting finite supplies of rhesus monkeys as laboratory animals has spurred efforts to perform careful surgical approaches that can be repeated with the same animal many times. *In situ* retrograde flushing of fallopian tubes for ovum recovery at laparotomy, described by Mastroianni and Rosseau (1965), can be repeated in the same animal six or more times without excessive interference of adhesions that result from fibrin deposition in response to surgical insult. This procedure, variously modified, has been useful in several studies (Suzuki and Mastroianni, 1966; Marston and Kelly, 1968; Marston *et al.,* 1969a; Eddy *et al.,* 1975; Batta *et al.,* 1978). As practiced by this author, a cellulose nitrate test tube is cut at an angle and inserted into the abdominal cavity under the fimbriated end of the oviduct and held in position by forceps attached to the long end. The oviduct is identified near its insertion into the uterus and gently held with forceps or by a blunt nerve hook. Then the oviduct is flushed with a 3-ml syringe fitted with a ½ inch 25-gauge needle. The needle is bent to facilitate alignment with the oviduct. After insertion of the needle into the oviduct, 0.1 ml saline is injected to verify proper positioning of the needle inside the lumen. Constant attention of an assistant is focused on correct positioning of the collecting tube beneath the fimbria. The flushing medium is forced retrograde through the oviductal lumen and recovered from the fimbriated end. Flushings obtained in this way are generally free of gross contamination by blood. A modification which involves cannulation of oviducts and collection into tubes held outside the abdominal cavity is frequently desirable when ovaries are hormonally hyperstimulated for superovulation (Fig. 1). Serial examination under a dissecting microscope (10–70 × magnification) of flushings, aspirated from the bottom of the collecting tube and placed in watch glasses (or commercially available beaker covers), lead to ovum recovery.

For recovery of eggs that might have passed into the uterine cavity, a thorough lavage of the uterus is performed (Seitz *et al.,* 1971). The approach used in the author's laboratory is diagrammed in Fig. 2. Both oviducts are clamped near the uterotubal junction to prevent the possibility of retrograde flushing (which in the rhesus monkey is not a prominent problem). The cervical canal is clamped with a right-angle gall bladder clamp and a 19-gauge needle on a 10-ml syringe barrel is inserted into the uterine cavity from the ventral surface. A second 19-gauge needle fitted on a 10-ml syringe filled with saline solution (or culture medium) is inserted into the fundic area of the uterus. The ends of the two needles are contacted inside of the uterine cavity to ensure correct positioning. Flushing is accomplished by forcing 10 ml saline through the needle inserted in the fundic region and recovering the flushings in the second syringe barrel. The fluid recovered from the oviducts and uterus is transferred to sterile petri dishes or watchglasses and examined under a dissecting microscope (7–70 ×) for the presence of ova. A modification of this technique has been useful for recovering

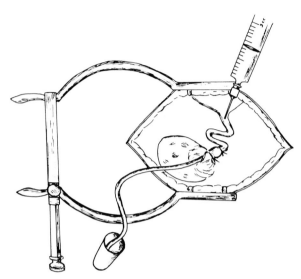

Fig. 1. Diagrammatic representation of a procedure for retrograde flushing of the rhesus monkey oviduct for recovery of tubal ova following hormonal treatments resulting in superovulation. Ovum recovery can also be done without catheterization of the oviduct with polyethylene or sialastic tubing as shown here (see text).

9 embryos, including blastocysts with and without zonae and one 22-cell morula stage embryo, and 2 unfertilized ova from 22 uterine flushes between days 17 and 19 of the menstrual cycle (Hurst *et al.*, 1976).

Using modifications of the techniques for tubal flushing (Mastroianni and Rosseau, 1965) and for uterine flushings (Seitz *et al.*, 1971) practiced in our laboratory, Eddy *et al.* (1975) confirmed tubal ovum transport time for untreated, spontaneously cycling rhesus monkeys to be approximately 72 hours, as estimated by Hartman (1944). In the recent work, laparotomies were performed approximately 24, 48, or 72 hours postovulation as estimated by plasma estrogen values rising to levels in excess of 200–300 pg/ml. The ampulla and isthmus of oviducts and the uterus were flushed separately, thereby allowing definition of the position of recovered ova within the tract. Ova were recovered from the tubal ampulla at 24 and 48 hours postovulation. By 72 hours, ova were recovered from both the oviduct and uterus.

Experiments have been carried out in our laboratory to recover rhesus monkey ova in varying stages of development. Initial experiments involved laparotomy near the estimated time of ovulation and upon identification of a fresh corpus hemorrhagicum, intrauterine insemination with washed monkey sperm (10^6 sperm cells) in 0.1 ml of medium was carried out. The ovum in Fig. 3 resulted from one of these experiments in which tubal flushing was 21¼ hours after

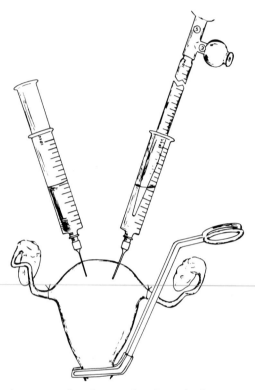

Fig. 2. Diagrammatic representation of a procedure for uterine lavage in the rhesus monkey. Uterotubal junctions may be occluded with ligatures (pictured here) or with small hemostats. After removal of clamps, tubal and cervical patency is reestablished by an additional flushing with warm saline.

intrauterine insemination at laparotomy. This 2-cell stage ovum appears to have very recently cleaved and represents the earliest 2-cell stage embryo recorded to date for this species.

Efforts to improve the numbers of ova and embryos obtainable from rhesus monkeys led to development of a means for superovulation of rhesus monkeys involving stimulation with pregnant mare serum gonadotropin (PMS) followed by human chorionic gonadotropin (HCG) and prostaglandin E_1 or E_2 (Batta and Brackett, 1974; Batta *et al.*, 1978). The best superovulation procedure from this work yielded mean ovulation responses (determined by ovulation points on the ovaries) of around 8 with 96–100% of treated animals ovulating. Animals were treated with this procedure in conjunction with intrauterine insemination for recovery of embryos (Batta *et al.*, 1978). In this work, ovulation timing was determined by a series of laparoscopic examinations, and subsequent experi-

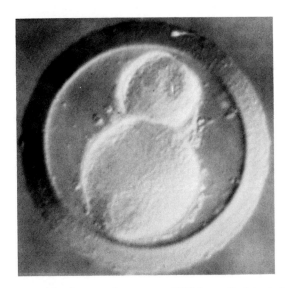

Fig. 3.   Recently cleaved 2-cell stage embryo recovered 21¼ hours after intrauterine insemination of a rhesus monkey with a fresh corpus hemorrhagicum.

ments involved intrauterine insemination at estimated intervals prior to and following the expected ovulation time. Although ova obtained in this study appeared normal under low-power magnification, more discriminating ultrastructural evaluations revealed many morphological aberrations. About 33–75% of the ovulated ova were recovered. At 86 hours after estimated ovulation time, ova were recovered from uterus and oviducts; while at 63 hours and earlier intervals after ovulation, almost all the recovered ova were from oviducts. A possible explanation for ovulation induction by prostaglandins of the E series in rhesus monkeys follows experiments revealing a release of LH by these agents (Batta *et al.*, 1976).

III. GAMETE RECOVERY, *IN VITRO* FERTILIZATION, EMBRYO CULTURE, AND EMBRYO TRANSFER

A. Sperm Capacitation and Penetration of the Zona Pellucida

Although not completely understood, the mechanism of sperm capacitation is known from experiments in the rabbit and in the mouse to involve removal of sperm surface antigens, at least one of which is inhibitory to the fertilization process (Oliphant and Brackett, 1973a,b; Reyes *et al.*, 1975; Brackett and Oliphant, 1975). This process can be rapidly effected by increasing the ionic strength of the medium in which sperm cells are held between washing procedures. In addition, capacitation of human, hamster, or mouse sperm can take place by preincubating sperm cells for varying intervals prior to *in vitro* insemination. Capacitation of human sperm can be experimentally accomplished in several ways, as determined by observations that treated sperm were able to penetrate ova *in vitro* (Edwards *et al.*, 1969; Bavister *et al.*, 1969; Seitz *et al.*, 1971; Yanagimachi *et al.*, 1976; Soupart and Morganstern, 1973; Soupart and Strong, 1974). Conditions similar to those effecting hamster sperm capacitation seem to be adequate for human sperm. Variability in proportions of ova penetrated by treated human sperm can be attributed to variability in condition or penetrability of the eggs as well as to the ability of the sperm. Soupart (1976) believes follicle cell stimulation by gonadotropins (FSH, LH, and HCG) significantly enhances sperm ability to penetrate through the zona pellucida in his human *in vitro* fertilization system (Soupart and Morgenstern, 1973). Additional work is indicated to assign accurately a precise role for steroids, although soluble estrogen was suggested to be a beneficial component of fertilization media used for early human experiments in our laboratory (Seitz *et al.*, 1971).

The penetration by human sperm of oocytes recovered from cadavers has been proposed as a test for assessing human sperm fertilizing ability *in vitro* (Overstreet and Hembree, 1976). Ovaries were obtained 8–45 hours postmortem from cadavers, 15–42 years of age. Oocytes were recovered in saline following puncturing of follicles under a dissecting microscope. Bavister's medium as modified (BMM) for use with human oocytes (Edwards *et al.*, 1970) was used. Within 3 hours of ejaculation, sperm cells were washed by centrifugation through 10% Ficoll (Sigma Chemical Co., St. Louis, Missouri) in saline. For the test, one to five oocytes in 0.05 ml BMM were incubated with an equal volume of medium containing spermatozoa in depression plates. In some experiments, half the sperm sample was from fertile donors and labeled with fluorescein isothiocyanate (FITC). Following incubation, oocytes were washed in saline and mounted between a glass slide and cover slip supported by Vaseline–paraffin dots. Examination was with a phase-contrast fluorescence microscope. The location of spermatozoa in the matrix of the zona pellucida and within the perivitelline space of each oocyte was of interest. In some cases, oocytes were fixed with acetic alcohol and stained with lacmoid (Chang, 1952) for evaluation of possible sperm entry into the ooplasm, which was not seen. Of 773 oocytes examined at 8 or 24 hours after insemination, 300 (38.8%) had spermatozoa in the zona pellucida, and 41 (5.7%) had spermatozoa in the perivitelline space. Oocyte zonae were penetrated to some extent by sperm from 11 of 16 infertile men, but a significantly lower proportion of penetration into zonae by these sperm samples was seen than by those from fertile donors, both when the respective sperm samples were incubated separately with oocytes (12.9% versus 46.4%) and when equal numbers of (FITC labeled and unlabeled) motile, donor-sperm samples were used in mixed insemination experiments (12.7% versus 50.0%). Lower sperm concentration and lower motility might be associated with lower penetration into the zona pellucida of nonliving oocytes *in vitro*. Overstreet and Hembree (1976) interpret their observations as indicating that the human zona pellucida remains similarly functional following death (of the ovum donor and ovum) and that sperm that penetrated into the matrix of the zona pellucida had undergone the capacitation and acrosome reaction processes *in vitro*. The latter conclusion followed comparison with previous reports of fertilization *in vitro* (Soupart and Strong, 1974) which showed similar timing and morphology— including ultrastructure—of sperm penetration, supporting the idea that the zona pellucida of nonliving oocytes retains characteristics essential for the early stages of fertilization and, further, that capacitation and the acrosome reaction do not require living follicle cells.

Overstreet and Hembree (1976) reported specificity of sperm adhesion to the zona pellucida following incubation of nonliving human and nonliving monkey oocytes together with human spermatozoa. Oocytes of the monkey were devoid of associated human spermatozoa, while the converse was true for human oocytes. Oocytes were distinguished in this experiment by FITC labeling of one group as described previously for rabbit oocytes (Overstreet, 1973). This study then demonstrates the usefulness of fluorescent labeling for primate studies, following previous reports in the rabbit and boar that suggest such treatments of spermatozoa (Mellish and Baker, 1970; Overstreet and Adams, 1971; Baker and Degen, 1972; Overstreet and Bedford, 1974b,c) or ova (Overstreet, 1973; Overstreet and Bedford, 1974a,c) do not interfere with gamete transport, fertilization, and early embryogenesis.

Since ova of laboratory animals are much more easily obtainable in adequate supply and with more uniformity of physiological condition, investigation of the use of eggs from lower species has been initiated as a means for assessing occurrence of changes in human sperm that are known prerequisites for fertilization. Yanagimachi and colleagues (1976) have recently found human sperm to undergo capacitation and the ultrastructurally observable membrane changes of the acrosome reaction during preincubation in Biggers-Whitten-Whittingham (BWW) medium. Such sperm can interact with zona pellucida-free hamster ova and undergo pronuclear development and even induce cleavage of naked hamster ova *in vitro*. Ovum penetration occurred with human oocytes exposed to sperm preincubated in this way (Yanagimachi *et al.*, 1976). This recent report promotes our understanding of how to achieve human sperm capacitation experimentally, supports the comparative experimental approach, and, when combined with knowledge from studies cited above, provides encouragement for developing *in vitro* fertilization in man and in species that have thus far escaped serious study.

B. Human Experiments and Efforts to Develop a Clinical Procedure

There is at present no standardization of methodology among laboratories around the world that are conducting human fertilization *in vitro*. The whole area remains experimental, and, aside from a recent undocumented verbal claim for successful application in overcoming infertility due to blocked oviducts (Bevis, 1974), the facility to obtain human embryos that are competent to continue normal gestational development remains to be established. It is agreed by scientists that certain criteria for the actual accomplishment of fertilization need be offered as documentation to preclude inappropriate conclusions following observation of activated or cleaved ova following various *in vitro* manipulations. It is well recognized that apparent fertilization can result from parthenogenetic or other activating influences, from enzymatic activity, or from degenerative changes within the ooplasm. The criteria for establishing the occurrence of fertilization have been extensively discussed on previous occasions (Bedford, 1971; Brackett, 1975). In brief, evidence for accomplishment of fertilization *in vitro* should include documentation of as many of the discrete events associated with fertilization as possible. These events include (1) sperm penetration; (2) ovum activation; (3) pronuclear formation and development; (4) pronuclear breakdown, chromosomal mixing, and initiation of mitosis resulting in orderly (in time and morphological appearance) cleavage stages of the early embryo. For indisputable achievement of fertilization *in vitro,* involvement of the sperm cell must be established. The best proof that fertilization can indeed occur under a certain set of experimental conditions, then, would involve direct observation such as time lapse microcinematography as done in the rabbit (Brackett, 1970) and hamster (Yang *et al.,* 1972) and in preliminary studies with human ova (unpublished), or the completion of normal gestational development of male offspring following transfer of *in vitro* fertilized embryos that are genetically distinguishable. The latter experiment has been successfully executed in the rabbit, mouse, and rat (for review, see Brackett, 1975). Societal ethical pressures dictate development of this technology first in animal species.

A limiting factor in human and nonhuman primate studies of fertilization has been the scarcity of "good" oocytes. The most abundant source of human oocytes has been from aspiration of follicles of ovarian tissue removed for surgical indications. One should expect almost all such oocytes to be atretic or immature even if the ovary is normal. Follicular aspiration has been done at surgery either via laparotomy (Morgenstern and Soupart, 1972) or at laparoscopy (Steptoe, 1973a,b; Steptoe and Edwards, 1970). One of the major difficulties, namely, induction of normal nuclear and cytoplasmic oocyte maturation *in vitro,* has been circumvented by scheduling of follicular aspiration to coincide with near completion of maturation *in vivo*. Best results were obtained in our laboratory with follicular oocytes obtained near midcycle in which maturation was presumably initiated *in vivo* and had only to be sustained *in vitro* prior to facilitating appropriate interaction with the sperm (Seitz *et al.,* 1971).

Accessibility of preovulatory oocytes was improved by treating women with gonadotropins to initiate maturation of oocytes in multiple follicles. Patients seeking help in overcoming infertility secondary to tubal disease have been so treated by several groups. The most extensive experience with human patients is that of Steptoe, Edwards, and colleagues (Steptoe *et al.,* 1976). These investigators reported that preovulatory oocytes could be collected undamaged from the ovaries by laparoscopy under three different conditions: (1) after priming the ovaries with gonadotropins, human menopausal gonadotropin, HMG (Pergonal, G. D. Searle and Co.), and HCG (Pregnyl Organon) so as to cause maturation of several oocytes *in vivo;* (2) after priming ovaries with clomiphene and HCG; and (3) after injecting HCG (Pregnyl Organon, 5000 units) alone in a natural cycle, a few hours before the anticipated LH surge. The anticipated LH surge was predicted from urinary hormone assays. Estrogens, pregnanediol, and LH were monitored during the preceding cycle and during the treatment cycle, urinary estrogens were followed to provide assurance that hormonal status was similar to that previously seen. HCG given just before the expected time of the LH surge should activate the preovulatory follicle without risk of natural ovulation occurring before laparoscopy. Preovulatory oocytes were usually not recovered unless the urinary output reached 50 μg/day. Treatment with HCG could be withheld for a day or two until the ovarian response was satisfactory, or a boost of HMG could be given. Good, large follicles with a high recovery rate of oocytes followed when estrogen output reached at least 100 μg on the day of laparoscopy. One to three preovulatory oocytes could be recovered via a 20-minute laparoscopy performed at 32 hours after HCG. The preferred gas mixture for pneumoperitoneum in this procedure was 5% O_2, 5% CO_2, and 90% N_2, the gas phase used successfully by the British scientists in their gamete and embryo cultures. Following laparoscopy, the abdomen was carefully flushed with CO_2 to remove all traces of N_2 which might give rise to upper abdominal and shoulder pain. In a good response to gonadotropins, each ovary became moderately enlarged by six to eight thin-walled, blue-pink follicles varying in size from 1 to 3 cm in diameter at the ovarian surface. Poor responses were characterized by normal to slightly enlarged ovaries with follicles less than 0.5 cm in diameter at the ovarian surface.

According to Steptoe and colleagues (1976) oocytes were collected from between one-half and two-thirds of the follicles aspirated, with a higher proportion being collected from larger follicles. Preovulatory oocytes from the largest follicles, will be in diakinesis, metaphase I, or metaphase II when recovered. These oocytes are typically surrounded by a thick viscous mass of mucus containing diffuse layers of cumulus cells. Such oocytes are capable of undergoing fertilization within a few hours after insemination. Nonovulatory oocytes are surrounded by several layers of tightly adhering corona cells, and oocytes are considered to be atretic if there are no attendant corona cells. A distinction between large preovulatory and large nonovulatory follicles has been made on the basis of follicular fluid steroid levels. Thus, progesterone, 17α-hydroxyprogesterone, estradiol 17-β, estrone, and pregnenolone were found in higher concentrations in fluids from preovulatory follicles, while androstenedione, dehydroepiandrosterone, testosterone, and 17α-hydroxypregnenolone were higher in fluids from follicles classified as nonovulatory (Steptoe, 1977a,b).

Human sperm have been prepared for *in vitro* fertilization by diluting an ejaculate with medium followed by gentle centrifugation and removal of the diluted seminal plasma. Sperm cells were resuspended for incubation at 37°C in an appropriate medium for at least 1½ hours for initiation of the capacitation process prior to ovum insemination. The medium used by Steptoe and Edwards (Steptoe *et al.*, 1976) was composed of Tyrode's solution with albumin, pyruvate, and penicillin added. The concentration of sperm during the preincubation interval varied between 5 and 20×10^6/ml and was reduced for insemination to around 10^6/ml. Oocytes were washed by passage through two or three changes of medium and placed into sperm-containing droplets within a few minutes of collection. Steptoe *et al.* (1976) reported a pH of 7.4 maintained by bicarbonate buffer; a gas phase of 5% CO_2, 5% O_2, and 90% N_2; and an osmotic pressure of approximately 285 mOsM/kg as excellent for fertilization.

In most recently described efforts of the Cambridge group (Steptoe *et al.*, 1976), approximately 12–15 hours after insemination pronucleate ova were transferred into Ham's F-10 medium supplemented with fetal calf serum, bovine serum albumin, or serum from the patient. Some development as far as the blastocyst stage has been observed *in vitro*. The temporal sequence of development was stated to be comparable to that found *in vivo* by Croxatto *et al.* (1972a).

Deposition of cleaved, *in vitro* fertilized embryos into the uterus was first attempted via the cervix (Steptoe, 1974). The embryo was deposited high in the uterus close to the fundus in around 0.2 ml of medium. An external catheter (2.1-mm diameter, Portex FG6) was positioned through the cervix and an internal, embryo-containing catheter (1.34-mm diameter, Portex FG4) was passed into the uterus while the unanesthetized patient was in the lithotomy position. Following threading of the inner catheter through the external catheter up to but not beyond the maximum extension of the external catheter, the external catheter was gently withdrawn, leaving the internal catheter exposed and extending into the uterine lumen for deposition of the embryo.

In absence of success with cervical transfers and from knowledge of better results with surgical transfer in the cow (Rowson and Moor, 1966; Testart and Leglise, 1971) recent efforts have bypassed the cervix for embryo transfer in a second laparoscopic procedure carried out 2–3 days after the initial laparoscopy for oocyte recovery. In this technique, a fine polyethylene cannula containing the embryo was passed into the uterine lumen through a needle introduced through the fundus and serving as a cannula.

Steptoe (1977a,b) reported recovery of preovulatory oocytes from each of 27 patients and development of 70% of the ova into embryos following *in vitro* fertilization. Transfer of one or more fertilized oocytes, in 8-cell to blastocyst stage, to a total of 60 women has resulted in some evidence of implantation in three or maybe four cases (Steptoe, 1977a,b) including one 7-week tubal pregnancy (Steptoe and Edwards, 1976). Beyond this, development of transferred human embryos has failed in spite of heroic clinical efforts (DeKretzer *et al.*, 1973; Steptoe *et al.*, 1976).

C. Ethical Considerations

Decisions regarding whether certain experimentation should be implemented and supported must come from knowledgeable representatives of society. In England and Australia, the embryo transplant procedure following *in vitro* fertilization as a means to overcome infertility has been made available to women, who, following exposure to facts regarding possible success and risks, have chosen or rejected the procedures, as in other surgical care. The clinical groups have offered such a procedure only in patients with fallopian tubes damaged beyond repair, with embryos obtained from the woman's oocytes and fertilized by her husband's sperm. During a Symposium on Antenatal Interference, Professor D. C. A. Bevis was reported to have presented the point of view that, as a biologist, he could not see that experimentation with germ cells differed from experimentation with somatic cells, nor could he accept that, to be moral, human reproduction must be coital (Medical World, 1974). Further, he allegedly mentioned that three children, apparently normal, were alive in the United Kingdom and Western Europe after embryo transplantation. Unfortunately, (or fortunately for the individuals involved if true), scientific documentation or additional clinical details were never forthcoming. Biologists would agree that more information is required to determine the risks of such clinical experimentation. In view of the dearth of information from animal experiments along these lines, it seems to be appropriate to place emphasis on animal studies in order to provide a more scientific basis for predicting risks and outcome following human clinical adaptation of *in vitro* fertilization and embryo transfer. Hopefully, *in vitro* fertilization in the cow (Brackett *et al.*, 1977) will lead to a practical and valuable procedure, and badly needed information will emanate from the cattle industry, as was the case for artificial insemination. Even so, ultimate answers must follow direct human involvement, and the rapidity with which such specific human information is forthcoming is, quite appropriately, tied to acceptance of such efforts in the moral and ethical sense. The latter considerations, then, lead to anticipation of various contributions along these lines by different societies of the world.

D. Progress in Experiments with Nonhuman Primates

Sperm in the perivitelline space, the second polar body, pronuclear formation, and cleavage of six ova to the 2-cell stage comprised initial evidence for fertilization of squirrel monkey (*Saimiri sciureus*) oocytes *in vitro* (Cline *et al.*, 1972; Gould *et al.*, 1973). In this work, ejaculated sperm were preincubated in a medium with follicular contents prior to insemination of follicular oocytes. Advancements have been made toward development of a predictable means for obtaining evidence for occurrence of fertilization *in vitro* in squirrel monkeys (Kuehl and Dukelow, 1975; Dukelow and Kuehl, 1975). Mature female squirrel monkeys were treated for ovulation induction without regard to their natural cycle status, by four daily im injections of follicle-stimulating hormone, FSH (1 mg, FSH-P, Armour-Baldwin Laboratories, Omaha, Nebraska) with an ovulation-inducing im injection of HCG (500 IU, A.P.L., Ayerst Laboratories, New York) early on the morning of the 5th day. Semen obtained by electroejaculation (Kuehl and Dukelow, 1974) was held in 1–2 ml of culture medium at room temperature 0.5–2 hours prior to use for insemination *in vitro*. Oocytes were recovered from follicles by aspiration at laparotomy 4–12 hours after the HCG injection and placed directly with the sperm suspension in TCM 199 or Ham's F-10, in either case supplemented with 20% heat-inactivated agamma calf serum and containing 50 units penicillin G/ml. Incubation was carried out in a moist 5% CO_2 in air atmosphere at 37°C. At intervals, ova were examined and stained with lacmoid (Iwamatsu and Chang, 1972). Oocytes (an average of 6.9 per animal) were obtained from 29% of aspirated follicles, and 79 or nearly 30% of the follicular oocytes developed to the first polar body stage. Of the 79 that matured, 32 exhibited some evidence of fertilization, including 21 with 2 polar bodies and 2 pronuclei and 11 that cleaved with 7 of these reaching the 4-cell stage (Kuehl and Dukelow, 1975). No difference in ovum maturation and fertilization was seen in the two media employed. Better results with maturation and with fertilization followed gamete incubation in smaller, less dilute volumes; hence, a greater concentration (two- or sixfold) of follicular fluid and a greater concentration (10–100 times) of sperm cells. This followed comparison of results using 30×13 mm sealable culture dishes (No. 4340, A. H. Thomas, Co., Philadelphia, Pennsylvania) with the larger volume of fluid under light viscosity silicone fluid (Dow Corning 200 fluid, Dow Corning Co., Midland, Michigan) and the small volume chamber-slide (tissue culture chamber/slide, No. 4808, Lab-Tek Products, Naperville, Illinois), having eight chambers and not covered with silicone fluid.

Additional data, including oocytes obtained by laparoscopy, further supported the case for achievement of *in vitro* fertilization in the squirrel monkey (Dukelow and Kuehl, 1975). The second polar body appeared 26.6 hours after insemination; 2-cell ova appeared at a mean time of 36 hours after insemination, but as early as 21.1 hours; and 4-cell ova were first seen at 43.7 hours and at an average of 49.1 hours after insemination. Dukelow and Kuehl (1975) further reported the 8-cell stage to appear at a mean time of 74.3 hours after insemination, with 71.6 hours being the earliest at which this stage was seen. No cleavage was seen following culture for 3 days without sperm in 36 oocytes (10 of which matured to the first polar body stage). Although it was not possible to positively identify sperm remnants within pronuclear ova in this work or to prove by embryo transfers that cleaved ova could continue development throughout gestation (Dukelow and Kuehl, 1975), it does appear that feasibility of *in vitro* fertilization studies in a nonhuman primate species is now established. Some encouragement has also followed initial experimentation with gametes of the senegal galago or bush baby (*Galago senegalensis*), a small prosimian (Keating *et al.,* 1974; L. Franklin, personal communication, 1977).

Rhesus monkey oocytes have been inseminated *in vitro* under a variety of experimental conditions, but, aside from sporadic occasions on which apparent pronuclei, 2- or 4-cell stage ova were obtained, inadequate encouragement in the way of consistent results has been achieved. A warning regarding unquestioning acceptance of morphological evidence for *in vitro* fertilization (including pronuclear development and cleavage) must be reiterated here. In this writer's experience, electron microscopic studies have been necessary for distinguishing apparent from actual fertilization in the rhesus monkey (Batta *et al.,* 1978). Persisting cortical granules, degenerative changes, absence of sperm remnants, and/or additional ultrastructural features not consistent with normal fertilization have characterized apparently fertilized rhesus monkey ova following *in vitro* insemination experiments in our laboratory (unpublished data).

Exciting progress has been reported by Kraemer *et al.* (1976) in their baboon embryo transfer experiments. A late morula stage embryo was surgically removed from a naturally ovulating, naturally inseminated *Papio cynocephalus* on day 5 of gestation and surgically transferred to a naturally synchronized non-mated female in which complete normal gestational development took place (Kraemer *et al.,* 1976). The embryo was recovered in TCM199 with Hanks' salts, 0.35 gm of sodium bicarbonate/liter, and 100 mg of neomycin solution/ml (Grand Island Biological Co.), and was held in a covered embryologic watch-glass for 20 minutes at 32°C. The recipient was selected by matching sex skin cycle with that of the donor. Ketamine hydrochloride and atropine were given preoperatively, and anesthesia was maintained with halothane during the transfer procedure. The uterus exposed by midventral laparotomy was first punctured with an 18-gauge Intracath (Jelco, Raritan, New Jersey) and followed with the embryo being deposited into the lumen via a Micro/pettor (Scientific Manufacturing Industries, Emeryville, California). Pregnancy was diagnosed on day 20 after ovulation by the monkey chorionic gonadotropin test on urine (Hodgen and Ross, 1974) and plasma (Hodgen *et al.,* 1974). Confirmation followed on days 20 and 52 by increases in plasma estrogen and progestin, and on day 100 by radiography and ultrasonic monitoring of the fetal heartbeat. The resulting neonate was male and weighed 875 gm following delivery by cesarean section 174 days after estimated ovulation time. This represented the initial successful embryo transfer in a primate species.

Recent successful term development has followed recovery of the single fertilized rhesus monkey ovum from an oviduct followed by replacement of the embryo into the contralateral oviduct (within 30 minutes of recovery) (Marston *et al.,* 1977). In this work, 13 ova were flushed from oviducts of mated rhesus females on menstrual cycle days 12–18. Ova varied in development from 1-cell to 7–8-cell stages. Dulbecco's phosphate-buffered saline was used at room temperature (20°–24°C). Upon location under a stereomicroscope, the ovum was taken up in a fine nylon iv cannula (0.63 mm O.D., Portex, Ltd.), which was attached to an Agla micrometer syringe filled with sterile liquid paraffin. The tip of the nylon cannula was passed through the tubal ostium to the point where there is usually a marked flexure of the ampulla, and each ovum was expelled in about 0.5 μl of medium with a similar volume of air. Five term offspring (three female, two male of which one was stillborn) resulted from 1-cell, 2-cell, and 6-cell stage ova. A question regarding significance of the notation of a ruptured blastomere in the 2-cell ovum that resulted in the stillborn must await more extensive observations. Following uterine transfers by the technique of Marston *et al.* (1969b), three embryos, in 5- to 8-cell stages, failed to sustain gestational development in this work (Marston *et al.,* 1977). Success from between-animal tubal transfers in the rhesus monkey might be expected to be difficult since Kraemer and his colleagues (1976) found with baboon uterine transfers, that the most crucial factor appears to be satisfactory synchronization of donor and recipient animals.

IV. *IN VITRO* TESTING OF POTENTIALLY TERATOGENIC AGENTS

Human material, especially that obtained following therapeutic abortion, has been recognized by scientists to be of potential value in tissue and organ culture testing of teratogenic agents (Shepard *et al.,* 1975). Although routine *in vitro* screening of various drug and environmental chemicals that might produce congenital defects would, at present, be an insurmountable task, much interest has recently been generated in development of new approaches for this purpose. The use of *in vitro* tests would certainly not replace the use of pregnant animal testing but might be an excellent adjunct for elucidation of mechanisms of teratogenesis.

With better understanding of the mechanisms, more intelligent ways can be devised for interruption of human embryopathy. Conduct of such work should be by developmental biologists after careful peer review and with fully informed consent of the donors (Shepard *et al.,* 1975).

Striking similarities exist in endocrine events of the normal menstrual cycle and during pregnancy for the chimpanzee and human being (Hobson *et al.,* 1976). Gonadotropin and steroid patterns of rhesus monkeys are quite different. Accurate assessment of safety for human use of compounds that might affect reproductive-endocrine events might be afforded by judicious use of great apes, *in vivo,* and their tissues *in vitro.*

V. CONCLUSIONS

Unfertilized ova and embryos have been recovered from oviducts and uteri of human and nonhuman primates. Refinements in methodology for flushing different segments of the female reproductive tract have led to definition of progression of the ovum along the tract and also in development if fertilized following ovulation.

Ovum recovery from ovarian follicles judged preovulatory has led to progress in efforts to produce viable embryos by *in vitro* fertilization. Although present *in vitro* methods are sufficient to enable primate (squirrel monkey, and human) ovum and sperm interaction to provide evidence for fertilization and early embryonic development, the presently employed methods are inadequate for supporting these processes in a way that is compatible with sustained gestational development following transfer. One possible reason for failure of the human embryos to proceed through gestation in the extensive efforts to date is the restriction imposed in returning embryos, held *in vitro* under conditions that retard development, to the patient's uterus during the same cycle. Asynchrony of *in vitro* embryonic development and of *in vivo* endometrial development may be one explanation for the incompatibility, but proper preparation, conditioning, and nourishment of gametes and early embryos might also not have been attained. If asynchrony of *in vitro* and *in vivo* conditions is the problem, it might at some future date be possible to store human embryos in a frozen state until a more appropriate time for introduction into the uterus. Such a direct human application of recent advances in mammalian reproductive biology is appropriately linked to prevailing ethical considerations.

Initial success with nonhuman primate embryo transfers provide encouragement toward realization of ideas for future applications, but, at the same time, calls attention to the need for much more extensive laboratory investigation in developing this technology. Although not constrained by ethical considerations, accessibility of nonhuman primates and expense of needed studies point to the importance of initial research in small laboratory and domestic species, with extension to nonhuman primates for definitive experiments.

Nonhuman primates, especially the apes, might also be useful in providing embryonic cell lines for use in detection of teratogenic influences on normal biochemical patterns. Direct study of human embryonic cells and alterations in biochemistry inflicted by teratogens might be of even greater value following analogous studies in animals closest to man on the evolutionary ladder.

Experimentation involving primates is dependent on scientific developments including embryologic methodology arising from observations and experimentation with laboratory and domestic species. Once worthwhile procedures are adequately exploited in lower animals, it may become appropriate to extend similar approaches to nonhuman primates and ultimately to human primates.

ACKNOWLEDGMENT

The author is thankful for the support of PHS Research Grant HD 09406 from the National Institute for Child Health and Human Development.

REFERENCES

Allen, E., Pratt, J. P., Newell, O. U., and Bland, L. (1928). *J. Am. Med. Assoc.* **91,** 1018–1020.
Allen, E., Pratt, J. P., Newell, O. U., and Bland, L. (1930). *Contrib. Embryol. Carnegie Inst.* **22,** 45.
Alliston, C. W., and Ulberg, L. C. (1961). *J. Anim. Sci.* **20,** 608–613.
Baker, R. D., and Degen, A. A. (1972). *J. Reprod. Fertil.* **28,** 369.
Batta, S. K., and Brackett, B. G. (1974). *Prostaglandins* **6,** 45–54.
Batta, S. K., Stark, R. A., and Brackett, B. G. (1978). *Biol. Reprod.* **18,** in press.
Batta, S. K., Brackett, B. G., and Niswender, G. D. (1976) *Curr. Topics in Molec. Endocrinol.* **3,** 477.
Bavister, B. D., Edwards, R. G., and Steptoe, P. C. (1969). *J. Reprod. Fertil.* **20,** 159–160.
Bedford, J. M. (1971). *In* "Methods in Mammalian Embryology" (J. C. Daniel, Jr., ed.), Vol. 1, pp. 37–63. Freeman, San Francisco, California.
Bevis, D. C. A. (1974). *Br. Med. J.* **3,** 238.
Brackett, B. G. (1970). *Fertil. Steril.* **21,** 169–176.
Brackett, B. G. (1975). *In* "Gynecologic Endocrinology" (J. J. Gold, ed.), pp. 621–644. Harper, New York.
Brackett, B. G., and Oliphant, G. (1975). *Biol. Reprod.* **12,** 260–274.
Brackett, B. G., Evans, J. F., Oh, Y. K., and Donawick, W. J. (1977). 10th Ann. Meet. Soc. Study Reprod. Abstract #86, 56–57.
Chang, M. C. (1952). *J. Exp. Zool.* **121,** 351.
Chattoraj, S. C., and Wottiz, H. H. (1967). *Fertil. Steril.* **18,** 342.
Clewe, T. H., Morgenstern, L. L., Noyes, R. W., Bonney, W. A., Burrus, S. B., and DeFeo, J. V. (1971). *Am. J. Obstet. Gynecol.* **109,** 313.
Cline, E. M., Gould, K. G., and Foley, C. W. (1972). *Fed. Proc., Fed. Am. Soc. Exp. Biol.* **31,** Abstr. No. 360.

Croxatto, H. B., Diaz, S., Fuentealba, B., Croxatto, H. D., Carrillo, D., and Fabres, C. (1972a). *Fertil. Steril.* **23**, 447–458.

Croxatto, H. B., Fuentealba, B., Diaz, M. S., Pastene, L., and Tatum, H. J. (1972b). *Am. J. Obstet. Gynecol.* **112**, 662.

Croxatto, H. B., Ortiz, M. E., Diaz, M. S., Hess, R., Balmaceda, J. P., Cheviakoff, S., and Llados, C. (1977). *Fertil. Steril.* **28**, 283.

Davajan, V., and Nakamura, R. M. (1975). *In* "Progress in Infertility" (S. J. Behrman and R. W. Kistner, eds.), pp. 17–46. Little, Brown, Boston, Massachusetts.

DeKretzer, D., Dennis, P., Hudson, B., Leeton, J., Lopata, A., Outch, K., Talbot, J., and Wood, C. (1973). *Lancet* **2**, 728.

Dickmann, Z., Clewe, T. H., Bonney, W. A., and Noyes, R. W. (1965). *Anat. Rec.* **152**, 293.

Doyle, L. L., Lippes, J., Winters, H. S., and Margolis, A. G. (1966). *Amer. J. Obstet. Gynec.* **95**, 115–117.

Dukelow, W. R., and Kuehl, T. J. (1975). *In* "La fécondation" (C. Thibault, ed.), pp. 67–80. Paris, Masson.

Eddy, C. A., Garcia, R. G., Kraemer, D. C., and Pauerstein, C. J. (1975). *Biol. Reprod.* **13**, 363–369.

Edwards, R. G., Bavister, B. G., and Steptoe, P. C. (1969). *Nature (London)* **221**, 632.

Edwards, R. G., Steptoe, P. C.. and Purdy, J. M. (1970). *Nature (London)* **227**, 1307.

Flechon, J. E., Panigel, M., Kraemer, D. C., Kalter, S. S., and Hafez, E. S. E. (1976). *Anat. Embryol.* **149**, 289–295.

Gould, K. G., Cline, E. M., and Williams, W. L. (1973). *Fertil. Steril.* **24**, 260–268.

Hamilton, W. J. (1949). *Ann. R. Coll. Surg. Engl.* **4**, 281.

Hartman, C. G. (1944). *West. J. Surg., Obstet. Gynecol.* **52**, 41–61.

Hendrickx, A. G. (1971). "Embryology of the Baboon." Univ. of Chicago Press, Chicago, Illinois.

Hendrickx, A. G., and Kraemer, D. C. (1968). *Anat. Rec.* **162**, 111–120.

Hertig, A. T., Rock, J., Adams, E. C., and Mulligan, W. J. (1954). *Contrib. Embryol. Carnegie Inst.* **35**, 199.

Hertig, A. T., Rock, J., and Adams, E. C. (1956). *Am. J. Anat.* **98**, 435.

Hobson, W., Coulston, F., Faiman, C., Winter, J. S. D., and Reyes, F. (1976). *J. Toxicol. Environ. Health.* **1**, 657–668.

Hodgen, G. D., and Ross, G. T. (1974). *J. Clin. Endocrinol. Metab.* **38**, 927.

Hodgen, G. D., Tullner, W. W., Vaitukaitis, J. L., Ward, D. N., and Ross, G. T. (1974). *J. Clin. Endocrinol. Metab.* **39**, 457.

Hurst, P. R., Jefferies, K., Eckstein, P., and Wheeler, A. G. (1976). *Biol. Reprod.* **15**, 429–434.

Iwamatsu, T., and Chang, M. C. (1972). *J. Reprod. Fertil.* **31**, 237–247.

Keating, R. J., Barros, C., and Franklin, L. E. (1974). *7th Annu. Meet. Soc. Study Reprod.* Abstract #104, 109.

Khvatov, B. P. (1959). *Arch. Anat.* **36**, 42.

Kraemer, D. C., and Hendrickx, A. G. (1971). "Embryology of the Baboon." Univ. of Chicago Press, Chicago, Illinois.

Kraemer, D. C., Moore, G. T., and Kramen, M. A. (1976). *Science* **192**, 1246–1247.

Kuehl, T. J., and Dukelow, W. R. (1974). *Lab. Anim. Sci.* **24**, 364–366.

Kuehl, T. J., and Dukelow, W. R. (1975). *J. Med. Primatol.* **4**, 209–216.

Lewis, W. H. (1931). *Bull. Johns Hopkins Hosp.* **48**, 368.

Lewis, W. H., and Hartman, C. G. (1933). *Contrib. Embryol. Carnegie Inst.* **24**, 187.

Lewis, W. H., and Hartman, C. G. (1941). *Contrib. Embryol. Carnegie Inst.* **29**, 7.

Marston, J. H., and Kelly, W. A. (1968). *Nature (London)* **217**, 1073.

Marston, J. H., Kelly, W. A., and Eckstein, P. (1969a). *J. Reprod. Fertil.* **19**, 149–156.

Marston, J. H., Kelly, W. A., and Eckstein, P. (1969b). *J. Reprod. Fertil.* **19**, 321–330.

Marston, J. H., Penn, R., and Sivelle, P. C. (1977). *J. Reprod. Fertil.* **49**, 175–176.
Mastroianni, L., and Rosseau, C. H. (1965). *Am. J. Obstet. Gynecol.* **93**, 416–420.
Medical World. (1974). **112**, 15–16.
Mellish, K. S., and Baker, R. D. (1970). *J. Anim. Sci.* **31**, 917.
Miller, M. F., Engel, G. C., and Reimann, S. P. (1938). *Growth* **2**, 381.
Morgenstern, L. L., and Soupart, P. (1972). *Fertil. Steril.* **23**, 751–758.
Newell, O. U., Allen, E., Pratt, J. P., and Bland, L. (1930). *Am. J. Obstet. Gynecol.* **19**, 180.
Noyes, R. W., Hertig, A. T., and Rock, J. (1950). *Fertil. Steril.* **1**, 3.
Noyes, R. W., Clewe, T. H., Bonney, W. A., Burrus, S. B., DeFeo, V. J., and Morgenstern, L. L. (1966). *Am. J. Obstet. Gynecol.* **96**, 157.
Oliphant, G., and Brackett, B. G. (1973a). *Biol. Reprod.* **9**, 73.
Oliphant, G., and Brackett, B. G. (1973b). *Fertil. Steril.* **24**, 945–955.
Overstreet, J. W. (1973). *J. Reprod. Fertil.* **32**, 291.
Overstreet, J. W., and Adams, C. E. (1971). *J. Reprod. Fertil.* **21**, 423.
Overstreet, J. W., and Bedford, J. M. (1974a). *Dev. Biol.* **41**, 185.
Overstreet, J. W., and Bedford, J. M. (1974b). *J. Exp. Zool.* **189**, 203.
Overstreet, J. W., and Bedford, J. M. (1974c). *J. Reprod. Fertil.* **39**, 393.
Overstreet, J. W., and Hembree, W. C. (1976). *Fertil. Steril.* **27**, 815–831.
Panigel, M., Kraemer, D. C., Kalter, S. S., Smith, G. C., and Heberling, R. L. (1975). *Anat. Embryol.* **147**, 45–62.
Pincus, G., and Saunders, B. (1937). *Anat. Rec.* **69**, 163.
Reyes, A., Oliphant, G., and Brackett, B. G. (1975). *Fertil. Steril.* **26**, 148–157.
Rock, J., and Hertig, A. T. (1944). *Am. J. Obstet. Gynecol.* **47**, 343.
Rowson, L. E. A., and Moor, R. M. (1966). *J. Reprod. Fertil.* **11**, 311.
Seitz, H. M., Jr., Rocha, G., Brackett, B. G., and Mastroianni, L., Jr. (1971). *Fertil. Steril.* **22**, 255–262.
Shepard, T. H., Nelson, T., Oakley, G. P., Jr., and Lemire, R. J. (1971). *In* "Monitoring Birth Defects and Environment—The Problem of Surveillance" (E. B. Hook, D. T. Janerich, and I. H. Porter, eds.), pp. 29–43. Academic Press, New York.
Shepard, T. H., Miller, J. R., and Marois, M. (1975). "Methods for Detection of Environmental Agents that Produce Congenital Defects." North-Holland Publ., Amsterdam.
Soupart, P. (1976). *Prog. Reprod. Biol.* **1**, 241–251.
Soupart, P., and Morgenstern, L. L. (1973). *Fertil. Steril.* **24**, 462–478.
Soupart, P., and Strong, P. A. (1974). *Fertil. Steril.* **25**, 11–44.
Steptoe, P. C. (1973a). *J. Reprod. Med.* **10**, 211–226.
Steptoe, P. C. (1973b). *IRCS Libr. Compend.* **4**, 73–75.
Steptoe, P. C. (1974). *In* "Gynecological Laparoscopy: Principles and Techniques" (J. M. Phillips and L. Keith, eds.), p. 309. Stratton Intercon.
Steptoe, P. C. (1977). *Fertil. Steril.* **28**, 313.
Steptoe, P. C., and Edwards, R. G. (1970). *Lancet* **1**, 683–689.
Steptoe, P. C., and Edwards, R. G. (1976). *Lancet* **1**, 880–882.
Steptoe, P. C., Edwards, R. G., Shulman, J., and Purdy, J. (1976). *In* "Recent Advances in Human Reproduction" (A. Campos da Paz *et al.*, eds.), pp. 285–295. Am. Elsevier, New York.
Stevens, V. C. (1969). *J. Clin. Endocrinol. Metab.* **29**, 904.
Streeter, G. L. (1942). *Contrib. Embryol. Carnegie Inst.* **30**, 211–245.
Streeter, G. L. (1945). *Contrib. Embryol. Carnegie Inst.* **31**, 27–63.
Streeter, G. L. (1948). *Contrib. Embryol. Carnegie Inst.* **32**, 133–203.
Streeter, G. L. (1951). *Contrib. Embryol. Carnegie Inst.* **34**, 165–196.
Suzuki, S., and Mastroianni, L., Jr. (1966). *Am. J. Obstet. Gynecol.* **96**, 723.
Testart, J., and Leglise, P. C. (1971). *C. R. Hebd. Seances Acad. Sci.* **272**, 2591.

Thomas, K., and Ferin, J. (1970). *Acta Endocrinol. (Copenhagen)* **141,** 75.
Yanagimachi, R., and Chang, M. C. (1961). *J. Exp. Zool.* **148,** 185.
Yanagimachi, R., Yanagimachi, H., and Rogers, B. J. (1976). *Biol. Reprod.* **15,** 471-476.
Yang, W. H., Lin, L. L., Wang, J. R., and Chang, M. C. (1972). *J. Exp. Zool.* **179,** 191-206.
Yussman, M. A., and Taymor, M. L. (1970). *J. Clin. Endocrinol. Metab.* **30,** 396.
Zamboni, L., Mishell, D. R., Bell, J. H., and Baca, M. (1966). *J. Cell Biol.* **30,** 579.

17

Transplanting and Explanting Organ Primordia

JEFFREY A. MacCABE

In our efforts to understand how the embryo develops, we frequently dissect it, not only structurally but functionally. We must see how the parts, at all levels of the organism's hierarchical organization, relate to one another structurally, how they behave under various experimental conditions, how they interact with one another, and, finally, how they coordinate their functions to give rise to the complete organism. To this end, many of us remove parts from the embryo, rearrange them or treat them in various other ways, and allow them to continue development so we can analyze the results of our tampering. The following is an account of some procedures designed to allow embryonic tissues and organs to continue development after removal and experimental manipulation.

I. TRANSPLANTING EMBRYONIC TISSUES AND ORGANS

The inaccessibility of developing mammalian embryos, although clearly to their benefit, poses some difficult problems for the experimenter undertaking a study of their developmental processes. One need only read the titles of the chapters in this volume to see that considerable effort goes into overcoming this disadvantage. Methods such as embryo transfer, embryo culture, organ and tissue culture, and transplantation allow the investigator direct access to the embryo for experimental purposes. This section will be concerned with transplantation to embryonic hosts, of necessity, avian hosts. The methods are not unique for the mammalian donor, but may offer, in some instances, an alternative to the *in vitro* culture of the entire embryo or its parts or having experimental treatments mediated by the maternal environment. Though not covered in this chapter, adult hosts are also used for the transplantation of embryonic tissues, the anterior chamber of the eye and the testis being particularly suitable sites.

A. Transplantation to the Chorioallantoic Membrane of the Chick Embryo

The allantois of the chick embryo develops as a diverticulum of the hindgut on the 3rd day of incubation (Hamilton, 1952). This diverticulum soon expands distally into an allantoic sac that will serve the embryo as a repository for metabolic wastes. More important for our present purpose, its outer wall fuses with the chorion on the 5th day, forming the chorioallantois, a highly vascular embryonic membrane that rapidly expands under the egg shell and shell membrane and serves as the embryo's respiratory organ. The chorioallantoic membrane (CAM) is composed of an outer ectodermal chorionic epithelium, underlying mesoderm from both the chorion and allantois, and the allantoic endoderm lining the inner surface of the allantoic sac. The blood vessels are at first embedded in the mesoderm, but later, by 10 days of incubation, begin pushing up through the ectoderm and come to lie directly under the shell membrane (Romanoff, 1960; Ausprunk *et al.*, 1974).

Because of its abundant network of vessels and capillaries, the CAM serves as an excellent site for the transplantation of embryonic tissues, most of which will readily vascularize within 12–24 hours of transplantation. The usefulness of the chick CAM in growing foreign tissues was first demonstrated by Rous and Murphy (1911) and Murphy (1912) for the growth of tumors and by Dantschakoff (1916) for the growth of normal embryonic tissue. The technique for transplantation to the CAM was developed further by Hoadley (1924) and Willier (1924), and it was used extensively for the study of embryonic development by Willier and many of his co-workers. It was first used for studying mammalian development by Hiraiwa (1927), who examined the development on the CAM of various tissues from the 11-day rat embryo. The technique has since been utilized for the growth of a wide variety of tissues from many different mammalian and nonmammalian species.

The most widely used procedure for transplanting embryonic tissues to the chick CAM is that described by Willier (1924), and in several subsequent reviews and experimental embryology laboratory manuals (Hamburger, 1960; Rugh, 1962; Coulombre, 1967; Johnson and Volpe, 1973). A modified technique first used by Martindale (1941) and described in detail by Zwilling (1959) may have an advantage in terms of host survival, at least in the hands of inexperienced operators. Both procedures will be described.

The ideal host age for transplanting to the chorioallantoic membrane is 9 or 10 days of incubation. Chick embryos younger than this do not have a sufficiently well-developed CAM, and older hosts will limit the length of time available for transplant growth and development, since the chorioallantoic circulation begins to dry up at about 18 days of incubation. Eggs should be incubated at 37.5°C in a modern forced-draft incubator and at a relative humidity of 58–60%. In an incubator with slow-moving air, the temperature should be slightly higher (38°C) and the relative humidity slightly lower (50–55%). The eggs should be turned in the incubator prior to preparing them as CAM hosts. This can be done manually, twice a day, or as often as every 2 hours if the incubator is equipped with an automatic turning device. At 9 or 10 days of incubation, host embryos are removed from the incubator and candled in order to see the vasculature of the CAM and the position of the air cell. Small, relatively inexpensive candlers are commercially available, but a makeshift candler can be just as effective. A microscope illuminator may be used, or a candler can be made by mounting a light bulb on a small platform and inverting over it a large tin can with a hole in the bottom. Using the candler, a highly vascular area on the side of the egg near a major blood vessel should be located, and a 1 cm² window marked on the shell at this site. If the air cell is not centered at the large end of the egg, it will be helpful to mark its position. The egg is swabbed with 70% ethanol and a small hole put through the shell into the air cell at the large end of the egg. Forceps or a probe (not delicate ones) can be used for this purpose. With the egg on its side on an egg flat or small dish (such as a 67-mm diameter Syracuse watchglass) lined with cotton, the window is carefully cut, penetrating the shell but not the underlying shell membrane. A piece of a hacksaw blade may be used, but the task will be easier if the teeth are made narrower by filing the sides. A thin Carborundum or diamond-grinding disc in a small hobbyist's or dental drill will do the job much faster. It is advisable to power the drill via a variable transformer or rheostat so it can be run slowly enough to avoid heating the shell and damaging the CAM. I have found a foot-pedal rheostat to be most convenient.

When the window has been cut, the piece of shell is lifted off very carefully to avoid penetrating the underlying membrane with its edges. A drop of sterile saline is placed on the egg shell membrane, and with sterile watchmaker's forceps, the membrane torn, allowing the saline to go between the shell membrane and the CAM. The CAM will usually drop away from the shell as the air cell in the large end of the egg collapses. If it does not, the egg can be rocked gently, and, if necessary, gentle suction applied to the hole in the large end of the egg with a pipette bulb. When the CAM has dropped away from the shell, the host is ready for the transplantation.

The tissue to be transplanted to the CAM must not be too large; approximately 1 mm^3 is the maximum size that will readily vascularize. The age of the donor embryo will, in most cases, be determined by the experiment being performed, but, generally, younger tissues vascularize and develop more readily. Some mammalian tissues or organs will develop well; others undergo rather aberrant morphogenesis. For example, physical constraints of the environment or abnormal vascularization may disrupt development. The hamster limb bud vascularizes when transplanted to the chick, but a normal vascular pattern never develops, and only limited morphogenesis occurs (J. A. MacCabe, unpublished). Mammalian skin, on the other hand, develops quite well on the chick CAM (cf. Briggaman and Wheeler, 1968; Sawyer et al., 1972).

Donor tissue should be dissected out using sterile procedures and put into sterile Tyrode's saline to await transplantation. It may be placed onto the CAM with a pipette or a small spatula or spoon, but if a pipette is used, as little saline as possible should be transferred with the tissue. Excess saline can be pipetted off or absorbed with small squares of sterile filter paper. Many authors suggest that the donor tissue be placed at the fork of a major vessel, though I have found that it makes little difference in the vascularization or development of the transplant, as long as it is placed on a region dense with capillaries. If the transplant consists of both mesenchymal and epithelial tissues, it should be oriented so the mesenchyme is against the surface of the CAM. Upon completion of the operation, the window in the host's shell must be covered with cellophane tape and the edges of the tape sealed with melted paraffin. Alternatively, a square of Parafilm can be placed over the window and the edges sealed to the shell with a soldering iron connected to a variable transformer (about 40–50 V gives the proper heat in a small pencil-type soldering iron). The host is returned to the incubator, taking care not to shake the donor tissue out of its position on the CAM. It is not necessary, and in most cases not desirable, to turn the eggs for the remainder of the incubation period. The egg should remain on its side, with the window and transplant uppermost. The transplants can be allowed to develop up to the 18th day of host incubation. At this time, the chorioallantoic circulation begins to slow and later will cease in preparation for hatching. The tape or Parafilm should be removed and the window enlarged by breaking away the shell. The transplant is removed by cutting the CAM around it with small scissors, and it can then be transferred to fixative for preservation and/or histological examination.

An alternative method for host preparation and one I have found to be more convenient in some instances has been described by Zwilling (1959). The hosts are prepared on the 3rd day of incubation, leaving more time available on the 9th or 10th day of incubation when the transplantations are performed. The 3-day egg should be placed on its side, swabbed with 70% ethanol, and a small hole put in the pointed end of the egg with forceps or a dental burr and drill. The hole should be slightly back from the end of the egg, so that a No. 18 needle attached to a syringe can be put vertically through the hole. This will place the needle into the albumin, rather than the yolk, and 2 ml of albumin can then be removed, discarded, and the hole sealed with paraffin. This will drop the level of the 3-day embryo (and subsequently the CAM) so that a window can easily be cut in the side of the egg and the small square of shell removed without risk to the embryo. Nevertheless, as before, the shell membrane should not be penetrated while sawing the window, but only afterwards with a sterile probe or scalpel. The window should immediately be covered with cellophane tape or Parafilm and sealed. The host embryos are then returned to the incubator and left without turning until needed on the 9th or 10th day of incubation. Under these conditions, there is a tendency for the chorionic epithelium to undergo slight proliferative metaplasia because of its exposure in the air pocket (Moscona, 1959). The area of the CAM to receive the transplant, therefore, should be gently scraped with a probe, small scalpel, or watchmaker's forceps before placing the tissue. The area should be slightly wet before scraping or the CAM may tear. After placing the transplant tissue on the prepared site and removing excess fluid, the window is covered, sealed, and the host incubated without turning until it is time to retrieve the graft.

1. Special Techniques for Growing Tissues on the Chorioallantoic Membrane

The transplanted tissue and surrounding CAM has a tendency to dry out because of its exposure to the air reservoir created when the CAM is dropped. In some cases, this may interfere with the development of the transplant. Rawles (1963) developed a method to prevent drying, thus obtaining more perfect morphogenesis of transplanted tissues. Beginning the day after transplantation, and each day thereafter, a few drops of a solution of albumin and saline (15:1) were dropped onto the transplant. The solution eventually gets under the CAM, raising its level in the egg. In order to continue these additions into the late stages of incubation, a "chimney" was constructed over the window in the shell. The chimney was constructed with cotton cord coated with paraffin and sealed to shell with paraffin. This allowed the continued daily addition of the albumin–saline solution until the time of graft recovery.

In addition to the nonspecific metaplasia that the chorionic epithelium undergoes upon exposure to air, it is capable of undergoing specific changes in response to various mesodermal inducers (Kato and Hayashi, 1963; Sawyer *et al.*, 1972). This, combined with its ability to grow over certain kinds of transplants, especially mesoderm that is without an epithelial covering, can lead to unwanted results with CAM-grown tissues. Kato (1969) devised a technique that prevents overgrowth of the transplant by the chorionic epithelium. He constructed a small chamber by gluing (Millipore MF cement, formulation No. 1) a 9.0-mm Millipore filter disc onto a ¼-inch section of plastic tubing with an outside diameter of 9.0 mm. A hole somewhat smaller than the tissue to be transplanted is put in the filter and the chamber sterilized in 70% ethanol. The unit with the hole in the filter is placed on the CAM over a blood vessel and the donor tissue placed in the chamber directly over the hole. This prevents overgrowth by the chorionic epithelium, but it allows vascularization through the hole in the bottom of the chamber. In addition, fluid may be added to the chamber with little loss during the remaining incubation time (Kato, 1970), obviating the need for daily additions. This avoids the problem of the CAM rising as fluids are added as in the method (Rawles, 1963) described above.

2. Summary of Methods of Transplantation to the Chick CAM (Method 1)

1. Candle the host eggs at 9 or 10 days of incubation, noting the positions of the air cell and a vascular area to receive the transplant tissue.

2. Swab the egg with 70% ethanol and put a small hole in the large end into the air cell.

3. Cut a 1 cm² window in the side of the egg, carefully penetrating the shell but not the underlying shell membrane.

4. Remove the piece of shell and place a drop of sterile saline on the shell membrane. Tear the shell membrane, being careful not to damage the underlying CAM. The saline will go between the shell membrane and CAM, and the CAM should drop down from the shell.

5. Place the transplant tissue, not larger than 1 mm³ onto a region rich with capillaries and near a major blood vessel.

6. Cover the window with tape or Parafilm and seal the edges. The host can then be returned to the incubator.

3. Summary of Methods of Transplantation to the Chick CAM (Method 2)

1. At 3 days of incubation swab the host with 70% ethanol and drill a hole in the pointed end of the egg, slightly back from the tip. Remove 2 ml of albumin with a syringe and No. 18 or larger needle.

2. Seal the hole with paraffin and cut a 1 cm² window in the side of the egg, penetrating the shell but not the shell membrane. Tear through the shell membrane

with a sterile probe, scalpel, or foreceps and remove the square of shell along with the shell membrane.

3. Cover the window with tape or Parafilm, seal the edges, and return the host to the incubator (without turning) for an additional 5 or 6 days.

4. For transplanting the donor tissue on day 9 or 10 of host incubation, remove the cover from the window, and gently scrape a region dense with capillaries near a major blood vessel. Place the donor tissue on the prepared site, cover and seal the window, and return the host to the incubator.

B. Transplantation to the Chick Embryo Coelom

Two methods have been described for transplanting embryonic tissues to the chick embryo coelom. The method introduced by Hamburger (1938) involves putting the transplant tissue through an incision in the body wall and is best performed with hosts ranging in age from 2½ to 4 days of incubation. With the modified procedure described by Dossel (1954), a hole is made only in the chorion and the tissue maneuvered into position. Slightly older hosts (4–5 days of incubation) can be used with this method (Philpott and Coulombre, 1965). Intracoelomic transplantation was first used with mammalian donors by Rawles (1940, 1947), who obtained convincing evidence that the neural crest is the source of melanoblasts in the mouse embryo. The technique continues to be useful for the studies of mammalian pigmentation (Mayer, 1973a,b).

Hamburger's (1938) method of intracoelomic transplantation can be used with hosts as early as 2 days of incubation, but the younger the host the smaller the transplant tissue must be. As with other transplantation procedures, a good rule of thumb is that the donor tissue be no larger than 1 mm^3. The hosts should be prepared by removing 2 ml of albumin through the small end of the egg and cutting a window in the side of the shell as described above for the Zwilling–modified CAM technique. This should be done at 2 or 3 days of incubation; if done earlier or later than this, there is greater risk to the host embryo. At the desired stage of incubation, the cover on the window is removed, and the vitelline membrane above the embryo is torn away. This membrane normally ruptures during the early stages of incubation, and, therefore, may not be present in older hosts. The amnion and chorion will not be covering the flank if the hosts are stage 16 (Hamburger and Hamilton, 1951) or younger—approximately 2¾–3 days of incubation. (The stages during the first few days of incubation will not exactly correspond to the incubation times given by Hamburger and Hamilton because, when they devised this staging series, the incubation temperature commonly used was slightly higher than we now know to be ideal for maximum viability.) For older hosts, the chorion and amnion should be torn open along the slightly opaque anteroposterior line of fusion of the lateral folds of the amnion.

These extraembryonic membranes are opened only enough to make the flank accessible. An anteroposterior incision is now made through the body wall between the leg and wing buds (or prospective buds, in the case of young hosts) just lateral to the somites on the right side of the embryo (Fig. 1). The incision can be made with an L-shaped needle made from glass (A 16-mm film by J. W. Saunders and M. Lange, entitled "Experiments on the Chick Embryo 1: Techniques and Tools," shows how these glass needles are made and is available from the Developmental Biology Film Program, BFA Educational Media, 2211 Michigan Avenue, Santa Monica, California 90404.) or tungsten (Dossel, 1958). The donor tissue is then transferred by pipette to a site near the incision and the tissue pushed through the hole in the body wall with forceps. It may be helpful to hold the slit open using a probe with a small hook in the end. The window in the shell is then covered with tape or Parafilm, sealed, and the host incubated without turning.

The modified procedure for intracoelomic transplantation described by Dossel (1954) differs from the one described above in that a hole, through which the

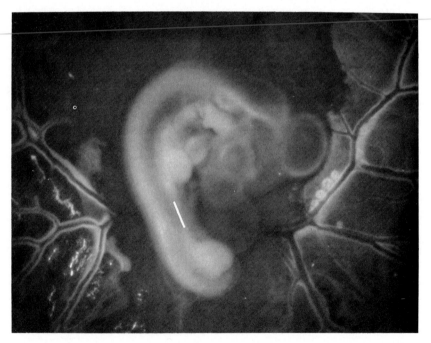

Fig. 1. A photograph of a 4-day chick embryo *in ovo*, showing the position of the incision (white line) in the body wall for intracoelomic transplantation and for transplanting to the flank. The white line represents an incision 1-mm long. In practice the cut should be just long enough to admit the donor tissue.

donor tissue passes, is made in the chorion, rather than the body wall. The host eggs are prepared with a window, as in the previous method, and a small hole torn in the chorion just anterior to the allantois. The donor tissue is transferred to the chorion and, with a blunt L-shaped instrument, the tissue is pushed through the hole and maneuvered through the umbilical opening and into the coelom (Fig. 2). The tissue should then be pushed slightly anterior or posterior so that it does not come out through the umbilicus. The window in the shell is covered and sealed as before and the host returned to the incubator. The host should not be turned for the remainder of the incubation period.

Tissues transplanted into the coelom will attach to the body wall or mesenteries of the viscera and can develop until well after hatching. Usually, however, the host embryo is killed just before hatching on the 18th or 19th day of incubation, the body cavity opened, and the transplant recovered.

Summary of Methods for Intracoelomic Transplantation

1. Prepare the hosts on the second or (preferably) the 3rd day of incubation. Place the egg on its side and remove 2 ml of albumin through a hole in the small end of the shell.

2. Cut a 1-cm square window in the shell, cover it with tape or Parafilm, and seal the edges with paraffin or a warm soldering iron. Return the host to the incubator if it is not to be used immediately.

3a. If the donor tissue is to be transplanted through the flank, cut a slit in the body wall just large enough to admit the transplant. If the host is beyond stage 16, the chorion and amnion will have to be torn for access. Place the transplant tissue on the embryo at a site near the slit in the body wall; maneuver the tissue into the coelom through the slit in the body wall.

3b. To transplant through the chorion, tear a small hole in this extraembryonic membrane just anterior to the allantois and place the transplant tissue nearby. With

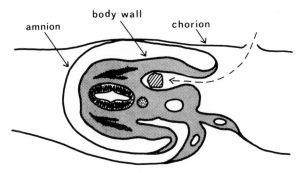

Fig. 2. A diagrammatic representation of a cross section through the umbilical region of a 4-day chick embryo. The dotted line shows the path of the donor tissue when transplanted to the coelom through a hole in the chorion.

a blunt instrument, push the transplant through the hole and into the coelom through the umbilical opening. Push the tissue slightly anterior or posterior so it will not come out through the umbilicus.

4. Cover and seal the window in the shell and return the host to the incubator.

C. Transplantation to the Flank and Other External Sites on the Chick Embryo

Embryonic tissues and organs can be transplanted to the flank of a 3- to 5-day chick embryo or to other external sites such as over the somites or on one of the limb buds. The choice of site may be determined by the nature of the experiment being performed, or, in some instances, simply the preference of the investigator. For example, in the study of dermal–epidermal interactions in the expression of agouti alleles in the mouse (Poole, 1974, 1975), any site suitable for the development of mouse skin and hair would suffice. However, in looking for a specific morphogenetic activity in the developing limb of the hamster (MacCabe and Parker, 1976) or mouse (Tickle et al., 1976), a limb site was required in order to provide the opportunity for the appropriate morphogenetic response. The principal advantages to these external transplantation sites over internal ones are that there is more room available for transplant growth and the donor tissue can be transplanted in a specific orientation relative to the host—a necessity in certain types of experiments.

Hamburger (1938) first described the procedure for transplanting tissues to the chick embryo flank, i.e., the body wall between the leg and wing buds. Hosts may be from 3 to 5 days of incubation and should be prepared on day 3 by removing albumin and cutting a window in the shell as described previously. If the host amnion is closed or nearly closed, it must be torn open to gain access to the flank. This should be done with care, keeping in mind that the amnion is continuous with the body wall, which should not be torn. An anteroposterior slit is then cut through the body wall between the leg and wing as for intracoelomic transplantation (Fig. 1). The donor tissue is transferred to the embryo by pipette. With forceps or a probe, the tissue can then be tucked into the slit, leaving it largely projecting out, rather than into the coelom.

Methods for transplanting to other external sites vary slightly, but basically any procedure that brings the vascular tissue of the host into contact with the donor tissue capable of becoming vascularized will succeed. This normally involves removing some of the host ectoderm at the transplantation site with a glass or tungsten needle to expose mesoderm and placing the donor tissue mesoderm in contact with this prepared site. In many cases, the donor tissue will stay in place only if the host is not moved or is set aside with extreme care for an hour or so after transplantation. During this hour, the window in the shell should be covered, but it is not necessary to seal it completely. Alternatively, the tissue may be held in place with very small glass or tungsten tacks (cf. Gasseling and Saunders, 1961; Tickle *et al.*, 1976). These tacks may be removed after about an hour or, in some instances, may be left in place. Obviously, you will not want to leave the tacks in place if the transplanted tissue is to be sectioned for histological examination later, however. Within an hour, even at room temperature, the transplanted tissue will be attached sufficiently that the host embryos may be returned to the incubator (incubate without turning) after first sealing the window in the shell.

A 16-mm film by J. W. Saunders, entitled "Experiments on the Chick Embryo 2: Grafting Limb Buds," shows procedures for chorioallantoic, intracoelomic, and flank transplantations and is available from the Developmental Biology Film Program, BFA Educational Media, 2211 Michigan Avenue, Santa Monica, California 90404.

D. Intraocular Transplantation

The eye has been used as a site for the transplantation of both embryonic and adult tissues, and both embryos and adults have been used as hosts. In adult animals, the anterior chamber of the eye is the preferred site for transplantation, with several mammalian species serving as hosts. Markee (1940) studied the cyclic changes in the endometrium of the adult rhesus monkey, using the same individual for both the donor and the host. Green (1941) transplanted tumors to the eyes of a variety of mammalian hosts. Many embryonic tissues develop well when transplanted to the adult eye (Runner, 1946; Grobstein, 1951; Levak-Suajger and Skreb, 1965), and entire embryos will undergo fairly normal development up to the time of implantation (Runner, 1947; Fawcett *et al.*, 1947). Coulombre and Coulombre (1964) described a procedure for the transplantation of tissues into the eye of the embryonic chick. Like the chorionic epithelium, the corneal epithelium of the chick embryo is capable of altering its course of differentiation in response to certain mesodermal inducers. Coulombre and Coulombre (1971), for example, found that the corneal epithelium could be induced to form feathers by transplanted chick or mouse dermis. Thus, as with transplantation to the chorioallantoic membrane, the possibility of donor and host tissue interactions must be borne in mind when using this technique. The potential for such interactions is, of course, present in any situation where inductive and responsive embryonic tissues can come into contact, but the chorionic and corneal epithelia seem to be responsive into rather late stages of their development. The following is an account of the procedure for transplanting tissues into the embryonic eye of the chick.

The technique is easiest with hosts of 4½–5 days of incubation whose right eye is not yet covered by the spreading allantois. The hosts should be prepared on the 3rd day of incubation by removing albumin and cutting a window in the shell as previously described. The windows should be covered, sealed, and the hosts returned to the incubator until they reach the desired age.

Access to the host eye is gained by tearing through the avascular chorion and amnion above the head, being careful not to tear or rupture vessels in the allantois. The tear in the chorion and amnion should be small enough to keep the head from slipping out of the amnion. The eye is penetrated at the margin of the lens and optic cup with a short, quick thrust of a sharp probe or forceps. The hole should be enlarged with forceps just enough to allow removal of the lens. The tips of watchmaker's forceps are then pushed through the hole in the eye, the back of the lens grasped, and the lens worked free by gently rocking it. The lens is removed through the hole and discarded. The tissue to be transplanted can be put directly into the eye through the same hole with a small-bore pipette, or placed on the chorion by pipette and pushed through the hole with forceps. The transplanted tissue should be maneuvered into the position previously occupied by the lens and the host window covered, sealed, and returned to the incubator. The tissue is recovered later by sacrificing the host and dissecting the eye.

II. THE SEPARATION AND RECOMBINATION OF EMBRYONIC TISSUES

The separation of embryonic mesoderm from epithelium or epithelium from epithelium, followed by the recombination of the isolated tissues from different sources or in different orientations, has provided a wealth of information on the nature of the communication occurring between tissues before and during organogenesis. While such methods have not yielded the answer to the difficult question of the physical nature of the communication, it has provided insights into such parameters as tissue specificity, spatial and temporal relationships, effects of tissue mass, site of gene action, reciprocity of inductive events, etc. In general, it must be concluded that these studies have impressed upon us the complexity of the interactions between tissues that lead, with an impressively high frequency, to the normal development of organs.

Most methods utilized for separating embryonic tissues rely on enzymatic digestion of intercellular materials or chelating divalent cations that have an important role in cell to cell associations. Medawar (1941) separated adult human skin into its dermal and epidermal components by incubating it in a 0.5% trypsin solution at 37°C. This procedure was used for embryonic tissues by Moscona (1952) to obtain single cell suspensions and by Zwilling (1955) to separate ectoderm from mesoderm. The technique was improved by incubating in trypsin for longer periods of time at 4°C (Szabo, 1955). This minimizes the curling of thin sheets of tissue and the dramatic shrinkage the epithelium undergoes during trypsinization. In my experience, it also yields tissues that stick together better when recombined, possibly because anionic binding sites are largely eliminated by trypsinization at 37°C, but not at 4°C (Caravita and Zacchei, 1974). Trypsin is used for the separation of mesoderm and epithelium in concentrations from 0.1 to 2.0%, and should be made up in calcium- and magnesium-free saline. The trypsinization time varies depending on the tissue and its stage of development; the older the tissue, the longer the incubation time need be. Generally speaking, 1–3 hours at 4°C is sufficient time for tissue separation. The trypsinization time should be no longer than the minimum required for successful separation. Crude trypsin preparations generally perform better than purified trypsin (Rinaldini, 1958), and, frequently, pancreatin or collagenase is added to the dissociation medium to aid separation. In some cases, particularly in the absence of pancreatin, trypsinization (or treatment with EDTA) can give tissues that are sticky and thus difficult to handle. This can probably be attributed to chromatin threads released from damaged cells, and the problem can be eliminated by passing the tissues through a saline rinse with 0.1% DNase after trypsinization (Steinberg, 1963). Tissues separated by trypsinization should be immediately and thoroughly rinsed in a solution of 25–35% horse serum in saline. This facilitates handling of the tissue and stops further digestion of extracellular material due to the antitryptic activity of the horse serum. There may be less damage to the tissue if they are transferred to the horse serum–saline before they are actually separated.

Zwilling (1954) introduced the use of EDTA (ethylenediamine tetraacetate, usually the disodium salt) for isolating mesoderm. EDTA separates cells and tissues by virtue of its ability to chelate divalent cations, which apparently have a role in intercellular attachments. Treatment with EDTA leaves mesoderm with much greater integrity than trypsin treatment, though epithelium is damaged considerably. This is in contrast to trypsin, which leaves epithelium in better condition than the mesoderm. For this reason, trypsin is frequently used for the isolation of epithelium, and EDTA is utilized for the isolation of mesoderm. The recombination of tissues so isolated is often easier than when both tissues are trypsin isolated because the tissues adhere more readily. This may be because the mesoderm has lost little of its extracellular material. The EDTA solution for tissue separation is usually made up at a concentration of 0.1–1.0% in calcium and magnesium-free saline. After separation, the tissues should immediately be transferred to complete saline (with calcium and magnesium, without chelating agents) to prevent further tissue damage after the isolated tissues are recombined. The reconstituted organ primordia may be cultured *in vitro* (cf. Lawson, 1972, 1974) or transplanted to a suitable host (cf. MacCabe *et al.,* 1974). In some cases, it may be necessary to culture the recombinant *in vitro* for a short period of time so the tissues can become coherent enough to withstand the rigors of transplantation (cf. Poole, 1975). The recombination of tissues has also been done with various filter barriers interposed between the interacting tissues (cf. Grobstein, 1955; Wartiovaara *et al.*, 1974).

The following is a protocol of the procedure that has been used in the author's laboratory for recombining 4-day chick limb bud mesoderm with 10-day hamster limb bud ectoderm.

1. After removing the hamster embryos from the uterus, excise the limb buds and rinse them in Tyrode's saline and then in cold (4°C) Moscona's solution (calcium- and magnesium-free Tyrode's saline).

2. Place the limbs in cold 1.0% trypsin (made up in Moscona's solution) and incubate for 3 hours at 4°C.

3. While the hamster limbs are trypsinizing, excise the chick limb buds, rinse them in Tyrode's saline and then in warm (37°C) Moscona's solution. Transfer the limbs to warm 1.0% EDTA in Moscona's solution and incubate at 37°C for 25 minutes.

4. After 25 minutes in the EDTA solution, carefully strip off the ectoderm under a dissecting microscope using watchmaker's forceps and rinse the limb mesoderms in a 33% solution of horse serum in Tyrode's saline. Place the mesoderms in fresh horse serum–Tyrode's solution, incubate for 15 minutes at room temperature, then cool them (still in horse serum–Tyrode's solution) to 4°C and keep them at this temperature until the ectoderm donors (hamster limbs) are ready.

5. After the hamster limbs have trypsinized for 3 hours, rinse them in horse serum–Tyrode's solution at 4°C and put them with the previously isolated mesoderms. It is helpful if at this point each mesoderm with an accompanying trypsinized hamster limb is in a separate dish (I find 37-mm Stendor dishes most convenient).

6. Keeping the mesoderm and trypsinized ectoderm donor bud at 4°C under a dissecting microscope with a cold stage or ice, remove the ectoderm from the hamster limb by working one side of the tip of the forceps between the ectoderm and mesoderm. Immediately place the hamster ectoderm over the mesoderm and adjust its position, being sure there is close contact between the mesoderm and ectoderm. Put the dish aside and allow it to warm to room temperature. Within minutes, the tissues will be so tightly adherent that they cannot be pulled apart. The recombinant limb is then ready for transplantation as in Section I,C.

A 16-mm film by J. W. Saunders and J. A. MacCabe entitled "Experiments on the Chick Embryo 3: Mesodermal Determination of Limb Type," shows the technique for the recombination of limb ectoderm and mesoderm and is available from the Developmental Biology Film Program, BFA Educational Media, 2211 Michigan Avenue, Santa Monica, California 90404.

III. A FEW COMMENTS ON THE *IN VITRO* CULTURE OF ORGAN PRIMORDIA

I will not attempt a complete review of organ culture methodology, since a recent review is available (Balls and Monnickendam, 1976). The methods vary with each organ and with the experiments being undertaken, and can only be determined empirically for each system. I will instead discuss a few topics of current concern to those using or contemplating the use of organ culture techniques.

One of the most important considerations when culturing organ primordia is the nutritional requirements. We, thus, must concern ourselves not only with the growth medium used, but also with the substrate to which the tissues attach and the size of the primordia cultured. As with the transplantation of tissues, 1 mm^3 is an approximate maximum size. In many instances, tissues must be considerably smaller than this, the size being influenced by such parameters as the density and shape of the tissue and whether or not it has an epithelial covering. Epithelium is relatively impermeable to many substances in the medium, so organ primordia with epithelium should be smaller and, in most cases, attached to a substrate, such as agar or a filter, which is permeable to nutrients. Unattached, the mesenchyme will quickly become encapsulated by epithelium, leaving it without sufficient nutrients. In some cases, very small tissues can be cultured on a solid substrate (cf. MacCabe and Parker, 1975) without starving the cells in the center of the culture. Under these conditions, however, the cells may migrate rapidly across the substrate affecting the morphogenesis of the tissue. In some cases, the substrate upon which the tissue is cultured may also affect the differentiation of the explant (Meier and Hay, 1974). In addition, the total mass of the tissue cultured may affect the developmental fate of the tissues (cf. Masters, 1976). In the past, the source of nutrients for organ culture has been largely serum or chick embryo extract (see Cahn et al., 1967, for preparation of embryo extract). However, there has been a recent trend toward defined media, designed primarily for cell cultures, supplemented with lower levels of serum or embryo extract. Some success has been achieved with totally defined media for organ culture (cf. Parsa and Flanchbaum, 1975) but, in general, tissues will develop better with these complex protein supplements. The sources of the embryo extract or serum and its age can significantly affect the usefulness of these additives. In general, cells will undergo more movement across solid surfaces with serum supplements than with unfractionated embryo extract.

The maintenance of the proper pH (7.2–7.4) is important for the survival of cultured tissues. For most systems, a $NaHCO_3$ buffer is best, particularly since cells need bicarbonate anyway, but CO_2 will be lost from the medium and the buffering capacity reduced unless the gaseous environment includes about 5.0%

CO_2 (see Loomis, 1959; Cahn *et al.*, 1967; Wessels, 1967). Recently, the use of complex organic buffers such as HEPES (*N*-2-hydroxyethylpiperazine-N'-2-ethanesulfonic acid), in conjunction with $NaHCO_3$, has increased, as it seems to help stabilize pH fluctuations (Fisk and Pathak, 1969; Eagle, 1971). It should not be assumed that HEPES will have no adverse effects on your culture system, however (cf. Daniel and Wolf, 1975), so this should be carefully checked.

Keeping organ cultures free of contaminating microbial growth is not much of a problem with short-term cultures (1 or 2 days), but may become a problem with long-term (weeks) cultures. Antibiotics such as a combination of penicillin and streptomycin are commonly added to the culture medium. In long-term cultures, it may be necessary to add a fungicide. Media are usually sterilized by pressure filtration, though some defined media can be autoclaved prior to the addition of $NaHCO_3$ and protein supplements. Some membrane filters used for filtration sterilization contain a small amount of detergent and should be washed before use by passing first hot, then cold sterile distilled water through it (Cahn, 1967).

The physical conditions for organ culture are fairly easy to satisfy. A constant temperature of around 37°C, and sufficient humidity to prevent significant evaporative water loss from the medium are required. A water-jacketed incubator is preferable, so that, after the door is opened and closed, the incubator will rapidly return to the desired temperature without overshoot. Either the atmosphere within the incubator should be nearly saturated with water (90–95% relative humidity) or the culture vessels themselves able to maintain a high humidity. This is particularly important for small volume cultures where even slight evaporation from the culture medium can make it hypertonic. Most tissue culture incubators have provisions for humidification. If a gas mixture is flowing into the incubator, it should be bubbled through distilled water at the bottom of the incubator for humidification.

Although considerable progress is being made in the techniques of tissue and organ culture, it must still be concluded that empiricism remains the only method for determining the requirements for particular cells or tissues. Also, though tissues may thrive *in vitro*, we must always question to what extent they are mimicking their *in vivo* behavior. Nevertheless, properly utilized, these methods can be of immeasurable benefit in the continuing battle to understand the complexities of biologic organization.

ACKNOWLEDGMENT

Author's work cited herein and tests of some procedures supported by NIH Grant HD07282.

REFERENCES

Ausprunk, D. H., Knighton, D. R., and Folkman, J. (1974). *Dev. Biol.* **38**, 237–248.
Balls, M., and Monnickendam, M., eds. (1976). "Organ Culture in Biomedical Research." Cambridge Univ. Press, London and New York.
Briggaman, R. A., and Wheeler, C. E., Jr. (1968). *J. Investebr. Dermatol.* **51**, 454–465.
Cahn, R. D. (1967). *Science* **155**, 195–196.
Cahn, R. D., Coon, H. G., and Cahn, M. B. (1967). *In* "Methods in Developmental Biology" (F. H. Wilt and H. K. Wessells, eds.), pp. 493–530. Crowell-Collier, New York.
Caravita, S., and Zacchei, A. M. (1974). *J. Embryol. Exp. Morphol.* **32**, 35–55.
Coulombre, A. J. (1967). *In* "Methods in Developmental Biology" (F. H. Wilt and N. K. Wessells, eds.), pp. 457–469. Crowell-Collier, New York.
Coulombre, A. J., and Coulombre, J. L. (1964). *J. Exp. Zool.* **156**, 39–47.
Coulombre, J. L., and Coulombre, A. J. (1971). *Dev. Biol.* **25**, 464–478.
Daniel, P. F., and Wolf, G. (1975). *In Vitro* **11**, 347–353.
Dantschakoff, V. (1916). *Am. J. Anat.* **20**, 255–308.
Dossel, W. E. (1954). *Science* **120**, 262–263.
Dossel, W. E. (1958). *Lab. Invest.* **7**, 171–173.
Eagle, H. (1971). *Science* **174**, 500–503.
Fawcett, D. W., Wislocki, G. B., and Waldo, C. M. (1947). *Am. J. Anat.* **81**, 413–444.
Fisk, A., and Pathak, S. (1969). *Nature (London)* **224**, 1030–1031.
Gasseling, M., and Saunders, J. W., Jr. (1961). *Dev. Biol.* **3**, 1–25.
Green, H. S. H. (1941). *J. Exp. Med.* **73**, 461–474.
Grobstein, C. (1951). *J. Exp. Zool.* **116**, 501–525.
Grobstein, C. (1955). *In* "Aspects of Synthesis and Order in Growth" (D. Rudnick, ed.), pp. 233–256. Princeton Univ. Press, Princeton, New Jersey.
Hamburger, V. (1938). *J. Exp. Zool.* **77**, 379–397.
Hamburger, V. (1960). "A Manual of Experimental Embryology." Univ. of Chicago Press, Chicago, Illinois.
Hamburger, V., and Hamilton, H. L. (1951). *J. Morphol.* **88**, 49–92.
Hamilton, H. L. (1952). "Lillie's Development of the Chick." Holt, New York.
Hiraiwa, Y. K. (1927). *J. Exp. Zool.* **49**, 441–457.
Hoadley, L. (1924). *Biol. Bull.* **46**, 281–315.
Johnson, L. G., and Volpe, E. P. (1973). "Patterns and Experiments in Developmental Biology." W. C. Brown, Dubuque, Iowa.
Kato, Y. (1969). *J. Exp. Zool.* **170**, 229–243.
Kato, Y. (1970). *Transplantation* **10**, 354–358.
Kato, Y., and Hayashi, Y. (1963). *Exp. Cell Res.* **31**, 599–602.
Lawson, K. A. (1972). *J. Embryol. Exp. Morphol.* **27**, 497–513.
Lawson, K. A. (1974). *J. Embryol. Exp. Morphol.* **32**, 469–493.
Levak-Suajger, B., and Skreb, N. (1965). *J. Embryol. Exp. Morphol.* **13**, 243–253.
Loomis, W. F. (1959). *Symp. Soc. Study Dev. Growth* **17**, 253–294.
MacCabe, J. A., and Parker, B. W. (1975). *Dev. Biol.* **45**, 349–357.
MacCabe, J. A., and Parker, B. W. (1976). *J. Exp. Zool.* **195**, 311–317.
MacCabe, J. A., Errick, J. E., and Saunders, J. W., Jr. (1974). *Dev. Biol.* **39**, 69–82.
Markee, J. (1940). *Contrib. Embryol. Carnegie Inst.* **28,** 219–308.
Martindale, F. M. (1941). *Anat. Rec.* **79**, 373–385.
Masters, J. R. (1976). *Dev. Biol.* **51**, 98–108.
Mayer, T. C. (1973a). *J. Exp. Zool.* **184**, 345–352.

Mayer, T. C. (1973b). *Dev. Biol.* **34,** 39–46.

Medawar, B. P. (1941). *Nature (London)* **148,** 783.

Meier, S., and Hay, E. D. (1974). *Dev. Biol.* **38,** 249–270.

Moscona, A. (1952). *Exp. Cell Res.* **3,** 535–539.

Moscona, A. (1959). *Dev. Biol.* **1,** 1–23.

Murphy, J. B. (1912). *J. Am. Med. Assoc.* **59,** 874–875.

Parsa, I., and Flanchbaum, L. (1975). *Dev. Biol.* **46,** 120–131.

Philpott, G., and Coulombre, A. J. (1965). *Exp. Cell Res.* **38,** 635–644.

Poole, T. W. (1974). *Dev. Biol.* **36,** 208–211.

Poole, T. W. (1975). *Dev. Biol.* **42,** 203–210.

Rawles, M. E. (1940). *Proc. Natl. Acad. Sci. U.S.A.* **26,** 673–680.

Rawles, M. E. (1947). *Physiol. Zool.* **20,** 248–265.

Rawles, M. E. (1963). *J. Embrol. Exp. Morphol.* **11,** 765–789.

Rinaldini, L. M. J. (1958). *Int. Rev. Cytol.* **7,** 587–647.

Romanoff, A. L. (1960). "The Avian Embryo." Macmillan, New York.

Rous, P., and Murphy, J. B. (1911). *J. Am. Med. Assoc.* **56,** 741–742.

Rugh, R. (1962). "Experimental Embryology." Burgess, Minneapolis, Minnesota.

Runner, M. N. (1946). *J. Exp. Zool.* **103,** 305–318.

Runner, M. N. (1947). *Anat. Rec.* **98,** 1–17.

Sawyer, R. N., Abbott, U. K., and Trelford, J. D. (1972). *Science* **175,** 527–530.

Steinberg, M. (1963). *Exp. Cell Res.* **30,** 257–279.

Szabo, G. (1955). *J. Pathol. Bacteriol.* **70,** 545.

Tickle, C., Shellswell, G., Grawley, A., and Wolpert, L. (1976). *Nature (London)* **259,** 396–397.

Wartiovaara, J., Nordling, S., Lehtonen, E., and Saxén, L. (1974). *J. Embrol. Exp. Morphol.* **31,** 667–682.

Wessells, N. K. (1967). *In* "Methods in Developmental Biology" (F. H. Wilt and N. K. Wessells, eds.), pp. 445–456. Crowell-Collier, New York.

Willier, B. H. (1924). *Am. J. Anat.* **33,** 67–103.

Zwilling, E. (1954). *Science* **120,** 219.

Zwilling, E. (1955). *J. Exp. Zool.* **128,** 423–441.

Zwilling, E. (1959). *Plast. Reconstr. Surg. Transplant. Bull.* **23,** 115–116.

18

The Regeneration of Mammalian Limbs and Limb Tissues

BRUCE M. CARLSON

I. INTRODUCTION

But if the above-mentioned animals, either aquatic or amphibious, recover their legs, even when kept on dry ground, how comes it to pass, that other land animals, at least such as are commonly accounted perfect, and are better known to us, are not endued with the same power? Is it to be hoped they may acquire them by some useful dispositions? and should the flattering expectation of obtaining this advantage for ourselves be considered entirely as chimerical?

Spallanzani (1769)

Ever since Spallanzani concluded his remarkable "Essay on Animal Reproductions" with these words, investigators in the field of limb regeneration have kept one eye upon the mammalian limb, while devising techniques for the stimulation of regeneration in lower vertebrates. To this date, however, the mammalian limb has remained stubbornly resistant to attempts to stimulate postamputational regeneration, and significant advances have been few. On the other hand, considerable progress has been made in our understanding of the natural regenerative capacities of the individual tissue components of mammalian extremities, and also in our ability to manipulate these regenerative processes to the advantage of the experimentalist or the clinician.

This chapter will describe techniques used in attempts to stimulate the regeneration of mammalian extremities. It will also summarize methods used in both the stimulation and control of regenerative processes in some of the major tissues that are found in limbs, specifically bone, muscle, and nerve. The main function will be to provide an overview and evaluation of existing techniques. Because the literature in this field is widely scattered, and much of it is sequestered in monographs and symposium reports that are not included in the standard literature retrieval services, one of the main purposes of this chapter will be to direct the reader to primary sources of information on techniques and experimental models used in the study of mammalian regeneration.

The subject is too broad to allow the inclusion of techniques used in studies on the regeneration of internal organs, but the interested reader can consult the following general references: Liozner (1960, 1974), McMinn (1969), Goss (1964), Bucher and Malt (1971), and Polezhaev (1972a,b).

II. EXTREMITIES

A. Limb Regeneration

In neither embryonic nor postnatal mammals do amputated limbs normally regenerate. Throughout the years, many methods have been used in attempts to stimulate epimorphic regeneration in mammals, but few of these have met with a significant degree of success. Most of these methods had been used previously in attempts to stimulate limb regeneration in frogs, which lose their capacity for epimorphic regeneration at metamorphosis.

For the proper interpretation of experimental attempts to stimulate limb regeneration in mammals, it is extremely important to recognize the morphological characteristics and developmental attributes of epimorphic regeneration, and to distinguish them from the quite different reactions that constitute a tissue regenerative response [see Carlson, (1970, in press) for more detailed comparisons of these processes]. The essence of epimorphic regeneration is the formation of a blastema from which the organized morphogenesis, differentiation, and growth of new limb structures occurs. Normally, the establishment of a regeneration blastema involves the coordinated interaction of nerve, wound epidermis, and damaged mesoderm of the amputated limb. Tissue regenerative reactions in mammals are often striking, but despite large amounts and often high degrees of organization of the regenerated structures, morphogenetic field activity, as seen in embryos or epimorphically regenerating limbs, is absent. The formation of entire muscles and bony nodules, complete with epiphyseal plates, can occur in the absence of a regeneration blastema by the tissue mode of regeneration (Carlson, 1972).

Working on the assumption that the capacity for epimorphic limb regeneration is lost during ontogenesis, several investigators amputated the digits of mammalian embryos *in utero* (Bors, 1925; Nicholas, 1926; Mitskevich, 1934, 1936; Aizupet, 1935, 1937). Although some outgrowth rarely occurred, the results were not spectacular, and the technique of intrauterine amputation has not been widely used since these early experiments. Improvements in *in utero* operative techniques would justify further investigation of the reactions of embryonic limbs to amputation.

Early attempts to stimulate limb regeneration in postnatal mammals met with relatively little success. These techniques will be only briefly mentioned. Some of the earliest stimulatory methods were designed to hasten the breakdown of distal skeletal tissue so that this reaction would correspond more closely in time to the breakdown of the soft tissues. Rogal (1951) accomplished this by subjecting newborn rats to avitaminosis A and D, whereas Umansky and Kudokotsev (1952) used parathyroid hormone to produce the same effect. Both treatments stimulated skeletal outgrowth, including the formation of new epiphyseal plates. Some outgrowth of amputated mouse digits treated with a preparation from the vitreous body was recently mentioned by Polezhaev (1972a), but no details of the experimental technique were given.

Scharf (1961, 1963) amputated the digits of 2-day-old rats and treated them with five or six alternating 3-minute applications of trypsin and 0.95% $CaCl_2$ solutions 1 day after amputation. This treatment removed the scab covering the wound. Distal outgrowth of the amputated phalanges, complete with epiphyses, occurred, but the more distal digital segments did not form. Scharf (1961) also described the formation of naillike outgrowths on the tips of the amputated digits.

Following the successful stimulation of limb regeneration in frogs by implants of additional adrenal tissue (Schotté and Wilber, 1958), Schotté and Smith (1961) attempted to stimulate digital regeneration in mice by injecting the animals with cortisone or ACTH. It was hoped that these agents would reduce the exuberant proliferation of scar tissue beneath the amputation surface and allow the epidermal–deep tissue contact that is necessary for dedifferentiation to occur. Pronounced modifications in the wound healing pattern occurred, but actual regeneration was minimal.

The electrical stimulation of limb regeneration in mammals (Becker, 1972;

Becker and Spadaro, 1972) is a controversial technique. The basis of this technique is the assumption that a "current of injury" is an integral feature of the events that initiate the normal epimorphic regenerative process in lower vertebrates. The electrical stimulation technique was applied in the hope of restoring the electrical factors that are presumably missing or greatly reduced in the amputated mammalian limb.

The seminal experiment involving this approach to the stimulation of limb regeneration was carried out by Smith (1967) on frogs. He constructed bimetallic rods by fusing 3-mm lengths of 28-gauge silver and platinum wires. After insulating a rod with Insl-X plastic, he scraped the tips and bent each end into a hook so that the rod would retain its position when implanted into a limb. The rod was then implanted alongside the shaft of the distal skeletal element of an amputated limb stump. In separate experiments, bimetallic rods were implanted with either the silver or the platinum ends located distally. Some outgrowth of cartilage and "mesenchymal" tissue occurred, but it was poorly organized.

Becker (1972) modified Smith's device by inserting a miniature 10 M ohm resistor between the silver and platinum wires and produced current levels of 3–6 nA in Ringer's solution. His device was about 35-mm long. In 21-day male rats, a forelimb was amputated at the midhumeral level, and the bimetallic implant was placed beneath the stump musculature, with the distal platinum portion bent and inserted into the open medullary cavity of the humerus (Becker and Spadaro, 1972). Greater outgrowth of bone was reported in experimental than in control limbs, and, in one case, a well-organized bone was formed alongside the stump of the original humerus. The bony outgrowths were in some cases accompanied by muscle fibers. No recognizable anatomic pattern of the regenerated muscle could be determined from the illustration (Becker and Spadaro, 1972, Fig. 5).

The degree of outgrowth in Becker's experiments was somewhat greater than that reported with other stimulatory techniques previously used on the rat, but, in essence, the reaction was similar. In none of these experiments is there compelling evidence that the induced outgrowth represents an epimorphic regenerative response of the type that occurs in amphibians. To this author, it seems more likely that tissue regeneration was stimulated. Much better documentation of the results of this type of experimentation must be done before it will be possible to interpret properly the efficacy of electrical stimulation techniques.

After Singer's (1954) demonstration that epimorphic regeneration in the frog can be stimulated by increasing the nerve supply to the forelimb, similar experiments were tried on mammals. Bar-Maor and Gitlin (1961) increased the innervation to the hindlimb in rats by deviating the sciatic nerve from one limb to the other. Amputation of these limbs, however, was not followed by regeneration.

The most significant step toward stimulating mammalian limb regeneration was taken by Mizell (1968; Mizell and Isaacs, 1970), who worked on newborn opossums. The newly born opossum is extremely immature, closely resembling a

12-day rat embryo. Yet, the limbs do not regenerate after simple amputation (McCrady, 1938; Mizell, 1968).

Mizell exploited the poorly developed immune system of newborn opossums and implanted pieces of brain tissue from other opossums into the limbs of the experimental animals. The donor material was small pieces of cerebral cortex taken from young opossums (age not specified). The pieces, suspended in chilled saline, were drawn up into a silicone-coated glass pipette with an inner diameter of 0.5 mm. Then, in hindlimbs of 1- to 2-day old host animals, a tunnel was made with watchmaker's forceps. The pipette was inserted into the channel, and the pieces of brain tissue were introduced into the limb. After a 2- to 4-day healing period, the limbs were amputated through the level of the brain implant. At the time of amputation, the mother opossum was anesthetized with Penthrane (Abbott), and under aseptic, but not sterile conditions, the limbs of the experimental animals, which are firmly attached to the mother's teats in the pouch, were amputated. In some cases, considerable outgrowth occurred, and grossly evident, but truncated digits occasionally appeared.

In summary, only after brain implantation in the opossum limb does it appear that a significant degree of epimorphic limb regeneration has been stimulated in mammals. Even in this case, there is a need for more material fixed at various stages after amputation in order to understand more fully the morphological nature of the regenerative process. The results obtained from virtually all of the other stimulatory techniques are roughly similar, except for degree, and it appears that they reflect an intrinsic self-organizational capacity of individual tissues, particularly the long bones, the growth of which was certainly stimulated in some experiments. One must remember, however, that most of the experimental animals have been young and rapidly growing, and that their bones have great growth potential. Even in young children with amputated limbs, one of the major clinical problems faced by orthopedic surgeons is the the continuing growth of the amputated skeletal elements past the level of the original amputation surface (Volkov, 1955). Thus, considerable caution must be exercised in the interpretation of attempts to stimulate limb regeneration in mammals.

B. Rabbit Earhole Regeneration

A potentially important model for the study of epimorphic regeneration in mammals is the filling in of holes punched in rabbit ears by a multitissue complex arising from what appears to be a regeneration blastema (Markelova, 1953, in Vorontsova and Liosner, 1960, pp. 377–379; Joseph and Dyson, 1966; Goss and Grimes, 1972). The time course, the morphology of the blastema and the developmental events preceding its establishment, and also the apparent necessity of some type of specific tissue interactions between ear epidermis and the cartilage beneath it (Goss and Grimes, 1972) constitute the main evidence in favor of its

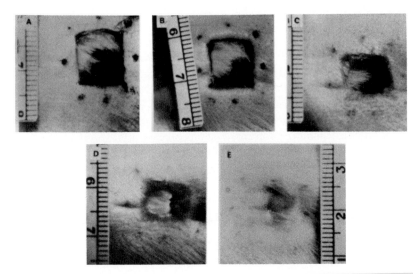

Fig. 1. Illustration of a punch wound in a rabbit's ear (from the inner surface) and the course of regeneration. (A) Immediately after the operation. (B) After 7 days. (C) After 14 days, a blastema is visible macroscopically. (D) After 35 days, the new tissue is highly vascularized, and the skin is smooth and thin. (E) After 98 days, most of the excised tissue has been replaced, and only a small hole remains. From Joseph and Dyson (1966).

being a true epimorphic regenerative process. Among the common laboratory animals, the ear of the rabbit seems unique in possessing this regenerative property.

The technique of producing the holes is not difficult. Both Joseph and Dyson (1966) and Goss and Grimes (1972) simply used punches, for example, a cork borer 1 cm in diameter, to make full-thickness holes through poorly vascularized regions of the ear (Fig. 1). No wound dressings were used after the hole was punched unless bleeding was excessive. Pressure or cotton sponges sufficed to bring hemorrhage under control.

This experimental model has proved useful in studying both tissue interactions involved in mammalian regeneration (Goss and Grimes, 1972), and the effects of male and female sex hormones on the rate and completeness of a complex regenerative process (Dyson and Joseph, 1968, 1971).

III. SKELETAL MUSCLE

For many years, the regenerative ability of mammalian skeletal muscle was considered to be minimal, particularly in clinical circles, but, as the result of a greatly increased amount of research during the last two decades, the regeneration of skeletal muscle is now generally recognized. A number of techniques have been devised for eliciting skeletal muscle regeneration for various purposes. Each has its advantages and disadvantages.

One of the earliest, and still most commonly used lesions is a simple transection or cut, either completely through or partly through a muscle. Research upon this type of lesion led to the concept of the "continuous" regeneration of a muscle fiber (review by Hudgson and Field, 1973; Hall-Craggs, 1974a). The major advantage of this type of lesion is that it demonstrates well the morphological transition between the normal and the regenerating part of the muscle fiber. The disadvantages are (1) that there is a very limited area of regeneration and (2) that the anatomic continuity between the regenerated portions of the muscle fibers is often lost.

The latter disadvantage can be eliminated by the use of local crush lesions. In many ways, crushing and transections are similar and would be complementary techniques, but, in most crush lesions, the continuity of the sarcolemmal sheaths is retained throughout the lesion. In addition, one can vary the width of the crush lesion to suit one's purposes. Many mechanical devices have been designed for producing uniform crush lesions (Allbrook *et al.*, 1966; Järvinen and Sorvari, 1975), but, for thin muscles, a firm pinch with a small hemostat suffices to produce a good crush lesion. With overlapping pinches, one can crush the entire muscle. This latter technique has recently been used on the levator ani muscle of the rat (B. M. Carlson and E. Gutmann, unpublished) to produce lesions that retain the afferent nerve and blood supply and cause minimal architectural disturbance to the muscle itself (Fig. 2).

One of the earliest techniques used to produce massive regeneration of skeletal muscle was ligature of the main blood vessels supplying the muscle (Le Gros Clark and Blomfield, 1945; Allbrook, 1951). One of the most important features of the devascularization model is the large amount of regeneration that can be elicited. In addition, the overall architecture of the muscle remains intact. Because the continuity of the blood supply is quickly restored by collateral vascular channels after the initial insult, sarcolysis of the degenerating muscle fibers and the subsequent regeneration of new muscle occur quickly. Unfortunately, this method does not result in degeneration of the entire muscle because, at both the proximal and distal ends, the muscle fibers are supplied by other blood vessels. As a result, varying amounts of muscle fibers remain intact in these regions.

Probably the most radical procedure for producing muscle regeneration is mincing. This technique was originally devised by Studitsky (1953) to demonstrate the validity of Lepeshinskaya's (1945) "new cell theory" on the origin of cells from a noncellular "living substance," but since that time it has come into use for a variety of purposes. The essence of the technique is to remove an entire muscle, for example, the gastrocnemius, mince it into 1 mm^3 fragments with

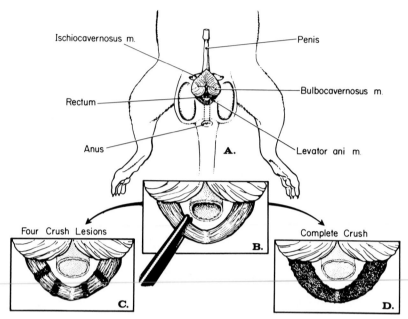

Fig. 2.   Technique of producing crush lesions of the levator ani muscle in the rat. (A) Location of the muscle. (B) Producing the crush with a hemostat. (C) Crushing the muscle in four places allows survival of segments of muscle fibers between two crush lesions. (D) Complete crush resulting in no intact muscle fibers or segments of muscle fibers.

scissors, and then replace the minced fragments into their original bed or into a heterotopic site (Fig. 3). The minced fragments then degenerate, and from their cellular remains, probably the satellite cells (Snow, 1977a,b), new muscle fibers are formed. The regenerating muscle fibers ultimately form a generalized model of a functional muscle (Fig. 4). Details of the technique and the regenerative process that follows are given in publications by Studitsky (1959; Studitsky *et al.*, 1956) and Carlson (1972).

More than any other experimental model, regeneration from minced fragments demonstrates the extent to which regenerating muscle fibers and their connective tissue stroma can reconstitute a grossly identifiable muscle in an adult mammal. In this regard, minced muscle regeneration has been particularly useful in studying tissue interactions (including revascularization and reinnervation) and morphogenetic mechanisms in regenerating muscle. Because complete destruction of all original muscle fibers is assured, the minced system has served as an early model for studying the developmental physiology (Salafsky, 1971; Carlson and Gutmann, 1972) and biochemistry (Gallucci *et al.*, 1966; Snow, 1973; Rifenberick *et al.*, 1974) of regenerating muscle. The exchange of minced mus-

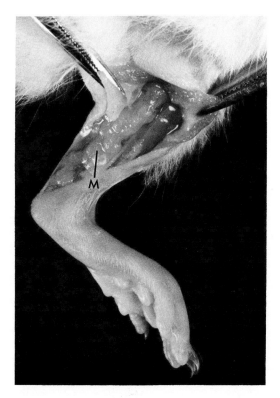

Fig. 3.   Implantation of minced muscle fragments (M) into the bed of the removed gastrocnemius muscle. The biceps femoris muscle (held in hemostats) and then the skin are sutured over the minced fragments. From Carlson (1968).

cles between normal and diseased mice has been used by several workers studying the pathogenesis and mechanisms of muscular dystrophy (Cosmos, 1973; Neerunjun and Dubowitz, 1974; Salafsky, 1971).

   On the negative side, minced muscle regenerates, more so in rats than in mice, are heavily bound down to surrounding tissues by connecting tissue adhesions. This reduces their utility in studies of contractile properties, and it creates problems in determining proper bases of comparison for biochemical studies. Because of the complete severance of neurovascular connections, regeneration proceeds more slowly in a mince than in system with an intact vascular supply. A further disadvantage is that some muscles, particularly thin ones such as the soleus, regenerate quite poorly after mincing.

   Another relatively new technique is the free grafting of entire muscles. A muscle is freely grafted if it is completely removed from its bed, with all ner-

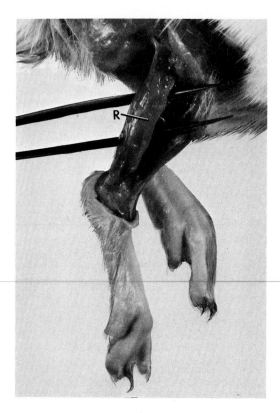

Fig. 4. Thirty-two-day minced gastrocnemius muscle regenerate (R) in the rat. The regenerate has normally positioned proximal and distal tendon connections and the site of entry of the tibial nerve is normal. The regenerate does not attain the bulk or exact form of the normal gastrocnemius muscle. From Carlson (1968).

vous, vascular, and tendinous connections severed. The muscle can then be replaced into its own bed (orthotopic graft) or into the bed of another muscle within the same animal (heterotopic graft). Most free grafts are replaced within the same animal (autografts), but isografts and allografts are also sometimes used in some experiments. Isografts between highly inbred animals are tolerated well, whereas allografts are ultimately rejected.

A predenervation technique (denervating a muscle from 14 to 28 days before grafting) for preparing muscles for free grafting (Fig. 5) was first reported from Studitsky's laboratory (Bosova, 1962) and independently by Thompson (1971a,b), who quickly applied it to man with considerable success (Thompson, 1974, review, with summary of techniques currently in clinical use). According

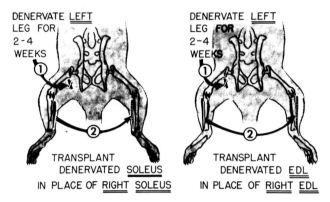

Fig. 5. Diagram of the technique used in grafting predenervated muscles in the rat. The left leg is denervated by severing the sciatic nerve high in the thigh and suturing the proximal stump of the nerve. After 2–4 weeks of denervation, the denervated left soleus or EDL (extensor digitorum longus) muscle is removed. The corresponding muscle in the right limb is removed, and the predenervated muscle is grafted into its place. In cross-transplantion experiments, the slow soleus muscle is grafted in place of the fast EDL muscle or vice versa.

to Thompson's initial hypothesis, predenervation changes the metabolism of the muscle fibers so that the original muscle fibers can survive the early avascular period of the free graft. The importance of regeneration was discounted. Now, it appears quite certain that regenerating muscle fibers comprise the bulk of a mature free graft (Carlson, 1976). In fact, recent studies on free muscle grafts in the cat (Faulkner *et al.*, 1976) have shown that predenervation is not a prerequisite for the successful free grafting of larger muscles. Studies on both the rat and cat have shown that in a graft of predenervated muscle, the early stages of degeneration and regeneration occur more rapidly than in a graft of normal muscle. However, there is normally little difference between mature grafts of predenervated versus normal muscle.

The free grafting technique has several advantages over the minced muscle technique, the main one being that the overall architecture of the muscle is preserved and a more fully functional regenerate is produced (Carlson and Gutmann, 1975; Faulkner *et al.*, 1976). The extent of adhesions to neighboring muscles is much less than in a minced muscle regenerate. For these reasons, free grafting of a muscle is acceptable clinical technique, whereas mincing is not. Another positive feature, shared by both free grafts and minces, is that the muscle can be grafted to another site. This is the normal clinical procedure. It has been shown that a cross-transplanted muscle takes on physiological and histochemical features appropriate to the site in which it is placed (Gutmann and Carlson, 1975a).

Drawbacks to free grafting are the interruption of the nerve and vascular supply. Probably because of the latter, grafts of muscles weighing more than 6–8 gm, are often not successful. Vascular anastomoses between the graft and host (Tamai *et al.*, 1970; Kubo *et al.*, 1976; Harii *et al.*, 1976) may be helpful clinically in this regard, but they may also eliminate the degeneration and subsequent regeneration of muscle fibers, thus making the graft less useful as a model for regeneration. As physiological and biochemical models, free grafts are "contaminated" by varying proportions of surviving muscle fibers (Table I). The accuracy of measurements would depend upon the percentage of surviving fibers.

To circumvent the problem of muscle fiber survival in free grafts, Gutmann and Carlson (1975b) devised a sliced graft model, in which a grafted muscle is cut into seven to eight transverse segments like a sausage. Although slicing eliminates all surviving muscle fibers, mature sliced grafts are smaller and contract more weakly than entire muscle grafts.

The more recent major technique used to produce muscle regeneration is the local application of the myotoxic local anesthetic, bupivacaine (Marcaine, Winthrop). In the first experiments, Marcaine was applied locally to the skin and resulted in the rapid degeneration and regeneration of the superficial muscle fibers beneath the site of application (Benoit and Belt, 1970; Jirmanová and Thesleff, 1972). Later, Hall-Craggs (1974b) described a technique of directly injecting a mixture of Marcaine and hyaluronidase into the rat tibialis anterior muscle over a period of several days. He reported that this regimen produced virtually complete degeneration and subsequent regeneration of the muscle.

TABLE I

Numbers of Muscle Fibers in Short- and Long-Term Free Grafts of the Rat Extensor Digitorum Longus Muscles after Various Treatments[a]

Treatment of graft	Short-term grafts (4 days)	No. of muscles	Long-term grafts (60 days)	No. of muscles
No pretreatment	132.0 ± 140.1[b]	4	3824.3 ± 571.1	3
14-day predenervation	1166.0 ± 332.1	5	3665.8 ± 153.0	4
Marcaine preinjection (−2 and 0 days)	8.2 ± 20.2	12	4071.0 ± 596.2	6
Marcaine injection (0 days)	2.2 ± 5.8	13	3508.6 ± 419.7	4

[a] The muscle fibers in 4-day grafts represent surviving original muscle fibers. The muscle fibers in long-term grafts could be either surviving original or regenerated muscle fibers, because they cannot be distinguished. The difference between the number of muscle fibers at 4 days and at 60 days gives an approximation of the number of regenerating muscle fibers in the graft.

[b] Standard deviation.

The most outstanding feature of Marcaine-treated muscles is that both the nerve and blood supplies to the muscle remain functionally intact, and the speed and synchrony of the regeneration are exceptional. The overall architecture of the muscle remains normal. The major disadvantage is that, with topical application of Marcaine, only the superficial layers of muscle fibers regenerate, and for deep muscles, like the soleus or extensor digitorum longus, direct injections, even into surgically exposed muscles do not lead to the degeneration of all muscle fibers (B. M. Carlson, unpublished). Making multiple injections over several days is also time consuming.

In our hands, the most satisfactory technique for obtaining the virtually complete degeneration and regeneration of muscle fibers within a muscle has been to combine a Marcaine injection with free grafting (Carlson, 1976; Carlson and Gutmann, 1976). In its most recent version, a muscle is removed from a rat and placed on a petri dish (Fig. 6). It is then injected with as much 0.75% Marcaine as it can hold [100–200 μl for the extensor digitorum longus in young (200-gm) rats]. It is best to insert the syringe needle (1 inch, 25-gauge) into one of the cut ends of the muscle and push it almost to the other end of the muscle. The Marcaine is then injected while the needle is being slowly withdrawn. If injected properly, the muscle swells up. The addition of hyaluronidase to the Marcaine is not necessary to produce good degeneration (B. M. Carlson, unpublished). The injected muscle is then soaked in a solution of Marcaine for 10 minutes to ensure that all superficial muscle fibers (those that most commonly survive in free grafts) are exposed. The muscle is then replaced into the animal by the usual free grafting technique. Almost no original muscle fibers survive (Table I). This model appears to be the most satisfactory one for studies on the physiology and biochemistry of early muscle regeneration and in studies on the regeneration of muscle in the absence of a nerve supply. For studies on long-term muscle regenerates, ordinary free grafts are often preferable because the operation takes only half as long as the combination of Marcaine plus free grafting.

In addition to the techniques mentioned above, a number of other models have been used to produce muscle regeneration. These have often been related to

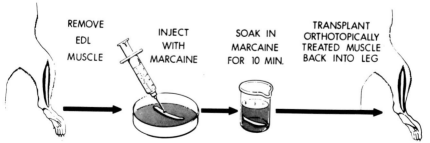

REMOVE EDL MUSCLE   INJECT WITH MARCAINE   SOAK IN MARCAINE FOR 10 MIN.   TRANSPLANT ORTHOTOPICALLY TREATED MUSCLE BACK INTO LEG

Fig. 6. Technique for Marcaine treatment of free muscle grafts in the rat. See text for details.

practical problems affecting humans in various occupations. Among these are radiant energy from incandescent lights on extraocular muscles (O'Steen *et al.*, 1975), local cold (Price *et al.*, 1964), or various chemicals (Standish, 1964).

The use of *in vitro* methods has recently been successfully applied to the study of mammalian muscle regeneration at the cellular level (Bischoff, 1975; Konigsberg *et al.*, 1975). Bischoff (1975) teased out single muscle fibers 2–3 cm long from adult rats. He cultured them in a fibrin clot in Eagle's medium with 10% chick embryo extract in an atmosphere of 95% air–5% CO_2. He was able to maintain the muscle fibers for up to 3 weeks *in vitro*. Konigsberg *et al.* (1975) isolated muscle fibers from the pectoralis profundus muscle of 3- to 6-week old Japanese quail. Their culture medium was similar to that used by Bischoff. In addition, Peterson and Crain (1972) have investigated interactions between nerves and regenerating muscle fibers in culture. Culture methods may be particularly useful in studies on membrane properties of regenerating muscle fibers.

IV. BONE

In most cases, studies on the regeneration of bone have been closely linked with practical problems in orthopedic surgery. Because of this link, countless specific experimental models have been devised to imitate as closely as possible certain classical types of fractures or methods involved in their treatment. It is beyond the scope of this chapter to deal with these clinical models. Many of these are summarized in detail in the monographs of Rusanov (1969) and Vinogradova and Lavrischeva (1974). Instead, I shall describe the major strategies that are used to manipulate the natural regeneration of bone or to stimulate the regeneration of new bone.

One item of terminology should be mentioned first. In the early phase of fracture healing, a mass of primitive-looking cells, whose origin is still debated, forms around the area of the fracture. This mass is commonly called a blastema, and from it arises the new cartilage or bone of the fracture callus. This "blastema" has sometimes been equated with the limb regeneration blastema of amphibians. Although skeletal tissue differentiates from both types of blastemas, they have few other points in common. The blastema surrounding a mammalian fracture appears to have none of the morphogenetic properties of the limb regeneration blastema, nor does it have the close relationship to epidermis, a necessity in the case of limb blastemas. "Blastemas," similar to those seen around mammalian bone, can be produced in urodelan amphibians as the result of fractures or the injection of irritating substances into the limb. This is a manifestation of a tissue regenerative process, rather than an epimorphic one. Although the newly deposited bone is gradually remodeled to approach more closely the form of the original bone, this appears to be an adaptation to the functional environment of the limb, rather than a primary morphogenetic process, which can proceed in the absence of ongoing function.

Clinical work in the field of bone regeneration makes use of the normal regenerative or healing capacity of fractured bone. Most research is designed to extend the natural healing capacity of bone or to stimulate osteogenesis where it is normally absent. A classical technique is to allow the natural healing reaction that occurs at the edge of a viable bone to cement a bone graft in place. This technique is oriented almost entirely toward practical orthopedic problems ranging from filling relatively small defects in bone to the replacement of entire joints with grafted material.

One of the major methods of stimulating osteogenesis *de novo* is the induction of new bone from competent connective tissue cells. A classic experiment in this area is the induction of new bone by implants of mucosa of the urinary bladder in dogs (Huggins, 1931). After determining that the vesical mucosa itself, rather than urine, is responsible for the induction of bone in connective tissues grafted to the urinary bladder, Huggins took pieces of mucosa from the urinary bladder (2 cm in diameter) and sutured these onto the sheath of the rectus abdominis muscle. The grafted mucosa commonly formed a cyst, and bone was deposited on the side of the cyst corresponding to the free surface of the original mucosal graft. Implantation of bladder scrapings within the rectus sheath resulted in cysts completely surrounded by bone. In experiments of this type, new bone is already forming around the implant within 2–3 weeks after the operation.

Over a long series of experiments, Friedenshtein has confirmed the results of Huggins on dogs and guinea pigs and has devoted much effort toward identification of the osteogenic precursor cells (Friedenshtein and Lalkina, 1973). He (Friedenshtein, 1962) demonstrated the humoral nature of the osteogenic activity of transitional epithelium by means of diffusion chamber experiments. He obtained bladder epithelial cells by treating urinary bladder mucosa with trypsin. Cells (5×10^4) suspended in Hanks' solution were placed into standard Millipore diffusion chambers (type HA filter), and the chambers were implanted beneath the skin of guinea pigs. After 30 days, bone was formed outside the chambers containing viable epithelium. Osteogenesis did not occur in the absence of viability and growth of the epithelium within the chamber.

In other early work, Levander (1964) developed an experimental model of bone induction involving the implantation of pieces of devitalized bone into loose connective tissue. He devitalized the inducing tissues by many means, such as boiling or fixation in absolute alcohol or formalin, but the most effective method was impregnation of the tissues with a 1% aqueous solution of trypan blue dye over a period of several hours to a few days. Levander also claimed to induce skeletal muscle and several other types of tissue by this method. Levander's model of tissue metaplasia remains highly controversial (Mitskevich *et al.,* 1970), and verification of his experiments is made difficult because only a certain old batch (No. 2691) of trypan blue made by the Gurr Company (London) seems to produce the inductive effects.

A more easily repeatable model of regeneration of bone by induction was developed in Polezhaev's laboratory (review by Polezhaev, 1972b, Chapter 2), with the specific aim of finding a means to fill in large normally nonregenerating defects in the mature skull with new bone. This method has been successfully tried in several species of adult laboratory animals. The first step is to create a rectangular defect, ranging from 5 × 10 mm in rats to 25 × 40 mm in dogs, in the parietal bone of the skull. Then pieces of bone are ground into the consistency of sawdust and mixed into a solution containing the recipient's blood and penicillin soaked in saline. The best results are obtained with autoplastic implants of "sawdust" made from the bone that was removed when the skull defect was created. Fresh or lyophilized bone also possesses inducing capacity, but somewhat less potent than that of fresh autologous bone. The bone sawdust preparation is then packed into the skull defect over the dura mater, which must be present for bone induction to occur. The galea aponeurotica and skin are then sutured over the sawdust-filled defect.

Within the 2nd week after the operation, spicules of new bone begin to form throughout the defect, and, after several months, the new bone is consistently well developed, with an architecture similar to that of the normal calvarium. According to Polezhaev, the bone sawdust acts as a specific inducer; immature connective tissue cells in the region of the skull defect constitute the reactive tissue; and the presence of dura mater underlying the defect is a condition necessary for the induction of new bone. In addition to laboratory animals, this method has been successfully applied to humans who have sustained severe trauma to the skull (Strebkov, 1966). This method of stimulating regeneration of bone deserves further attention.

A very similar method of bone regeneration by induction has been developed by Urist (1965), although the emphasis here was turned toward long bones. He prepared a dead, decalcified bone matrix by removing 1–2 cm diaphyseal segments of long bone from rabbits, other laboratory animals, or humans. These segments were decalcified by soaking them in a sterile solution of 0.6 N HCl for 5 days. The acid was removed by prolonged washing in 0.15 M NaCl. The decalcified bone matrix was then implanted into soft tissue pockets in several locations in mice, rats, rabbits, and guinea pigs. After several weeks, new bone was formed around up to 95% of the implants. Similarly, decalcified segments of bone were implanted into artificially created spaces of approximately one-third the length of the ulna in rabbits. The HCl-treated bone implants stimulated the formation of more new bone that was better integrated with the bone ends of the host than did undecalcified bone segments of the same size. Many other experiments involving modifications of this basic induction system, as well as properties of the bone induction principle, are given in later papers by Urist's group (Urist *et al.,* 1967, 1968).

In some cases, such as the ribs, large amounts of bone can be removed, but if the periosteum remains, it will ultimately fill in the empty space with new bone. This phenomenon has long been recognized and exploited by surgeons. In some early experimental work, Studitsky (1954) found that after the removal of the diaphysis of a long bone, a tissue interaction between the epiphysis and diaphyseal periosteum was necessary for the formation of new bone. In the absence of the epiphyseal cartilage, new bone failed to occur.

The electrical stimulation of fracture healing has aroused considerable interest over the last decade. This field is still in the early stages of development, and there are a number of different techniques used to attempt to stimulate bone regeneration. At this point, it is still not possible to identify a single stimulatory technique that would be preferable to the others. A recent symposium report (Liboff and Rinaldi, 1974) provides a good summary of current techniques and hypotheses in this field.

There is still not uniform agreement on the physiological basis for electrical stimulatory techniques, but a widely accepted hypothesis is that normal bone exhibits piezoelectric properties that act like a transducer to translate mechanical changes in the functional environment to electrical signals (Bassett, 1971). The electrical signals, in turn, exert their effect on osteoblastic and osteoclastic cells, which one then stimulated to resorb old or deposit new bone. In this way, mechanical stress is translated into a structural adaptation in the bone.

Many attempts to influence the structure of normal bone or to accelerate the healing of fractures have involved the implantation under the skin of the back of small coated battery packs suitably connected with resistors and transistors to deliver a constant current. The leads from the batteries are insulated wires of platinum–iridium or stainless steel. The bare tips of the wires are placed on the bone or, more commonly, into holes drilled into the bone on either side of a fracture site (Friedenberg *et al.,* 1971).

According to Bassett *et al.* (1974a), several factors should be taken into consideration when attempting to stimulate bone regeneration electrically: (1) With a dc current, osteoblastic activity and bone deposition occur at the cathode, whereas bone resorption takes place at the anode. (2) The optimal current is in the range of 10–25 μA. A minimum current 2–5 μA must be applied to stimulate osteogenesis. (3) Currents over 50 μA produce deleterious effects upon the system. (4) A polarity-dependent cellular response (osteoblastic activity at cathode and osteoclastic activity at the anode) does not occur under pulsed or ac conditions. In earlier attempts at electrostimulation, bone was deposited at the cathode, whereas bone was resorbed around the anode. Other experimental models (Lavine *et al.,* 1971) have attempted to stimulate the deposition of bone

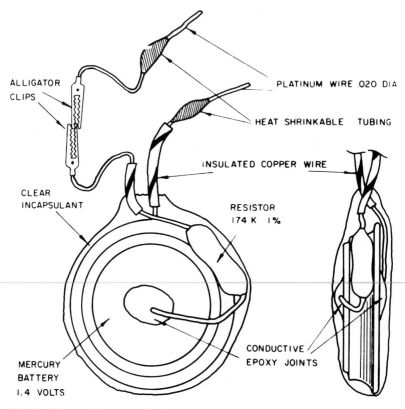

Fig. 7. Diagram of one type of unit used to produce weak electrical currents in bone healing experiments. The battery capsule is implanted beneath the skin. The insulated wire leads are brought to a bone, and the terminal platinum wires are inserted into drill holes made in the cortex of the bone. This unit produces a direct current of 2–4 μA. From Lavine *et al.* (1971).

between the implanted electrodes (Fig. 7). Recently, Bassett *et al.* (1974a,b) have used externally applied electromagnetic fields to stimulate fracture repair without surgical invasion of the tissue at the fracture site. At this point, there is not yet agreement on what constitutes the most effective method of electrostimulation of bone regeneration.

V. PERIPHERAL NERVE

The regeneration of peripheral nerves is one of the best known and most extensively documented of the regenerative phenomena that occur in mammals. In essence, peripheral nerve regeneration is an intracellular process in which a partially destroyed axon or dendrite grows out to reestablish functional contact with an end organ. Because of the high natural regenerative potential of peripheral nerves, the main problem for both research and clinical practice is how to control and direct the regenerating nerve. Although peripheral nerve regeneration is normally considered to be a response to direct trauma applied to the nerve trunk, the phenomenon of collateral sprouting (Edds, 1953) can be looked upon as a form of supernumerary regeneration within the nerve fiber. Both processes probably share a common underlying mechanism, namely, axoplasmic flow (Weiss and Hiscoe, 1948). Only the basic techniques used in studies of nerve regeneration will be presented here. For additional details, the reader is referred to a review by Gutmann (1973); to monographs by Gutmann (1958), Kaverina (1975), and Sunderland (1968); and to a recent symposium (Simeone, 1972).

The main techniques used to elicit the posttraumatic regeneration of nerves are crushing or severing some point along a nerve. Nerve crushing is normally done by gently lifting a nerve with a fine glass hook and crushing it at one site with a fine pair of watchmaker's forceps (No. 5) or with fine artery forceps. The crushing of a nerve causes the degeneration of all neuronal processes distal to the lesion, but the endoneurial sheaths remain intact. Structural and functional regeneration of the nerve fibers is virtually complete. This method is ideally suited for studies in which repeated denervation of the same end organ is required.

Nerve section is commonly used when one wishes to denervate an end organ, but it is also used when one wishes to direct the regenerating nerve fibers to heterotopic sites. In this type of experimentation or in the clinical repair of traumatized nerves, suturing, or some other method (e.g., arterial sleeves) of joining the proximal and distal ends of severed nerve trunks is normally required. Nerve section is easily accomplished by lifting a nerve and cutting it perpendicularly with fine scissors. The nerve should not be greatly stretched, nor should it be compressed proximal to the lesion. Unnecessary trimming of the nerve stumps should also be avoided because this could lead to excessive stretching of the nerve trunk when it is sutured. The level at which the nerve lesion is made can be very important, particularly when changes in some parameter of the end organ are to be measured. The trophic effects of degenerating distal nerve segments of different lengths from the end organ are discussed in detail by Gutmann (1973).

The object of nerve suturing is to allow the regenerating terminals of a peripheral nerve the greatest opportunity to reach the desired end organ. In clinical practice and in some research applications, the proximal and distal ends of the same nerve are sutured together. In this procedure, one attempts to approximate as closely as possible the corresponding nerve fascicles of the proximal and distal stumps, for if they enter the wrong funiculus, the regenerating nerve fibers will be directed to an incorrect location. If the ends of the nerves are too far apart to be sutured without excessive stretching, the gap between them can be bridged by an implanted segment of another nerve, which acts as a substrate to guide the regenerating nerve fibers into the distal stump (Freilinger, 1975). Commonly, a segment of autogenous sural nerve is used for the ''bridge,'' but pieces of lyophilized homografted nerve can be used as well.

In larger nerves, the surgeon commonly uses the pattern of superficial blood vessels on the surface of the nerve as a guide for realigning the two ends of a severed nerve. The suturing of nerves is commonly done by passing several 10-0 sutures through the perineural sheath. A new technique for rapidly rejoining the ends of severed nerves without suturing is being developed by Hall and Kuhn (1975) and Kuhn and Hall (1975). They have made small cylinders of varying diameters out of a powder of type 216-L stainless steel. The walls of these cylinders are porous and allow the interchange of fluids and oxygen. One-third of the way along its length, a hole is bored through the wall of the cylinder (Fig. 8). This hole is attached to a suction apparatus. The two ends of a severed nerve are led into the holes at each end of the cylinder, and suction is applied through the small hole in the wall. The two ends of the nerve are then pulled together at the center of the cylinder by means of the applied suction (pressure differential between 50- and 75-mm Hg). The slight roughness of the inner wall of the cylinder prevents the ends of the nerve from pulling apart. The cylinders have been left around the nerves of experimental animals for long periods (up to 41 months) without adverse tissue reactions, but it is possible to produce cuffs that could be

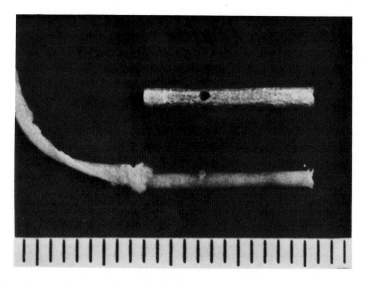

Fig. 8.   Photograph showing the porous tube (above) used in the nerve approximation technique, and (below) a segment of severed rat sciatic nerve that had been joined within the tube. From Hall and Kuhn (1975).

removed after the ends of the nerve are united. In early trials, both the speed of rejoining the cut ends of the nerves and the degree of functional return have compared favorably with suturing methods (Figs. 8 and 9).

For many experimental purposes, the proximal half of the severed nerve is sutured to the distal part of another, leading to a "cross-innervation" effect by the regenerating nerves. The most common use of the cross-innervation effect is in the study of the neural control of muscle structure and function, where the nerve to a fast muscle is directed toward a slow muscle or vice versa (Buller *et al.*, 1960). The cross-innervation technique is used, as well, in studies on sense organs, such as taste buds (Oakley, 1967).

Some assessment of the rate, the most distal extent, or the distribution of regenerating nerve fibers is frequently desirable. An early method for demonstrating the extent of regeneration of sensory nerve fibers after a crush lesion was to elicit simple sensory reflexes in the skin in the originally denervated zone (Gutmann *et al.*, 1942). By mapping the ever shrinking asensory zone, one can follow the advance of the regenerating nerve fibers. A more indirect method uses the rate of axoplasmic flow as an indicator of the rate of regeneration. Cockett (1972) has described a direct method involving removal of a large nerve trunk at a given interval after pinching and counting the number of silver-stained nerve fibers at various distances distal to the pinch lesion. This allows one to determine

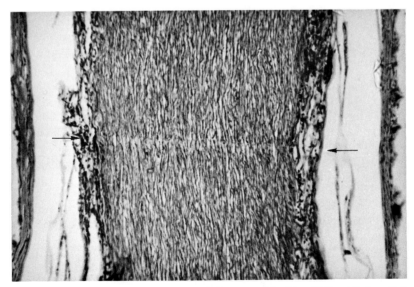

Fig. 9. Microscopic section of severed rat sciatic nerve rejoined in a Hall and Kuhn cylinder. The level of sectioning is indicated by the arrows. (Photomicrograph courtesy of Dr. James L. Hall).

the average length of the regenerated nerve fibers at a specific postoperative time.

Interest in the collateral sprouting of peripheral nerves has increased during recent years, particularly with respect to research on sensory nerve fields (Diamond *et al.,* 1976) and in the clinical application of free muscle transplantation (Holle, 1976). A common method of eliciting the collateral sprouting of sensory nerves is to sever the sensory nerve on either side of the nerve under investigation. In the case of muscle grafts, collateral sprouting is commonly stimulated by damaging the fascial coverings of a normal muscle lying alongside the free graft. Recent work, however, suggests that direct traumatization of neither surrounding muscles nor neighboring nerves is necessary to stimulate the collateral sprouting of nerve fibers into a grafted rat muscle (Gutmann and Carlson, 1976).

VI. CONCLUDING REMARKS

Although relatively little progress has been made toward the stimulation of limb regeneration in mammals, recent research has resulted in a substantial increase in our ability to manipulate the regeneration of some of the individual tissues that comprise the limb. The regeneration of tissues, even to the point of forming complete morphofunctional units, such as bone or muscles, appears to be based largely upon the mechanisms that these tissues normally use to adapt to changes in the functional environment of the limb. Significant techniques for improving or controlling the regeneration of limb tissues will, to a great extent, depend upon identifying these normal control mechanisms.

The stimulation of limb regeneration is a far more difficult task. Much more background information on the reactions to amputation of amphibian and, particularly, mammalian limbs, will be needed to provide a rational basis for techniques designed to stimulate the epimorphic regenerative process in mammals. One must keep in mind the complexity of the regenerating limb and not expect that the stimulation of limb regeneration in mammals will necessarily be accomplished by manipulating a single variable or applying a single stimulatory technique.

REFERENCES

Aizupet, M. P. (1935). *Biol. Zh.* **4,** 233–236.
Aizupet, M. P. (1937). *Biol. Zh.* **6,** 779–786.
Allbrook, D. B. (1951). Ph.D. Thesis, University of London (University College).
Allbrook, D. B., Baker, W. de C., and Kirkaldy-Willis, W. H. (1966). *J. Bone Joint Surg., Br. Vol.* **48,** 153–169.

Bar-Maor, J. A., and Gitlin, G. (1961). *Transplant. Bull.* **27**, 460–461.

Bassett, C. A. L. (1971). *Biochem. Physiol. Bone, 2nd Ed.* **3**, 1–76.

Bassett, C. A. L., Pawluk, R. J., and Pilla, A. A. (1974a). *Ann. N. Y. Acad. Sci.* **238**, 242–261.

Bassett, C. A. L., Pawluk, R. J., and Pilla, A. A. (1974b). *Science* **184**, 575–577.

Becker, R. O. (1972). *Nature (London)* **235**, 109–111.

Becker, R. O., and Spadaro, J. A. (1972). *Bull. N.Y. Acad. Med.* [2] **48**, 627–641.

Benoit, P. W., and Belt, W. D. (1970). *J. Anat.* **107**, 547–556.

Bischoff, R. (1975). *Anat. Rec.* **182**, 215–236.

Bors, E. (1925). *Wilhelm Roux' Arch. Entwicklungsmech. Org.* **105**, 655–666.

Bosova, N. N. (1962). *Byull. Eksp. Biol. Med.* **53**, 88–92.

Bucher, N. L. R., and Malt, R. A. (1971). "Regeneration of Liver and Kidney." Little, Brown, Boston, Massachusetts.

Buller, A. J., Eccles, J. C., and Eccles, R. M. (1960). *J. Physiol. (London)* **160**, 417–439.

Carlson, B. M. (1968). *J. Morphol.* **125**, 447–472.

Carlson, B. M. (1970). *Am. Zool.* **10**, 175–186.

Carlson, B. M. (1972). "The Regeneration of Minced Muscles." Karger, Basel.

Carlson, B. M. (1976). *Exp. Neurol.* **52**, 421–432.

Carlson, B. M. *In* "Muscle Biology" (A. M. Pearson, ed.) (in press).

Carlson, B. M., and Gutmann, E. (1972). *Exp. Neurol.* **36**, 239–249.

Carlson, B. M., and Gutmann, E. (1975). *Pflügers Arch.* **353**, 215–225.

Carlson, B. M., and Gutmann, E. (1976). *Exp. Neurol.* **53**, 82–93.

Cockett, S. A. (1972). *Exp. Neurol.* **37**, 635–638.

Cosmos, E. (1973). *Physiologist* **16**, 167–177.

Diamond, J., Cooper, E., Turner, C., and Macintrye, L. (1976). *Science* **193**, 371–377.

Dyson, M., and Joseph, J. (1968). *J. Anat.* **103**, 491–505.

Dyson, M., and Joseph, J. (1971). *J. Endocrinol.* **51**, 685–697.

Edds, M. V. (1953). *Q. Rev. Biol.* **28**, 260–276.

Faulkner, J. A., Maxwell, L. C., Mufti, S. A., and Carlson, B. M. (1976). *Life Sci.* **19**, 289–296.

Freilinger, G. (1975). *Plast. Reconstr. Surg.* **56**, 44–48.

Friedenberg, Z. B., Roberts, P. G., Didizian, N. H., and Brighton, C. T. (1971). *J. Bone Joint Surg., Am. Vol.* **53**, 1400–1408.

Friedenshtein, A. Ya. (1962). *Nature (London)* **194**, 608–699.

Friedenshtein, A. Ya., and Lalkina, K. S. (1973). "The Induction of Bone and Osteogenic Precursor Cells." Izd. Med., Moscow (in Russian).

Gallucci, V., Novello, F., Margreth, A., and Aloisi, M. (1966). *Br. J. Exp. Pathol.* **47**, 215–227.

Goss, R. J. (1964). "Adaptive Growth." Academic Press, New York.

Goss, R. J., and Grimes, L. N. (1972). *Am. Zool.* **12**, 151–157.

Gutmann, E. (1958). "Die funktionelle Regeneration der peripheren Nerven." Akademie-Verlag, Berlin.

Gutmann, E. (1973). *Methods Neurochem.* **5**, 189–254.

Gutmann, E., and Carlson, B. M. (1975a). *Pflügers Arch.* **353**, 227–239.

Gutmann, E., and Carlson, B. M. (1975b). *Experientia* **31**, 848–849.

Gutmann, E., and Carlson, B. M. (1976). *Life Sci.* **19**, 649–656.

Gutmann, E., Guttmann, L., Medawar, P. B., and Young, J. Z. (1942). *J. Exp. Biol.* **19**, 14–42.

Hall, J. L., and Kuhn, W. E. (1975). *Natl. Bur. Stand. (U.S.), Spec. Publ.* **415**, 99–101.

Hall-Craggs, E. C. B. (1974a). *J. Anat.* **117**, 171–178.

Hall-Craggs, E. C. B. (1974b). *Exp. Neurol.* **43**, 349–358.

Harii, K., Ohmori, K., and Torii, S. (1976). *Plast. Reconstr. Surg.* **57**, 133–143.

Holle, J. (1976). *Wien. Klin. Wochenschr.* **88**, Suppl. 48, 1–21.

Hudgson, P., and Field, E. J. (1973). *Struct. Funct. Muscle, 2nd Ed.* **2**, Part 2, 311–363.

Huggins, C. (1931). *Arch. Surg. (Chicago)* **22**, 377–408.

Järvinen, M., and Sorvari, T. (1975). *Acta Pathol. Microbiol. Scand., Sect. A* **83**, 259–265.

Jirmanová, I., and Thesleff, S. (1972). *Z. Zellforsch. Mikrosk. Anat.* **131**, 77–97.

Joseph, J., and Dyson, M. (1966). *Br. J. Surg.* **53**, 372–380.

Kaverina, V. V. (1975). "The Regeneration of Nerves in Neuroplastic Operations." Izd. Med., Leningrad (in Russian).

Konigsberg, U. R., Lipton, B. H., and Konigsberg, I. R. (1975). *Dev. Biol.* **45**, 260–275.

Kubo, T., Ikuta, Y., and Tsuge, K. (1976). *Plast. Reconstr. Surg.* **57**, 495–501.

Kuhn, W. E., and Hall, J. L. (1975). *Natl. Bur. Stand. (U.S.), Spec. Publ.* **415**, 91–98.

Lavine, L. S., Lustrin, I., Shamos, M. H., and Moss, M. L. (1971). *Acta Orthop. Scand.* **42**, 305–314.

Le Gros Clark, W. E., and Blomfield, L. B. (1945). *J. Anat.* **79**, 15–32.

Lepheshinskaya, O. B. (1945). "The Origin of Cells from Living Substance and the Role of Living Substance in the Organism." Izd. Akad. Nauk SSSR, Moscow (in Russian).

Levander, G. (1964). "Induction Phenomena in Tissue Regeneration." Williams & Wilkins, Baltimore, Maryland.

Liboff, A. R., and Rinaldi, R. A., eds. (1974). "Electrically Mediated Growth Mechanisms in Living Systems," Ann. N. Y. Acad. Sci., Vol. 238. N. Y. Acad. Sci., New York.

Liozner, L. D., ed. (1960). "Organ Regeneration in Mammals." Medgiz, Moscow (in Russian).

Liozner, L. D. (1974). "Organ Regeneration." Consultants Bureau, New York.

McCrady, E. (1938). "The Embryology of the Opossum," Am. Anat. Mem., No. 16. Wistar Inst. Press, Philadelphia, Pennsylvania.

McMinn, R. M. A. (1969). "Tissue Repair." Academic Press, New York.

Mitskevich, M. S. (1934). *Biol. Zh.* **3**, 20–29.

Mitskevich, M. S. (1936). *Biol. Zh.* **5**, 1055–1072.

Mitskevich, M. S., Stroeva, O. G., and Mitashov, V. I., eds. (1970). "Tissue Metaplasia." Izd. Nauka, Moscow (in Russian).

Mizell, M. (1968). *Science* **161**, 283–286.

Mizell, M., and Isaacs, J. J. (1970). *Am. Zool.* **10**, 141–156.

Neerunjun, J. S., and Dubowitz, V. (1974). *J. Neurol. Sci.* **23**, 505–519.

Nicholas, J. S. (1926). *Proc. Soc. Exp. Biol. Med.* **23**, 436–439.

Oakley, B. (1967). *J. Physiol. (London)* **188**, 353–371.

O'Steen, W. K., Shear, C. R., and Anderson, K. V. (1975). *J. Cell Sci.* **18**, 157–177.

Peterson, E. R., and Crain, S. M. (1972). *Exp. Neurol.* **36**, 136–159.

Polezhaev, L. V. (1972a). "Organ Regeneration in Animals," pp. 28–31. Thomas, Springfield, Illinois.

Polezhaev, L. V. (1972b). "Loss and Restoration of Regenerative Capacity in Tissues and Organs of Animals." Harvard Univ. Press, Cambridge, Massachusetts.

Price, H. M., Howes, E. L., and Blumberg, J. M. (1964). *Lab. Invest.* **13**, 1264–1278.

Rifenberick, D. H., Koski, C. L., and Max, S. R. (1974). *Exp. Neurol.* **45**, 527–540.

Rogal, I. G. (1951). *C. R. Acad. Sci. URSS* **78**, 161–164.

Rusanov, G. A. (1969). "The Restoration of Bone after Transverse Resection of the Diaphysis." Izd. Med., Leningrad.

Salafsky, B. (1971). *Nature (London)* **229**, 270–273.

Scharf, A. (1961). *Growth* **25**, 7–23.

Scharf, A. (1963). *Growth* **27**, 255–269.

Schotté, O. E., and Smith, C. B. (1961). *J. Exp. Zool.* **146**, 209–230.

Schotté, O. E., and Wilber, J. F. (1958). *J. Embryol. Exp. Morphol.* **6**, 247–269.

Simeone, F. E., ed. (1972). *Surg. Clin. North Am.* **52**, 1097–1355.

Singer, M. (1954). *J. Exp. Zool.* **126**, 419–471.

Smith, S. D. (1967). *Anat. Rec.* **158,** 89–98.
Snow, M. H. (1973). *Anat. Rec.* **176,** 185–204.
Snow, M. H. (1977a). *Anat. Rec.* **188,** 181–200.
Snow, M. H. (1977b). *Anat. Rec.* **188,** 201–218.
Spallanzani, A. (1769). "An Essay on Animal Reproductions." London.
Standish, S. M. (1964). *Arch. Pathol.* **77,** 330–339.
Strebkov, V. S. (1966). *In* "Conditions of Regeneration of Organs and Tissues in Animals" (A. A. Voitkevich *et al.,* eds.), pp. 277–281. Moscow (in Russian).
Studitsky, A. N. (1953). *Zh. Obshch. Biol.* **14,** 177–197.
Studitsky, A. N. (1954). *In* "Problems of Restoration of Organs and Tissues in Vertebrates" (G. K. Khruschov, ed.), pp. 138–157. Izdatel. Akad. Nauk SSSR, Moscow (in Russian).
Studitsky, A. N. (1959). "Experimental Surgery of Muscles." Izd. Akad. Nauk SSSR, Moscow (in Russian).
Studitsky, A. N., Zhenevskaya, R. P., and Rumyantseva, O. (1956). *Česk. Morfol.* **4,** 331–340.
Sunderland, S. (1968). "Nerves and Nerve Injuries." Livingstone, Edinburgh.
Tamai, S., Komatsu, S., Sakamoto, H., Sano, S., Sasauchi, N., Hori, Y., Tatsumi, Y., and Okuda, H. (1970). *Plast. Reconstr. Surg.* **46,** 219–225.
Thompson, N. (1971a). *Plast. Reconstr. Surg.* **48,** 11–27.
Thompson, N. (1971b). *Transplantation* **12,** 353–363.
Thompson, N. (1974). *Clin. Plast. Surg.* **1,** 349–403.
Umansky, E. E., and Kudokotsev, V. P. (1952). *Dokl. Akad. Nauk. SSSR* **86,** 437–440.
Urist, M. R. (1965). *Science* **150,** 893–899.
Urist, M. R., Silverman, B. F., Büring, K., Dubuc, F. L., and Rosenberg, J. M. (1967). *Clin. Orthop. Relat. Res.* **53,** 243–283.
Urist, M. R., Dowell, T. A., Hay, P. H., and Strates, B. S. (1968). *Clin. Orthop. Relat. Res.* **59,** 59–96.
Vinogradova, T. P., and Lavrischeva, G. I. (1974). "The Regeneration and Transplantation of Bones." Izd. Med., Moscow (in Russian).
Volkov, M. V. (1955). "Amputation of Limbs in Children." Izd. Med., Moscow (in Russian).
Vorontsova, M. A., and Liosner, L. D. (1960). "Asexual Propagation and Regeneration." Pergamon, Oxford.
Weiss, P., and Hiscoe, H. B. (1948). *J. Exp. Zool.* **107,** 315–395.

19

Pheromones, Estrus, Ovulation, and Mating

WESLEY K. WHITTEN AND ARTHUR K. CHAMPLIN

I. INTRODUCTION

Successful embryologic experiments require a supply of eggs or embryos. Gates (1971) described how to obtain the maximum yield from some strains of mice (*Mus musculus*) by the administration of the gonadotropins PMSG and

HCG. However, for various reasons, some projects require naturally ovulated eggs, and some workers prefer to use natural embryos because they exhibit fewer chromosomal errors (Takagi and Sasaki, 1976). In addition, the response to injected gonadotropins appears to vary with the strain of mouse, as judged by inquiries received at the Jackson Laboratory, as well as with the age and the environment. Some workers report difficulty standardizing the response to gonadotropins, which is not surprising, since there are several variables involved. The variation may be due to the gonadotropins themselves, which, under some conditions, are quite labile. It seems most likely that the hormones are standardized by radioimmunoassays, rather than by ovulation, in mice, which may depend on a different property of the molecule. It should also be remembered that previous treatment with gonadotropins may produce antibodies which could neutralize subsequent doses of the hormones. Perhaps better results will be obtained when synthetic gonadotropin-releasing factors become readily available.

Some of the variation following the administration of gonadotropins may be related to the observation made by Zarrow and his associates (1970) that the response to both gonadotropins may be augmented by a pheromone produced by males. Thus, the response is greater in the females of some strains if they are housed near an adult male.

In this chapter, we will be concerned primarily with mice and will discuss some of the variation that occurs with natural mating as the result of genetic and environmental differences. Our aim is to help select conditions that will produce the greatest number of natural eggs from each strain at times suitable for use. In some strains, these methods may prove to be more efficient than induction by hormones, and, in some, they may be considerably less. We will describe how to recognize animals in estrus, animals that have mated, and animals that will not mate. We will also describe how to determine the time of ovulation and of fertilization, so that stages of embryologic development can be related to the latter and not to the more variable time of copulation.

II. PATTERNS OF REPRODUCTION IN LABORATORY MAMMALS

Most experimental mammals are polyestrous, and so have recurrent short cycles throughout the year. However, this certainly is not the case in natural populations where, for example, the European rabbit (*Oryctolagus cuniculus*) breeds only during those months with lengthening hours of daylight. Other factors such as temperature, humidity, and food supply may restrict breeding in feral animals. The loss of seasonality in breeding in captivity may be due in part to the constant artificial environment of animal houses or to the unwitting selection of animals that are not genetically restricted to seasonal breeding. For example, several strains of laboratory rodents are homozygous for the gene causing retinal degeneration, which could reduce their dependence on light cycles. At the same time, it could make them easier to catch and, thus, appear more tractable.

Continuous breeding in animal houses may be due to the environmental effects acting on both sexes, but, as we become more aware of the dialogue of signals that goes on between the sexes, we may find that the environmental change is acting only on members of one sex and the other sex is reflecting that change.

Asdell (1946) considered that there were two distinct patterns of mammalian reproduction: spontaneous ovulation and induced or reflex ovulation. The golden hamster (*Mesocricetus auratus*) is an example of the former, because under normal diurnal light cycles it ovulates and exhibits estrus every 4 days. The model for induced ovulation is the rabbit because most females that have been in isolation copulate soon after pairing with a male, and ovulation ensues about 10½ hours later. A similar sequence takes place in the ferret (*Mustela putorius furo*) and the cat (*Felis domestica*).

These patterns of ovulation are not as fixed as was originally thought, and induced ovulation may be an artifact resulting from the isolation. Most rats (*Rattus norvegicus*) living in the normal light–dark sequence ovulate spontaneously every 4 or 5 days. However, some strains can be converted to induced ovulators by exposure to constant light (Everett, 1964). A similar change may occur in some mice following blinding.

Even in spontaneously ovulating rodents, copulation or artificial cervical stimulation induces a change in the pattern of release of hormones from the pituitary. Prolactin is released with a semicircadian rhythm, apparently to initiate and maintain functional corpora lutea (Freeman *et al.*, 1974; Butcher *et al.*, 1974). The next crop of follicles is prevented from maturing at 4 or 5 days, and the endocrine state of pregnancy or pseudopregnancy is established.

Much of the stimulus for the hormone release is provided by the penis, and it may be difficult to induce an equivalent release by artifical probes in mice, even when electrically vibrated (Diamond, 1970). Therefore, if one wishes to obtain suitable pseudopregnant foster mothers as recipients for cultured embryos, it is advisable to use vasectomized or genetically sterilized males of a vigorous strain or hybrid. Presumably, these animals cause sufficient arousal by other tactile, visual, or olfactory pathways to effect an adequate release of hormones.

From the foregoing, it should be apparent that rats, mice, and hamsters do not normally have a luteal phase in their short 4–6 day cycles, and that fully functional corpora lutea depend on mating and occur only during pregnancy and pseudopregnancy. However, in some instances, pseudopregnancies are observed in grouped females, and may result from mutual stimulation, such as the "riding" seen with females of some strains.

The light–dark sequence is the major modulator in spontaneously ovulating animals, and the critical periods of hypothalmic activity have been worked out for the rat (Everett, 1964). Whitten and Dagg (1961) showed that ovulation took place 3–5 hours after the midpoint of the dark period in BALB/c and 129 mice. Fertilization should follow soon after, but, in some strains, it is delayed several hours. We maintain 14 hours of light and 10 hours of dark in our animal rooms. The lights come on at 5 A.M. and go off at 7 P.M. unless we wish to obtain ovulation and fertilization during normal working hours. In this case, we delay the cycle for 3 hours and use a room without any windows.

It is not known whether stimuli from the male, especially those received during copulation, alter the time of ovulation in rats or mice. One could expect that it would speed up the process and perhaps even increase the clutch size. Copulation could theoretically advance ovulation by a whole 24 hours, or perhaps it would be more correct to say that, in its absence, ovulation may be delayed 1 or even 2 days.

III. THE ROLE OF PHEROMONES

Pheromones were first studied and identified in insects, and their importance in mammals has only recently become established [see Whitten (1966) and Whitten and Champlin (1973) for reviews and references]. Even so, the role of pheromones that attract partners or initiate behavioral responses is very difficult to establish in such complex animals that learn to associate stimuli remarkably quickly. This is particularly true in primates. However, some recent work has shown that male hamsters only approach females after receiving an olfactory cue from dimethyl disulfide, which is a constituent of the vaginal pouch secretion only during estrus (Singer et al., 1976). In addition to their role in mating, pheromones are also important for the recognition and retrieval of young, and for stimulating mothering in several species.

As far as we know, the mouse is the only common laboratory mammal in which primer pheromones—those which act directly on the endocrine system—are important in reproduction. Two pheromones, one stimulating and the other depressing the reproductive cycles, appear to be important in many strains. There may also be a pheromone in both rats and mice which stimulates hormone production in males (Macrides et al., 1975; Maruniak and Bronson, 1976).

A. Pheromones Produced by Males

Male mice produce a pheromone in their urine which causes the release of gonadotropins from the pituitaries of females of some strains of mice (Bronson and Stetson, 1973). The action of this pheromone is not to cause the rupture of existing large follicles, but rather to stimulate the growth of smaller follicles. Thus, depending on the condition of the females that receive the pheromone, it may shorten their cycles, advance the appearance of the first cycle of immature animals, or under special circumstances, induce a new crop of follicles in recently mated animals and, thus, block an established pregnancy. We will consider the importance of each of these phenomena in later sections. Much remains to be learned about the stability and structure of pheromones. For some reason, it appears that the females must be exposed to the substance or substances for a considerable portion of the time (48 hours) during which the response develops. Thus, repeated application is necessary to obtain any responses with urine preparations.

B. Pheromones Produced by Females

Several workers have found that females housed in groups, remote from males, exhibit various degrees of inhibition of their estrous cycles. This may take the form of an extension of the diestrous phase of the cycle (Lamond, 1959; Champlin, 1971), the spontaneous induction of pseudopregnancy (van der Lee and Boot, 1955, 1956; Dewar, 1959; Mody, 1963). or the occurrence of anestrus throughout the entire experimental period of 40 days (Whitten, 1958).

Vandenbergh and his associates (1971) showed that puberty was delayed in young females housed with only female cage partners. The reasons for concluding that these effects are produced by pheromones are discussed by Whitten and Champlin (1973). One of the important findings is that females with suppressed cycles are very susceptible to the action of the pheromone from males. Thus, when the two pheromones act in sequence, a peak in the incidence of estrus occurs on the 3rd night after exposure to the male pheromone. This will be discussed in the next section.

IV. THE EXPLOITATION OF PHEROMONAL EFFECTS

In suitably designed animal quarters with light control and small individually ventilated rooms, it is possible to exploit the effects of pheromones to obtain large enough batches of eggs, at any desired stage, for experiments during normal working hours. Likewise, it is possible to arrange for suitable numbers of pseudopregnant females to act as hosts for embryos when required.

A. Synchronization of Mating and Ovulation on the Third Night

A number of studies have demonstrated a peak incidence of fertile mating on the 3rd night after females are paired with males (Whitten, 1956, 1959). This apparent synchrony of estrus has been shown to be due to an acceleration of estrous cycling induced by the presence of a male mouse (Whitten, 1958), and more specifically to a pheromonal component of his urine (Marsden and Bronson, 1964). Although a significant peak of mating on the 3rd night can be obtained by pairing individually caged females with males, a peak of greater magnitude can be achieved by caging the females in groups away from male odors for several days prior to pairing (Fig. 1).

Not all strains of mice show this kind of estrous synchrony. Table I gives a listing of the strains from the production colonies at the Jackson Laboratory in which significant 3rd night peaks in mating and ovulation have been found when previously grouped females are paired with males. SJL/J females give the best response of any of the inbred strains tested. It is probable that the lack of synchrony in other strains is not due to the absence of the accelerating pheromone(s) in the urine of the males of those strains, but to the inability of the females to perceive or react physiologically to the pheromonal stimulus (W. K. Whitten and W. G. Beamer, unpublished).

Although few of the inbred strains respond with a 3rd night peak, peaks are evident in several of the noninbred strains in common use. Land and McLaren (1967) reported up to 75% of Q mice mated on the 3rd night, and Ross (1961, 1962) observed about 50% with Parkes TO and Dutch mice. Similar proportions

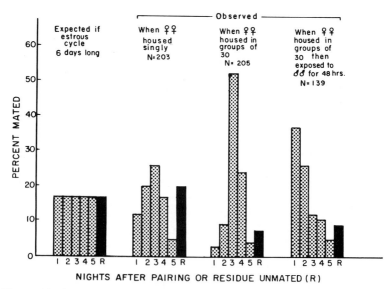

Fig. 1. The frequency distribution of mating for the first 5 nights after pairing of Walter and Eliza Hall mice. (From Whitten, 1956, 1959.)

TABLE I

**Breeding Data from Jackson Laboratory Production Colony Showing Synchrony
of Mating on the Third Night after Pairing[a]**

Strain	No.	Night 1		Night 2		Night 3		Night 4	
		Mated (%)	Pregnant (%)	Mated (%)	Pregnant (%)	Mated (%)	Pregnant (%)	Mated (%)	Pregnant (%)
SJL/J	98	5.1	60.0	13.3	53.9	41.8	58.5	5.1	40.0
BALB/cJ	238	25.6	39.3	14.3	44.1	29.4	44.3	10.9	30.8
RF/J	58	20.7	66.7	15.5	66.7	25.9	60.0	6.9	0.0
AKR/J	810	8.8	80.3	10.3	78.3	21.1	70.8	11.9	46.9
C3H/HeJ	142	12.7	83.3	9.9	100.0	17.6	76.0	20.2	62.1

[a] From Jax Notes, No. 416, November, 1973.

were obtained by Whitten with (SJL × SWR)F$_1$ and with Walter and Eliza Hall mice, and by Beilhartz (1968) with an unidentified strain.

B. Synchronization of Mating and Ovulation on the First Night

The peak of mating activity can be shifted to the 1st night after pairing by exposing grouped females to confined males or their urine for 2 days before pairing (Whitten, 1956; see Fig. 1). By using this technique, an investigator can obtain a large number of recently mated females with naturally ovulated eggs on the 1st night after pairing with males, and the unmated females can be returned to stock for use in 10–14 days (Ross, 1962).

C. Advancement of Puberty

Castro (1967) and Vandenbergh (1969) observed that female mice exhibited their first estrus and ovulated at an earlier age in the presence of a male or his urine. This appears to be another and, perhaps, the main action of the male pheromone in wild animals. In a manner probably similar to the suppression of cycles by females in a group, puberty is delayed when young females are housed only in the presence of females. In those strains that are susceptible to the pheromonal action of males, it is often necessary to wean the young before they are 28 days old; otherwise, they are inseminated by their fathers.

Early insemination may be an advantage under certain conditions. For example, the mutation *an* causes anemia and a progressive depletion of germ cells, and, unless homozygous females become pregnant early, the store of germ cells is reduced to levels incompatible with fertility (see Green, 1966).

D. Production of Regular Short Cycles

Whitten (1956) showed that the cycles of Walter and Eliza Hall mice were shorter and much more regular in the presence of a male. When one is selecting females in estrus for mating with stud males or for artificial insemination, one can get a constant supply of such animals from a smaller colony if the females are housed with confined males or exposed to male urine (Ross, 1961, 1962). This procedure will, of course, only work in those strains which respond to the male pheromone.

E. Increasing the Clutch Size

Beilhartz (1968) examined the litter size of mice and observed that those which could be related to mating on the 3rd night were larger by approximately one. From this, he argued that the male induced surge of gonadotropin induced estrus and also increased the clutch size. We (W. K. Whitten and P. A. Chisholm, unpublished) confirmed this finding when we counted the eggs shed by mice caged in groups and then paired with males at metestrus or proestrus. Further work needs to be done with this phenomenon, but our results indicated an additional two eggs were shed by those paired in metestrus and, thus, exposed to the male pheromone for the longest period before ovulation.

F. Pregnancy Block and Related Phenomena

Bruce (1959) observed that when a recently mated female mouse of the Parkes strain was exposed to an alien male, the female continued to cycle as though she had not been inseminated. The embryos of the first mating were transported rapidly through the reproductive tract and probably lost to the exterior with secretions accompaning estrus. This interesting phenomenon, which she called pregnancy block, is rare among mouse strains, but Chapman and Whitten (1969) and Hoppe and Whitten (1972) observed something similar in SJL and BALB/c females. Pregnancy block was not present in C57BL/10 animals or in (SJL × C57BL/10)F_1 hybrids, which suggested genetic control of the phenomenon, but the role of heterosis was not excluded. Hoppe and Whitten (1972) showed that the effect could be imitated by a small dose of gonadotropin (PMSG) and that susceptible animals required a smaller dose. Runner (1959) and Chipman and Fox (1966) observed that handling could upset pregnancy, and experience with timed pregnancies at the Jackson Laboratory supports this finding. Many pregnancies were lost in mice shipped during early pregnancy.

The findings indicate that mice should be handled as little as possible during the first 10 days of pregnancy and not placed near males of other strains. We prefer to leave the females with the stud as long as possible unless the males are particularly randy. The findings also suggest that strains or hybrids resistant to pregnancy block and handling effects should be used as hosts for transferred embryos.

V. MATING AND OVULATION SOON AFTER PAIRING

In recent years, it has become clear that the females from some strains of inbred mice show a marked peak in mating activity, accompanied by ovulation on the 1st night after pairing with a male mouse. This has been examined in our laboratories using BALB/cWt and C57BL/10Wt females with SJL/Wt males (Champlin and Whitten, 1977), and is summarized here.

Mature females of both strains were housed either individually or in groups of four for a period of 2 weeks in a room free of male mouse odors before pairing with males. Pairing was done during the midafternoon, and the females were checked for the presence of a vaginal plug, indicating mating, each morning for 5 days. When mating had occurred, the female was left with her mate until the next day, when she was killed and her oviducts flushed with physiological saline to obtain ovulated eggs and embryos. The developmental stage of the embryos obtained allowed the investigators to determine the date on which the eggs had been ovulated.

In both strains, a significant number of females both mated and ovulated on the 1st night after pairing (Fig. 2). Individual caging of the females before pairing resulted in a marked increase in the size of the 1st night peak of both mating and ovulation in BALB/cWt females when compared to those housed in groups. Such an increase in mating activity was not observed in singly caged C57BL/10Wt females when compared to grouped females of the same strain. The physiological basis for this rapid induction of mating and ovulation, which is particularly apparent in singly caged BALB/cWt females, and the nature of the inducing stimulus, have yet to be determined. This observation recalls the reflex ovulation known to take place when isolated female rabbits or ferrets are paired with males.

Data from the production colonies at the Jackson Laboratory (Table II) show that the 1st night peak in reproductive activity is found in strains other than those studied in our laboratory. These data were gathered from previously grouped females mated to males of the same strain. The magnitude of the 1st night peak is, in all cases, less than that seen in previously grouped BALB/cWt or C57BL/10Wt females in our laboratory. These differences may be due to procedural differences in the way the animals were housed prior to mating. The production colony females were housed in groups of up to 20 females per cage in colony rooms containing males. Our females were caged either individually or in groups of four in a room free of males and their odors. Further, the production data measures ovulation at mating in terms of the number of females that were

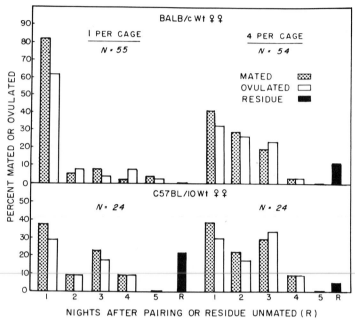

Fig. 2. The frequency distribution of mating for the first 5 nights after pairing of BALB/cWt and C57BL/10Wt mice held singly or in groups of four. SJL/Wt males were used. (From A. K. Champlin and W. K. Whitten, 1977.)

TABLE II

Breeding Data from Jackson Laboratory Production Colony Showing Spontaneous Synchrony of Mating on the First Night after Pairing[a]

		Night 1		Night 2		Night 3		Night 4	
Strain	No.	Mated (%)	Pregnant (%)	Mated (%)	Pregnant (%)	Mated (%)	Pregnant (%)	Mated (%)	Pregnant (%)
BALB/cJ	238	25.6	39.3	14.3	44.1	29.4	44.3	10.9	30.8
C57BL/6J	520	25.4	46.2	6.9	38.9	15.0	69.2	9.2	68.8
C57BL/10J	84	25.0	38.1	9.5	62.5	16.7	64.3	3.6	0.0
C57BL/10Sn	126	20.6	65.8	10.3	69.3	12.7	50.0	4.0	20.0
C58/J	162	23.5	57.9	13.6	59.1	13.6	15.1	13.6	40.9
C57BR/cdJ	218	16.1	91.4	6.4	85.7	7.3	87.5	4.1	55.6

[a] From Jax Notes, No. 416, November, 1973.

pregnant by palpation, while our study judged ovulation time by the condition of the eggs obtained from each female on the day after a vaginal plug was found.

We have yet to determine whether the time of ovulation in these animals that mate on the 1st night is directly related to copulation, rather than to the end of the dark phase of the diurnal cycle. Mice normally commence to mate in the early evening, but we have indications that the BALB/c animals may copulate soon after pairing.

VI. OTHER USEFUL TECHNIQUES

A. Staging of the Estrous Cycle

Naturally ovulated eggs from timed matings can be obtained by selecting females that are in proestrus from a colony and pairing them individually with males. The determination of estrous stage can be accomplished by one of two methods.

The vaginal smear technique has been the accepted procedure for determining the estrous state in mammals since the initial study of the estrous cycle in the guinea pig by Stockard and Papanicolaou in 1917. The technique utilizes the changes in cell type and their relative frequencies that occur in the vaginal walls during a normal estrous cycle. A small sample of cells from the vaginal epithelium and contents is obtained by lavage or gentle scraping. The cell types and relative frequencies are then identified microscopically to determine the stage of estrus. This technique and the cellular changes observed have been described in a number of publications, including Snell (1941) for the mouse.

We prefer to take a single scraping gently from the dorsal wall of the vagina as described by Emmens (1950). This has the advantage of being a biopsy, rather than a sample of the cellular debris in the vagina, as is the case with the vaginal lavage methods. We examine the smears dry and unstained because mucin, which is the best indicator of diestrus or pseudopregnancy, may be lost during processing.If the spatula fails to collect any significant amount of material, the process is not repeated because of the risk of inducing cornification and because the absence of cells is a good sign of diestrus.

Although widely used, the technique is not without disadvantages. Frequent vaginal smearing has been found to result in an abnormally high incidence of estrouslike smears (Wade and Doisy, 1935), and may induce pseudopregnancy or abnormally long estrous cycles in some species. Although basically a simple technique, vaginal smearing does involve several steps between the obtaining of a sample from the vagina and the identification of the estrous stage. Clearly, an error in identification of a given sample could be made between any of the steps, particularly when smears are being obtained from a large number of females.

Allen (1922) first reported that gross changes in the appearance of the vagina during the estrous cycle were readily observed in the mouse. These easily observable changes have been further described by Champlin *et al.* (1973) and serve as the basis for a visual method of identification of the estrous stages in mice. This technique has been used in our laboratories for a number of years and has proven to be as reliable as vaginal smearing. It does not involve mechanical manipulation of the vaginal tract and, thereby, avoids the possibility of inducing cornification of the vaginal epithelium. Furthermore, it is more rapid than the smearing technique, is a single-step process, and eliminates the possiblity that bacteria, pheromones, or other components of the vaginal tract will be transferred from one animal to the next.

The visual method utilizes changes in the size of the vaginal opening, the degree of vaginal swelling, the color and moistness of the tissues, and the presence or absence of obvious cellular debris within the vagina to determine the estrous stage. The appearance of the vagina at each stage of the estrous cycle is described in Table III, and photographs in color can be seen in the original article (Champlin *et al.*, 1973).

Similar vaginal changes are seen in all strains of mice that have been examined. Some differences do exist between strains, particularly with respect to vaginal size and coloration. The latter criterion is more easily observed in albino or lightly pigmented strains than in heavily pigmented strains, where pigmentation of the skin tends to slightly mask the color changes described in Table III.

We have found this visual method to be extremely useful in the selection of female mice in proestrus to be mated on a given night for timed matings, the collection of naturally ovulated eggs, and for the routine determination of estrous stages in mice.

TABLE III
Appearance of the Vagina at Various Stages of the Estrous Cycle[a]

Estrous stage	Appearance
Diestrus	Vagina has a small opening and the tissues are bluish-purple in color and very moist.
Proestrus	Vagina is gaping and the tissues are reddish-pink and moist. Numerous longitudinal folds or striations are visible on both the dorsal and ventral lips.
Estrus	Vaginal signs are similar to proestrus, but the tissues are lighter pink and less moist, and the striations are more pronounced.
Metestrus 1	Vaginal tissues are pale and dry. Dorsal lip is not as edematous as in estrus.
Metestrus 2	Vaginal signs are similar to metestrus 1, but the lip is less edematous and has receded. Whitish cellular debris may line the inner walls or partially fill the vagina.

[a] Champlin *et al.* (1973).

Estrus or receptivity can, of course, be determined by observing whether or not the female will permit a male to mount her. This applies to laboratory species other than mice, and a typical lordotic response has been described for the rat by Boling and Blandau (1939). This response can be evoked in suitable animals simply by stroking the female's back. In guinea pigs, the vagina is normally closed, and vaginal opening takes place at or near estrus. The female hamster produces an malodorous secretion from the lateral pouches of the vagina containing a pheromone that releases sex-related activity in males (Singer *et al.*, 1976). In the rabbit, the vaginal mucosa of a receptive female is engorged, and she is more apt to spray the quarters with urine when disturbed.

B. Finding Copulation Plugs

The finding of a copulation plug is the criterion commonly used to infer that pregnancy has commenced, and from which gestation time is calculated. The plug results from the cross-bonding of proteins derived from the seminal vesicles and catalyzed by enzymes from the coagulating gland. The plug is a hard horny mass that may be seen or felt with the aid of a probe in the vagina. We use a dentist's plastic instrument with a blade 5-mm long or a moistened toothpick. The latter can be used once and discarded and, thus, does not transfer secretions from one mouse to the next. It is possible that, in many mice, one or even two plugs are superimposed upon the first, so that a third plug is seen to overfill the vaginal orifice. Occasionally, one finds a misplaced plug in the anus. Some males are not capable of producing plugs, or perhaps even of mating on successive nights (see Section VII below), and even vigorous males may be overextended if caged with two or more females. Plugs may not occur in females with imperforate vagina or thick vertical bands of tissue dividing the vaginal orifice (Cunliffe-Beamer and Feldman, 1977).

C. Timing Ovulation and Fertilization

Ovulation of a clutch of eggs probably takes about 1 hour, and can be determined by slaughtering groups of estrous animals at various times after the middle of the dark period or after copulation and examining the ampullae for eggs. There will be variation between individual animals and between eggs within the same animal. Nevertheless, a meaningful estimate of the time of ovulation can be obtained in this manner (Whitten and Dagg, 1961).

It is obvious that fertilization is the start of embryonic development, and its use as the reference point, with the time given in hours, would eliminate the confusion resulting from the disagreement as to whether the plug is found on day 0 or day 1. The time of fertilization can be determined by collecting clutches of eggs as described above, removing the cumulus cells with hyaluronidase, washing them thoroughly to remove any adherent sperm, and then setting up the clutch in culture (Whitten, 1971). Those eggs that develop two pronuclei and discharge polar bodies can be considered fertilized, or at least to have been penetrated by sperm. By plotting the proportion of each clutch fertilized against the time of collection, an estimate of the time of fertilization can be obtained.

VII. MALE PERFORMANCE

Males of the SJL inbred strain are capable of producing vaginal plugs on each of 5 successive nights if presented with estrous females. In contrast, C57BL/10 males will not mate more frequently than every 4th night (P. C. Hoppe, unpublished). In contrast, vigorous F_1 hybrid males will torment inbred females, and frequent deaths have been observed. Some male mice will rape females, particularly if they have been conditioned to receive into their cage only receptive proestrous females. Mating records from these animals must be checked for evidence of ovulation. In practice, we try to use our inbred males once a week, and we house stud males or males to be used for sperm studies individually for at least 2 weeks because the sperm quality appears better.

VIII. SUMMARY

Methods for the detection of estrus, mating, ovulation, and fertilization in mice have been described. Genetic and environmental factors that influence the estrous cycle have been discussed. Particular emphasis has been placed on pheromones and on the way in which these can be exploited to provide embryos for experiments on one of several desired schedules.

ACKNOWLEDGMENTS

This research was supported by NIH Research Grant HD 04083 from the National Institute of Child Health and Human Development, and a National Sciences grant from Colby College.

REFERENCES

Allen, E. (1922). *Am. J. Anat.* **30**, 297–371.
Asdell, S. A. (1946). *In* "Patterns of Mammalian Reproduction," 1st ed., pp. 15–16. Comstock,
Beilharz, R. G. (1968). *Aust. J. Biol. Sci.* **21**, 583–585.
Boling, T. L., and Blandau, R. T. (1939). *Endocrinology* **25**, 359–364.
Bronson, F., and Stetson, M. H. (1973). *Biol. Reprod.* **9**, 449–459.

Bruce, H. M. (1959). *Nature (London)* **184,** 105.
Butcher, R. L., Fugo, N. W., and Collins, W. E. (1974). *Endocrinology* **90,** 1125–1127.
Castro, B. M. (1967). *An. Acad. Bras. Cienc.* **39,** 289–291.
Champlin, A. K. (1971). *J. Reprod. Fertil.* **27,** 233–241.
Champlin, A. K., and Whitten, W. K. (1977). In preparation.
Champlin, A. K., Dorr, D. L., and Gates, A. H. (1973). *Biol. Reprod.* **8,** 491–494.
Chapman, V. M., and Whitten, W. K. (1969). *Genetics* **61,** S9 (abstr.).
Chipman, R. K., and Fox, K. A. (1966). *J. Reprod. Fertil.* **12,** 233–236.
Cunliffe-Beamer, T. L., and Feldman, B. D. (1977). *Lab. Anim. Sci.* **26,** 895–898.
Dewar, A. D. (1959). *J. Endocrinol.* **18,** 186–190.
Diamond, M. (1970). *Science* **169,** 995–997.
Emmens, C. W. (1950). In ''Hormone Assay'' (C. W. Emmens, ed.), pp. 391–417. Academic Press, New York.
Everett, J. W. (1964). *Physiol. Rev.* **44,** 373–431.
Freeman, M. E., Smith, M. S., Nazion, S. J., and Neill, J. D. (1974). *Endocrinology* **94,** 875–882.
Gates, A. H. (1971). In ''Methods in Mammalian Embryology'' (J. C. Daniel, Jr., ed.), pp. 64–75. Freeman, San Francisco, California.
Green, M. C. (1966). In ''Biology of the Laboratory Mouse'' (E. L. Green, ed.), 2nd Edit., pp. 87–150. McGraw-Hill, New York.
Hoppe, P. C., and Whitten, W. K. (1972). *Biol. Reprod.* **7,** 254–259.
Lamond, D. R. (1959). *J. Endocrinol.* **18,** 343–349.
Land, R. B., and McLaren. A. (1967). *J. Reprod. Fertil.* **13,** 321–327.
Macrides, F., Bartke, A., and Dalterio. S. (1975). *Science* **189,** 1104.
Marsden, H. M., and Bronson, F. H. (1964). *Science* **144,** 1469.
Maruniak, J. A., and Bronson, F. H. (1976). *Endocrinology* **99,** 963–969.
Mody, J. K. (1963). *Anat. Rec.* **145,** 439–447.
Ross, M. (1961). *J. Anim. Tech. Assoc.* **12,** 1–8.
Ross, M. (1962). *J. Anim. Tech. Assoc.* **13,** 1–4.
Runner, M. (1959). *Anat. Rec.* **133,** 330–331.
Singer, A. G., Agosta, W. C., O'Connell, R. J., Pfaffmann, C., Bowen, D. V., and Field, F. H. (1976). *Science* **191,** 948–950.
Snell, G. D. (1941). In ''Biology of the Laboratory Mouse'' (G. D. Snell, ed.), pp. 55–88. McGraw-Hill (Blakiston), New York.
Stockard, C. R., and Papanicolaou, G. N. (1917). *Am. J. Anat.* **22,** 225–283.
Takagi, N., and Sasaki, M. (1976). *Nature (London)* **264,** 278–281.
Vandenbergh, J. G. (1969). *Endocrinology* **84,** 658–660.
Vandenbergh, J. G., Drickamer, L. C., and Colby, D. R. (1971). *J. Reprod. Fertil.* **28,** 397–405.
van der Lee, S., and Boot, L. M. (1955). *Acta Physiol. Pharmacol. Neerl.* **4,** 442–443.
van der Lee, S., and Boot, L. M. (1956). II. *Acta Physiol. Pharmacol. Neerl.* **5,** 213–214.
Wade, N. J., and Doisy, E. A. (1935). *Proc. Soc. Exp. Biol. Med.* **32,** 707–709.
Whitten, W. K. (1956). *J. Endocrinol.* **13,** 399–404.
Whitten, W. K. (1958). *J. Endocrinol.* **17,** 307–313.
Whitten, W. K. (1959). *J. Endocrinol.* **18,** 102–107.
Whitten, W. K. (1966). *Adv. Reprod. Physiol.* **1,** 155–177.
Whitten, W. K. (1971). *Adv. Biosci.* **6,** 317–340.
Whitten, W. K., and Champlin, A. K. (1973). *Handb. Physiol., Sect. 7: Endocrinol.* **2,** Part 1, 109–123.
Whitten, W. K., and Dagg, C. P. (1961). *J. Exp. Zool.* **148,** 173–183.
Zarrow, M. X., Estes, S. A., Denenberg, V. H., and Clark, J. H. (1970). *J. Reprod. Fertil.* **23,** 357–360.

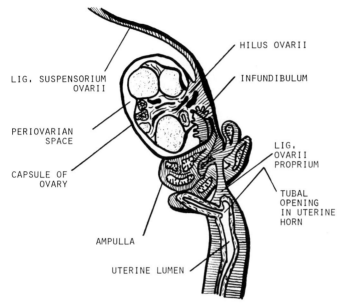

HILUS OVARII

INFUNDIBULUM

LIG, SUSPENSORIUM
OVARII

PERIOVARIAN
SPACE

LIG,
OVARII
PROPRIUM

CAPSULE OF
OVARY

TUBAL
OPENING
IN UTERINE
HORN

AMPULLA

UTERINE LUMEN

Fig. 1. Anatomy of the ovarian region in the mouse. The uterine horn with tubal opening on the tubal collicle is seen in the lowermost part of the drawing. Note entrance of the infundibular end of the tube into the ovarian capsule (bursa ovarii) lying freely around the ovary.

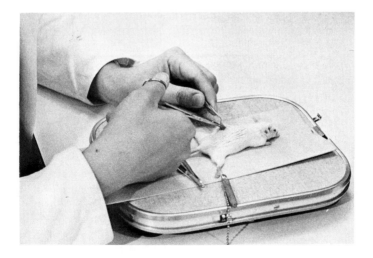

Fig. 2. A midline dorsal incision is cut, and the abdominal cavity is reached lateral to the back muscles, whereby the periovarian fat is easily grasped.

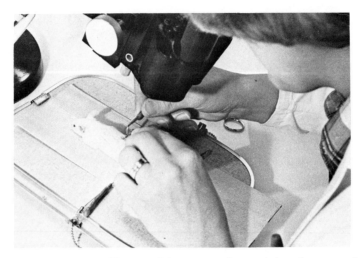

Fig. 3. The ovary is then lifted out of the torn capsule, care being taken not to disturb the infundibular region of the tube as it enters into the periovarian (subcapsular) space. Of utmost importance is the complete removal of the ovary, since even very minute remnants of ovarian tissue may be sufficient to yield estrogen-inducing implantations.

of the tube, particular attention should be paid not to stretch the ovarian bursa adjacent to the fimbrial opening. After removal of the ovary, the grasped uterine horn is cautiously dropped into the abdominal cavity from the dorsal aspect, and the same procedure is carried out in the other horn. The back skin is then closed with agraffes. The animal is never visibly disturbed by the dorsal incision or by the agraffes.

Postoperatively, the mouse is given progesterone, around 1 mg subcutaneously, or a long-acting progestagen (e.g., medroxyprogesterone). The former drug is repeated daily in the same dose, while the latter is given only once if the desired delay is not unusually long (within day 10 or so). In long-standing delay, a complementary dose of medroxyprogesterone is advisable (Dickson, 1969a). The critical dose level for the maintenance of implantation delay seems to be around 0.8 mg progesterone daily (Smith, 1968). There is no evidence of implantation-inducing effect of progesterone in this dose range, while some evidence indicates that there may be an implantation induction with higher doses (McLaren, 1971). Data are, however, contradictory on this point (Humphrey, 1967). Certainly, as we have noted, some commercially available progesterone preparations are crude and may contain estrogenic contaminations in concentrations that are far beyond the minimum dose for implantation induction. Progesterone preparations designed for use in the human are usually not pure enough for the maintenance of implantation delay. Omission of progesterone postopera-

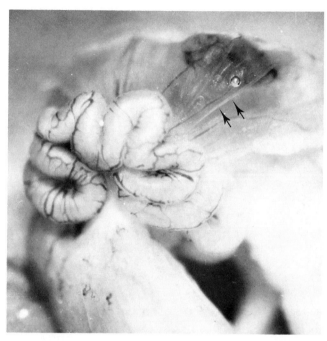

Fig. 4. Microscopic view of the periovarian anatomy in the mouse. Uppermost the ovary lies in close connection with the adjacent tube. Folds in the ovarian capsule (arrows) expose the thin capsule, through which the ovarian surface is barely visible. The coiled appearance of the tube conceals the uterotubal junction. The uterine horn is lowermost.

tively means a risk of viability decline. No maintenance of delay nor steady-state delay is achieved if progesterone is omitted temporarily. Viability decline of blastocysts is significant rather soon after omission of progesterone (Kirby, 1971). The decline in viability can be followed by a nearly parallel change in blastocyst surface ultrastructure. By observations of the imprint pattern of the trophoblast cell surfaces, the viability decline can be followed in terms of vanishing "craterlike" imprints (Bergström, 1972a). The physiological events reflected in the altered blastocyst morphology may be related to a deficient luminal environment due to the disappearance of apical protrusions from the uterine epithelium (Bergström and Nilsson, 1972), cf. Figs. 5 and 6.

Tube-locking in combination with experimental delay will make it possible to study the influence of the tubal environment upon morula/blastocyst. The uterine influence can then be ruled out, and systemic administration of hormones may reveal the extent to which the hormonal effects upon the blastocyst are mediated via the endometrium. Technical precautions in this type of experimental delay involve hypophysectomy, since surgical removal of the ovaries will make scar-

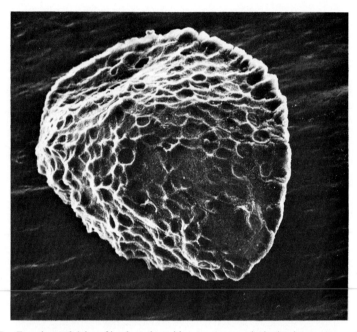

Fig. 5. Experimental delay of implantation with progesterone substitution in a mouse on day 7 of pregnancy. Scanning electron micrograph of mouse blastocyst. Note numerous imprints covering the trophoblast surface and representing a negative replica of the apical area of the apposing uterine epithelium. × 850.

ring and adhesions inevitable around the tubes. Tube-locked embryos can then hardly be rinsed out of the tube. On the other hand, there may be minute hormonal release from the ovaries reaching the tube, thereby making the contralateral side unsuitable for control purposes (Weitlauf, 1971).

B. Experimental Aspects

The availability of experimental implantation delay has had an obvious impact on our knowledge of the hormonal regulation of implantation. Functionally—by way of metabolic studies—and structurally—by way of morphologic studies—experimental delay has been used for detailed hour-by-hour studies of the effects of various hormones on the dormant blastocyst.

Protein synthesis has been studied in detail by Weitlauf and his co-workers in blastocysts both during "normal" pregnancy and during delayed implantation. By incorporation studies of labeled amino acids, they could show that little or no protein is synthesized in the blastocyst during implantation delay in relation to

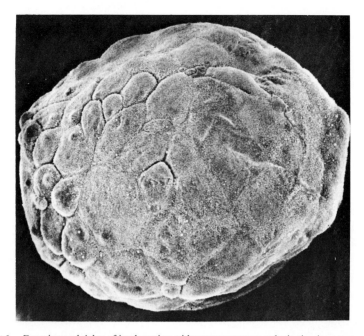

Fig. 6. Experimental delay of implantation without progesterone substitution in a mouse on day 18 of pregnancy. Scanning electron micrograph of mouse blastocyst. Note absence of imprints and visible individual trophoblast cells. (cf. Fig. 5). × 750. From Bergström and Nilsson (1972) by permission.

normal pregnancy (Weitlauf and Greenwald, 1965, 1968). The depressed metabolic activity during delay is obvious also in various *in vitro* experiments demonstrating a much slower incorporation of label in delayed than in "normal" blastocysts upon explantation (Weitlauf, 1973). The dependency of the blastocyst *in utero* upon the uterine environment concerning amino acid incorporation was shown by transfer of normal blastocysts to spayed recipients, in which "incorporation dormancy" could be induced by the transfer (Weitlauf, 1969). In relation to morphological surface changes, the attainment of a "steady state" seems to occur earlier during implantation delay concerning the level of embryonic protein, the latter reaching a fairly steady level already in the afternoon of day 5 (Weitlauf, 1973), while the corresponding constancy in morphology occurs about 2 days later (Bergström, 1972a).

Carbohydrate metabolism has been studied by measuring the production of CO_2 labeled by ^{14}C after incubation of blastocysts in medium containing ^{14}C-labeled glucose. Assuming that this rate of production reflects the rate of aerobic carbohydrate metabolism, CO_2 measurements indicate that delayed blastocysts decline in carbohydrate metabolism fairly soon after ovariectomy (Menke and

McLaren, 1970a). Progesterone administration to such mice decrease the metabolic rate still further (Menke and McLaren, 1970b). A significant difference of this kind in spayed mice could not be reproduced by others (Torbit and Weitlauf, 1974). The deletion of progesterone upon spaying (Fig. 6) may have more evident late effects than early ones, since both viability and morphology differences appear 1–2 weeks after the attainment of the steady state in surface morphology (Bergström, 1972a).

Structural changes in the blastocyst accompanying the first days after spaying (with concomitant progesterone) essentially parallel the changes occurring in normal pregnancy. The first sign of delayed development is a delayed shedding of the zona pellucida. Late on day 4, about half of the blastocysts in normal pregnancy have shed their zonae, while none or very few blastocysts from experimentally delayed animals have done so (Bergström, 1972c). As late as in the afternoon of day 5, about one-tenth of delayed blastocysts are still zona-encased, while none or very few blastocysts from normal pregnancy are so. The pattern of zona-shedding appears otherwise to be similar to that of normal pregnancy as followed by light and scanning electron microscopy. The cracked zonae in delayed implanting mice seem to remain unaffected but empty in the vicinity of its blastocyst in a closed uterine lumen. The attainment of a luminal closure upon progesterone treatment after spaying (Martin *et al.,* 1970; Hedlund and Nilsson, 1971) is the basis for the morphological features characteristic for the steady state in blastocyst surface ultrastructure. Strangely enough, studies still appear on uterine fluid during delayed implantation in spite of the well-established fact that there is no such fluid whatsoever because of the luminal attachment reaction, whereby a complete obliteration of the lumen takes place.

Ultrastructural changes of trophoblast cells specific of implantation delay can be observed soon after zona pellucida shedding on day 5. Interestingly, this blastocyst category—on its way to the steady state in ultrastructure from about day 7 onward—is morphologically similar to the blastocyst category on its way from the steady state under early influence of estrogen. Thus, "deactivation" and "reactivation" of blastocysts seem to mean similar changes in surface morphology of trophoblast cells. The constancy in morphology attained a couple of days later (Fig. 5) is preceded by transition stages of blastocyst development with features in common with both deactivation and steady-state blastocysts (Bergström, 1972a,b). The gradually more closely apposing epithelia force the malleable trophoblast cell membranes to approach the outline of the apical surface of the endometrium, thereby giving the enclosed blastocyst the character of a replica of the luminal crypt, in which it is firmly grasped by the tightly closed lumen surrounding it (Bergström and Nilsson, 1973). The findings obtained by scanning electron microscopy could later be confirmed in all details by parallel studies with transmission electron microscopy (Bergström, 1974).

IV. REVERSAL OF IMPLANTATION DELAY AND INDUCTION OF BLASTOCYST ACTIVATION

A. Technical Aspects

At the time of implantation in normal pregnancy, the peripheral levels of estrogen are higher than during implantation delay (Whitten, 1955, 1958). Reversal of delay can be achieved by exogenous estrogen, provided sufficient progesterone priming is at hand; the key substance for delay reversal thus seems to be estrogen, even if recent evidence indicates that messengers for estrogen may also induce similar changes directly.

A single dose of estrogen is usually sufficient to trigger the cellular events finally resulting in the implanted embryo. Several investigations have demonstrated that there is an optimum dose interval for estrogen in this respect (Humphrey, 1967; Smith, 1968; Smith and Biggers, 1968). Most evidence indicates that there is an all-or-none response to estrogen in the blastocyst during delay. When a dose range from 0.001 to 5.0 μg of estradiol-17β was tested, a low dose threshold was found between 0.001 and 0.01 μg, while a high dose (5.0 μg) gave some effect, but very few implantations (Bergström, 1972b). An optimum dose in the mouse seems to be between 0.01 and 0.1 μg.

Triggering the blastocyst with estrogen can be used also in the study of the hormonal control of zona pellucida shedding (Bergström, 1972c). By early spaying and combined estrogen and progesterone substitution, these experiments aimed at mimicking the "normal" shedding rate by exogenous hormones. In summary, it was demonstrated that the zona loss is an estrogen-dependent event like implantation and that the zona-shedding rate of normal pregnancy could be provoked by 0.01 or 0.1 μg estradiol-17β, either late on day 4 or early on day 4, but not early on day 3. If subimplantation doses were used (0.001 μg), no influence on the shedding rate was seen. If pretreatment with progesterone was omitted, 0.1 μg estradiol-17β could not mimic the shedding rate of normal pregnancy. Of a certain interest was the finding that a zona-shedding rate similar to that of normal pregnancy could be seen with treatments not giving implantations, suggesting that the estrogen "peak" is not a discrete and short release, but rather extended to cover various preimplantation events (Bergström, 1972c).

B. Experimental Aspects

Reversal of experimental delay is accompanied by early metabolic changes in the blastocyst. At 6 hours after a single estrogen dose, a significant increase in amino acid uptake occurs (Weitlauf and Greenwald, 1968). In these experiments, it was also demonstrated that neither progesterone nor estrogen influence alone had any effect on the uptake. A few hours later, the first sign of morphological reaction is obvious, pointing to an expansion of the blastocyst concomitant with an increase in trophoblast cell volume (Bergström, 1972b). These early changes run parallel to an activation of the endometrium, with an early reversal of luminal closure due to the appearance of secretion separating trophoblast cells and uterine epithelium from each other (Bergström and Nilsson, 1975).

The functional changes demonstrable with uptake of labeled amino acids are later followed by various changes related to membrane properties of trophoblast cells. Such changes occur in antigenicity and in protein-binding capacity of blastocysts, and also concerning enzymatic and surface coat properties of trophoblast cells. Blastocysts examined during delay and after 14 hours of estradiol-17β show a marked reduction in alloantigenicity, as measured by isotope antiglobulin technique or by a modified mixed hemadsorption technique (Håkansson and Sundqvist, 1975). These experiments conducted with more specific antisera demonstrated that delayed blastocysts express paternal H-2 antigens, while, after 14 hours of estradiol activation, no specific H-2 antigens could be detected by isotope antiglobulin technique (Håkansson et al., 1975). Though also studied under other conditions (Searle et al., 1974), the switch in blastocyst expression of antigens with this experimental design is clearly related to the influence of a specific combination of progesterone and estrogen influence, thereby yielding a direct clue to the regulation of antigenic determinants by exogenous sex hormones. More detailed investigations on the character of this switch in antigenic expression revealed that β_2-microglobulin is present both on delayed and on 14-hour activated blastocysts, thereby indicating a different response in relation to H-2 antigens and a probable difference in the loci by which the different proteins are coded (Håkansson and Peterson, 1976).

In further experiments on differences in antigenicity in delayed and activated blastocysts, it was found that a strong protein-binding tendency occurs after the attachment stage has been passed. The results indicate that there may be specific protein receptors situated mainly in the abembryonic part of the blastocyst, indicating the possibility of a selective utilization of available protein sources in the uterus (S. Håkansson and K. G. Sundqvist, unpublished). In the series of experiments designed to elucidate estrogen influence on blastocyst immunology, the mixed hemadsorption technique has been used also to visualize erythrocyte markers in scanning electron microscopy. By way of such particulate labeling of tissue surfaces, a quantitative estimation of changes in antigenicity can be obtained (Bergström and Håkansson, 1975).

Structural changes in the blastocyst after the reversal of delay can be used as indicators of events preceding implantation, with some exceptions. One of the first uses of the experimental delay system in the mouse was made by Dickson (1969b), who noted accumulation of sudan III-stainable trophoblast droplets, particularly in the abembryonic pole after 24 hours of estradiol when compared to delayed implanting blastocysts. Many concomitant events take place during estrogenic influence and may somehow be related to preparation of trophoblast ingrowth. Activation of both acid phosphatases (Dickson, 1969b) and tyrosine aminotransferase (Holmes and Dickson, 1973) occur as an expression of the altered membrane function. The surface coat characteristics change, and negative surface charge during delay tends to decrease prior to implantation (Nilsson *et al.*, 1975).

In terms of ultrastructure, this experimental model allows the useful hour-by-hour investigation of hormonal effects prior to implantation. After the earliest recognizable ultrastructural changes at about 8 hours after estradiol, the reappearing uterine secretion yields a detachment reaction and a reversal of the luminal closure (Fig. 7). The secretion seems to be involved in the blastocyst activation, and presumably it conveys a triggering message for the blastocyst (Bergström and Nilsson, 1976). The luminal opening is gradually followed by another luminal closure starting between 16 and 24 hours after estradiol. This second attachment of apposing epithelia is obvious immediately preceding the abembryonic proliferation of trophoblast cells, giving the first ultrastructural signs of impending invasion of trophoblast cells into the sensitized endometrium. These events occur prior to a more generalized polar specialization with the virtually inactive embryonic pole apposed to the adjacent uterine epithelium and the abembryonic pole penetrating between degenerating epithelial cells (Bergström and Nilsson, 1976). Most evidence from these studies indicates that there is an increase in multivesicular bodies, possibly involving a release of hydrolytic enzymes. This is in accordance with the finding of naphtylamidase activity, mostly in the antimesometrial half of the periembryonic area (Bergström, 1972d).

Reversal of implanting delay can be achieved not only by conventional estrogens but also by various anti-estrogenic compounds. Most of them display estrogenic properties, but they are unable to mimic the implantation-inducing effect of several other estrogens. As ''impeded estrogens'' (Emmens, 1965), these compounds bring about estrogenic activation of trophoblast cells but fail to induce the complete preparation for polar differentiation and abembryonic proliferation (Bergström, 1972e). As anti-estrogens, these compounds prevent the implantation induction of conventional estrogens, rendering the blastocyst an ''activated'' appearance, but no further differentiation.

Messengers for estrogens like cyclic AMP seem to mimic most of the effects obtained with estrogens during implantation delay and to induce implantation followed by a normal gestation (Holmes and Bergström, 1975). Detailed investigations on the early blastocyst response to the secondary messenger for estrogen show that the ultrastructural characteristics of early estrogenic influence are expressed in the blastocyst surface (Holmes and Bergström, 1976). Initiation of normal gestation by cyclic AMP and the inability of this compound to maintain the gestation until term suggest that its action is incomplete in a single dose and

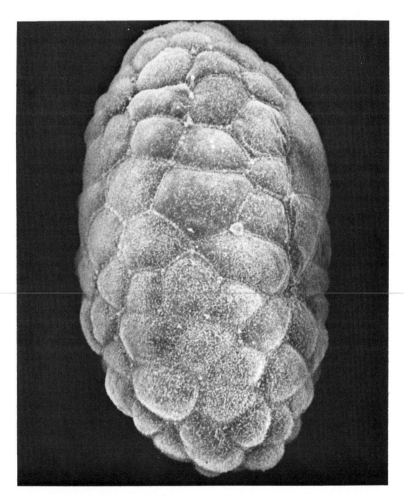

Fig. 7. Experimental delay of implantation with progesterone substitution in a mouse reversed by 0.1 μg estradiol-17β for 16 hours. Note bulging trophoblast cells with distinct polygonal intercellular borders carrying knotlike junctions. The microvillous lining is obvious, and no imprints can be seen. Expansion of the blastocyst has occurred, rendering the trophoblast cells less malleable than before estrogen was given. cf. Fig. 5. × 1200.

that it differs from estrogen in this aspect. Its reported contraceptive effect in mice (Ryan and Coronel, 1969), together with the findings mentioned, make it similar to impeded estrogens like some anti-estrogens.

Testing of blastocyst activation during delay can be performed ultrastructurally and metabolically. The trigger effect of estrogens upon the delayed blastocyst has also been demonstrated upon explantation without estrogen *in vitro* (Naeslund and Lundkvist, 1977). Steady-state blastocysts harvested from delayed mice display a certain outgrowth pattern upon explantation *in vitro*. If delayed mice are induced by estrogen and blastocysts flushed out for *in vitro* cultivation, activated blastocysts show an accelerated outgrowth in relation to delayed blastocysts. If invading blastocysts are explanted, outgrowth starts almost immediately. These experiments indicate that the reversal of implantation delay attained upon explantation *per se* is accelerated by the trigger effect of added estrogen.

V. IMPLANTATION DELAY *IN VITRO*

Attempts to mimic *in vivo* implantation delay under experimental conditions *in vitro* were first made by Gwatkin (1966) by omitting various amino acids from the medium. These experiments did not, however, arrive to a conclusive statement on the chemical basis of implantation delay in terms of environmental uterine compounds. Since then, few attempts appear to have been made to elucidate this issue. In recent experiments in our laboratory (Naeslund, 1978), the findings reported by Gwatkin (1966) were extended. In addition to the earlier tested omission of arginine and leucine, Naeslund also omitted glucose. By comparing expansion and outgrowth in blastocysts deprived *in vitro,* either of arginine and leucine or of arginine, leucine, and glucose, it could be shown that the latter combination is more efficient in delaying blastocyst outgrowth. All cultured blastocysts were expanded and seemingly normal, but none had grown out after 5 days *in vitro*. By adding the missing compounds to the medium used, outgrowth could be induced in 2 days in a normal way. Ultrastructural investigations on the achievement of delay "by omission" and its reversal "by addition" display similarities between blastocysts cultured *in vitro* and those *in vivo*. Thus, by omitting arginine, leucine, and glucose, depletion of glycogen and scattered ribosomes were observed, features also observed during experimental delay *in utero*. By adding the omitted components, outgrowth was obtained within 2 days with seemingly normal outgrowth pattern. Already at 24 hours after addition of glucose and arginine-leucine to an incomplete medium, polyribosomes were formed, and glycogen appeared, as in the case of reversed delay *in utero* (Naeslund, 1978).

ACKNOWLEDGMENT

The technical assistance of Mrs. Barbro Einarsson is gratefully acknowledged. This work was supported by Grant 12-X-70 of the Swedish Medical Research Council to Professor Ove Nilsson.

REFERENCES

Bergström, S. (1972a). *Fertil. Steril.* **23**, 548–561.
Bergström, S. (1972b). *Arch. Gynaekol.* **212**, 285–307.
Bergström, S. (1972c). *Z. Anat. Entwicklungsgesch.* **136**, 143–167.
Bergström, S. (1972d). *J. Reprod. Fertil.* **30**, 177–183.
Bergström, S. (1972e). *Contraception* **5**, 215–236.
Bergström, S. (1974). *Proc. 7th Annu. SEM Symp., 1974,* pp. 605–612.
Bergström, S., and Håkansson, S. (1975). *J. Reprod. Med.* **14**, 210–212.
Bergström, S., and Nilsson, O. (1972). *J. Endocrinol.* **55**, 217–218.
Bergström, S., and Nilsson, O. (1973). *J. Reprod. Fertil.* **32**, 531–533.
Bergström, S., and Nilsson, O. (1975). *J. Reprod. Fertil.* **44**, 117–120.
Bergström, S., and Nilsson, O. (1976). *Anat. Embryol.* **149**, 149–154.
Bergström, S., Lundkvist, Ö., Naeslund, G., and Pettersson, B. (1976). *In* "Scanning Electron Microscopy Atlas of Mammalian Reproduction" (E. S. E. Hafez, ed.), pp. 318–333. Igaku Shoin, Tokyo.
Dickson, A. D. (1969a). *J. Reprod. Fertil.* **18**, 227–233.
Dickson, A. D. (1969b). *J. Anat.* **105**, 371–380.
Emmens, C. W. (1965). *J. Reprod. Fertil.* **9**, 277–283.
Enders, A. C., and Nelson, D. M. (1973). *J. Anat.* **138**, 277–300.
Gwatkin, R. B. L. (1966). *J. Cell. Physiol.* **68**, 335–344.
Håkansson, S., and Peterson, P. (1976). *Transplantation* **19**, 479–484.
Håkansson, S., and Sundqvist, K. G. (1975). *Transplantation* **19**, 479–484.
Håkansson, S., Heyner, S., Sundqvist, K. G., and Bergström, S. (1975). *Int. J. Fertil.* **20**, 137–140.
Hedlund, K., and Nilsson, O. (1971). *J. Reprod. Fertil.* **26**, 267–269.
Holmes, P., and Bergström, S. (1975). *J. Reprod. Fertil.* **43**, 329–332.
Holmes, P., and Bergström, S. (1976). *Am. J. Obstet. Gynecol.* **124**, 301–306.
Holmes, P., and Dickson, A. D. (1973). *J. Embryol. Exp. Morphol.* **29**, 639–648.
Humphrey, K. W. (1967). *Steroids* **10**, 591–600.
Kirby, D. R. S. (1971). *In* "Biology of the Blastocyst" (R. J. Blandau, ed.), pp. 393–411. University of Chicago Press, Chicago, Illinois.
McLaren, A. (1971). *J. Endocrinol.* **50**, 515–526.
Martin, L., Finn, C. A., and Carter, J. (1970). *J. Reprod. Fertil.* **21**, 461–469.
Menke, T. M., and McLaren, A. (1970a). *J. Reprod. Fertil.* **23**, 117–127.
Menke, T. M., and McLaren, A. (1970b). *J. Endocrinol.* **47**, 284–294.
Naeslund, G. (1978). *Upsala J. Med. Sci.* (In press).
Naeslund, G., and Lundkvist, Ö. (1978). *Upsala J. Med. Sci.* (In press).
Nilsson, O., Lindqvist, I., and Ronquist, G. (1975). *Contraception* **11**, 441–450.
Parr, M. B., and Parr, E. L. (1974). *Biol. Reprod.* **11**, 220–233.
Ryan, W. L., and Coronel, D. M. (1969). *Am. J. Obstet. Gynecol.* **105**, 125–134.
Searle, R. F., Johnson, M. H., Billington, W. D., Elson, J., and Clutterbuck-Jackson, S. (1974). *Transplantation* **18**, 136–145.
Smith, D. M. (1968). *J. Endocrinol.* **41**, 17–29.
Smith, D. M., and Biggers, J. D. (1968). *J. Endocrinol.* **41**, 1–9.
Torbit, C. A., and Weitlauf, H. M. (1974). *J. Reprod. Fertil.* **39**, 379–386.
Weitlauf, H. M. (1969). *J. Exp. Zool.* **171**, 481–486.
Weitlauf, H. M. (1971). *J. Exp. Zool.* **176**, 35–40.

Weitlauf, H. M. (1973). *J. Exp. Zool.* **183,** 303–312.
Weitlauf, H. M. (1974). *J. Reprod. Fertil.* **39,** 213–224.
Weitlauf, H. M., and Greenwald, G. S. (1965). *J. Reprod. Fertil.* **10,** 203–208.
Weitlauf, H. M., and Greenwald, G. S. (1968). *J. Exp. Zool.* **169,** 463–472.
Whitten, W. K. (1955). *J. Endocrinol.* **13,** 1–11.
Whitten, W. K. (1958). *J. Endocrinol.* **16,** 435–443.

21

Laparoscopic Research Techniques in Mammalian Embryology

W. RICHARD DUKELOW

In recent years, the use of laparoscopy (also termed endoscopy or pelviscopy) in research has greatly increased. Initial application in the field of human gynecology has led to a variety of observational and sampling techniques which employ laparoscopy and avoid the stress and complication of laparotomies. Application in the area of mammalian biological research has also developed at a rapid pace. It is now possible to observe and sample from a wide variety of abdominal organs, as well as to recover ova from ovarian follicles, embryos from uterine cavities, or to place substances (including early preimplantation stage embryos) into the oviductal or uterine lumen.

I. HISTORICAL ASPECTS OF LAPAROSCOPY

The earliest known report of laparoscopy is that of Bozzini (1806), who projected candlelight through a double-lumen urethral cannula. It was not until 61 years later that the term "endoscopy" was coined by Segelas and Desormeaux in 1867 (cited by Benedict, 1951). They described the passage of light through a genitourinary speculum to observe the internal organs.

The first successful viewing of an internal body cavity (the bladder), using an incandescent light source, is credited to von Nitze (1894). He also was the first to take internal photographs through the prismatic cystoscope.

The first laparoscopic visualization of the general peritoneal cavity can be traced to the contributions of Kelling (1902) and Jacobaeus (1910); the work of these individuals resulted in the development of a safe technique for insertion of an optical telescope through a small abdominal incision. Kelling, a surgeon from Dresden, observed the abdominal organs of a dog by inserting a cystoscope through a small incision in the anterior abdominal wall. Jacobaeus, of Sweden, was the first to apply the procedure to humans and coined the term "laparoscopy."

In the United States, Bernheim (1911) was the first to report the use of laparoscopy. A year later, Nordentoeft (1912) of Copenhagen made observations of the pelvic region after insufflation of the abdomen and adoption of Trendelenburg's position for observation.

Ruddock (1937) described the results of 500 laparoscopies carried out under local anesthesia to investigate upper abdominal pathology. In the same year, Hope (1937) reported the value of laparoscopy for the diagnosis of ectopic pregnancy.

The next significant development was the endoscope of Fourestier, which eliminated several of the disadvantages of distal bulb illumination by the use of proximal light projection (see Fourestier et al., 1952). In this procedure, light was transmitted from the proximal to the distal end of a clear rod of fused quartz. Heating and drying effects of distal bulb illumination were avoided by this "cold light" projection method. Thus, this procedure removed the threat of heatburn and also furnished more brilliant illumination than had previously been possible.

During this time, there were several attempts to construct fiber optic endoscopes. The construction of such devices was based on the transmission of light along a transparent fiber cylinder as a result of internal reflectance. Extensive clinical testing of these laparoscopic systems was reported by Fear (1968). He described the results of 134 such examinations performed under general anesthesia, with emphasis on the safety and convenience of laparoscopy in gynecologic procedures.

At this time in the development of laparoscopic procedures, many investigators were contributing refinements which lead to the current popularity of the technique. Semm (1969, 1970), in particular, made major contributions to the development of the instrumentarium for a variety of procedures, such as uterine biopsy and tubal sterilization. He also outlined the surgical procedure in detail and cautioned about potential hazards.

In 1970, Smith and Dillon compiled a comprehensive list of indications, contraindications, complications, and case studies involving the use of the laparoscope. They noted that laparoscopy could be performed in cases where contraindication due to disease or abnormal anatomy preclude culdoscopy.

The repertoire of ancillary techniques that can be performed in human gynecologic laparoscopy has vastly expanded from the earliest first crude attempts at observation. These have been chronicled by Siegler and Garret (1970). These techniques now include aspiration, insufflation, lysis of adhesions, and coagulation (Fig. 1). Additional procedures have been developed with special application to research situations and will be described later.

In 1957, the first 16-mm color cinematography and television recordings were made with laparoscopy. In 1964, the first international symposium on laparoscopy

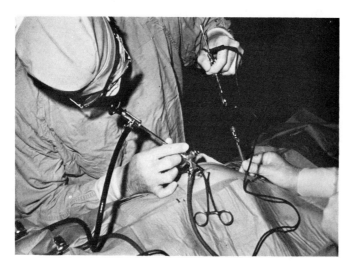

Fig. 1.   Laparoscopic techniques in the human with electrocoagulation being performed through a second puncture site.

was held in Italy, and, in 1967, the first English textbook on laparoscopy was produced by Steptoe.

Traditionally, basic scientists have made discoveries and developed techniques which were then applied to clinical problems. In the field of laparoscopy, the developmental procedure has been reversed with the extensive development of practical, clinically important techniques relating to biopsy, electrocautery, and tubal sterilization. The contributions of Palmer, Semm, Frangenheim, Megale, Steptoe, and other pioneers have allowed relatively easy adaptation of the techniques to controlled studies of mammalian embryonic and fetal development. In the following sections, arranged by species, a brief review of published work with each species is followed by a detailed description of the technique and special adaptations that have been made for specific areas of research study.

II. GENERAL COMMENTS

Several generalizations can be made relative to the laparoscopic procedure. The procedure is rapid and simple. It allows rapid observation and provides for simple procedures with minimal stress to the animal. No adverse effects have been reported from the laparoscopic procedure itself that might be reflected in a blockage of ovulation, change in cycle length, or early termination of pregnancy. It is, of course, possible that varying anesthetic regimens, drugs, and unusual surgical techniques (such as exceptionally long fasting periods) could exert an effect on these parameters.

Initial attempts at laparoscopy can be frustrating. The anatomy is being examined from a new dimension and in changing magnification. Practice and experience soon overcome this problem.

Very few complications arise from laparoscopy if normal precautions are taken. While completely sterile technique may be desirable with very valuable animals, this does not seem to be required with most species. Our own experience, with 23 species, has resulted in only 1 case of peritonitis. That case was with an African pygmy goat early in our experimental program. Normal cleanliness of the instruments, care in the abdominal wall puncture, and careful postlaparoscopic care greatly decrease the possibility of complications.

In recent years, a wide variety of laparoscopic instruments have appeared on the market. While certain sizes and angles of light projection can be adapted to specific situations, there does not appear to be any "best" general instrument. Sizes range from 1.7-mm "needlescopes" to 5–6-mm pediatric laparoscopes to 8–10-mm adult gynecologic laparoscopes. As an indication of adaptability, we have routinely used the 5-mm pediatric laparoscope on animals ranging in size from a mouse to a cow (Fig. 2). Given a large armoratorium of instruments, the 1.7-mm laparoscope would be preferable for small rodents and birds; the 5-mm for rabbits, monkeys, dogs, cats, sheep, and swine; and the 8- to 10-mm laparo-

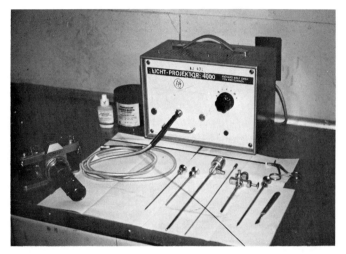

Fig. 2. Laparoscopy equipment used in mammalian embryo research. (Left to right) camera, flexible fiber optic cable, second puncture 3-mm trocar, second puncture cannula, 5-mm pediatric laparoscope, tactile probe, laparoscopic cannula, trocar, and scapel. At the base of the light projector is the 3-mm grasping forceps.

scope for large swine, cattle, and horses. The larger domestic animals generally require a longer (60-cm) laparoscope. The selection of the proper angle of view from the distal end of the laparoscope (usually 130°, 160°, or 180°) is dependent on the preference of the laparoscopist and is usually predicated on the type of instrument with which he has had the most experience.

The choice of a light projector is usually dependent on the type of research being done and the need for quality photographs. Suitable photos can be obtained merely with the normal light transmitted through the fiber optic system of most projectors. The best quality pictures, however, require transmission of a high-intensity flash. Originally, this was accomplished by means of a distal flash bulb unit on the tip of the laparoscope. More recent equipment provides for generation of the flash from a proximal location, i.e., the light projector itself.

Operating laparoscopes are available for a single insertion (puncture) site. These are routinely used in human gynecologic procedures and have some application to research situations. Other procedures (especially those that require extensive manipulation within the abdominal cavity) will require a second entry site, which necessitates a second trocar. Regardless of the size of the viewing laparoscope, second entry sites usually admit instruments of 4–5 mm in size. With earlier equipment, the trocars were made of stainless steel, whereas new models have fiberglass sleeves to prevent accidental transmission of current to the abdominal wall and organs. If electrocautery is to be used, the sleeves should definitely be of the fiberglass variety. Trocar points can be either of the pyramidal (cutting edge) or conical type. Here, as with the angle of laparoscopic view, the choice is primarily based on laparoscopist preference. Laparoscopes are now available which are autoclavable (Richard Wolf Medical Instruments Corporation, Rosemount, Illinois).

Abdominal insufflation is routinely used with most experimental animals. This can be accomplished either by an automatic insufflator that maintains constant abdominal pressure, or by periodical introduction of gas manually through the value located on the primary puncture cannula. The latter suffices with most species but some, such as the rabbit, require continual insufflation. We have routinely used 5% CO_2 in air for insufflation but have used other gases on some occasions. This gas passes through a water bath to moisten it, and others have used warmed water for this purpose. Interestingly, a recent study reported the use of air alone for insufflation, in women, without adverse effects. Some individual animals can be laparoscoped without insufflation, but the procedure does greatly enhance the ease of laparoscopy.

In humans, insufflation is normally accomplished through the Verres cannula needle separate from the laparoscopic cannula, and this procedure can be used in research animals as well if desired. The choice of the route of insufflation is not critical.

III. LABORATORY RODENTS, RABBITS, BIRDS, AND EXOTIC ANIMALS

A. Anesthesia and Restraint

General anesthesia is usually used for laparoscopy with all but the larger domestic animals. Mice and hamsters can be anesthetized with ether or halothane inhalant devices or chambers and maintained in the anesthetized state with a small anesthesia face cone. Mice can also be anesthetized with pentobarbital administered at a rate of 50–80 mg/kg body weight ip. Rats and wild rodents can be easily anesthetized with ip pentobarbital at a level of 25–40 mg/kg. Rabbits can be brought to a deep plane of anesthesia with iv administration of pentobarbital at a rate of 24 mg/kg. Mink can be adequately anesthetized with administration of Ketamine (Parke-Davis Co.) at a level of 10 mg/kg im. In the case of birds, either pentobarbital (30 mg/kg, iv) or, for longer effect, phenobarbital (130–170 mg/kg, iv) is satisfactory. An endotracheal tube should be used with birds to prevent breathing problems caused by regurgitation from the crop sac when the bird is in the head down position.

All small rodents and rabbits should be restrained on an appropriately sized surgery restrain board or table in the dorsal recumbent position. This board or table should be tilted to an angle of 30°–45°. Figure 3 illustrates one such table

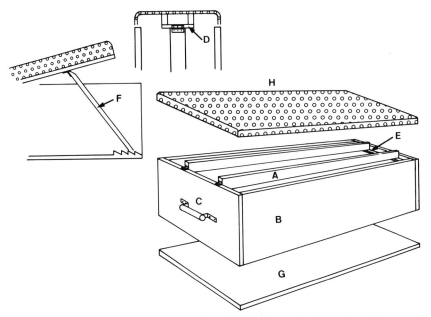

Fig. 3. Variable-angle laparoscopy stage. Description of pieces, their quantity and size: A × 2, 26⅓ × 1⅝ × 3½ inch; B × 2, 26⅛ × 9⅜ inch; C × 2, 13 × 19⅜ × ⅝ inch; D × 1, 26½ × 9½ × ⅝ inch; E × 1, 10 × ⅝ × 1 inch; F × 1, 15 × 5 × ⅝ inch; G × 1, ¼ × 14¼ × 28½ inch; H × 1, surgical table. (From Jewett and Dukelow, 1973.)

that has been effective for animals ranging in size from laboratory rats to small dogs.

Birds are restrained, head down on their right side with a strap around both legs. The laparoscope is inserted at a point midway between the posterior sternum and posterior ribs above the abdominal muscles.

B. Basic Laparoscopic Procedure

1. Anesthetize animal and place in dorsal recumbent, head down position.
2. Clip the hair, fur, or feathers from the abdominal area and scrub with surgical soap. Rinse and swab with iodine solution or equivalent.
3. With a scalpel, make a small skin incision (not through the abdominal wall). This procedure is necessary with conical-pointed trocars, but not with trocars having pyramidal (cutting edge) points.
4. Slowly push trocar slightly under the skin, and then downward (dorsally) through the abdominal wall. This allows a nonalignment of skin and abdominal

wall when the instruments are removed, precluding the need for suturing. With the animal restrained head down on a sloped surface, the same effect is accomplished by inserting the trocar at a dorsal–posterior angle.

5. Attach gas line to the trocar and slightly insufflate the abdomen. Alternatively, one can insert the Verres cannula first and attach the gas line for insufflation before trocar insertion.

6. Slowly withdraw the trocar (too rapid withdrawal will result in a suction action pulling abdominal contents against, or into, the cannula).

7. Insert the telescope and attach it to the light source.

8. Insert ancillary probe (Verres or larger, dependent on species) several centimeters to the right (left if you are left handed) of the telescope.

9. Manipulate the organ you wish to view into position while observing through the telescope.

10. If an ancillary port is needed for the insertion of biopsy or surgical instruments, insert the smaller trocar lateral to the telescope. The chance of damage to internal organs and vasculature is greater, and the abdomen should be distended with gas.

11. At the conclusion of the procedure, all instruments are slowly withdrawn, a suture is used to close the wound, if desired, and the animal receives a prophylactic injection of antibiotic.

C. Photography

While the basic technique of laparoscopy is easily learned, photography is more difficult because of the changing intensity of light and focus as the animal's internal organs move during respiration. Special flash systems, either at the light projector source or on the tip of the telescope, are available which allow the best photographs. Satisfactory photos and movies can be taken with standard laparoscopic light projectors using special telescope camera adaptors available from most suppliers (Fig. 4). Distal and proximal flash generators are equipped with synchronizing attachments that allow the flash to occur at the same time that the shutter is opened. If no flash generator is used, adequate pictures can be made with most equipment at ⅛- to ¼-second exposure with the projector set for the brightest level of exposure. A variety of films can be used in photolaparography. In our own laboratory, we routinely use Kodak EHB film (ASA 125). Infrared film can also be used advantageously with the laparoscope (Jewett and Dukelow, 1972a), recognizing that this is not true infrared photography, since the image does pass through an optical system (the laparoscope) before being exposed on the film. In such procedures, Kodak Ektachrome infrared film can be used in combination with three filters, CC20-C, Corning CS-1-59(3966), and a Kodak Wratten No. 12.

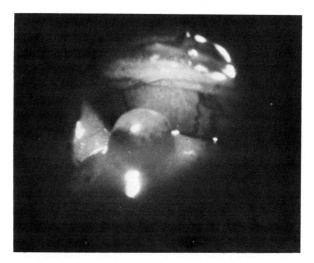

Fig. 4. Ovarian follicle 30 minutes before ovulation in the squirrel monkey (*Saimiri sciureus*). (From Harrison and Dukelow, 1974.)

D. Special Considerations with the Rabbit

Because of the flaccid nature of the abdominal contents of the rabbit, laparoscopy is difficult. This necessitates nearly continual insufflation of the abdominal contents. In addition, it is difficult to elevate and hold, for close observation, the ovaries in an exposed position. Accordingly, a technique was developed (Fujimoto *et al.*, 1974) to allow periodic examination of the rabbit ovaries

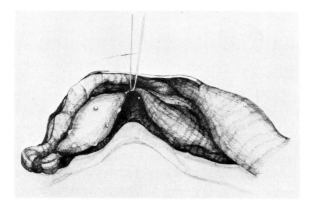

Fig. 5. Diagrammatic representation of the ovarian suspension technique used to facilitate ovarian observation during laparoscopy in the rabbit. (From Fujimoto *et al.*, 1974.)

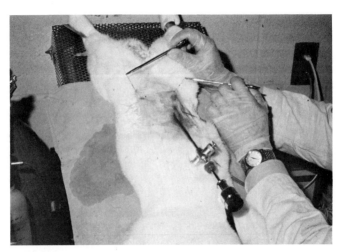

Fig. 6. Elevation of the external portion of sutures laparoscopically placed around the ovarian ligaments to facilitate suspension and observation of the ovaries in a rabbit. (From Fujimoto *et al.,* 1974.)

without excessive manipulation. A large, curved needle, with 3–0 gut suture, is passed through the skin and abdominal wall. As one individual holds the needle in firm position, the laparoscopist elevates the ovary so that the needle point passes under, or through, the ovarian ligament (Fig. 5). The needle is then brought back through the abdominal wall and skin, where it is tied loosely or clamped with a hemostat. The same procedure is carried out with the opposite ovary. When examination is needed, manual elevation of the sutures bring the ovary into view (Fig. 6). At the conclusion of the procedure, the suture is cut and withdrawn.

IV. DOGS AND CATS

A. Anesthesia and Restraint

Procedures for laparoscopy in the dog have recently been developed by Dr. David E. Wildt (Wildt *et al.,* 1977a) of the Institute of Comparative Medicine at Baylor College of Medicine in Houston, Texas. Dogs can be anesthetized with ketamine hydrochloride (11 mg/kg) and xylazine (2.2 mg/kg) im. Alternatively, pentobarbital can be given iv at a level of 30–35 mg/kg or, phenobarbital at a level of 80 mg/kg.

Cats can be anesthetized with pentobarbital at a level of 25–36 mg/kg either iv or ip. Alternatively, phenobarbital can be administered ip at a level of 180 mg/kg or thiopental at a level of 28 mg/kg. As with the rodents, the animal should then be restrained on a surgical table at an angle of 30°–45°. The laparoscopic table shown in Fig. 3 is adequate for cats and smaller dogs, whereas a regular veterinary surgical table can be used for larger dogs.

B. Basic Laparoscopic Procedure

Laparoscopic observation of the dog ovaries is complicated by the presence of an ovarian bursa. This bursa has a slitlike opening ventrally, which prevents direct examination of the ovary. This slit is 1–2 cm in length and is of insufficient size to allow extrusion of the ovary for observation. Accordingly, Wildt *et al.* (1977a) have developed the following procedures to make direct ovarian observations. Following the normal preoperative procedures described in the previous section, the abdomen is insufflated through a Verres needle inserted 4 cm lateral to the midline. A skin incision is then made approximately 4 cm posterior to the xiphoid process and the trocar inserted as previously described for rodents and rabbits. An accessory trocar assembly is inserted and then the trocar is replaced with an electrocautery hook scissors. The jaws of the scissors are inserted into the posterior edge of the bursal slit nearest the anterior terminus of the uterine horn. The animal is grounded using a clip or ground plate and the lead wire attached to the laparoscopic hook scissors. Following a period of electrocautery discharge (50 W) ranging from 3 to 30 seconds, the tissue is cut to lengthen the bursal slit to 1.0–1.5 cm, allowing complete ovarian exposure. During the recovery period, it is often necessary to laparoscopically break away tissue adhesions (with a manipulatory probe) forming in the incised area. This procedure allows a preparation suitable for frequent sequential laparoscopic examinations without a detectable effect on ovarian cyclicity or animal health. Laparoscopy in the cat is similar to that described earlier with rodents and rabbits.

V. NONHUMAN PRIMATES

A. Previous Studies

Most of the earlier experimental research in laparoscopy was carried out either with nonhuman primates or with large domestic animals rather than the more traditional laboratory animals. Balin *et al.* (1969) described the use of laparoscopic equipment in studying ovulation in the rhesus monkey (1969). In 1971, Dukelow *et al.* described the basic technique for laparoscopy in nonhuman primates (cynomolgus macaque and the squirrel monkey) and the goat. Since that time, our own studies have covered eight different species of nonhuman primates and the application of laparoscopy to studies on ovulatory mechanism (Jewett and Dukelow, 1971b, 1972b; Rawson and Dukelow, 1973a,b; Harrison and Dukelow, 1974); testing of contraceptive agents (Harrison and Dukelow, 1971; Harrison et al., 1974; Rawson and Dukelow, 1973c), seasonality and adaptation (Harrison and Dukelow, 1973), and in vitro fertilization (Kuehl and Dukelow, 1975; Dukelow and Kuehl, 1975; Dukelow, 1975). Graham et al. (1973) have described the surgical technique for laparoscopy in the chimpanzee and have produced an instructional film of the technique. A similar film has been produced showing laparoscopic technique in primates by Mahone and Dukelow (1976a). Wildt et al. (1977b) have described the use of laparoscopy in studying follicular development in the baboon.

B. Anesthesia and Restraint

The two most popular anesthetic agents used with nonhuman primates in recent years have been phencyclidine hydrochloride (Bio-ceutic Laboratories) and ketamine hydrochloride. The former is usually administered im at a dose of from 0.5 to 3.0 mg/kg to macaques and South American species. The baboon and chimpanzee require lower doses of 0.5–1.0 mg/kg. Ketamine hydrochloride is usually given im at a dose of 5–10 mg/kg for rhesus monkeys. Slightly higher levels (12–15 mg/kg) are recommended for cebus, squirrel, cynomolgus, and bonnet monkeys. For complete anesthesia in chimpanzees, Graham et al. (1973) followed phencyclidine or ketamine with intubation and a mixture of 1–2% halothane, 60% nitrous oxide, and 40% oxygen. This mixture was administered through a semiclosed system at 4 liters/minute.

Small primates can be anesthetized ip (the procedure has been used with both squirrel monkeys and greater and lesser galagos) with pentobarbital at a level of approximately 22 mg/kg of body weight.

C. Basic Laparoscopic Procedure

As described above with laboratory animals, cats, and dogs, the same basic procedure is used. The primates are prepared for surgery and placed on a sloped table (Fig. 7). A 5-mm laparoscope is adequate for all but the larger primates and is inserted in a dorsal–posterior position in such a manner that, upon removal, the skin and abdominal entry punctures are not aligned. This prevents herniation and reduces the chance of abdominal infection.

The stress involved with laparoscopy is minimal. In our colony of cynomolgus macaques, nearly 45% of all cycles have been subjected to laparoscopy over a 5-year period. An average cycle, where laparoscopy is carried out, entails two to three laparoscopic examinations for a 3-day period near the time of ovulation. No effect has been noted on ovulation, menstrual cycle length, or gestation. In fact, the procedure has been used to predict ovulation time for timed-mating studies

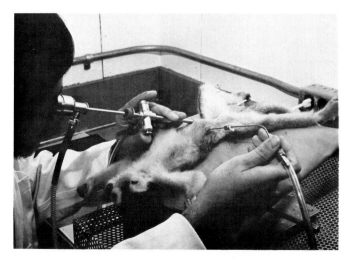

Fig. 7. Laparoscopic technique in the squirrel monkey with follicle aspiration through a second puncture site.

(Jewett and Dukelow, 1971a). Some animals in our colony have been "scoped" as many as 83 times without apparent ill effects, and macaques laparoscoped as many as 49 times have subsequently become pregnant and borne normal young.

After laparoscopy, a single suture is placed in the skin. In smaller primates, this further lowers the chances of herniation and serves cosmetic purposes.

D. Ancillary Techniques in Nonhuman Primates

In recent years, many ancillary procedures have been developed for laparoscopic application in human patients. Most of these procedures can be adapted for research with nonhuman primates. These include aspiration, biopsy, insufflation, lysis of adhesions and coagulation, suturing and ligation, and the application of surgical clips. These techniques are not immediately applicable to studies in mammalian embryology, but the reader is referred to the works of Siegler and Garret (1970), Smith and Dillon (1970), Clarke (1972), Hulka and Omran (1972), and Fishburne *et al.* (1974) for a more detailed description of these techniques.

Several other ancillary laparoscopic techniques do have application to studies of mammalian embryology and are discussed in the sections below.

1. Follicular Aspiration and Injection

To aspirate the ovarian follicles in nonhuman primates, a 25-gauge needle (⅝ inch long) is passed through the skin and abdominal wall at a point 2–3 cm lateral to the laparoscopic entry point. The needle is then pushed gently (bevel side down) into the follicle and slight suction applied with a 1-ml tuberculin syringe to aspirate the contents into 0.1 ml of culture medium in the syringe. A more complex system for follicular aspiration, eliminating the necessity for aspiration into medium, has previously been described (Jewett and Dukelow, 1973). Similar systems have been described by Steptoe and Edwards (1970), and Morgenstern and Soupart (1972) for recovering human oocytes. For intrafollicular injections, smaller needles (32-gauge) are used to prevent leakage at the site of puncture. In this case, a 24-gauge 0.5 inch needle is inserted through the lower abdominal wall as a cannula for the smaller injection needle. For precise injection, the needles can be attached to a 10-μl Hamilton syringe equipped with a

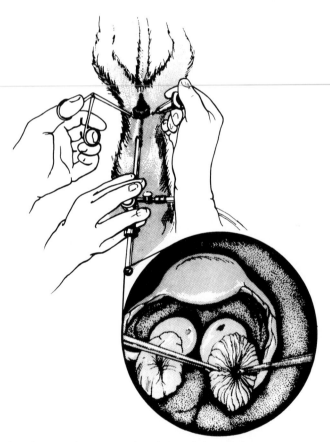

Fig. 8. Diagrammatic representation of the technique for laparoscopic embryo transfer in the squirrel monkey. (From Kuehl and Dukelow, 1977.)

Chaney adaptor (Hamilton Co., Whittier, California). In our experiments, volumes of 1 μl are routinely injected. India ink or trypan blue (0.05%) can be used to assess the reliability of the delivery technique.

2. Topical Application of Compounds to the Ovarian Surface

Using the laparoscope, one can place 2-mm discs on the surface of the ovary (or on the follicle) and recover them from the anesthetized monkey 2 hours later. These can be made of No. 42 filter paper (Whatman Co.) or Gelfoam (Upjohn Co.), and can be saturated with various test compounds. They are placed in position with a 3-mm grasping laparoscopic forceps inserted through a 6-mm cannula inserted lateral to the laparoscope entry point.

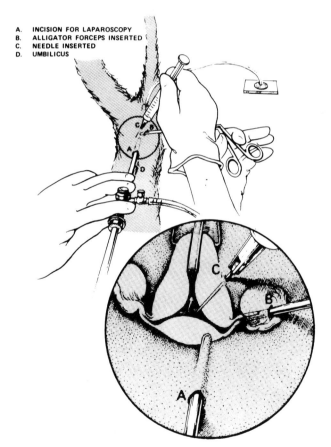

A. INCISION FOR LAPAROSCOPY
B. ALLIGATOR FORCEPS INSERTED
C. NEEDLE INSERTED
D. UMBILICUS

Fig. 9. Diagrammatic representation of uterine flushing technique from the squirrel monkey. (From Ariga and Dukelow, 1977.)

3. Oviductal Deposition

It is possible to deposit test solutions (including ova in medium) into the oviductal fimbria in primates as small as squirrel monkeys (Kuehl and Dukelow, 1977). The organs are first manipulated into position with the Verres cannula. Then a Kingman alligator forceps is inserted and used to spread the fimbrial tissue. Finally a micropipettor (Micro/petter, Scientific Manufacturing Industries, Emeryville, California) is inserted and the tip placed 1–2 mm into the oviduct (Fig. 8). Upon injection, 1 μl of fluid is deposited into the oviduct. As with follicular injections, dyes or stains can be used to verify the site of deposition.

4. Uterine Flushing in Primates

Using the laparoscope, one can recover uterine flushings from nonhuman primates as small as the squirrel monkey (Ariga and Dukelow, 1977). The laparoscope is inserted in the normal, midventral position and the Verres needle used laterally to locate the uterus. A 3.5-inch Kingman alligator forceps (Fig. 9) is then inserted through the needle puncture hole. The round ligament is grasped to steady the uterus, while a 25-gauge needle, attached to a 3-ml syringe, is passed, midventrally, through the skin and abdominal wall. The needle is gently pushed through the fundus to the lumen and 2.0–2.5 ml of flushing medium is injected. The fluids are recovered through a piece of polyethylene tubing (PE 200, Clay-Adams) previously passed through the vagina and cervix. In the case of the squirrel monkey, the polyethylene tube can be attached to a Pasteur pipette and the large end of the pipette inserted into the vagina and pressed against the cervical os. This procedure has been used in squirrel monkeys to recover uterine

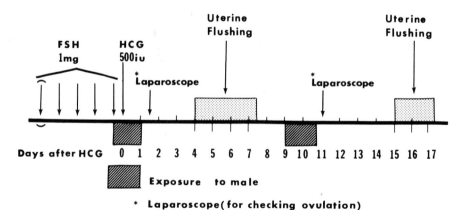

Fig. 10.   Schedule for ovulation induction and laparoscopic uterine flushing in the squirrel monkey.

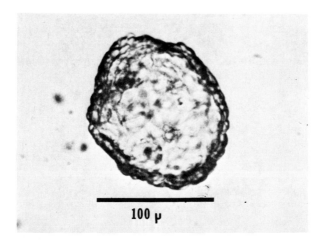

Fig. 11.   Blastocyst recovered laparoscopically from the squirrel monkey uterus 5 days (93–109 hours) after fertilization.

fluid flushing, ova, and preimplantation blastocysts. The scheme to recover blastocysts is indicated in Figs. 10 and 11. One can expect to recover an average of 70–80% of the flushing fluid, and recoveries approaching 100% are not uncommon.

VI. DOMESTIC ANIMALS

A. Previous Studies

In 1956 Megale, Fincher, and McEntee carried out very original studies on laparoscopy in the cow through the vaginal fornix and by way of the paralumbar fossa. This was further described by Megale (1967) and also adapted to the sheep and goat. The light source used was a small incandescent lamp powered by a 6-V pocket battery.

Lamond and Holmes (1965) used a laparoscope inserted into a cow through a chronically implanted cannula in the paralumbar fossa and with a distal light source. A similar technique (chronically implanted cannula) was used by Betteridge and Raeside (1962) for ovarian observation in the pig.

Laparoscopy in the pig through midventral incision was first described by Wildt *et al.* (1973).

In mares, Witherspoon and Talbot (1970) used fiber optic light transmission and both 135° and 180° laparoscopes to describe ovarian changes in the mare.

Heinze *et al.* (1972) and Heinze and Klug (1973) have described a laparoscopic technique in both the horse and donkey. Inserting the laparoscope just caudal to the last rib, they entered the muscle layer. With visual guidance, they inserted a cannula for abdominal insufflation before complete insertion of the laparoscope. This procedure reduced the danger of cecal puncture.

Rapid laparotomy procedures have been developed in the sheep. Lamond and Urguhart (1961) developed a sheep laparotomy table and procedure which involved an incision just anterior to the mammae and lateral to the midline. Hulet and Foote (1968) modified the table and procedure, using a plastic speculum and long spoon to facilitate examination. Dierschke and Hyatt (1969), using a chronically implanted cannula in the right paralumbar fossa, did periodic peritoneoscopic examinations for as long as 424 days in one animal. Corticosteroid and enzyme treatments were necessary to prevent granuloma and adhesion formation and maintain a clear route of examination.

In 1968, Roberts employed Lamond and Urguhart's laparotomy table and a laparoscope with a proximal light source to examine ovaries of sheep through a midventral approach.

Thimonier and Mauléon (1969) also used the midventral approach. The insertion was 15 cm cranial to the mammae through a 1-cm midline incision. This procedure allowed as many as 40 examinations of one animal, over a 2-year period, to detect ovulation for characterization of the estrous cycles and for assessment of hormonal treatments in ewes (Land *et al.*, 1973; Pelletier and Thimonier, 1973).

Phillippo *et al.* (1971) used laparoscopy through a midventral approach to diagnose early pregnancy in sheep. Boyd and Ducker (1973) also used a midventral approach in sheep under general anesthesia with etorphine hydrochloride and acepromazine.

Seeger (1973) utilized Hulet and Foote's laparotomy table for laparoscopy in the sheep. Although local anesthesia had been used, general anesthesia was preferred because of the anesthetic effect on internal organ movement. Seeger and Humke (1974) used this technique to monitor ovulation in sheep stimulated with gonadotropin-releasing hormone. Similar procedures were used by Snyder and Dukelow (1974).

B. Anesthesia and Restraint

Swine, sheep, and goats are best laparoscoped in the supine position on a sloped table such as that described by Hulet and Foote (1968). Cattle and horses, on the other hand, are normally laparoscoped in the standing position with the hindquarters slightly higher than the forequarters and with local anesthesia.

Swine can be anesthetized by iv injection of pentobarbital (18–22 mg/kg) into the anterior vena cava. This is best done with a 3-inch, 18-gauge needle inserted into the pocket formed by the junction of the first rib and the sternum. Tranquilizing agents can be given im prior to this if desired. Another anesthesia procedure consists of administration of thiopental (im) and then placing the animal on a halothane-breathing apparatus. Sheep can be anesthetized with an injection of 250–350 mg of promazine hydrochloride (for an adult sheep), followed 5–10 minutes later with an iv injection of pentobarbital at a level of 9–10 mg/kg. Alternatively, there are many current anesthetic methods for large domestic animals. The above represent those used in our own laboratory for laparoscopic examination. Cattle and horses are usually anesthetized locally with lidocaine after tranquilization.

C. Basic Laparoscopic Procedure

With swine, after surgical preparation and proper restraint described above, a ventral midline incision, 1 cm in length, is made just anterior to the position of the ovaries. In an adult, this is usually about 30 cm posterior and 5–10 cm lateral to the xiphoid process of the sternum. The trocar is inserted subcutaneously (Fig. 12) and posterior 2 cm, then dorsally through the musculature of the abdominal wall. This procedure precludes the necessity for suturing the incision. The abdominal cavity is then insufflated with gas as previously described. A second incision is made 4 cm posterior and 10 cm lateral to the midline incision for inserting of a tactile (manipulatory) probe into the abdomen. In about 40% of the examinations of nonpregnant animals, the ovaries can be immediately located. In

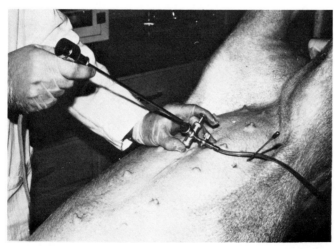

Fig. 12. Insertion of 5-mm pediatric laparoscope in the pig (with tactile probe already in place). (From Wildt *et al.*, 1973.)

other cases, the ovaries can be easily located following minor manipulation of the uterine horn.

In sheep, the trocar is inserted immediately anterior to the mammary gland with the tactile probe entry site located 5–6 cm lateral to the midline incision. A movie showing the laparoscopic technique in swine and sheep has been made by Mahone and Dukelow (1976b).

Both swine and sheep can be laparoscoped with standard length (30 cm) laparoscopes. Very large swine, cattle, and horses are most easily done with longer (60 cm) instruments of 8–10 mm diameter. In cattle, the laparoscope can be inserted into the vagina and through the vaginal wall, but this approach offers technical difficulties that are easily overcome by insertion in the paralumbar fossa.

The following procedure has been used with good success by Karl Seeger of Hoechst, AG, of Frankfurt, Germany. After an initial incision through the skin and muscle of the right paralumbar fossa, the trocar is inserted in a median, horizontal, and slightly caudal direction. With a short push, the peritoneum is punctured, and gas is allowed to flow into the abdominal cavity. If the peritoneum separates from the abdominal wall, a common problem with this species, one observes an artificial cavity with fatty and foamy appearance. In this case, a puncture of the peritoneum can be accomplished with a long, sharp needle followed by insertion of the laparoscope (Fig. 13). An assistant who manipulates the reproductive tract rectally or with a forceps grasping the cervix is helpful with the procedure and also a laparoscopic forceps, inserted through a

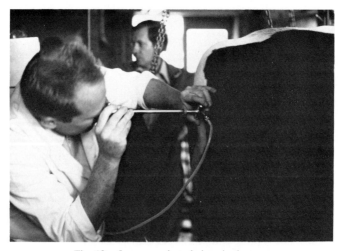

Fig. 13. Laparoscopic technique in the cow.

second puncture site about 10 cm anterior to the laparoscopic incision is helpful. The procedure in horses (Heinze *et al.*, 1972) is similar to that used with cattle.

D. Ancillary Techniques

Follicular aspiration can be easily accomplished in swine and sheep using the technique described earlier for nonhuman primates, but with appropriately larger syringes and needles.

We have used laparoscopy to collect uterine fluid throughout the estrous cycle of the pig (Wildt *et al.*, 1973; Morcom and Dukelow, 1976). An accessory cannula is inserted laterally from the midline, and the uterus held in position with laparoscopic grasping forceps. A 15-gauge, 7.6-cm needle is inserted through the abdominal wall at a site anterior to the point of cannulation (Fig. 14). After the needle passes into the uterine horn, polyethylene tubing (PE90; Clay Adams), with the terminal end sealed and small perforations along 4 cm of its length, is inserted through the shaft of the needle and into the uterine lumen. The cannulation needle is then withdrawn. By then lowering the animal to a level position (to

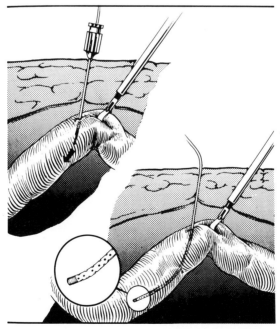

Fig. 14. Diagram (left) of the uterus of a gilt being grasped with forceps and the insertion of a 15-gauge needle. Diagram (right) showing the needle removed, leaving only the polyethylene tubing *in utero*. (From Wildt *et al.*, 1975.)

allow pooling of the flushing medium), fluids can be injected and aspirated. The laparoscope has also been used for oviductal insemination in swine, with resultant pregnancy and delivery.

VII. SUMMARY

Laparoscopy offers a simple and easily learned technique for the observation and manipulation of the reproductive tract in a wide variety of animals. Tract biopsies can be taken, fluids can be recovered, and substances injected into a variety of locations without major surgical intervention. In the field of gamete handling, sperm, ova, and developing embryos can be recovered and transferred using laparoscopic techniques.

The laparoscopic technique has a tremendous potential for biomedical research; its limitations are determined only by limitations of skill and ingenuity of the laparoscopist.

ACKNOWLEDGMENTS

The author wishes to express his appreciation to Drs. R. M. Harrison, D. A. Jewett, D. E. Wildt, J. M. R. Rawson, S. J. Jarosz, S. Fujimoto, S. Ariga, T. J. Kuehl, J. P. Mahone, and C. B. Morcom for their many contributions to the development of laparoscopic techniques at the Endocrine Research Unit over recent years.

REFERENCES

Ariga, S., and Dukelow, W. R. (1977). *Primates* **18,** 453–457.
Balin, H., Wan, L. S., Rajan, R., Kaiser, A., and McMann, R. H. (1969). *Clin. Obstet. Gynecol.* **12,** 534–552.
Benedict, E. B. (1951). "Endoscopy as Related to Diseases of the Bronchus, Esophagus, Stomach and Peritoneal Cavity." Williams & Wilkins, Baltimore, Maryland.
Bernheim, B. M. (1911). *Surgery* **13,** 764.
Betteridge, K. H., and Raeside, J. I. (1962). *Res. Vet. Sci.* **3,** 390–398.
Boyd, J. S., and Ducker, M. J. (1973). *Vet. Rec.* **93,** 40–43.
Bozzini, P. (1806). *J. d. pract. Arznk, u. Wundarznk.* **24,** 107–124.
Clarke, H. C. (1972). *Fertil. Steril.* **23,** 274–277.
Dierschke, D. J., and Hyatt, J. L. (1969). *J. Anim. Sci.* **28,** 645–649.
Dukelow, W. R. (1975). *J. Reprod. Fertil., Suppl.* **22,** 23–51.
Dukelow, W. R., and Kuehl, T. J. (1975). *La Fécondation* (Masson et Cie, Publishers, Paris, France) pp. 67–80.
Dukelow, W. R., Jarosz, S. J., Jewett, D. A., and Harrison, R. M. (1971). *Lab. Anim. Sci.* **21,** 594–597.
Fear, R. E. (1968). *Obstet. Gynecol.* **31,** 297–304.

Fishburne, J. I., Omran, K. F., Hulka, J. F., Mercer, J. P., and Edelman, D. A. (1974). *Fertil. Steril.* **25,** 762–766.

Fourestier, N., Glader, A., and Vulmiere, J. (1952). *Presse Med.* **60,** 1292.

Fujimoto, S., Rawson, J. M. R., and Dukelow, W. R. (1974). *J. Reprod. Fertil.* **38,** 97–103.

Graham, C. E., Keeling, M., Chapman, C., Cummins, L. B., and Haynie, J. (1973). *Am. J. Phys. Anthropol.* **38,** 211–216.

Harrison, R. M., and Dukelow, W. R. (1971). *J. Reprod. Fertil.* **25,** 99–101.

Harrison, R. M., and Dukelow, W. R. (1973). *J. Med. Primatol.* **2,** 277–283.

Harrison, R. M., and Dukelow, W. R. (1974). *Primates* **15,** 305–309.

Harrison, R. M., Rawson, J. M. R., and Dukelow, W. R. (1974). *Fertil. Steril.* **25,** 51–56.

Heinze, V. H., and Klug, E. (1973). *Blauen Hefte Tierartz.* **50,** 555–560.

Heinze, V. H., Klug, E., and von Lepel, J. D. (1972). *Dtsch. Tieraerztl. Wochenschr.* **79,** 49–51.

Hope, R. (1937). *Surg., Gynecol. Obstet.* **64,** 229.

Hulet, C. V., and Foote, W. C. (1968). *J. Anim. Sci.* **27,** 142–145.

Hulka, J. F., and Omran, K. F. (1972). *Fertil. Steril.* **23,** 633–639.

Jacobaeus, H. E. (1910). *Muench. Med. Wochenschr.* **57,** 2090.

Jewett, D. A., and Dukelow, W. R. (1971a). *Lab. Primate Newsl.* **10,** 16–17.

Jewett, D. A., and Dukelow, W. R. (1971b). *Folia Primatol.* **16,** 216–220.

Jewett, D. A., and Dukelow, W. R. (1972a). *J. Med. Primatol.* **1,** 193–195.

Jewett, D. A., and Dukelow, W. R. (1972b). *J. Reprod. Fertil.* **31,** 287–290.

Jewett, D. A., and Dukelow, W. R. (1973). *J. Med. Primatol.* **2,** 108–113.

Kelling, G. (1902). *Muench. Med. Wochenschr.* **49,** 21.

Kuehl, T. J., and Dukelow, W. R. (1975). *J. Med. Primatol.* **4,** 209–216.

Kuehl, T. J., and Dukelow, W. R. (1977). *J. Med. Primatol.* (submitted for publication).

Lamond, D. R., and Holmes, J. H. G. (1965). *Aust. Vet. J.* **41,** 324–325.

Lamond, D. R., and Urguhart, E. J. (1961). *Aust. Vet. J.* **37,** 430–431.

Land, R. B., Pelletier, J., Thimonier, J., and Mauléon, P. (1973). *J. Endocrinol.* **58,** 305–317.

Mahone, J. P., and Dukelow, W. R. (1976a). "Laparoscopy of Laboratory Animals" (16 mm movie). Endocrine Research Unit, Michigan State University, East Lansing.

Mahone, J. P., and Dukelow, W. R. (1976b). "Laparoscopy of Domestic Animals" (16 mm movie). Endocrine Research Unit, Michigan State University, East Lansing.

Megale, F. (1967). *Vet. Med. & Small Anim. Clin.* **62,** 555–557.

Megale, F., Fincher, M. G., and McEntee, K. (1956). *Cornell Vet.* **46,** 109–121.

Morcom, C. B., and Dukelow, W. R. (1976). *Proc. Int. Pig Vet. Soc. Congr., 1976,* p. D27.

Morgenstern, L. L., and Soupart, P. (1972). *Fertil. Steril.* **23,** 751–758.

Nordentoeft, S. (1912). *Verh. Dtsch. Ges. Chir.* **42,** 78.

Pelletier, J., and Thimonier, J. (1973). *J. Reprod. Fertil.* **33,** 310–313.

Phillippo, M., Swapp, G. H., Robinson, J. J., and Gill, J. C. (1971). *J. Reprod. Fertil.* **27,** 129–132.

Rawson, J. M. R., and Dukelow, W. R. (1973a). *Lab. Primate Newsl.* **12,** 4–5.

Rawson, J. M. R., and Dukelow, W. R. (1973b). *J. Reprod. Fertil.* **34,** 187–190.

Rawson, J. M. R., and Dukelow, W. R. (1973c). *Pharmacologist* **15,** 256.

Roberts, E. M. (1968). *Proc. Aust. Soc. Anim. Prod.* **7,** 192–194.

Ruddock, J. C. (1937). *Surg., Gynecol. Obstet.* **65,** 623.

Seeger, K. (1973). *Tiererztl. Prax.* **1,** 295–299.

Seeger, K., and Humke, R. (1974). *Blauen Hefte Tieraerzt.* **52,** 40–48.

Semm, K. (1969). *Acta Eur. Fertil.* **1,** 81–97.

Semm, K. (1970). *Endoscopy* **2,** 35–42.

Siegler, A. M., and Garret, M. (1970). *Fertil. Steril.* **21,** 763–773.

Smith, B. D., and Dillon, T. F. (1970). *Fertil. Steril.* **21,** 193–200.

Snyder, D. A., and Dukelow, W. R. (1974). *Theriogenology* **2**, 143–148.

Steptoe, P. C. (1967). "Laparoscopy in Gynecology." Livingstone, Edinburgh.

Steptoe, P. C., and Edwards, R. G. (1970). *Lancet* **1**, 683–689.

Thimonier, J., and Mauléon, P. (1969). *Ann. Biol. Anim., Biochim., Biophys.* **9**, 233–250.

von Nitze, M. (1894). *In* "Cystographic Atlas" (J. F. Bergmann, ed.), pp. 140–143. Wiesbaden.

Wildt, D. E., Fujimoto, S., Spencer, J. L., and Dukelow, W. R. (1973). *J. Reprod. Fertil.* **35**, 541–543.

Wildt, D. E., Morcom, C. B., and Dukelow, W. R. (1975). *J. Reprod. Fertil.* **44**, 301–304.

Wildt, D. E., Levinson, C. J., and Seager, S. W. J. (1977a). *Anat. Rec.* **189**, 443–450.

Wildt, D. E., Doyle, L. L., Stone, S., and Harrison, R. M. (1977b). *Primates* **18**, 261–270.

Witherspoon, D. M., and Talbot, R. B. (1970). *J. Am. Vet. Med. Assoc.* **157**, 1452–1457.

22

The Use of Amniocentesis in Prenatal Diagnosis

CARMEN B. LOZZIO

I. INTRODUCTION

Amniocentesis for prenatal diagnosis of genetic disorders is a diagnostic procedure that has contributed valuable information to the knowledge of human fetal development. It is useful for early detection of various genetic defects and could help reduce the incidence of some genetic conditions such as Down's syndrome if it were offered to all pregnant women with an increased risk for these disorders. The procedure has been used for many years (Menees *et al.*, 1930), with its main application being in the management of Rh disease (Freda, 1965; Queenan and Adams, 1965). Recently, the number of pregnancies with Rh incompatibility has decreased, and the referrals for prenatal diagnosis have increased significantly. Studies of sex chromatin (Nelson and Emery, 1970; Valenti *et al.*, 1972; Nadler, 1971), of the Y chromosome body fluorescence (Khudr and Benirschke, 1971), and chromosome analyses (Steele and Breg, 1966) have made possible the determination of the fetal sex and the detection of chromosomal disorders in amniotic fluid cells and cell cultures. Chromosomal disorders (Jacobson and Barter, 1967; Valenti *et al.*, 1969; Gertner *et al.*, 1970; Nadler and Gerbie, 1971; Milunsky *et al.*, 1972), hereditary biochemical disorders (Nadler, 1968; Milunsky *et al.*, 1970; Milunsky and Littlefield, 1972), and neural tube defects (Brock and Sutcliffe, 1972; Milunsky and Alpert, 1976a; Lindsten *et al.*, 1976) are detectable by this procedure at a stage of gestation that is early enough for active intervention if an abnormality is discovered.

Several books (Milunsky, 1973, 1975; Boué, 1976) and many review articles dealing with amniocentesis have been published. The techniques employed have been reported in many publications and cannot be summarized comprehensively. Thus, a selective analyses of the most common procedures is presented.

II. AMNIOCENTESIS

A. Technique

This procedure is performed by an obstetrician in an outpatient clinic under strictly aseptic conditions. Local anesthesia is employed, and the fluid is aspirated with a spinal needle through the midline of the abdominal wall (Freda, 1965; Queenan, 1966; Queenan and Adams, 1965; Fuchs, 1971; Gerbie *et al.*, 1971). Most centers perform the amniocentesis when the patient's bladder is empty in order to avoid aspiration of maternal urine. This is checked further by testing one drop of the fluid with a Multistix reagent strip (AMES) which shows alkaline pH and positive proteins if the sample is amniotic fluid, and acid pH and negative proteins if it is urine. Approximately 20–25 ml of fluid are sufficient for the different types of studies. Ultrasound studies should be performed routinely prior to amniocentesis in order to localize the placenta, determine fetal age, and select an optimal site for the amniocentesis.

B. Safety and Accuracy of the Procedure

The safety and accuracy of midtrimester amniocentesis was investigated by a cooperative study performed at nine institutions in the United States, under a contract with the National Institute of Child Health and Human Development (NICHD National Registry for Amniocentesis Study Group, 1976). This was a prospective study of 1040 women undergoing amniocentesis and 992 controls matched as closely as possible for race, gravity, and family income. More women older than 35 were included in the amniocentesis group because the control group was formed by those who elected not to have amniocentesis. The results of this cooperative study showed that approximately 2% of the women had immediate complications after amniocentesis (vaginal bleeding or amniotic fluid leakage). The diagnostic accuracy was high (99.4%), and there was no statistically significant increase in the rate of fetal loss or in the complications of pregnancy or delivery. The Canadian collaborative study of 1223 amniocenteses performed in 1020 pregnancies of 990 women also demonstrated that this is a safe and accurate procedure (Simpson *et al.,* 1976). The European experience included 1674 cases in the review by Lindsten *et al.* (1976) and 6121 cases from 46 centers in 8 Western European countries in the survey reported by Galjaard (1976). These studies showed a percentage of "spontaneous" abortions of 1.4% following early amniocentesis. This percentage does not exceed the normal rate of spontaneous abortions for this period of pregnancy. Other fetal or maternal complications did not differ significantly from other prospective studies of pregnancies without amniocentesis. Follow-up studies of 3777 children born after amniocentesis were reviewed by Murken (1976), who agreed with the general conclusion that practically no detrimental effect to the newborn child was caused by amniocentesis.

C. Timing for Prenatal Genetic Diagnosis

The optimal time to schedule an amniocentesis for prenatal genetic diagnosis depends on the volume of amniotic fluid. The procedure is usually performed at 16 weeks of gestation (Nadler, 1969; Nadler and Gerbie, 1970). At this time, the amount of amniotic fluid is usually of a sufficient volume to permit an adequate sampling, and it is early enough in the pregnancy to obtain results while a therapeutic abortion of an abnormal fetus is still possible. There is very little amniotic fluid before 11 weeks of gestation, whereas the volume increases 25 ml/week between 11 and 15 gestational weeks (Monie, 1953; Rhodes, 1966; Wagner and Fuchs, 1962) and 50 ml/week from 15 to 28 weeks (Wagner and

Fuchs, 1962; Elliott and Inman, 1961; Charles *et al.,* 1965). At 14–16 weeks of gestation, the volume of amniotic fluid ranges between 100 and 285 ml (Fuchs, 1966) and at 20 gestational weeks the average volume is 400 ml. The volume required for prenatal diagnosis ranges between 10 and 25 ml; thus, it is not safe to attempt the amniocentesis before the 14th week of gestation when less than 50–100 ml of total fluid is present.

The amniotic fluid circulates rapidly between fetus and mother, and total replacement of the fluid occurs in a 3-hour period (Cox and Chalmers, 1953; Hutchinson *et al.,* 1955; Plentl and Hutchinson, 1953). At term, the exchange of fluid approaches 500 ml/hour (Hutchinson *et al.,* 1955, 1959). The exact origin of the fluid is unknown, and it may be considered as a transudate of maternal serum across the placenta or fetal membranes, with a contribution of the fetal tracheobronchial tree and fetal skin. Fetal urine is also present in the amniotic fluid after the 20th week (Jeffcoate and Scott, 1959). Pathological decrease in the amount of amniotic fluid (oligohydramnios) has been observed in fetuses with bilateral renal agenesis, probably as the result of lack of fetal urine in the amniotic fluid (Jeffcoate and Scott, 1959). However, this is not seen in all the cases with urinary tract obstruction or bilateral renal agenesis (Ostergard, 1970). On the other hand, increases in the amount of amniotic fluid (polyhydramnios) have been observed in fetuses with anencephaly, probably due to the lack of antidiuretic hormone formed by the posterior pituitary (Benirschke and McKay, 1953). In other congenital malformations, such as esophageal or duodenal atresia, polyhydramnios is the result of defective fetal swallowing. It appears that the normal fetus swallows about 20 ml of amniotic fluid/hour or 500 ml/day, and this swallowing is one of the most important mechanisms of disposal of the amniotic fluid (Pritchard, 1965, 1966).

D. Indications

The indications for midtrimester amniocentesis for prenatal diagnosis are: (1) increased incidence of chromosomal disorders due to maternal age over 35 years; (2) previous birth of a child with a chromosomal syndrome or positive family history for chromosomal syndromes; (3) parental chromosome translocations; (4) increased risk for metabolic disorders due to previous birth of an affected child or demonstration that the parents are heterozygous carriers of a hereditary biochemical disorder; (5) previous offspring with neural tube defects; (6) determination of the sex in pregnancies at risk for recessive sex-linked disorders; and (7) a miscellaneous group including maternal ingestion of high doses of teratogens and other drugs, such as LSD; exposure to X-irradiation during early pregnancy; abnormal karyotype of one of the parents, such as XYY, XXX, mosaicism, or increased number of satellite associations; maternal hyperthyroidism; or parental anxiety. In the cases labeled as parental anxiety, the risk is the same as in the general population, (0.56% for chromosomal disorders, and 1–2%/oo for neural tube defects), but the parents want to assure themselves that their child will not suffer one of these conditions. They must understand that they still carry the average risk for other congenital defects (Polani and Benson, 1973; Milunsky, 1973; NICHD National Registry for Amniocentesis Study Group, 1976; Simpson *et al.*, 1976; Lindsten *et al.*, 1976).

III. ULTRASOUND

A. Technique

Ultrasound is based on the use of sound waves whose frequency is above the audible range (greater than 18,000 cps). These high frequency ultrasound waves are generated by naturally occurring crystals, such as quartz and Rochelle salt, or polycrystalline ceramics, such as barium titanate and lead zirconate-titanate (Sundén, 1964). The equipment used for ultrasound scanning utilizes a crystal of lead zirconate-titanate, which both generates the sound and receives the echoes. The sounds are generated by applying short electrical pulses to the crystal which is contained in a probe. The probe is applied to the skin of the patient, with a thin film of olive oil used to improve the contact. The examination is performed by moving the probe both longitudinally and transversally at various levels of the abdomen (midline, right, and left longitudinal scans; transverse umbilical plane; or cranial and caudal of the umbilical plane). The pregnant woman usually lies on her back and has the bladder well filled to avoid gas-filled bowels interfering with the echoes generated by the placenta, amniotic fluid, and fetus. The echoes are received by the crystal in the probe and are transformed into electrical pulses which are then amplified. These pulses give an image which is observed on the oscilloscope screen and photographed on Polaroid film type 107C.

B. Placenta Localization and Fetal Age Determination

Preamniocentesis ultrasonic placental localization and fetal age determination are used to improve the safety of amniocentesis. The information as to the location of the placenta helps the obstetrician avoid this area, if at all possible, when making the puncture. The ultrasound pictures are also helpful in estimating the depth required to reach the fluid in obese patients (Scrimgeour, 1976). Our own experience and reports from others (Arger *et al.*, 1976) show that most problems occur when the placenta is in an anterior position. In this case, multiple transverse scans are usually done to localize the site of the thinnest segment of placenta, as well as to locate the most amniotic fluid. When the placenta is completely anterior and there is no thin site, the benefit versus the risk of

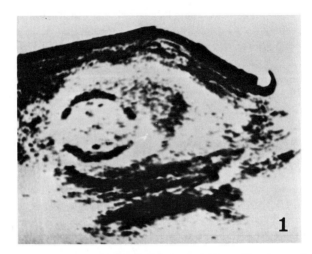

Fig. 1. Normal sonography with a biparietal diameter of 44 mm. The placenta lies on the right side extending anteriorly as well as posteriorly.

transplacental amniocentesis should be discussed with the patient. In cases with low genetic risk and complete anterior placenta, most patients decide not to undergo the procedure. On the other hand, in cases with high genetic risk, such as carriers of chromosomal translocations or metabolic disorders, the benefits clearly outweigh the risk of transplacental amniocentesis, and most patients elect to go on with the amniocentesis.

TABLE I

Estimated Gestational Age According to Biparietal Diameters Measured by Sonar and to Length of Human Fetuses Studied as Pathological Specimens

Duration of pregnancy (weeks)[a]	Biparietal diameter (mm)	Length of fetus (mm) (Streeter)
13	23	74
14	28	87
15	32	101
16	36	116
17	40	130
18	44	142
19	48	153
20	51	164

[a] Estimation of gestational duration from the fetal bitemporo-parietal diameter according to Ron Brown, M.D., "Ultrasono-graphy," Table 8-1, p. 116.

The age of the fetus is determined by measurement of the biparietal diameter of the skull (Brown, 1975). The fetal head can be recorded at the 13th week of pregnancy. At this time, the biparietal diameter is on the average 23 mm, and the fetus has a length of about 74 mm (Sundén, 1964). At 16 weeks, the biparietal diameter is 36 mm, and the length of the fetus is 116 mm. From 13 to 20 weeks (Fig. 1) of gestation, the biparietal diameter is a very good measure of the gestation age (see Table I). This information is important, not only in determining the best time for amniocentesis, but also in clarifying the significance of the values obtained in studies of α-feto proteins.

C. Ultrasound Diagnosis of Fetal Malformations, Twins, and Intrauterine Growth Retardation

Ultrasound studies are useful in diagnosing some fetal malformations. For example, the absence of echoes from the head (Fig. 2) on sonar scans performed between 14 and 18 weeks of gestation establishes the diagnosis of anencephaly (Campbell *et al.*, 1972), and this diagnosis is confirmed by the finding of elevated levels of α-feto proteins in the amniotic fluid (Milunsky and Alpert, 1976b). Ultrasound diagnosis is also useful in determining whether a fetus is present in threatened abortions during the 3rd and 4th months of pregnancy. Absence of fetal parts is seen in cases of "blighted ovum" (Fig. 3) when a gestational sac is present, but there is a complete absence or only a remnant of an

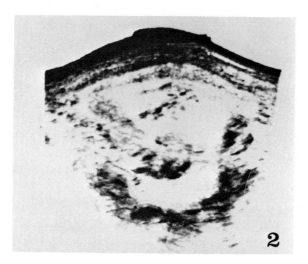

Fig. 2. Sonogram of the anencephalic fetus shown on Figs. 7 and 8. This sonogram was performed at approximately 16 gestational weeks, and no head can be identified. There also appears to be excessive fluid representing hydramnios.

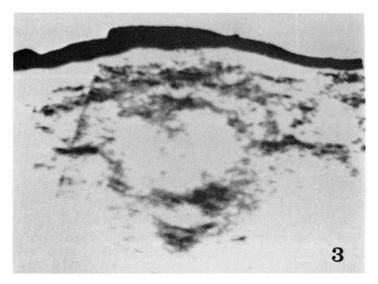

Fig. 3.   Pelvic ultrasound of a pregnancy in approximately the 12th week of gestation. No fetal parts were identified.

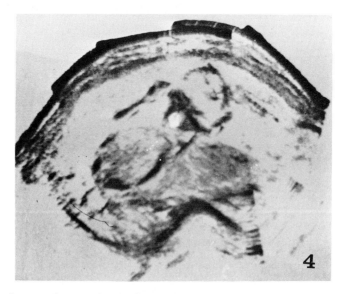

Fig. 4.   Sonogram demonstrating two fetuses. They both lie in a somewhat transverse position, one in the upper uterus and one in the lower uterus. The largest has a biparietal diameter of 45 mm, corresponding to a fetal age of 18.3 weeks. The placenta lies on the posterior wall.

embryo within it (MacVicar, 1976). Absence of fetal echoes and a typical ultrasound picture are observed in cases of hydatid mole (Sundén, 1964). Twin pregnancies are also diagnosed by ultrasound early in pregnancy (Fig. 4). It is important to study both fetuses when prenatal chromosomal diagnosis or α-fetal protein studies are indicated. In advanced pregnancy, the ultrasound diagnosis of hydrocephaly and microcephaly is possible. A biparietal diameter greater than 11 cm when the fetus is near to term is presumptive evidence of hydrocephaly (Campbell, 1972, 1974; Donald, 1972). Another indication is a head significantly larger than the fetal trunk (MacVicar, 1976). Microcephaly is suspected when the head size is significantly smaller than the chest size (MacVicar, 1976). A small head with a small chest may indicate an error in the gestational age and maturity of the fetus or intrauterine growth retardation (MacVicar, 1976). Serial measurements of the biparietal diameter throughout pregnancy can detect a "low growth profile" (Campbell, 1974), which is associated with an increased incidence of fetal abnormalities.

D. Safety of Sonography and Comparison to Prenatal Diagnosis by X-Rays

Ultrasound studies performed late in pregnancy are useful in diagnosing cephalic or breech presentations, twin pregnancies, and the presence of hydramnios without exposing the fetus to X-irradiation. Before the discovery of sonar, the use of X-rays was indicated to estimate fetal maturity, to determine the presenting part, and to detect fetal malformation such as anencephaly. The possibility of damaging the fetus by X-rays while *in utero* (Stewart *et al.*, 1956, 1958) has made many obstetricians reluctant to use X-rays during pregnancy unless it is necessary for the management of the case (MacVicar, 1976). It now appears that sonar diagnosis is a safer procedure than X-rays for use during pregnancy. The review of the literature (Donald, 1974) and the results of experimental studies performed by Sundén (1964) demonstrate that exposure to pulsed ultrasound applied with a scanning technique does not provoke abortion, intrauterine death, premature birth, malformation, or any other fetal damage, and subsequent fertility is unimpaired.

Sonar diagnosis is also more accurate than X-rays in diagnosing cases with anencephaly, since, at 15–16 weeks of pregnancy, the small fetal skull may appear absent on X-rays if it is overshadowed by the mother's vertebral column. Placental localization by X-rays is possible, but the risks of the technique is such that it outweighs the benefits. On the other hand, sonar localization of the placenta is a simple, quick, and safe procedure that reduces the complications of amniocentesis. This procedure should precede all amniocentesis performed in midtrimester pregnancies. The combination of sonar prenatal diagnosis and amniocentesis has significantly increased the possibilities of antenatal detection of fetal abnormalities, and both procedures are currently used extensively in obstetrical practice.

IV. CELL CULTURE TECHNIQUES

Several techniques and multiple modifications of these techniques have been described for the culture of amniotic fluid cells (Steele and Breg, 1966; Jacobson and Barter, 1967; Valenti et al., 1969; Ferguson-Smith et al., 1971; Gray et al., 1971; Cederqvist et al., 1973). The success rates and the number of days from the inoculation of the cells until chromosome preparations can be obtained varies with the method employed and the experience of the laboratory. All laboratories follow some basic, general principles and specific modifications introduced by each group. It has been generally agreed that experience in the field of tissue culture, with particular emphasis on techniques used for cultures of human fibroblasts and/or embryonic cells, is more important than the type of culture media and percent or type of serum used (Lindsten et al., 1976).

A. Transportation of the Amniotic Fluid

The best results are obtained when the fluid is drawn in a clinic located at the same institution as the tissue culture laboratory and when the amniotic fluid cultures are started soon after amniocentesis. If the fluid must be transported to the laboratory, it is best to use sterile glass tubes without any pretreatment and keep the fluid at room temperature.

B. Effects of Grossly Bloody Fluids on the Rate of Cell Growth

The presence of blood in the amniotic fluid may inhibit the rate of growth of amniotic cell cultures. To avoid this problem, various techniques for the elimination of red blood cells have been described (Lee et al., 1970; Milunsky, 1973). These techniques are modifications of the method of Dioguardi et al. (1963), which utilizes ammonium chloride (NH_4Cl) to lyse erythrocytes and platelets. The modification described by Milunsky (1973) involves treating the sediment of centrifuged cells with a cold (4°C) solution of 0.83% of ammonium chloride after one rinse in Eagle's minimum essential medium (MEM). The effect of the NH_4Cl is stopped after 3 minutes at 4°C by the addition of 1 ml of fetal calf serum. The suspension of amniotic fluid cells is rinsed once or twice in MEM. The procedure may be repeated if excess blood is still present. When the cell pellet is relatively free of red cells, the amniotic cells are resuspended in fresh medium and incubated at 37°C in an atmosphere of 5% CO_2 in air.

In our laboratory, the presence of blood in the amniotic fluid does not affect the rate of growth or the success of the cultures when we incubate the cells for 30 minutes with 2 ml of fetal bovine serum prior to the addition of the culture media. Grossly bloody samples were received in 22% of the cases when the amniocentesis was performed without prior sonogram localization of the placenta. Only 5% of the amniocentesis performed with ultrasound studies resulted in visible red blood cell contamination. Moderate to small amounts of red blood cells were present in 70% of the fluids that appeared to be clear. The presence of large numbers of red blood cells in highly contaminated fluids was probably the cause of slow growth in 25% of the 40 cultures in which the amniotic fluid was incubated in culture media without prior centrifugation and resuspension of the cells in fetal bovine serum. These results suggest that the presence of red blood cells in the initial culture interferes with the attachment of sufficient amniotic cells to start the growth of a good monolayer. This problem is avoided when the amniotic cells are incubated in a small amount of fetal bovine serum until they attach to the glass surface. Using this method, the cells grow fast and form a good monolayer even in the presence of large amounts of blood.

C. Choice of Culture Media

The selection of basal culture medium does not seem to be a critical factor. Good results were reported with Eagle's BME and MEM, RPMI-1640, F-10, and Parker 199 (Lindsten *et al.*, 1976, Table V). The same media may be considered good by one laboratory and very poor in another laboratory. For example, Hoehn *et al.* (1974) used Dulbecco's modification of Eagle's medium with good results, and Kaback and Leonard (1972) reported that this was a very poor medium compared to others. We use Eagle's MEM supplemented with 1% nonessential amino acids or McCoy's 5a with very good results.

Most laboratories supplement the basal medium with 20–30% fetal calf serum, although Felix *et al.* (1974) demonstrated that concentrations higher than 15% do not improve the results. It is very important to test each batch of fetal calf serum with cultured amniotic cells which are known to grow well with a previous lot of fetal calf serum (Therkelsen, 1976). We have found significant differences in growth rates using different batches of the same type of fetal bovine serum ordered from the same commercial source. We also keep the serum frozen until we use it, and we inactivate the media containing fetal bovine serum by incubation at 56°C for 1 hour. Some laboratories supplement media with 10% human AB serum (Therkelsen, 1976) or 20% pooled human serum (Hasholt, 1976). Human serum should not be added when the culture is done to detect a mucopolysaccharidosis because this serum contains the specific enzymes (Neufeld, 1973), and the uptake by the cells of the corrective factor (Lindsten *et al.,* 1976) could affect the interpretation of the results. In addition to the type of serum, other factors such as the type of basal medium, the time of culture, the frequency of medium change, the pH of the medium, the degree of confluency, growth phase, etc., may influence the enzyme activity of cultured cells. Thus, the culture conditions should be standardized for biochemical studies of hereditary metabolic disorders.

D. Techniques for Primary Cultures of Amniotic Cells

1. In Situ *Karyotyping of Primary Cultures*

The cells may be cultured in 30-mm petri dishes or Leighton tubes containing cover glasses. This technique is called *in situ* karyotyping of primary amniotic fluid cell cultures, and the details of one of these methods has been published by Schmid (1975, 1976). This author prepares two Leighton tubes with 1 ml AF and 1 ml of EMB or Ham's F10 plus 30% fetal calf serum or 20% human serum. He also centrifuges aliquots of 3–5 ml AF and resuspends the cells in 2 ml of medium. The Leighton tubes are closed after they are gassed, or they are incubated in an open system with 5% CO_2 in air. After 6–12 days in culture with change of medium every 2 or 3 days, 5–10 clones of 1–4 mm are present, and the cells are ready to harvest. The medium is changed on the next day, and the cover slip is transferred for 4–5 hours to another Leighton tube with 2 ml of medium and 2 μg of colcemid. Then, the cover glass is transferred to one of the compartments of a petri dish 100×15 mm style Y (Falcon Plastics No. 1004) containing prewarmed hypotonic solution (NaCl, 0.08%), and incubated at 37°C for 20 minutes. The hypotonic solution is gradually replaced by fixative (methanol–acetic acid 3:1) during 15 minutes, fixed for 10 minutes, and air-dried.

Boué *et al.* (1976) have described a similar *in situ* technique using 30-mm petri dishes and round cover glasses. Aliquots of 1.5 ml AF are added to 1.5–2 ml of medium, which contains RPMI 1640, 20% fetal calf serum, 5 ml of a solution of 1.4% sodium bicarbonate and antibiotics. Other dishes are inoculated with the sediment of 3–5 ml of AF centrifuged at 600–900 rpm. The dishes are incubated at 37°C in a CO_2 incubator at pH 7.3. The medium is changed after 4–5 days and later on every 2 days until enough clones have grown. When the cells are ready to be harvested, the cover glasses are transferred to another petri dish with fresh medium without addition of colchicine. After 20–22 hours, the medium is replaced by an hypotonic solution containing 5 ml of Hanks' and 95 ml of normal distilled water at pH 7. The cells are treated with this hypotonic solution for 10 minutes and fixed with Carnoy chloroform for 1 hour and air-dried.

Chromosome preparations are obtained with these *in situ* techniques in 9–12 days, and the morphology of the clones can be correlated to the karyotypes observed. The disadvantage of these methods is the difficulty of handling the fragile cover glasses. In addition, in our experience, the quality of the metaphases obtained is not as good as with preparations of cells trypsinized and resuspended in hypotonic solution.

2. Monolayer Cultures of Amniotic Cells

Many laboratories use petri dishes without cover slips for the primary cultures. After 10–20 days in culture with changes of medium twice a week, the cells are trypsinized. These cells may be harvested immediately, or transferred to other petri dishes or flasks. They may be harvested 24 hours after transfer to dishes with cover slips or grown until an increased number of cells is available for studies (Milunsky, 1973). Other laboratories prefer to start the primary cultures in 30-ml plastic T flasks, 250-ml plastic culture flasks, or milk dilution glass bottles. The advantages of flasks over the petri dishes include: (1) lower incidence of contamination, and (2) greater yield of cultured cells for chromosome analysis and biochemical studies.

In the method described by Cederqvist *et al.* (1973), the amniotic fluid is incubated for 15 minutes without centrifugation. After this incubation, an equal amount of a highly enriched culture medium is added. This medium contains 30% fetal calf serum, 2.0 mM glutamine, and 100 μg/ml gentamicin. The pH is adjusted to 7.2–7.4 by the addition of sodium bicarbonate. The cells are incubated at 37°C in an atmosphere of 5% CO_2 and left without disturbance for 4 days. At this time, 15 ml of fresh medium is added without removing the old medium. According to the authors, sufficient cells for karyotyping are obtained in 5–14 days. Colcemid at a final concentration of 0.6 μg/ml is added, and the hypotonic treatment is performed with 4 ml of 0.075 M potassium chloride for 20 minutes.

The cell culture technique used at our laboratory (C. B. Lozzio and J. Kim unpublished) is based on the same general procedures followed by other laboratories with modifications that have improved our results. The details of this method are the following:

1. Aliquots of 5 ml AF are centrifuged for 5 minutes at 500–600 rpm.

2. The supernatant fluid is removed and used to study α-feto proteins. The sediment is resuspended in 2 ml of fetal bovine serum (GIBCO) and inoculated into glass milk dilution bottles. These bottles are incubated for 30 minutes at 37° in a CO_2 incubator.

3. Ten milliliters of medium (inactivated McCoy 5a with 20% fetal bovine serum) are added to each bottle. These are incubated at 37°C in a CO_2 incubator at pH 7.2–7.4 for 5 days without disturbance.

4. Ten additional milliliters of fresh medium (20% inactivated McCoy 5a) are added to each bottle on the 5th day without removing the old medium.

5. On the 6th day, the cell growth and cell density are checked. If the cells are growing fast and many floating cells are present, one-third of the medium is transferred and replaced with a similar amount of fresh medium (McCoy 5a with

15% fetal bovine serum). If the cell density is low and the growth is not heavy, the medium is not changed until 2 or 3 days later.

6. Half the medium is changed every 2 or 3 days until a monolayer of good growing colonies of fibroblasts are observed. If two or three bottles have good growth, one of the primary cultures is harvested for chromosome analyses and the others are subcultured after trypsinization. If each bottle has several slow growing clones, the cells from two or three bottles are pooled into a new bottle. On the other hand, if the growth is fast and heavy, the cells are split into two bottles.

7. The medium is changed 20 hours prior to the harvest, and colcemid at a final concentration of 0.025 μg/ml is added during the last 4 hours of incubation.

8. At the time of harvest, the medium is discarded, 1.5 ml of trypsin (0.2%) is added for a few seconds to rinse off any medium left into the bottle. This trypsin is replaced by 3.5 ml of fresh trypsin, and the bottle is incubated at 37°C. After 3 minutes, the cells are observed with an inverted microscope, and 10 ml of fresh medium is added to stop the action of the trypsin as soon as the cells begin to detach from the glass surface. The cells are then resuspended in the medium and transferred to centrifuge tubes.

The following harvest method (C. B. Lozzio, M. B. Klepper, and J. Kim, unpublished) is used in our laboratory:

1. The cells are spun down for 5 minutes at 500–600 rpm. The supernatant is removed and 6 ml of warmed Hanks' solution is added. The cells are resuspended slowly in this solution and centrifuged again for 5 minutes.

2. The supernatant is removed, and a warmed hypotonic solution is added drop by drop while the cells are resuspended slowly. After addition of a total of 10 ml of hypotonic solution, the cells are incubated at 37°C for a total of 10 minutes, including the time of resuspending the cells when the hypotonic solution is added. The first bottle of a given culture ready to harvest is treated with a hypotonic solution of 2 gm KCl and 2 gm Na citrate in 1000 ml distilled water. This hypotonic treatment gives a good number of well-spread metaphases suitable for banding studies. The second bottle of the same culture is treated with a mixture of 95% of a solution of 0.075% KCl and 5% of the KCl–Na citrate solution. With this hypotonic solution, the chromosomes are elongated and show more details with banding techniques, but we find less well-spread metaphases. In most cases, we have good growth in enough bottles to use both types of hypotonic solutions, and we study the cells with both methods.

3. A few drops of fixer (absolute methanol–glacial acetic acid 3:1) are added to the cells in hypotonic solution. The cells are resuspended again and then centrifuged for 5 minutes.

4. The supernatant is discarded and the fixer is added up to 6 ml without disturbing the cell pellet.

5. After 30 minutes, the cells are resuspended slowly in the fixer and spun down for 5 minutes. The supernatant is removed, fresh fixer is added, the cells are resuspended again, and centrifuged for 5 minutes. This process is repeated three times.

6. A small amount of fixer is added to the cell sediment, the cells are resuspended, and a drop of the cell suspension is spread on wet slides which are allowed to air dry without flaming. The first slide is checked with phase contrast, and the amount of fixer is adjusted before the other slides are prepared. Usually 8–10 good quality slides are obtained from each bottle.

V. CHROMOSOME ANALYSES WITH BANDING TECHNIQUES

A. Characteristics of the Different Types of Bands

1. The Q Bands

These are bright, faint, or dark fluorescent regions with a specific consistent sequence along the length of each chromosome (Caspersson *et al.,* 1968, 1970).

2. The C Bands

They are dark centromeric areas of constitutive heterochromatin obtained by alkali denaturation and reassociation (Pardue and Gall, 1970; Arrighi and Hsu, 1971).

3. The G Bands

These bands are dark regions of intercalary constitutive heterochromatin which correspond to the bright fluorescent Q bands. The G-banding techniques derived from Pardue and Gall's method (1970) use various denaturation treatments followed by Giemsa staining (Sumner *et al.,* 1971; Drets and Shaw, 1971; Patil *et al.,* 1971). Trypsin pretreatment with Giemsa staining is a widely used method for G banding (Seabright, 1972; Pathak, 1976). After trypsin pretreatment, the chromatids are smaller in the lighter bands, and apparent constrictions are seen at the dark bands stained with Giemsa.

4. The R Bands

These bands are the reverse counter type of the G bands. The euchromatin is darkly stained at the terminal regions of most chromosomes, and the intercalary constitutive heterochromatin remains as negative bands. Giemsa staining after mild denaturation by heat (Dutrillaux and Lejeune, 1971) acridine orange and fluorescence studies after heat treatment (Verma and Lubs, 1975, 1976) direct staining with acridine orange (Couturier *et al.,* 1973) or BUdR pretreatment plus acridine orange staining (Dutrillaux *et al.*, 1973) are different procedures for R banding.

5. The T Bands

These are darkly stained terminal bands of the chromosomes which show different intensities from one chromosome to another. They represent the most resistant R bands to the denaturation process with only the tips of the chromatids showing intense fluorescence (Dutrillaux, 1973).

B. Chemical Properties of the Bands

It is known that the bands observed after staining with various special techniques are not artifacts and are not due to the staining alone. A faint banding pattern is seen on unstained slides studied by phase contrast microscopy (Dutrillaux and Lejeune, 1975). However, the biochemical nature of these bands is not known, and two main hypotheses have been postulated and are discussed below.

1. The DNA Hypothesis

The sequences of DNA especially rich in particular bases appears to be the reason for the differential banding. The specificity of quinacrine to A-T (adenine–thymine)-rich DNA segments (Weisblum and de Haseth, 1972) could explain the typical Q-banding pattern. The heat denaturation of A-T-rich segments would allow the staining of G-C (guanine–cytosine)-rich DNA segments by acridine orange at the R bands (Dutrillaux and Lejeune, 1975). Further evidence for this interpretation was provided by the induction of characteristic reverse fluorescence bands with the G-C-specific DNA binding antibiotics oligomycin, chromomycin A_3 and mithramycin (van de Sande *et al.*, 1977). This hypothesis does not explain why the repetitive DNA of the secondary constrictions of chromosomes 1, 9, and 16 that are not resistant to denaturation give a faint red fluorescence with acridine orange (Dutrillaux and Lejeune, 1975).

2. The Protein Hypothesis

The demonstration that proteolytic treatments induce G bands (Dutrillaux *et al.*, 1971) suggests that the chromosome proteins play a role in G banding. Some proteins may be more tightly bound to DNA after G- or R-banding treatment of the chromosomes, and differences in nonhistone proteins in the Q and R bands may account for the reversal of patterns seen after changes in the banding conditions (Comings and Avelino, 1975; Comings, 1976).

C. Techniques for Chromosome-Banding Analyses

The following procedures are the modifications of the original methods which are used with good results at our laboratory.

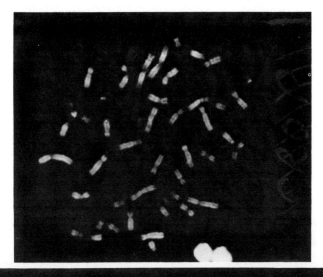

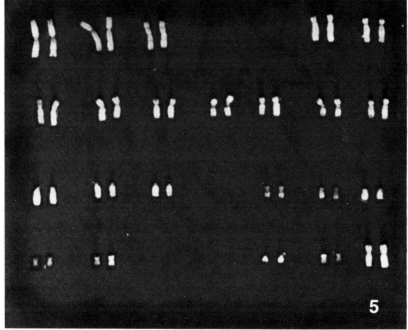

Fig. 5. Female karyotype studies with fluorescence Q-banding technique.

1. Fluorescence Q Bands

This technique is essentially the same as described by Caspersson *et al.* (1970) with very slight modifications.

    a. Fixed slides are hydrated in alcohol of decreasing concentrations:

    1. 95% Methyl alcohol—15 minutes

    2. 70% Methyl alcohol—2 minutes

    3. Distilled water—2 minutes

    b. The slides are stained for 5–20 minutes in the dark with a solution of 1 ml quinacrine mustard in 20 ml of distilled water. (This solution is kept in the refrigerator in the dark, and can be reused several times.)

    c. Rinse in running tap water for 5 minutes.

    d. Immerse in citric acid–phosphate buffer McIlvaine for 3 minutes.

    e. Rinse twice in citric acid–phosphate buffer. This buffer is prepared as two separate solutions:

    1. 0.2 M phosphate (35.6 gm Na_2HPO_4 2 HO per liter)

    2. 0.1 M citric acid (21.01 gm $C_8H_8O_7$ HO per liter)

They are mixed in the proportion of 58 ml of (1) plus 42 ml of (2) for a pH of 6.5. The slides are mounted with a cover slip in the same buffer.

    f. The metaphases are photographed with an epifluorescence microscope using Kodak Tri-X film. The film is developed in Microdol-X for 13–14 minutes (Fig. 5).

2. Giemsa Banding (G Bands)

There are many variations of this technique. Two main types are used by different laboratories: one is based on denaturation by partial heat and/or alkaline solutions (Sumner *et al.,* 1971; Drets and Shaw, 1971); the other involves partial digestion by proteolytic enzymes, such as pronase (Dutrillaux *et al.,* 1971) or trypsin (Seabright, 1972).

The modification of the ASG (acid–saline–giemsa) technique described by Sumner *et al.* (1971) which is used at our laboratory (C. B. Lozzio and M. B. Klepper, unpublished) is described below:

    a. Incubate the slides for 1 hour at 62°C in SSC × 2 (0.3 M NaCl and 0.03 M trisodium citrate). Best results are obtained if the slides are warmed prior to this incubation.

    b. Rinse three times in distilled water and let the slides air-dry.

    c. Rinse twice in phosphate buffer at pH 6.8 (This buffer is prepared with 9 ml of 0.2 M Na_2HPO_4, 3 ml of 0.1 M citric acid and 100 ml distilled water.)

    d. Rinse twice in 70% methyl alcohol and then in absolute methyl alcohol.

    e. Stain for 1 hour, 40 minutes in a mixture of 8.5 ml Giemsa Gurr R-66, 5.8 ml of absolute methyl alcohol, and 192 ml of phosphate buffer at pH 6.8, if the slides were prepared with the 95% KCl hypotonic treatment. For cells harvested with the hypotonic mixture of KCl and Na citrate, use 9 ml of Giemsa for

192 ml of buffer and 6 ml absolute methyl alcohol. The stain should be mixed just prior to use to avoid precipitation.

　　f. Rinse three times in distilled water. Let the slides dry and mount the next day.

　　g. Photograph metaphases with Panatomic X and develop the film with Kodak D-76. (Fig. 6)

The Giemsa trypsin method used at our laboratory for G-T bands is a slight modification of the technique described by Pathak (1976). The steps of this technique are the following:

　　a. Incubate the slides for 35 seconds to 2 minutes in a working solution of trypsin prepared by dilution of 5 ml of a stock solution (0.25%) with 95 ml of Hanks' balanced salt solution BSS.

　　b. Rinse quickly in Hanks'.

　　c. Rinse in 70% ethyl alcohol.

　　d. Rinse in 95% ethyl alcohol and air-dry.

　　e. Stain for 5–7 minutes in a solution of 2 ml Giemsa Harleco and 98 ml of 0.01 M phosphate buffer at pH 7 (mix 39.2 ml of 0.01 M KH_2PO_4 = 1.36 gm per 1000 ml distilled water and 60.8 ml of 0.01 M Na_2HPO_4 = 1.42 gm per 1000 ml distilled water.)

　　f. Rinse in distilled water.

The quality of these bands may be improved by incubating the dry slides at 62°C for 1 hour prior to the treatment with the trypsin solution.

The reverse banding method described by Dutrillaux and Lejeune (1971) has been improved (Dutrillaux and Lejeune, 1975), and it is used as follows:

　　a. Incubate the slides in Earle's BBS (pH 6.5) at 87°C for 45–60 minutes. Old slides need a shorter incubation (10 minutes), and fresh smears may be denatured for longer periods of time (up to 2 hours).

　　b. Rinse in phosphate buffer at pH 6.5.

　　c. Stain for 10 minutes in a mixture of 4 ml Giemsa (GT Gurr R66), 4 ml phosphate buffer, and 92 ml of distilled water or for 60 minutes in a mixture of 2 ml Giemsa, 8 ml buffer at pH 6.7, and 90 ml distilled water.

　　d. Rinse in buffer at pH 6.7.

　　e. Rinse in a solution of 8 ml buffer pH 6.7 and 92 ml of distilled water.

The modification described by Sehested (1974) is also used as follows:

　　a. Incubate the slides at 88°C in a solution of 1 M NaH_2PO_4 (pH 4–4.5) for 10 minutes.

　　b. Rinse briefly in distilled water.

　　c. Stain for 10 minutes in a solution of 2–3 ml of Giemsa (G. T. Gurr R66) and 50 ml of distilled water.

　　d. Rinse briefly with tap water and air-dry.

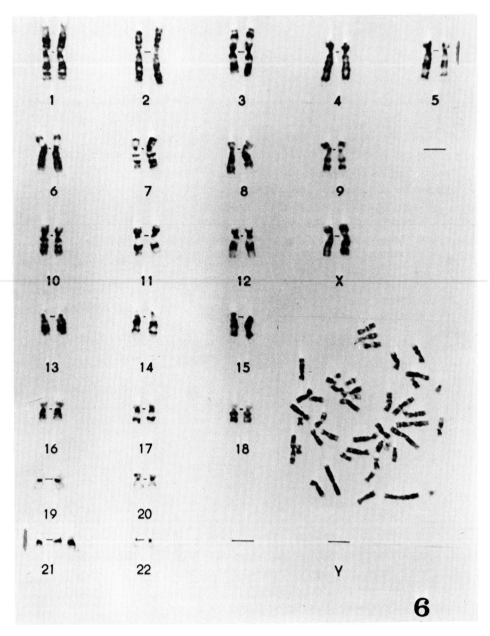

Fig. 6. Female karyotype analyzed with ASA Giemsa banding technique.

D. Chromosome Banding in Prenatal Diagnosis

Routine use of banding techniques is recommended in prenatal chromosome studies because structural chromosomal abnormalities may be present in cases studied for indications other than parental translocations. The nomenclature of the various types of chromosomal abnormalities has been described in the reports of the 1971 Paris Conference (1972) and its supplement (1975). Boué (1976) detected five structural chromosomal aberrations in parents with normal karyotype among 800 prenatal diagnoses. Two of these cases (46,XX,18p- and 46, XX,5p-) were detected in mothers over 40. Two other cases with karyotypes 46,XX,rD and 46,XY,13p- were studied because the pregnancy was abnormal, and one case 46,XY t(21q21q) +21 was investigated for detection of a neural tube defect.

Banding studies are important to avoid mistakes in diagnosis caused by lack of information on the sex and phenotype of the fetus and by poor identification of chromosomes stained with conventional techniques. In some cases, the differentiation between two possible karyotypes is only academic because both are seen in abnormal fetuses. For example, a male with Klinefelter's syndrome can be diagnosed by G bands and confirmed by autopsy and sex chromatin findings, but the same karyotype could be misinterpreted as a female with Down's syndrome on conventional staining studies (Murken et al., 1974; Stengel-Rutkowski et al., 1976). Another misinterpretation between two abnormal karyotypes was reported by Boué et al. (1976) in a male with Down's syndrome who was a balanced carrier of an inherited translocation with karyotype 47,XY,+21,t(6;22)(q16;q13)pat. This karyotype appeared to be a trisomy D with classical staining techniques. In other cases, a fetus with a karyotype of unknown or questionable clinical significance (e.g., XYY) is misinterpreted as a male with Down's syndrome when classical staining techniques are used (Stengel-Rutkowski et al., 1976). The mistake may have severe consequences in a case with a clinically normal phenotype and a balanced translocation that is aborted because the karyotype is misinterpreted as unbalanced. The use of banding techniques prevented this mistake in one case with balanced translocation 46,XY,t(1,10)(p36q24) who appeared to be a male with mongolism due to translocation G/G on conventional staining (Stengel-Rutkowski et al., 1976).

Unbalanced and balanced translocations in the offspring of balanced carriers of chromosomal translocations were studied with banded techniques at our laboratory. One of these cases was an anencephalic fetus (Fig. 7, 8) with an unbalanced translocation t(2;9) (q37,p11) 15p+ as the result of partial trisomy for the short arm of chromosome number 9 (Fig. 9). This partial trisomy is most likely due to crossing over at the proximal region of the short arm of chromosome 9. The studies of α-feto protein showed extremely high values in the amniotic fluid and maternal serum. The father of this fetus was the balanced carrier of the transloca-

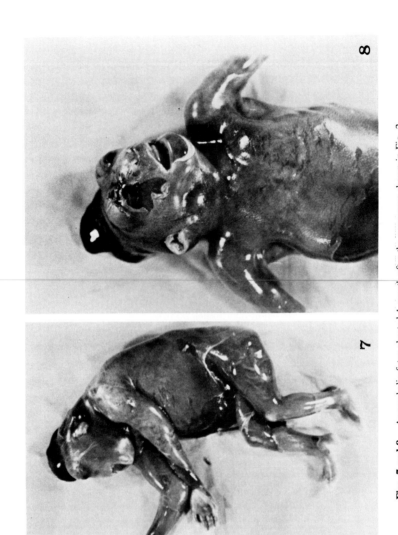

Figs. 7 and 8. Anecephalic fetus aborted 1 month after the sonogram shown in Fig. 2.

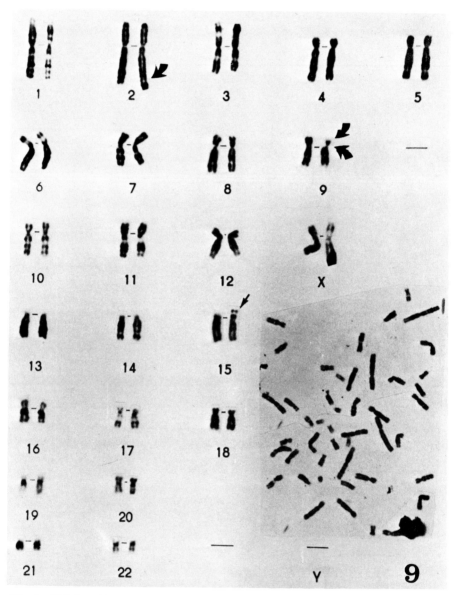

Fig. 9. Unbalanced karyotype 46,XY,t(2,9)(q37 p11), 15p+pat found in the anencephalic fetus shown in Figs. 7 and 8. A very small partial trisomy for the proximal region of the short arm of the translocated chromosome 9 is observed. The large arrows show the bands where breakage and rejoining have occurred. The small arrow demonstrates the familial variant chromosome 15p+ inherited from the father (pat = paternal).

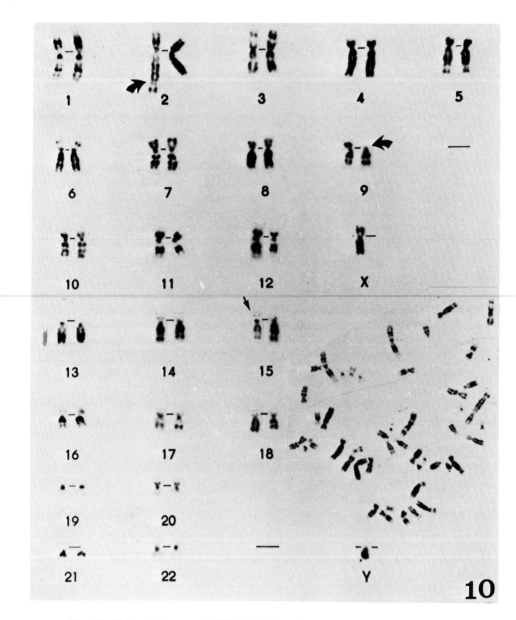

Fig. 10. Balanced karyotype 46,XY,t(2,9)(q37 p11)15p+ observed in the father of the fetus shown in Figs. 7 and 8. Note that the entire short arm of chromosome 9 is missing, and it is translocated to the distal end of one chromosome number 2. The points where breakage and rejoining have occurred are marked by big arrows. The small arrow shows the variant chromosome 15 p+.

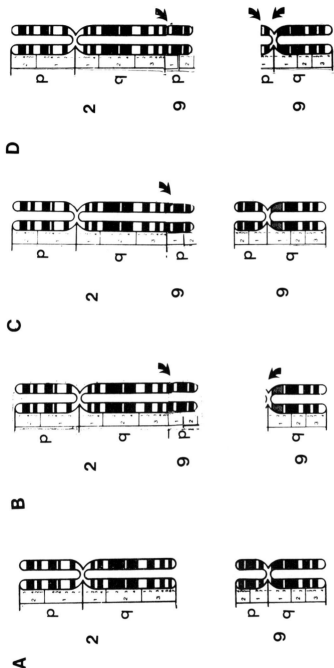

Fig. 11. Diagramatic representation of chromosomal translocation t(2,9) (q37 p11). The nomenclature is as follows: p, short arm; q, long arm; p11, the break of the short arm at region 1 band 1, q37, the break at region 3 band 7. (A) Normal chromosomes number 2 and 9. (B) Balanced translocation with most of the short arm of one chromosome number 9 translocated to the distal end of one chromosome number 2. This diagram corresponds to the karyotype shown in Fig. 10. (C) Unbalanced translocation with complete trisomy for the short arm of one chromosome number 9. This derivative chromosome was observed in the first child with hydrocephaly. (D) Unbalanced chromosome translocation with partial trisomy for the proximal region of the short arm of one chromosome number 9. This derivative chromosome translocation with partial trisomy for the proximal region of the short arm of one chromosome number 9. The diagram corresponds to Fig. 9 and was observed in the anencephalic fetus.

Carmen B. Lozzio

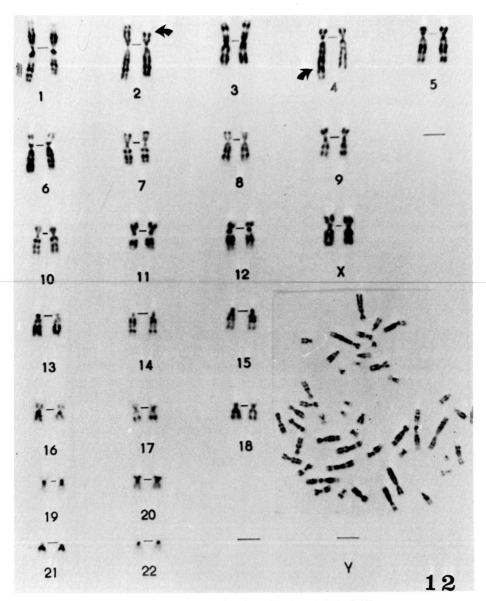

Fig. 12. Balanced carrier of translocation t(2;4) (p16q33).

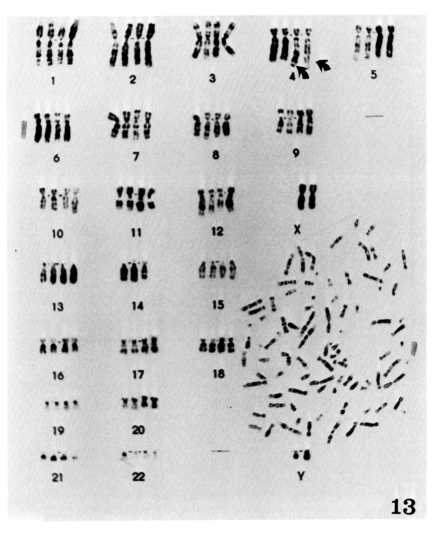

Fig. 13. Polyploid cell showing the unbalanced form of the translocation t(2,4) (p16 q33). The fetus miscarried spontaneously and had multiple congenital anomalies.

tion (Fig. 10) and his first child, by another marriage, was a stillborn hydro-cephalic with an unbalanced karyotype and complete trisomy for the short arm of chromosome number 9 (Lozzio and Kattine, 1969). Diagrammatic representa-tion of these chromosomes are shown in Fig. 11. Two other cases were the offspring of two sisters who are carriers of a balanced translocation t(2;4) (p16,q33) (Fig.12). One of the sisters had a normal female fetus with the same balanced translocation as the mother. The other sister had a fetus with multiple congenital anomalies who aborted spontaneously approximately 4–5 weeks after the amniocentesis. The chromosome studies in amniotic fluid cultures showed several abnormal clones probably derived from the unbalanced derivative 4 karyotype. One clone was tetraploid (Fig. 13) and showed two normal chromosomes number 4 and two derivative 4 translocations. Additional chromosomal rearrangements, including an extra band in the short arm of one chromosome number 1 and various new translocations and other structural rearrangements, were seen. We could not determine whether or not they had developed *in vitro*. Unfortunately, after miscarriage, the tissues from the fetus were not submitted to our laboratory for chromosomal analyses.

VI. REPORTED EXPERIENCE IN HUMAN PRENATAL DIAGNOSIS

The cumulative experience of many laboratories in the United States was reviewed by Milunsky (1973, 1975), and the most recent data (Milunsky, 1977)

TABLE II
Results of Prenatal Diagnoses for Chromosomal and Non-Chromosomal Indications

| Indications | United States | | | | Canadian study | |
| | (Milunsky, 1977)[a] | | (NICHD Study 1976) | | (Simpson et al., 1976) | |
	Tested	Abnormal	Tested	Abnormal	Tested	Abnormal
Maternal age > 35	3097[a]	83 (2.68%)	489	10(2%)	466	18(3.9%)
Maternal age 35–39	1109	17 (1.53%)			249	5(2%)
Maternal age > 40	1164	53 (4.5%)			217	13(6%)
Previous trisomy	1722	25 (1.45%)	273	4(1.5%)	283	5(1.76%)
Parental translocation	101[a]	19[a](18.8%)	18	3(16.7%)	14	7(50%)
with unbalanced fetuses					14	1(7.1%)
with balanced offspring					14	6(42.9%)
History of other chromosomal disorder			35	1(2.9%)	66	1(1.5%)
Miscellaneous			114	1(0.9%)	191	3(1.5%)
X-linked disorders[b]			21	11(52.4%)	33	23(69.7%)
Metabolic disorders			90	15(16.7%)	35	8(22.9%)
Neural tube defects	4739	66 (1.5%)			90	6(6.7%)

[a] This data was reported by Milunsky in 1975. The other values were presented at the Vth International Congress of Human Genetics at Mexico City, October, 1976.

(in press) plus results of the NICHD cooperative study from the United States (1976), the Canadian collaborative study (Simpson *et al.,* 1976), and the European experience (Lindsten *et al.,* 1976; Galjaard, 1976) are summarized in Tables II–IV.

A. Cytogenetic Indications

1. Advanced Maternal Age

An average of 2.8% abnormal fetuses was observed in the offspring of mothers older than 35 years. Significant differences in the risk were detected, however, if the results observed for mothers 35–39 years old was compared to those from mothers older than 40 years. The mean risk for the 35–39 age group was 1.45% and the risk for the older group was 4.78%. In fact, the risk increases every year both at the time of amniocentesis and at term, as shown by comparing the results of prenatal diagnosis to chromosome surveys in newborn (Hamerton, 1977). At 35–36 years, the approximate incidence of chromosomal disorders is 1 in 78 at 16 weeks of gestation and 1 in 169 at birth. At 40 years, the risk increases up to 1 in

TABLE II (Continued)

European experience							
Cumulative (Galjaard, 1976)		West of Scotland (Ferguson-Smith, 1976)		West Germany (BRD Study 1975)		Total	
Tested	Abnormal	Tested	Abnormal	Tested	Abnormal	Tested	Abnormal
2269	63(2.8%)	252	8(3.1%)	660	21(3.2%)	7233	203(2.8%)
410	5(1.2%)	105	1(1%)	332	4(1.2%)	2205	32(1.45%)
883	41(4.6%)	147	7(5.4%)	328	17(5.2%)	2739	131(4.78%)
1047	14(1.3%)	112	1(0.9%)	254	2(0.8%)	3691	51(1.38%)
179	57(31.8%)	18	9(50%)			330	95(28.8%)
179	12(6.7%)	18	1 (5.5%)	36	3(8.3%)	247	17(6.9%)
179	45(25%)	18	8(44.5%)			211	59(28%)
		48	1(2.1%)			149	3(2%)
711	12(1.7%)	74	4(5.4%)			1090	20(1.83%)
280	124(44.3%)	22	11(50%)	16	9(56.2%)	372	178(47.8%)
206	54(25.7%)	17	4(24%)	42	11(26.2%)	390	92(23.6%)
2708	82(3%)	357	15(5.6%)			7894	168(2.1%)

[b] All male fetuses were included as abnormal, although only half of them will be affected.

TABLE III

Results of α-Feto Protein (AFP) Assay in Amniotic Fluid (AF) for Detection of Open Neural Tube Defects (NTD)

Publication[a]	No. of AF	Cases of NTD	Other elevated AFP					False negatives	Cases at risk for NTD		No history of NTD	
			+ Fetal blood	Other defects	Borderline values	False positive	Total		No. of AF	NTD	No. AF	NTD
Milunsky and Alpert, 1976 (a)	2495	49(1.96%)		27			122	1	637	43(6.75%)	1858	6(0.3%)
Milunsky and Alpert, 1976 (b)	3536		9		11	15(0.4%)	35	1			2694	8(0.3%)
Milunsky, 1977 (c)	4739	66(1.5%)	11	46	2	4(0.1%)	63	1	1100	55(5%)	3639	11(0.3%)
Brock, 1976 (d)	997	31(3.1%)	12	2		0	45		452		545	
Lindsten et al., 1976 (e)	3565	79(2.2%)		14		3(0.1%)	17	7				
Galjaard, 1976 (f)	2708	81(3%)										
Simpson et al., 1976 (g)	1020	5(0.5%)							89	3(3.4%)	931	2(0.2%)

[a] This table includes information described in several publications, and the aspects not reported in a given publication were left blank, although the author may address that point in another publication. The results in (a), (b), and (c) overlap and represent different publications of the same population studied by the same group. The criteria for considering AFP values elevated was above 2 SD in (a) and > 3 SD in (b) and (c). The values reported as true false positives in (b) were reassayed (Milunsky and Kimball, 1976), and only five cases remained with AFP values > 3 SD. The data reported in (c) were presented at the Vth International Congress of Human Genetics in Mexico City on October 10–15, 1976. (d) Data presented in Paris on June 3–5, 1976 (Inserm 61, 221–226). Termination of the pregnancy was recommended only in the 33 cases without fetal blood contamination. The following outcome was reported: 16 anencephaly, 15 spina bifida, 1 intrauterine death, 1 exomphalos. No information was given on the outcome of the 12 cases with fetal blood contamination. (e) and (f) Represents the European experience in various centers—some of the data overlap and include part of the data described in (d). The published and unpublished data in (e) were reported to the Stockholm conference in June 1975 and includes 9 European centers. The results given in (f) were published in 1976 as a survey of 46 European centers from 8 countries, although this information is mainly based on data provided by 20 centers.

TABLE IV

Results of Prenatal Diagnosis for Hereditary Disorders of Metabolism

Metabolic disorder	American studies				European experience (Galjaard, 1976)		Total	
	National survey (Milunsky, 1973)		NICHD study (1976)					
	Tested	Affected	Tested	Affected	Tested	Affected	Tested	Affected
Tay-Sachs-Gm$_{2a}$ gangliosidosis type 1	68	16	36	4	31	5	135	25
Sandhoff-Gm$_2$ gangliosidosis type 2					8	2	8	2
Generalized gangliosidosis type 1	4	2			6	0	10	2
Pompe's glycogenosis II	24	6	7	0	25	8	56	14
Gaucher's disease	6	1			3	1	9	2
Galactosemia	5	3	5	2	8	2	18	7
Mucopolysaccharidoses	19	2	—	—	54	10	73	12
Metachromatic leukodystrophy	6	1	5	0	10	2	21	3
Krabbe's disease	4	1			12	3	16	4
Cystinosis	6	0			10	1	16	1
Maple syrup disease	7	1			11	5	18	6
Niemann-Pick disease	6	1			1	1	7	2
Miscellaneous disorders	25	3	37	9	27	14	89	26
Total	180	37	90	15	206	54	476	106(22.3%)

20 at 16 gestational weeks and 1 in 38 at birth. At 43 years and over, the frequency of Down's syndrome is 1 in 13 at 16 weeks and 1 in 20 at birth (Hamerton, 1977, in press). The increase in the risk of having a child with Down's syndrome has been detected for maternal ages 39–41 even in reports of birth-certificates of liveborn infants (Hook, 1976). Of course, the estimated rates are lower than those observed in chromosome surveys because many cases are not reported at birth. The frequencies of abnormal karyotypes detected by amniocentesis is double that usually reported in series of consecutive live births (Ferguson-Smith, 1976; Polani et al., 1976). Approximately 13.6% of the trisomic fetuses abort spontaneously after 16 weeks of gestation and 6.4% are stillborn (Polani, et al., 1976). It is obvious that the differences between prospective amniocentesis studies and retrospective studies are only due in part to fetal wastage. It is possible that the women having amniocentesis for maternal age are at higher genetic risk than other women of the same age because many have positive family history, abnormal obstetrical history, or were exposed to diagnostic X-rays. Trisomy 21 is the most common chromosomal aberration found in the advanced maternal age group. However, other chromosomal syndromes such as trisomy 18 and 13 or sex chromosome aberrations, such as Klinefelter's syndrome, are also detected at a much higher frequency in mothers older than 35 years (Simpson et al., 1976; Galjaard, 1976).

2. Positive Family History for Down's Syndrome

A mean recurrence risk of 1.38% was estimated (Table II) for chromosome abnormalities in mothers with a previous child with nondisjunction type of trisomy 21. An additive effect of advanced maternal age and positive family history was observed (Simpson et al., 1976). The mothers younger than 35 years who had a previous child with Down's syndrome had a recurrence risk of 1 in 100, whereas those mothers older than 35 years with positive family history appeared to have a greater rate of chromosomal abnormalities (Simpson et al., 1976).

3. Parental Translocations

Pregnancies at high risk because one of the parents was a carrier of a balanced translocation were a relatively small group. All the results, however, show that only 6.9% of the fetuses had an unbalanced karyotype, while 28% were balanced carriers (Table II).

4. Miscellaneous Indications

This is a group formed by cases studied for various reasons such as maternal exposure to drugs or X-rays, parental anxiety, abnormal karyotype in one parent, and history of abortions or other malformations. The frequency of abnormal karyotypes observed in this group was 1.83%.

5. *Sex Determination in X-Linked Disorders*

In a large proportion of X-linked disorders, the only test available for prenatal diagnosis is the determination of the sex of the fetus. If a male is found, an abortion is indicated, although one-half of these fetuses will be normal. This information should be clearly explained to the mother, and the technique used for sex determination should be reliable. The sex of the fetus may be studied with three techniques: (1) demonstration of positive Barr-body sex chromatin, (2) study of Y chromosome fluorescence, and (3) chromosome analyses. Sex chromatin and the Y chromosome body are demonstrable in noncultivated amniotic fluid cells, but accurate results are not always obtained. Sex chromatin studies predict the sex of the fetus in 87–88% of the cases (Nelson and Emery, 1970; Valenti *et al.,* 1972) and should be used only to obtain a rapid preliminary report. The results of these tests should be confirmed by chromosome analyses in cultured amniotic cells before an abortion is recommended. In a relatively small proportion of cases, the amniocentesis is performed for sex determination in a pregnancy at risk for X-linked disorders. The psychological effects of terminating a pregnancy with 50% chance of being normal is a factor to take into consideration before recommending this procedure, and studies to detect whether or not the fetus is abnormal should be attempted in all the cases with X-linked disorders due to a known metabolic defect. This is possible in the Lesch-Nyhan syndrome and Hunter's syndrome. It is not feasible yet for hemophilia, and only very preliminary data is available for Duchenne muscular dystrophy.

B. Diagnosis of Neural Tube Defects (NTD)

The study of amniotic fluid α-feto protein (AFP) concentrations is a reliable method for prenatal diagnosis of open neural tube defects (NTD). The results of AFP studies in pregnancies at increased risk for NTD showed a 3–6% recurrence risk (Table III). These studies also confirmed the empirical calculations of 10–12% recurrence risk (Carter, 1976; Carter and Fraser, 1967) for parents who have had two previous children affected by NTD. (Milunsky and Alpert, 1976a). Routine studies of AFP in cases with negative family history for NTD have shown a 0.2–0.3% affected fetuses. These results support the need to investigate AFP in all the amniotic fluids obtained before 24 weeks of gestation. False positive results have been observed with different frequencies due to the changes in the criterion used to label a given AFP value as abnormal. This criterion has changed in the same laboratory in a short period of time (Table III **a,b,c**). In an earlier publication, Milunsky and Alpert (1976a) used 2 SD as the upper limit of normal, although all the cases of NTD detected had values higher than 3 SD. The purpose of including fluids with values over 2 SD as false positives was to assure that no case of open NTD would be missed by this assay. The danger of this criterion is that abortion may be recommended in some normal pregnancies. To avoid this, an upper limit of 3 SD was established, and the reasons for high AFP values in pregnancies with normal outcome was investigated. It is generally agreed that a large percentage of the cases with high AFP values in normal pregnancies are due to contamination of AF with fetal blood (Ward and Stewart, 1974; Brock, 1974, 1976). For this reason, Brock does not recommend termination of the pregnancy when a high AFP value is found in a fluid where studies on fetal hemoglobin show the presence of fetal blood. Following this criterion, Brock has a 0 rate of false positives. It has been pointed out, however, that fetal blood is present in 47% of the fluids obtained from cases with anencephaly (Milunsky and Alpert, 1976a; Milunsky and Kimball, 1976). Therefore, it is not advisable to disregard all the high AFP values in fluids containing fetal blood. A better approach seems to be the correlation of AFP results with ultrasound studies. When the ultrasound study shows a normal biparietal diameter for the estimated gestational age, the high AFP value of a fluid containing fetal blood may be considered to be of little clinical significance. On the other hand, the lack of head echoes in a pregnancy with an estimated gestational age over 14 weeks and high AFP in the presence of fetal blood are strong indications that the fetus is anencephelic. Routine ultrasound studies and close correlation of AFP values to gestational age are required because the AFP values decrease significantly in a few weeks, and normal values for 16 weeks of gestation would be interpreted as abnormal if the gestational age is estimated as 18–20 weeks. Another parameter that could help interpret the results of high AFP in amniotic fluids containing fetal blood is the routine investigation of AFP in maternal serum. Maternal serum studies of AFP are usually done as a screening test for NTD (Cowchock and Jackson, 1976; Macri et al., 1975; Lindsten et al., 1976; Wald, 1976), and a normal value in serum will not rule out the presence of a NTD. A high serum value for the corresponding gestational age, however, would be supportive of the presence of an affected fetus if the blood serum was collected before amniocentesis. The need to draw blood for AFP before amniocentesis is based on the observation made by Chard et al. (1976) that 11 of 65 cases (17%) showed elevation of maternal serum AFP after amniocentesis when AFP values were compared in samples collected before and after amniocentesis. The increase in serum AFP after amniocentesis is explained by fetomaternal transfusion due to minor degrees of damage to the placenta, especially in cases with anterior localization of the placenta. Thus, collection of maternal blood for serum AFP determination prior to each amniocentesis is recommended. It is important to correlate the results of serum AFP and the values of AFP in the amniotic fluid with the gestational age established by the ultrasound.

C. Diagnosis of Inherited Metabolic Disorders

Prenatal detection of specific biochemical defects has been performed in approximately 70 different inborn errors of metabolism (Milunsky and Littlefield, 1972; Milunsky, 1973; Littlefield et al., 1974; Lindsten et al., 1976; Nadler, 1977). The majority of these disorders are inherited as autosomal recessive conditions, and the parents of an index case have a recurrence risk of 25%. A few of these disorders are X-linked (Lesch-Nyhan syndrome, Hunter's syndrome, Fabry's disease, and Menkes's disease) with a 50% risk in the male offspring of a carrier mother. The results of a survey of 41 centers from United States and Canada (Milunsky, 1973) of a collaborative study of nine American centers [NICHD (National Registry for Amniocentesis), Study Group 1976], and of 36 European centers (Galjaard, 1976) are summarized in Table IV. The data of the NICHD study may overlap in part with the survey published by Milunsky (1973) because the same nine institutions were included in both reports and the data of the NICHD study was collected from July 1, 1971 to June 30, 1973. This overlapping does not change the interpretation of the results, which confirm the theoretical expectation for recessive inheritance (Table IV). Many inborn errors of metabolism are severe diseases with poor prognosis and no available treatment. For these reasons, the parents with high genetic risk for one of these conditions elect more often to risk another pregnancy if they have the alternative of selective abortion of an abnormal fetus. Thus, the accuracy of the prenatal diagnosis is very important because it leads to a therapeutic decision, and tragic mistakes may be made by either overlooking a deficiency or concluding that low enzyme values are due to an affected fetus when the baby is normal or heterozygous (Dreyfus and Poenaru, 1976). Errors are more frequent with uncultured amniotic cells or fluid. Uncultured amniotic cells have detectable levels of enzymes and have been used for prenatal diagnosis (Nadler and Gerbie, 1969). Variations in the number of cells and their viability may lead to results that are interpreted as due to the presence of an abnormal fetus. In these cases, an abortion should not be indicated until the results are confirmed in cultured amniotic fluid cells. Enzyme assays in amniotic fluid are also dangerous when they are not compared to results in cultured amniotic cells. Maternal blood contamination of the fluid, frequent changes in the content of proteins, and lack of information on the amount of fetal urine present in the amniotic fluid are factors that affect the results and make their interpretation very difficult (Golbus, 1976). Enzyme assays in cultured amniotic cells are considered the most reliable source of information. They are not exempt, however, from the risk of errors caused by variations in enzyme-specific activity at various phases of growth in culture (Henkels-Dully and Niermeyer, 1976), changes related to the type of media (Ryan et al., 1972; Butterworth et al., 1974), or to the pH (Eagle, 1973; Lie et al., 1973). Thus, biochemical studies in amniotic cell cultures should be performed by laboratories with experience in the assay of the specific enzyme defect, using standardized techniques. Good controls should include cultures of normal amniotic cells of the same gestational age and cultures of fibroblasts from cases with confirmed diagnosis. If possible, cultures of skin fibroblasts obtained from the index case should be studied before prenatal diagnosis in order to identify the specific enzymatic defect and the level of any residual enzymatic activity present in the affected homozygote. Cultured fibroblasts from the parents are also useful in establishing the level of enzyme activity in heterozygote carriers. Samples of these cultures should be stored frozen and placed in culture again at the time of prenatal diagnosis using similar culture conditions. In this form, the enzyme assay is performed in the cultured amniotic cells and in known normal, heterozygous, and homozygous control cultures. The values obtained are compared to those of the different controls, and the results can be interpreted more accurately.

VII. PROBLEMS, ETHICS, AND FUTURE OF PRENATAL DIAGNOSIS

The interpretation of the results of prenatal studies may be difficult. Occasionally, the clinical significance of the findings is not known or the values are borderline, and the parents are presented with dilemmas, rather than definite conclusions.

The most frequent problem that occurs in prenatal chromosome analysis is the finding of mosaicism. In many cases, the abnormal clone was induced *in vitro* or it was derived from a few amniotic cells that are not present in the baby at the time of birth. Examples of these pseudomosaics are the cultures with variable proportion of polyploid cells, which are frequently seen in pregnancies with normal offspring (Milunsky *et al.*, 1971; Cox *et al.*, 1974). Other examples are cases with aneuploidy in the first culture and normal karyotype on the second culture or in cultures derived from fetal tissues (Kardon *et al.*, 1972; Kajii, 1971). "Spontaneous" translocations occur in cell cultures (Kohn *et al.*, 1974) or may be induced by mycoplasma contamination (Schneider *et al.*, 1974) or by exposure of the cells to alkaline culture media (Ford, 1973) or to pH ranges between 6.7 and 6.9 (Ingalls and Shimada, 1974). Hypo- or hyperdiploid cells with random losses and gains of chromosomes are also frequently observed in cultures of pregnancies with a normal outcome (Milunsky, 1975). As shown by these examples, prenatal detection of true mosaics is difficult. To avoid misinterpretations, it is advisable to study at least 30 metaphases from amniotic cultures started in two or three different bottles or dishes (Milunsky, 1973). Cases with true mosaicisms should give similar results in different samples, and termination of the pregnancy should not be considered unless consistent results are found in repeated studies. True mosaicism has been detected prenatally by

Bloom *et al.* (1974) and may be found occasionally. Even in these cases, however, it is difficult to predict the severity of the case, since a wide range of clinical manifestations is expected, depending on the proportion of normal versus abnormal cells present in different tissue. Discovery of karyotypes such as XYY or XXX may raise questions concerning the possibility of a normal phenotype in individuals with those karyotypes. "Marker" chromosomes may be difficult to differentiate from chromosome translocations, and studies of chromosomes in the blood of the parents are often used to differentiate between these two possibilities.

One of the most frequent problems found in biochemical studies is the overlapping of values between heterozygote carriers with low activity and the homozygous affected individuals. Examples of pseudodeficiencies with very low activity in clinically normal carriers has been reported for Tay-Sachs disease (Vidgoff *et al.*, 1973), Sandoff's disease (Dreyfus and Poenaru, 1976), Krabbe's disease (Wenger *et al.*, 1974), and metachromatic leukodystrophy (Dubois *et al.*, 1975). These cases may be differentiated by using natural substrates and by studies of the enzyme activity in the parents. The frequency of false-positive diagnoses is reduced by the use of well-controlled studies and standardized culture conditions. These studies should be performed at laboratories with experience in the enzyme assay, and, if possible, the enzyme levels should be compared to those observed in culture of the propositus, the heterozygous parents, and normal controls.

Problems in the detection of neural tube defects have been discussed in Section VI,B, and are mainly related to the presence of fetal blood in the amniotic fluid or to errors in the determination of the gestational age.

The problems of interpretation described in the previous paragraph may be reduced by improved techniques and the use of good controls. Other problems related to moral and ethical issues are more difficult to resolve. Among these issues are the approval or disapproval of abortion when the fetus is found to be abnormal, the legal rights of the fetus, the question of fetal viability versus fetal life, the degree of severity of the birth defect in cases recommended for abortion, the psychological effects of prenatal diagnosis, genetic counseling and therapeutic abortion, the rights of privacy and confidentiality of the individual, and the needs of society to reduce the incidence of genetic defects. These problems have been extensively discussed by philosophers, ethicists, theologians, lawyers, and biologists, who ask many questions but who have not found the answers.

The basic principle of prenatal diagnosis and the most common result in over 95% of the cases is the assurance to parents with increased risk for specific genetic disorders that their unborn child is not affected. This assurance reduces the anxiety of the mother during the last 4 months of pregnancy and contributes to the improvement of her mental health. The possibility of selective abortion also encourages the continuance of pregnancies in couples at high genetic risk for disorders detectable by amniocentesis. Thus, instead of increasing the number of abortions, the possibility of prenatal diagnosis reduces the number of early abortions and allows for postponing this decision until the fetus is known to be abnormal.

The future will bring new progress in the prenatal diagnosis of genetic disorders. New techniques with fewer problems of interpretation and availability of amniocentesis to all pregnant women at risk will be the major advances expected in the near future.

ACKNOWLEDGMENTS

The original cytogenetic studies reported in this publication have been performed by the author in collaboration with Mary Beth Klepper, M.S., and Jinhi Kim, M. S. The excellent work of these collaborators is acknowledged. The studies were supported in part by Grant C-22 from the National Foundation March of Dimes.

The sonogram studies shown in Figs. 1–4 were performed at the Radiology Department, University of Tennessee Memorial Hospital, under the direction of E. Buonocore, M.D. The reports were interpreted by Paul T. Wooten, M.D. This contribution is greatly appreciated.

REFERENCES

Arger, P. H., Freiman, D. B., Komins, J. I., and Schwarz, R. H. (1976). *Radiology* **120,** 155–157.

Arrighi, F. E., and Hsu, T. C. (1971). *Cytogenetics* **10,** 81–86.

Benirschke, K., and McKay, D. C. (1953). *Obstet. Gynecol.* **1,** 638–649.

Bloom, A. D., Schmickel, R., and Barr, M. (1974). *J. Pediatr.* **84,** 732.

Boué, A., ed. (1976). "Prenatal Diagnosis." INSERM, Paris.

Boué, J., Boué, A., Girard, S., Thépot, F., Barickard, F., Deluchat, C., Nicolesco, H., and Yvert, F. (1976). *In* "Prenatal Diagnosis" (A. Boué, ed.), Vol. 61, pp. 105–116. INSERM, Paris.

Brock, D. J. H. (1974). *Clin. Chim. Acta* **57,** 315–320.

Brock, D. J. H. (1976). *In* "Prenatal Diagnosis" (A. Boué, ed.), Vol. 61, pp. 221–226. INSERM, Paris.

Brock, D. J. H., and Sutcliffe, R. G. (1972). *Lancet* **2,** 197–199.

Brown, R. (1975). "Ultrasonography," p. 116. Warren H. Green, Inc., New York.

Butterworth, J., Sutherland, G. R., Broadhead, D. M., and Bain, A. D. (1974). *Clin. Chim. Acta* **53,** 239–247.

Campbell, S. (1972). *Br. J. Hosp. Med.* **8,** 541–555.

Campbell, S. (1974). *Birth Defects. Proc. 4th Int. Conf., 1973,* pp. 240–247.

Campbell, S., Johnstone, F. D., Holt, E. M., and Emay, P. (1972). *Lancet* **2,** 1226–1227.

Carter, C. O. (1976). *Br. Med. Bull.* **32,** 21–26.

Carter, C. O., and Fraser, J. A. (1967). *Lancet* **1,** 306–308.

Caspersson, T., Farber, S., Foley, G. E., Kudynowski, J., Modest, E. J., Simonsson, E., Wagh, U., and Zech, L. (1968). *Exp. Cell Res.* **49,** 219–222.

Caspersson, T., Zech, L., and Johansson, C. (1970). *Exp. Cell Res.* **62,** 490–492.

Cederqvist, L. L., Wennerstrom, C., Senterfit, L. B., Baldridge, P. B., and Rothe, D. J. (1973). *Am. J. Obstet. Gynecol.* **116,** 871–874.

Chard, T.. Kitau, M. J.. Ledward, R., Coltart, T., Embury, S., and Seller, M. (1976). *J. Obstet. Gynaecol. Br.* **83**, 33–34.

Charles, D., Jacoby, H. E., and Burgess, F. (1965). *Am. J. Obstet. Gynecol.* **93**, 1042–1047.

Comings, D. E. (1976). *J. Reprod. Med.* **17**, 19–20.

Comings, D. E., and Avelino, E. (1975). *Chromosoma* **51**, 365–381.

Couturier, J., Dutrillaux, B., and Lejeune, J. (1973). *C. R. Acad. Sci.* (Paris) **276**, 339–342.

Cowchock, F. S., and Jackson, L. G. (1976). *Obstet. Gynecol.* **47**, 63–68.

Cox, D. M., Niewczas-Late, V., Riffell, I., and Hamerton, J. L. (1974). *Pediatr. Res.* **8**, 679.

Cox, L. W., and Chalmers, T. A. (1953). *J. Obstet. Gynaecol. Br. Emp.* **60**, 222–225.

Dioguardi, N., Agostani, A., Fiorelli, G., and Lomanto, B. (1963). *J. Lab. Clin. Med.* **61**, 713–723.

Donald, I. (1972). *Obstet. Gynecol. Annu.* **1**, 245–271.

Donald, I. (1974). *Am. J. Obstet. Gynecol.* **118**, 299–309.

Drets, M. E., and Shaw, M. W. (1971). *Proc. Natl. Acad. Sci. U.S.A.* **68**, 2073–2077.

Dreyfus, J. C., and Poenaru, L. (1976). *In* "Prenatal Diagnosis" (A. Boué, ed.), Vol. 61, pp. 155–162. INSERM, Paris.

Dubois, G., Turpin, J. C., and Bauman, N. (1975). *N. Eng. J. Med.* **293**, 302.

Dutrillaux, B. (1973). *Chromosoma* **41**, 395–402.

Dutrillaux, B., and Lejeune, J. (1971). *C. R. Acad. Sci.* (Paris) **272**, 2638–2640.

Dutrillaux, B., and Lejeune, J. (1975). *Adv. Hum. Genet.* **5**, 119–156.

Dutrillaux, B., de Grouchy, J., Finaz, C., and Lejeune, J. (1971). *C. R. Acad. Sci.* (D) (Paris) **273**, 587–588.

Dutrillaux, B., Laurent, C., Couturier, J., and Lejeune, J. (1973). *C. R. Acad. Sci.* (Paris) **276**, 1379–1381.

Eagle, H. (1973). *J. Cell. Physiol.* **82**, 1–8.

Elliott, P. M., and Inman, W. H. W. (1961). *Lancet* **2**, 835–840.

Felix, J. S., Doherty, R. A., Davis, H. T., and Ridge, S. C. (1974). *Pediatr. Res.* **8**, 870–874.

Ferguson-Smith, M. F., Ferguson-Smith, M. A., Nevin, N. C., and Stone, M. (1971). *Br. Med. J.* **4**, 69–74.

Ferguson-Smith, M. F. (1976). *Lancet* **2**, 252.

Ford, J. (1973). *Lancet* **1**, 54.

Freda, V. J. (1965). *Am. J. Obstet. Gynecol.* **92**, 341–374.

Fuchs, F. (1966). *Clin. Obstet. Gynecol.* **9**, 449–460.

Fuchs, F. (1971). *Birth Defects, Orig. Artic. Ser.* **7**, 18.

Galjaard, H. (1976). *Cytogenet. Cell Genet.* **16**, 453–467.

Gerbie, A. B., Nadler, H. L., and Gerbie, H. V. (1971). *Am. J. Obstet. Gynecol.* **109**, 765.

Gertner, M., Hsu, L. Y., Martin, Y. F., and Hirshhorn, K. (1970). *Bull. N.Y. Acad. Med.* **46**, 916–921.

Golbus, M. S. (1976). *Obstet. Gynecol.* **48**, 497–506.

Gray, C., Davidson, R. G., and Cohen, M. M. (1971). *J. Pediatr.* **79**, 119–122.

Hamerton, J. H. (1977). *Proc. 5th Int. Cong. Hum. Genet.* (Mexico City, October 10–15, 1976) (in press).

Hasholt, L. (1976). *J. Med. Genet.* **13**, 34–37.

Henkels-Dully, N. J., and Niermeyer, M. F. (1976). *Exp. Cell Res.* **97**, 304–312.

Hoehn, H., Bryant, E. M., Karp, L. E., and Martin, G. M. (1974). *Pediatr. Res.* **8**, 746–754.

Hook, E. B. (1976). *Lancet* **2**, 33–34.

Hutchinson, D. L., Hunter, C. B., Neslen, E. D., and Plentl, A. A. (1955). *Surg., Gynecol. Obstet.* **100**, 391–396.

Hutchinson, D. L., Gray, M. J., Plentl, A. A., Alvarez, H., Calaeyro-Barcia, K., Kaplan, B., and Lind, J. (1959). *J. Clin. Invest.* **38**, 971–980.

Ingalls, T. H., and Shimada, T. (1974). *Lancet* **1**, 872.

Jacobson, C. B., and Barter, R. H. (1967). *Am. J. Obstet. Gynecol.* **99,** 796–807.

Jeffcoate, T. N. A., and Scott, J. S. (1959). *Can. Med. Assoc. J.* **80,** 77–86.

Kaback, M. M., and Leonard, C. O. (1972). *In* "Autenatel Diagnosis" (A. Dorfman, ed.), pp. 81–94. Univ. of Chicago Press, Chicago, Illinois.

Kajii, T. (1971). *Lancet* **2,** 1037.

Kardon, N. B., Chernay, P. R., Hsu, L. Y., Martin, J. L., and Hirschhorn, K. (1972). *J. Pediatr.* **80,** 297–299.

Khudr, G., and Benirschke, K. (1971). *Am. J. Obstet. Gynecol.* **110,** 1091–1095.

Kohn, G., Aronson, M., and Mellman, W. J. (1974). *Clin. Genet.* **5,** 113.

Lee, C. L. Y., Gregson, N. M., and Walker, S. (1970). *Lancet* **2,** 316–317.

Lie, S. O., Schofield, B. H., Taylor, H. A., Jr., and Doty, J. B. (1973). *Pediatr. Res.* **7,** 13–19.

Lindsten, J., Zetterström, R., and Ferguson-Smith, M. (1976). *Acta Paediatr. Scand., Suppl.* **259,** 1–99.

Littlefield, J. W., Milunsky, A., and Atkins, L. (1974). *In* "Birth Defects" (A. Motulsky and W. Lenz, eds.), pp. 221–225. Am. Elsevier, New York.

Lozzio, C. B., and Kattine, A. (1969). *J. Med. Genet.* **6,** 174–179.

Macri, J. N., Weiss, R. R., Starkovsky, N. A., Elligers, K. W., and Berger, D. B. (1975). *Lancet* **2,** 719–720.

MacVicar, J. (1976). *Br. Med. Bull.* **32,** 4–8.

Menees, T. O., Miller, J. D., and Holly, L. E. (1930). *Am. J. Roentgenol. Radium Ther.* [N.S.] **24,** 363–366.

Milunsky, A. (1973). "The Prenatal Diagnosis of Hereditary Disorders," pp. 22–28. Thomas, Springfield, Illinois.

Milunsky, A. (1975). "The Prevention of Genetic Disease and Mental Retardation." Saunders, Philadelphia, Pennsylvania.

Milunsky, A. (1977). *Proc. 5th Int. Congr. Hum. Genet.* (Mexico City, October 10–15, 1976) (in press).

Milunsky, A., and Alpert, E. (1976a). *Lancet* **1,** 1015.

Milunsky, A., and Alpert, E. (1976b). *Obstet. Gynecol.* **48,** 1–5.

Milunsky, A., and Kimball, M. E. (1976). *Lancet* **2,** 209.

Milunsky, A., and Littlefield, J. W. (1972). *Annu. Rev. Med.* **23,** 57–76.

Milunsky, A., Littlefield, J. W., Kanter, J. N., Kolodny, E. H., Shih, V. E., and Atkins, L. (1970). *N. Engl. J. Med.* **282,** 1370, 1441, and 1498.

Milunsky, A., Alkins, L., and Littlefield, J. M. (1971). *J. Pediatr.* **79,** 303.

Milunsky, A., Atkins, L., and Littlefield, J. W. (1972). *Obstet. Gynecol.* **40,** 104–108.

Monie, I. W. (1953). *Am. J. Obstet. Gynecol.* **66,** 616–625.

Murken, J. D. (1976). *In* "Prenatal Diagnosis" (A. Boué, ed.), Vol. 61, pp. 273–282. INSERM, Paris.

Murken, J. D., Stengel-Rutkowski, S., Walther, J. D., Westenfelder, S. R., Remberger, K. R., and Zimmer, F. (1974). *Lancet* **2,** 171.

Nadler, H. L. (1968). *Pediatrics* **42,** 912–918.

Nadler, H. L. (1969). *J. Pediatr.* **74,** 132–143.

Nadler, H. L. (1971). *Birth Defects, Orig. Artic. Ser.* **7,** 5.

Nadler, H. L. (1977). *Proc. 5th Int. Congr. Hum. Genet. 1976* and Excerpta Med. Found. Int. Congr. Ser. No. 397, pp. 13–14.

Nadler, H. L., and Gerbie, A. B. (1969). *Am. J. Obstet. Gynecol.* **103,** 710.

Nadler, H. L., and Gerbie, A. B. (1970). *N. Engl. J. Med.* **282,** 596–599.

Nadler, H. L., and Gerbie, A. B. (1971). *Obstet. Gynecol.* **38,** 789–799.

Nelson, M. M., and Emery, A. E. H. (1970). *Br. Med. J.* **1,** 523–526.

Neufeld, E. (1973). *In* "Medical Genetics" (V. A. McKusick and R. Claiborne, eds.), pp. 141–147. H. P. Publishing Co., Inc., New York.

NICHD National Registry for Amniocentesis Study Group. (1976). *J. Am. Med. Assoc.* 1471–1476.

Ostergard, D. R. (1970). *Obstet. & Gynecol. Surv.* **25**, 297–319.

Pardue, M. L., and Gall, J. G. (1970). *Science* **168**, 1356–1358.

Paris Conference. 1971 "Standardization in Human Cytogenetics." (1972). Birth Defects, Orig. Artic. Ser., Vol. 8, No. 7. Natl. Found., New York.

Paris Conference, Supplement. (1975). "Standardization in Human Cytogenetics, 1971." Birth Defects, Orig. Artic. Ser., Vol. 9, No. 9. Natl. Found., New York.

Pathak, S. (1976). *J. Reprod. Med.* **17**, 25–28.

Patil, S. R., Merrick, S., and Lubs, H. A. (1971). *Science* **173**, 821–822.

Plentl, A. A., and Hutchinson, D. L. (1953). *Proc. Soc. Exp. Biol. Med.* **82**, 681–684.

Polani, P. E., and Benson, P. F. (1973). *Guy's Hosp. Rep.* **122**, 65–89.

Polani, P. E., Alberman E., Berry, A. C., Blunt, S., and Singer, J. D. (1976). *Lancet* **2**, 516–517.

Pritchard, J. A. (1965). *Obstet. Gynecol.* **25**, 289–297.

Pritchard, J. A. (1966). *Obstet. Gynecol.* **28**, 606–610.

Queenan, J. T. (1966). *Clin. Obstet. Gynecol.* **9**, 491–496.

Queenan, J. T., and Adams, D. W. (1965). *Obstet. Gynecol.* **25**, 302–307.

Rhodes, P. (1966). *J. Obstet. Gynaecol. Br. Commonw.* **73**, 23–26.

Ryan, C. A., Lee, S. Y., and Nadler, H. L. (1972). *Exp. Cell Res.* **71**, 388–393.

Schmid, W. (1975). *Humangenetik* **30**, 325–330.

Schmid, W. (1976). *Acta Paediatr. Scand., Suppl.* **259**, 57–59.

Schneider, E. L., Stanbridge, E. J., Epstein, C. J., Abbo-Halbaseh, G., and Rodgers, C. (1974). *Science* **184**, 477–479.

Scrimgeour, J. B. (1976). *In* "Prenatal Diagnosis" (A. Boué, ed.), Vol. 61, pp. 39–44. INSERM, Paris.

Seabright, M. (1972). *Chromosoma* **36**, 204–210.

Sehested, J. (1974). *Humangenetik* **21**, 55–58.

Simpson, N. E., Dallaire, L., Miller, J. R.. Siminovich. L., Hamerton, J. L., Miller, J., and McKeen, C. (1976). *Can. Med. Assoc.* **115**, 739–746.

Steele, M. W., and Breg. W. R. (1966). *Lancet* **1**, 383–385.

Stengel-Rutkowski, S., Wirtz, A., Hahn, B., Hofmeister, A., and Murken, J. D. (1976). *Hum. Genet.* **31**, 231–234.

Stewart, A., Webb, J., Giles, D., and Hewitt, D. (1956). *Lancet* **2**, 447.

Stewart, A., Webb, J., and Hewitt, D. (1958). *Br. Med. J.* **1**, 1495–1508.

Sumner, A. T., Evans, H. J., and Buckland, R. A. (1971). *Nature (London), New Biol.* **232**, 31–32.

Sundén, B. (1964). *Acta Obstet. Gynaecol. Scand.* **43**, Suppl. 6, 7–179.

Therkelsen, A. J. (1976). *In* "Prenatal Diagnosis" (A. Boué, ed.), Vol. 61, pp. 55–66. INSERM, Paris.

Valenti, C., Schutta, E. F., and Kehaty, T. (1969). *J. Am. Med. Assoc.* **207**, 1513–1515.

Valenti, C., Lin, C. C., Baum, A., Hasso briou, and Carbonara, A. (1972). *Am. J. Obstet. Gynecol.* **112**, 890–895.

van de Sande, J. H., Lin, C. C., and Jorgenson, K. F. (1977). *Science* **195**, 400–402.

Verma, R. S., and Lubs, H. A. (1975). *Am. J. Hum. Genet.* **27**, 110–117.

Verma, R. S., and Lubs, H. A. (1976). *Can. J. Genet. Cytol.* **18**, 45–50.

Vidgoff, J., Buist, N. R. M., and O'Brien, J. S. (1973). *Am. J. Hum. Genet.* **25**, 372.

Wagner, G., and Fuchs, F. (1962). *J. Obstet. Gynaecol. Br. Commonw.* **69**, 131–136.

Wald, N. J. (1976). *In* "Prenatal Diagnosis" (A. Boué, ed.), Vol. 61, pp. 227–238. INSERM, Paris.

Ward, A. M., and Stewart, C. R. (1974). *Lancet* **2**, 345–346.

Weisblum, B., and de Haseth, P. L. (1972). *Proc. Natl. Acad. Sci. U.S.A.* **69**, 629–632.

Wenger, D. A., Sattler, M., and Hiatt, W. (1974). *Proc. Natl. Acad. Sci. U.S.A.* **71**, 854.

23

Collection and Analysis of Female Genital Tract Secretions

FULLER W. BAZER, R. MICHAEL ROBERTS, AND D.C. SHARP, III

I. INTRODUCTION

A. Historical Perspectives

According to Bonnet (1882), the concept that "uterine milk" exists for nourishment of the embryo was discussed by Aristotle (384–322 B.C. and William

Harvey (1578– 1657 A.D.). Both scientists recognized that blood, milk from mammary glands, and uterine fluids were of different composition, but were all involved with nutrition. Early studies of uterine milk, again as described by Bonnet (1882), indicated that uterine milk contained 87.9% water, 12.09% solids, 10.40% protein (including cells), 0.02% alkaline albumin, 0.37% organic salts, and 1.22% fat in the cow. In sheep, uterine milk was reported to contain 88.3% water, 1.2% solids, 11.7% fat, 9.5% protein (including cells), 0.47% alkaline albumin, and 0.45% salts.

Bonnet (1882) considered uterine milk to represent products of disintegration of maternal tissues and secretion of the glands of the uterine endometrium. According to Amoroso (1952), Grosser (1921) introduced the term "histotroph" to refer to secretions from the endometrium (histopoietic materials) and detritus from the degeneration of endometrial cells (histolytic materials); Meyer (1925) proposed the term "embryotroph" to describe all material available to the embryo *in utero*. The term "uterine milk" was introduced by W. Needham in 1667 and, according to Amoroso (1952), it was first analyzed by Prevast and Morin (1842) and then by Schlossberger (1855) and Gamgee (1864).

It should also be pointed out that uterine milk is not unique to mammals, but has also been described in ovoviviparous selachians. In these animals, as in mammals, uterine milk is believed to serve in nourishment of the embryos (Amoroso, 1952). Scientists have been interested in the role of uterine secretions in mammals and ovoviviparous animals for over 100 years. In the following sections, an attempt will be made to describe events that occur during the estrous cycle and early pregnancy which may be affected by uterine milk or, as described hereafter, female genital tract (uterine and oviductal) secretions.

B. Critical Events during the Estrous Cycle and Pregnancy

1. Sperm Capacitation and Fertilization

According to Austin (1972), sperm cells must undergo "capacitation" in the female reproductive tract before they achieve the capacity to fertilize the egg. The time required for this process ranges from 1.5 hours (sheep) to 7 hours (human). The precise nature of the capacitation process is unknown. However, according to Hafez (1974), the process may involve, in part, removal of inhibitors from proteolytic enzymes, e.g., acrosin and hyaluronidase, located in the acrosome. These enzymes then allow digestion of and penetration through the membranes of the ovum and subsequent fertilization.

2. Luteolytic Agents

It is well established that the uterus, specifically the endometrium, is the source of a luteolytic factor that causes corpus luteum (CL) regression in subprimate mammals (Anderson *et al.*, 1969). The CL produces progesterone, which inhibits recurrence of the estrous cycle. Therefore, in the absence of pregnancy, a uterine secretion is necessary to cause CL to regress. Considerable data are available to indicate that the uterine luteolysin is prostaglandin $F_{2\alpha}$ (PGF) [see reviews by McCracken (1971) and Goding (1974)]. The PGF is produced by epithelial cells of the oviduct (Ogra *et al.*, 1974) and uterus (McCracken *et al.*, 1972; Patek and Watson, 1976).

3. Blastocyst Development

a. Shedding of Zona Pellucida. The precise mechanism(s) involved in shedding of the zona pellucida prior to expansion of the mammalian blastocyst are not known. However, available data suggest that loss of the zona pellucida may be affected by factors associated with the blastocyst and the uterine environment. For example, Denker (1972) suggested lysis of the zona pellucida by a protease localized in the trophoblast, and Kirchner *et al.* (1971) indicated that the rabbit uterine β-glycoprotein, a protease, is responsible for shedding of this membrane. In support of the position of Kirchner *et al.* (1971), Beier *et al.* (1971) reported that the zona pellucida of rabbit blastocysts is not shed if β-glycoprotein secretion is delayed by estradiol treatment of does.

b. Intermediary Metabolism. It is not within the scope of this chapter to review the very extensive data on intermediary metabolism of the mammalian embryo. The review of Biggers and Borland (1976) deals with this subject in some detail. They indicate that 2-cell mouse embryos develop best when pyruvate is the energy source and, at the morula stage, lactate may be utilized more readily. By the blastocyst stage, there is a marked increase in glucose utilization. Biggers and Borland (1976) also discuss amino acid metabolism, electrolyte concentrations, generation of adenosine triphosphate, protein synthesis, and other anabolic and catabolic processes that are critical to embryonic development. It would appear that the oviductal and uterine fluids provide the nutrients and regulatory agents, e.g., enzymes and hormones, which are essential for embryonic development.

Hamner (1971) reported the numerous constituents of rabbit, sheep, sow, and monkey oviductal secretions that have been identified. In the rabbit, for example, oviductal fluid contains oxygen, sodium, chloride, potassium, magnesium, zinc, calcium, phosphate, bicarbonate, lactate, pyruvate, glucose, inositol, phospholipid, urea, amino acids, sialic acid, acid mucopolysaccharide, numerous enzymes, albumin, and other, as yet unidentified, proteins. Uterine fluids appear to provide an equally complex milieu. All of the carbohydrates, amino acids, and electroytes that appear to be essential for embryonic development seem to be present in the oviductal and uterine fluids. Data concerning the concentrations of lipid-soluble and water-soluble vitamins in genital tract secretion are not available. However, Chytil *et al.* (1975) have reported retinol and retinoic acid-binding proteins in human endometrium, and ascorbic acid has been found in sow uterine flushings (F. W. Bazer, W. Clark, and R. M. Roberts, unpublished data).

From available data, it is obvious that oviductal and uterine fluids contain substances known to be essential for embryonic development. However, there are even more components for which there is no known role.

c. Blastocyst Expansion. It is well recognized that expansion of the blastocyst occurs and that it is associated with fluid accumulation (Gamow and Daniel, 1970). Evidence presented by Gamow and Daniel (1970) and Biggers and Borland (1976) suggest that fluid accumulation in the blastocoel of rabbit blastocysts is due to active, i.e., sodium-dependent, transport of water across the trophoblast. However, the precise mechanisms controlling fluid accumulation are not known.

Fluid accumulation and blastocyst expansion are of considerable importance in species having either eccentric or interstitial types of implantation. However, this phenomenon would appear more critical in species having central type of implantation, e.g., the cow, ewe, mare, and sow. In the cow, ewe, and sow, blastocysts undergo elongation to threadlike organisms of several hundred to over 1000 mm in length. After the blastocyst has elongated, the allantoic sac begins to accumulate water at a very rapid rate to allow for concomitant expansion of the allantois and chorion and the achievement of apposition between those membranes and the uterine endometrium. In the sow, for example, allantoic fluid volume increases rapidly from day 20 (about 5 ml) to day 30 (250 ml), decreases to day 45 (75 ml), increases again to day 60 (350 ml), and then decreases to term (50 ml). Again, the precise mechanisms controlling these events are not known, but available data suggest active transport processes (Goldstein *et al.,* 1976).

d. Initiation of Steroidogenesis. The onset of steroid production by mammalian embryos may begin at the blastocyst stage. For example, Heap *et al.* (1975) have demonstrated that pig blastocysts develop the capability of converting dehydroepiandrosterone and androstenedione to estrone and estradiol. However, their results indicate that pregnenolone, progesterone, and testosterone cannot be converted to estrogens to any significant extent. Pack and Brooks (1970) have demonstrated the presence of sulfotransferase in the endometrium. Collectively, these data suggest that estrogens produced by the blastocyst may exert a local effect on the uterine vasculature and endometrium and possibly on the blastocyst itself, but, before entering the maternal circulation, the estrone is converted to estrone sulfate (Heap and Perry, 1974). This concept is consistent with the fact that the placental estrogens only affect certain tissues, i.e., those tissues that have the sulfatase enzyme to allow for conversion of estrone sulfate to estrone, which would be biologically active. Consequently, the female would not exhibit such phenomenon as estrous behavior, since the centers in the nervous system associated with such behavior would only be exposed to the biologically inactive estrone sulfate.

The possibility exists that components of genital tract secretions may influence steroid production by the trophoblast; however, data are not now available to support or reject this notion.

e. Placentation or Implantation.   Kirchner *et al.* (1971) has suggested that protease activity in rabbit uterine secretions is associated with the period of implantation in rabbits. However, there is another aspect of implantation/ placentation which should be considered. Daniel (1972) reported that the endometrium continues to produce blastokinin at the implantation site. Chen *et al.* (1975) and Bazer (1975) have reported that the porcine uterine purple acid phosphatase is produced by the uterine glands, transported by the areolae, and sequestered in the allantoic fluid. Therefore, attention should also be given to tissues and fluids of the maternal-fetal unit as a source of uterine secretion for study.

II. METHODS FOR COLLECTION OF FEMALE GENITAL TRACT SECRETIONS

A. General Background

The desire to study uterine and oviduct function has prompted development of a variety of techniques for collection of genital tract secretions. The evolution of methodology has generally reflected special needs of individual researchers. Therefore, care should be exercised in selecting a technique for collection of female genital tract secretions to assure that the method is appropriate for the research needs. The first consideration is usually whether to collect fluids continually with the aid of a collecting device (chronic collection) or to collect the fluids at a discrete time in the reproductive cycle (acute collection). This decision involves consideration of the necessity of obtaining secretory pattern information, possible alteration of secretion by the presence of the collecting apparatus, volume of material obtainable, availability of research animals, and other factors.

B. Chronic Collection of Oviductal and Uterine Secretions

The suggestion that the oviduct actively secretes fluid came from Woskressensky (1891), who ligated the uterine and ovarian ends of oviducts and observed the subsequent accumulation of fluids. Bond (1898) also observed fluid accumulation following ligation of a uterine horn in rabbits, guinea pigs, and sheep. Thus, early workers utilized the technique of ligation to collect uterine and tubal fluids.

Studies on the biologic properties of murine uterine fluid (uterone) were conducted after harvesting sufficient material by ligating the uteri and withdrawing the fluid with a syringe at monthly intervals (Homberger and Tregier, 1957; Homberger et al., 1957). These authors reported that 50–200 ml of fluid/mouse could be collected during the course of a year. The amount of fluid present in ligated uteri was affected by hormonal status of the animal. Highest amounts of fluid were found during estrus, and the lowest amounts of fluid were observed during diestrus or following castration (Homberger and Tregier, 1957). Among the biologic properties observed after administration of (128 mg) lyophilized uterone to mice were: increased uterine size and weight, increased adrenal weight, inhibition of accelerated tumor growth following hysterectomy in mice, and a necrotizing ophthalmia. The long accumulation time in the collection of these fluids could have resulted in disproportionate concentrations of certain materials. Brackett and Mastroianni (1974) reported that ligation of the rabbit oviduct resulted in decreased total protein content of the accumulated fluid as distention of the oviduct impaired the circulation and, thus, reduced transudation of serum proteins. Similarly, Heap (1962) reported changes in the relative proportions of certain constituents of uterine fluids collected by ligation when compared with fluids collected by flushing the uterus. Total nitrogen, for example, was increased tenfold in the ligated uteri. Sodium and carbohydrate content were also altered. Vishwakarma (1962) ligated the uterine horns and oviducts of New Zealand rabbits and collected the accumulated fluid 12 hours to 5 days later. In this report, uterine and oviductal fluids contained more bicarbonate and were more basic than plasma (HCO_3^- = 50.10, 52.19, and 24.0 mEq/liter for uterus, oviduct, and plasma, respectively; pH 7.857, 7.713, and 7.522 for uterus, oviduct, and plasma, respectively).

A microsurgical technique that resulted in only minimal disturbance of the blood supply was used to divide rabbit oviducts into four segments (David et al., 1969). This technique appears to provide oviductal fluid that is comparable in many respects to fluid collected via an indwelling catheter. Fluid was accumulated for 3 days and collected by aspiration with a syringe. The rate of accumulation of fluid in the segmented oviduct (0.25–1.25 ml/24 hours), assuming uniform accumulation over the 3-day period, was comparable to the volume of fluid recovered with indwelling catheters (0.9 to 1.4 ml/24 hours) (Mastroianni and Wallach, 1961; Hamner and Williams, 1965). Total protein content of the fluid in microsurgically ligated rabbit oviducts (3.3 mg/ml/72 hours; David et al., 1969) was comparable to total protein content of rabbit oviductal fluid obtained with continuous collection devices (2.1–2.7 mg/ml; Hamner and Williams, 1965; Holmdahl and Mastroianni, 1965). Segmentation of the rabbit oviduct with the microsurgical technique (David *et al.,* 1969) and analysis of the fluid from each segment revealed differences in chemical constituents from different segments. The concentration of sodium, bicarbonate, inorganic phosphate, protein, and lactic acid increased from the fimbriated end to the tubouterine portion of the oviduct. Chloride concentration was decreased in the isthmic segment (David *et al.,* 1969).

The use of cannulation techniques, especially for the collection of oviductal fluid, developed largely from the report of Bishop (1956), who demonstrated active secretion in the rabbit oviduct with the aid of a pressure manometer and a cannula inserted into the fimbriated end of the oviduct. Bishop (1956) reported that rabbit oviducts secreted fluid against a pressure of up to 71 cm of water, and at a rate of nearly 0.8 ml/24 hours. The report of Bishop (1956) clearly established the active nature of oviduct secretion and set a precedent for collection of oviduct fluids with indwelling cannulae. Most techniques that utilize indwelling cannulae include a collecting chamber located inside or outside of the body cavity of rabbits (Clewe and Mastroianni, 1960; Hamner and Williams, 1965; Holmdahl and Mastroianni, 1965), sheep (Black *et al.,* 1963; Perkins *et al.,* 1965; Restall, 1966), cows (Carlson *et al.,* 1970), horses (Engle *et al.,* 1970), sows (Edgerton *et al.,* 1966), monkeys (Mastroianni *et al.,* 1961), and humans (Moghissi, 1970; Lippes *et al.,* 1972). These devices permit fluid to accumulate in the oviduct and to be collected as needed (Feigelson and Kay, 1972). The use of an intraabdominal chamber (Hamner and Williams, 1965) has the advantage of reduced risk of contamination and reduced access to the chamber by the animal; hence, less chance of a displaced or destroyed chamber. A consideration of the extraabdominal collection chamber, however, is the ease of visual appraisal of volume collected and quality of material collected (Clewe and Mastroianni, 1960). A second consideration of the extraabdominal chamber is the option of temperature control. Holmdahl and Mastroianni (1965) devised an external collecting device with refrigeration coils incorporated into it so that the oviduct fluid would be stored at 2°–4°C as it accumulated in the collecting device. This was expected to minimize bacterial and/or enzymatic degradation of oviduct fluid constituents. Comparison of rabbit oviduct fluid collected "warm" (ambient) or "cold (2°–4°C) revealed that at least two constituents, calcium and glucose, were different under the two collection temperatures (Holmdahl and Mastroianni, 1965). Glucose concentrations were three- to fivefold higher $P < .005$ (5.0–8.5 versus 25.7–28.9 mg/100 ml), and calcium levels were slightly reduced when the fluids were collected in refrigerated chambers. A similar experiment in sheep, however, failed to indicate any difference in constituents of oviductal fluid collected in ambient temperature chambers or refrigerated collecting chambers. Calcium, glucose, protein, chloride, potassium, and dry matter were all similar under the two collecting conditions (Black *et al.,* 1970). Since the length of cannula required to carry oviduct fluid from the oviducts to the site of storage is necessarily long in large animals, it is possible that enzymatic or bacterial degradation could occur prior to the effects of refrigeration.

Restall and Wales (1966) examined major constituents of sheep oviductal fluid collected throughout the estrous cycle and reported changes in content. Total protein was increased during the luteal stage of the cycle; 0.93 gm/100 ml (estrus) versus 1.59 gm/100 ml (diestrus). A similar finding in the cow was reported by Carlson *et al.* (1970). In this report, total protein increased from 0.99 to 1.17 mg (estrus) to 3.74 to 5.26 mg (after estrus). Total glucose in oviductal fluid of cows increased from 8.89 to 24.92 μg (estrus) to 29.5 to 87.4 μg (after estrus).

Oviductal fluid collected by a short-term (1–2 hours) cannulation technique was subjected to microchemical analysis (Brackett and Mastroianni, 1974). For this technique, mated rabbits were anesthetized with sodium pentobarbital, the oviducts were cannulated at the fimbriated end, and respiration was maintained with an artificial respirator to keep plasma pCO_2, pH, and bicarbonate levels constant. Oviductal fluid collected in this manner contained higher concentrations of potassium and bicarbonate than did plasma (K = 9.2 mEq/liter oviductal fluid versus 3.7 mEq/liter plasma; HCO_3^- = 43.5 mEq/liter oviduct fluid versus 23.3 mEq/liter plasma). Sodium and chloride were essentially the same in oviduct fluid and plasma.

Collection of uterine fluids by chronic cannulation has also been accomplished using essentially similar techniques (Perkins *et al.*, 1965; Iritani *et al.*, 1969; Black *et al.*, 1963). These workers placed polyethylene or silicone rubber tubing through oviducts and into the uterine lumen via a stab puncture near the tubouterine junction. The uterine horn was usually ligated near the bifurcation. Edgerton *et al.* (1966) cannulated the uterine horns and oviducts of sows in a similar fashion. Iritani *et al* (1971) also cannulated the uterus and oviducts of rabbits, but the uterus was not ligated. Instead, both horns were cannulated, and uterine secretions from both horns were emptied into a common intraabdominal collecting chamber.

A common finding in most of these studies was an increase in volume of both uterine and oviductal fluids secreted at estrus and 24–48 hours after estrus. Oviductal and uterine secretion rates of sheep during peak production were approximately 1–1.6 ml/24 hours and 5–8 ml/24 hours, respectively, but were 0.3–0.7 ml/24 hours and less than 1.0 ml/24 hours, respectively, during diestrus (Black *et al.*, 1963; Iritani *et al.*, 1969; Perkins *et al.*, 1965). Oviductal and uterine fluid volumes were highest on day 2 postestrus in sows with one collection of 29 ml/two uterine horns and 5 ml/two oviducts over a 24-hour period (Edgerton *et al.*, 1966). Similar secretory rates of oviductal fluid were reported in rabbits ($\bar{x}$ = 0.89 ml/24 hours) by Iritani *et al.* (1971), Clewe and Mastroianni (1960), and Hamner and Williams (1965), although rabbit uterine secretory rate was considerably lower ($\bar{x}$ = 0.37 ml/24 hours). In one report in which oviductal and uterine fluids were collected from a pseudopregnant rabbit, secretion rates were greatly reduced; 0.07 and 0.19 ml/24 hours, respectively (Iritani et al., 1971).

A unique technique for the collection of uterine fluid and estimation of uterine secretory rates in monkeys (Sturgis, 1942, 1957) and in dogs (Marco, 1930) involved the use of a uteroabdominal fistula similar to the technique described by Van Wagenen and Morse (1940). In this technique, a cannula could be inserted into the uterine lumen through the fistula opening whenever collection of fluids was desired. Secretory rates were generally higher near the time of presumed ovulation and during the early luteal phase. A possible drawback to this method is the likelihood of bacterial contamination of the uterine lumen.

Studies of uterine secretory rates in monkeys and dogs receiving cardiovascular-affecting drugs (Sturgis, 1942; Marco, 1930) indicated that alterations in cardiovascular function (cardiac output, blood pressure, pulse rate) were associated with alterations in uterine secretory rate. Epinephrine administration, for example, resulted in an increase in pulse rate, blood pressure, and uterine secretory rate (Sturgis, 1942). Thus, factors which influence blood flow to the genital tract may influence the quantity or quality of the genital tract secretions.

C. Acute Collection of Female Genital Tract Secretions

1. Rabbit

Numerous reports have described the technique for recovery of rabbit uterine secretions. The procedure most commonly used has been described by Murray et al. (1972b).

2. Pig

A technique for collection of uterine secretions from the uterine lumen of nonpregnant pigs has been described by Murray et al. (1972a). This technique is carried out with the pigs under general anesthesia. Anesthesia is induced with 1 gm (5% solution) of thiopental sodium and maintained with methoxyflurane. Since pigs do not breathe through their mouth except during respiratory distress, Nos. 34–36 French intranasal tubes can be placed in each nasal passage and connected to a closed or open circuit anesthetic unit. In the pig, therefore, intubation of the trachea is not necessary.

The reproductive tract is exposed by midventral laparotomy, and a small (2mm) incision made in an avascular area of the oviduct using a surgical needle with a cutting edge. The incision should be about 1 cm above the tubouterine junction. A polyvinyl catheter (i.d. = 1.25 mm), with two to four side holes in the last 3 cm of the end of the catheter to be inserted, is then passed through the incision in the oviduct, through the tubouterine junction and to a point 4–6 cm into the uterine lumen (see Fig. 1). The surgical assistant should then secure the catheter at its point of entry into the oviduct with the thumb and forefinger of one hand. With the other hand, the thumb and forefinger should be used to restrict the lumen of the uterine horn being flushed. The surgeon then introduces 20 ml of 0.33 M NaCl into the uterine horn via the catheter. The saline is forced toward the body of the uterus to the point at which the uterine horn is being restricted. The fluid should then be forced back toward the oviduct and out through the catheter into a sterile serum bottle.

The flushings from each uterine horn may then be processed individually or after being pooled. First, the volume of uterine flushing recovered should be measured. In most cases, 21–25 ml of fluid are recovered following introduction of 20 ml of 0.33 M NaCl. Fluid volume recovered has not been shown to be significantly affected by day of the estrous cycle. The flushings should then be centrifuged at 10,000 g to remove cellular debris and the supernatant filtered through a 0.45-μm filter and stored frozen until analyzed. The uterine flushings can then be analyzed for enzymatic activity, sugars, prostaglandins, steroids, protein, etc., on a per milliliter basis. The total recoverable activity or amount of each constituent can then be expressed by multiplying those values by total fluid volume recovered. Comparisons of differences in the total amount of the various constituents recovered due to treatment effects or day of the estrous cycle depends upon the assumption that the same proportion of intraluminal fluid and constituents is recovered from each animal.

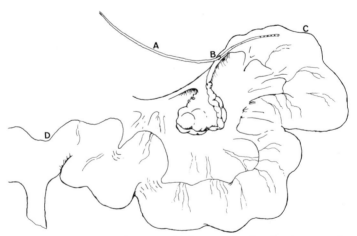

Fig. 1. Diagrammatic sketch of pig reproductive tract showing the placement of a polyvinyl catheter (A) through a small incision in the isthmus of the oviduct (B) and into the uterus (C). The uterine horn joins the uterine body at the point designated by D. The technique for flushing the uterus is described in the text.

The procedure described can also be used for collection of uterine secretions from pregnant pigs up to day 12 of pregnancy (day of onset of estrus = day 0). After day 12 of pregnancy, the blastocysts undergo rapid elongation, i.e., from about 2 mm in diameter on day 12 to a length of about 1000 mm on day 15. Consequently, the mass of tissue becomes such as to occlude the lumen of the catheter. Therefore, uterine secretions collected from days 13 to 18 of pregnancy are obtained immediately following hysterectomy. The ovaries, oviduct, uterus, and about 4 cm of the cervix are removed and immediately placed in an ice bath. The uterus is then dissected free of the mesometrium and washed extensively in cold water to remove blood. Forceps are then placed at the junction of each uterine horn and uterine body and 20 ml of 0.33 M NaCl is introduced into each uterine horn via a catheter, as previously described, and forced to the position of the forceps by hand pressure. The catheter is then removed and the oviduct and ovary is removed. Two clean mosquito forceps are then introduced about 1 cm into the uterine horn along the antimesometrial border, and an incision is made between the forceps to expose the uterine lumen. The saline and blastocysts are then forced out of the uterus through the incision and collected in sterile petri dishes.

The uterine flushings from pregnant pigs are processed as previously described for flushings from nonpregnant gilts. The blastocysts in the precipitate can be resuspended in a suitable buffer for homogenization and further study.

The procedure described has the obvious disadvantage of not allowing for repeated collection of uterine secretions from the same animal on consecutive days of the estrous cycle or pregnancy. However, the length of the uterine horns in swine precludes the possibility of obtaining meaningful results from secretions obtained via indwelling cannulae. Also, this procedure is very laborious and expensive, since surgery must be performed on each animal in appropriate facilities.

In spite of these possible disadvantages, the pig has proved to be an excellent animal model for studying uterine secretions (see review by Bazer, 1975).

3. Mare

Description of a technique for collecting uterine fluids from the mare is not available in the literature. However, a nonsurgical technique for collection of mare uterine fluids has been developed in our laboratory (M. T. Zavy, F. W. Bazer, and D. C. Sharp, unpublished data).

The design of the catheter is based on a modification of the apparatus used by Fahning et al. (1966). The catheter consists of a No. 26 to 30 French Foley catheter with an inflatable 30 ml cuff. The Foley catheter serves as a casing for a 16-gauge stainless steel inner catheter. Attached to the anterior end of the inner catheter is a 10-cm long silastic catheter with several side holes. The complete catheter can be autoclaved.

The sterile catheter is placed transcervically into the uterus (Fig. 2) by hand manipulation of the catheter through the external os of the cervix and body of cervix to a point internal to the internal os cervix. The inflatable cuff is then inflated with 60 ml of air and pulled back against the internal os of the cervix to provide a block to the leakage of the flushing medium.

Eighty milliliters of sterile 0.33 M NaCl are then infused through the inner catheter into the uterine lumen. The uterus is then massaged gently per rectum for 5 minutes to ensure adequate mixing of the contents of the uterine lumen and flushing medium. The fluid is then withdrawn, centrifuged at 10,000 g for 20 minutes, filtered through a 0.45 micron filter, and stored frozen until analyzed.

Based on data from 41 mares, an average of 85.0 ml of fluid was recovered after 80 ml of saline was introduced. Recovery volume was not affected by day of the estrous cycle. Total recoverable protein ($\overline{X}$) ranged from a 39.1 mg on day 4 to 118.9 mg on day 16 of the estrous cycle. Only one of the 41 uterine flushings was obviously contaminated with blood. Removal of the uterus from four mares

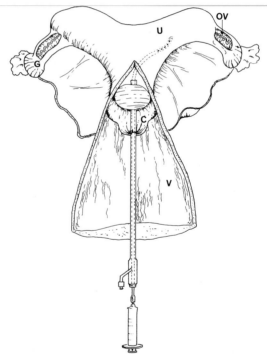

Fig. 2. Diagrammatic sketch of mare reproductive organs, i.e., the vagina (V), cervix (C), uterus (U), oviduct (OV), and ovary (G) with the device developed by M. T. Zavy and D. C. Sharp in position for obtaining a uterine flushing. A detailed description of this device is provided in the text.

immediately after obtaining a uterine flushing indicated that less than 1.5 ml of fluid was not recovered.

This procedure may also be used to recover uterine flushings from pregnant mares for at least the first 20 days of gestation.

4. Ewe

Acute collection of uterine secretions may be carried out *in situ* or following hysterectomy. G. P. Roberts *et al.* (1976a) have described a technique for removal of the reproductive tract and flushing each uterine horn three times with 3 ml of 0.15 M NaCl.

Uterine secretions may also be obtained by flushing the uterine horn *in situ* in the same manner as described for pigs. However, F. W. Bazer (unpublished data) used 5 ml of 0.33 M NaCl to flush each uterine horn. In these studies, surgical anesthesia was induced and maintained in the ewes with methoxyflurane.

5. Cow

Fahning *et al.* (1966) have described a procedure for collecting uterine fluids from cows. This procedure involves vacuum aspiration of uterine fluid through a cannula passed through the cervix and into the uterine lumen.

Roberts and Parker (1974b) have described a procedure for obtaining fluid from uteri obtained following slaughter of the cattle.

In our laboratory (F. W. Bazer, W. W. Thatcher, and A. C. Mills, unpublished data), attempts to obtain uterine flushings in live cows using a technique similar to that of Fahning *et al.* (1966) were unsatisfactory. The flushings were often contaminated with blood and/or cervical mucus and were, therefore, unsuitable for analysis. Subsequently, uterine flushings have been obtained from cattle following slaughter.

The ovaries, oviducts, uterus, and cervix are removed within 15 minutes after slaughter and placed in an ice bath. The reproductive tract is then dissected free of supporting connective tissue, and the intercornual ligament is dissected to permit clamping of each uterine horn at a point proximal to the uterine body. Each uterine horn is then flushed with 20 ml of 0.33 M NaCl, following the same procedure as that described for pigs.

It appears that concentration of bovine uterine flushings must be done by ultrafiltration procedures. Vacuum dialysis results in loss of low molecular weight proteins ($< 10,000$ MW), and lyophilization causes considerable denaturation of the proteins (F. W. Bazer and W. W. Thatcher, unpublished results).

6. Human

Procedures for obtaining uterine flushings from women have been described by Shirai *et al.* (1972) and Wolf and Mastroianni (1975), and involve lavaging the uterine lumen with sterile normal saline.

7. Rats and Mice

A technique for collection of uterine secretions by flushing each uterine horn of rats (Surani, 1976) and mice (Gore-Langton and Surani, 1976) has been described.

D. Short-Term *in Vitro* Culture of Endometrium

The synthesis of specific proteins and their appearance in the reproductive tract can be demonstrated in intact animals by introducing radioactively labeled precursors either into the blood stream or directly into the uterine lumen. The protein components in the flushings may then be analyzed for radioactivity. However, in large animals, swine in particular, these methods of labeling can lead to a considerable dilution and redistribution of both the labeled precursor and the final protein product. More recently, therefore, attempts have been made to examine the effects of steroid hormones on the synthesis of endometrial proteins *in vitro* (Garcia *et al.,* 1970; Joshi and Ebert, 1976). In these experiments, endometrium was scraped from the animals, e.g., rabbits, which had been appropriately primed with hormone. This tissue was incubated with a buffer containing radioactive amino acids or D-glucosamine. The latter compound acts as a general precursor of the carbohydrate groups of most glycoproteins. The medium is usually fortified with antibiotics and the tissue shaken for relatively short periods (not longer than 36 hours) to preclude metabolic contributions by microorganisms. Proteins secreted in soluble form into the medium may then be analyzed. Only those components synthesized during the incubation will of course be radioactive. The effects of exogenous hormones or other drugs, such as inhibitors of protein synthesis, may also be tested by simply adding the compounds to the culture medium and noting any change in the spectrum or amount of secretory products.

A related technique that might permit investigation of factors controlling endometrial protein synthesis is to employ explants of endometrium maintained in culture over longer periods than in the experiments described above. Such explants have been used to study the early events of implantation in the rabbit and hamster (Glenister, 1971) and mouse (Biggers *et al.,* 1962) and, conceivably, could be equally useful to investigate the formation of secretory products under a variety of hormonal regimens.

E. Endometrial Cell Cultures

1. General Background

An approach likely to assume increasing importance in research on female genital tract secretions is *in vitro* culture of endometrial cells. Such experimental material has a number of potential advantages over whole animal or excised organ preparations, particularly for studying the molecular effects of sex steroids on their target tissues and the secretory activities of epithelial cells, in general. Thus, tissue culture can provide uniform populations of cells that can be maintained under defined hormonal and nutritional conditions. Because of this, many of the problems associated with interspecimen variability and experimental design inherent in whole animal or organ studies will be avoided. Unfortunately, the use of cultured endometrial cells has so far had limited application, and results have been somewhat disappointing. Further, a number of problems have become evident in attempts to culture epithelial cells, whatever their origin. These may be summarized as listed below:

1. Cells of mesenchymal origin proliferate well in culture, while epithelial cells do not thrive. Therefore, since the initial tissue biopsy is usually contaminated with connective tissue, any epithelial outgrowths become rapidly overgrown by fibroblasts.

2. Another consequence of propagating a mixed initial population of cells has been to obscure the tissue origin of a final cloned line. For example, cultures with an "epitheliallike" morphology have been derived from endometrial tissue, but it is not clear whether they correspond to the secretory cells of the surface or glandular epithelium.

3. The epithelial cultures in many instances do not retain their hormonal responsiveness and lose their differentiated functional properties.

4. The primary cultures demonstrate only a short life span in culture. That is, they can only be maintained through a limited number of passages in culture. Under these conditions, it is impossible to obtain a large population of cells for experimental purposes. It is not clear whether this is due to intrinsic lower level limitations on division potential or to medium inadequacy.

Bearing in mind these problems, we shall now review some of the methods that have been employed successfully or appear to have potential for success for obtaining endometrial epithelial cell cultures.

2. Isolation of Cells from Tissue

Cells have been obtained from normal tissue or from tumors (Kuramoto *et al.*, 1972). They are usually scraped from the epithelial lining or removed in a small biopsy cut from the endometrial surface. The tissue is then treated with either dilute trypsin solution (0.25% w/v in buffered salt solution) or with a number of other enzymes or mixtures of enzymes. This procedure serves to free the cells from each other and from underlying connective tissue. They are then suspended in tissue culture medium and dispersed into growth vessels (usually sterile plastic dishes). If collagenase or other proteases are used to disrupt the epithelial sheets, care has to be taken to centrifuge the cells before plating them out in medium, since, unlike trypsin, the activities of these enzymes are not inhibited by serum (Gwatkin, 1973; Hilter, 1973).

There are some indications that the stage in the estrous cycle at which the biopsy is taken is important in determining the subsequent proliferative capacity of the cells. For example, the use of animals in estrus has been stressed (Whitson and Murray, 1974; Bouillant et al., 1973). In our experiments with pigs (R. M. Roberts and F. W. Bazer, unpublished), we have obtained best results with animals a few days (up to day 6) after estrus. This corresponds with the proliferative stage of the estrous cycle. Even so, we have only managed to maintain the cells through approximately 10 population doublings in culture.

Rather than use scrapings or biopsies, we have obtained our primary cultures by flushing the uterine horns of the pigs with tissue culture medium. This seems to loosen a few cells, which can be transferred directly to cell growth vessels. The surgical technique is the same as that used for obtaining the uterine secretions as described previously (Section II,C,2). The method seems to minimize contamination by fibroblasts.

An apparently permanent cell line has been established from a minced sample of human endometrial adenocarcinoma (Kuramoto et al., 1972; Shapiro et al., 1975). Cells derived from such tumors could have certain advantages over normal epithelial cells, since they might be expected to show many of the typical characteristics of transformed cells when cultured (i.e., prolonged or infinite life span, rapid growth from low density inocula, less fastidious nutrient requirements, low adhesion to the substratum and to each other). On the other hand, it is possible that transformation results in loss of some of the differentiated characteristics of the normal epithelial cell. Thus, the human line does not appear to show a marked responsiveness to either estrogen or progesterone (Shapiro et al., 1975).

3. Cell Maintenance

Cultures are normally maintained at 37°C in a moist incubator in an atmosphere of air and 5% CO_2. Several kinds of culture medium have been employed, supplemented with a variety of types and concentrations of sera. However, no general rules have become evident to provide a consistent methodological guide to the beginner. It is also unclear whether the exogenous addition of hormones such as insulin, hydrocortisone, or estrogens are necessary for continued proliferation of the cells (Whitson and Murray, 1974). The levels of these and other hormones (such as progesterone) in serum might become an important consideration in this type of work. During maintenance of our porcine cultures, we routinely add insulin (1 $\mu g/ml$), but we have no quantitative data to prove its value.

Various methods have been used to select epithelial populations in mixed cultures, although there are no published reports for endometrial cells. A recent paper has indicated that, whereas fibroblasts will not proliferate in medium in which the essential amino acid L-valine is replaced by its D-enantiomer, epithelial cells from a variety of tissues continue to grow (Gilbert and Migeon, 1975). We have recently shown that epithelial cells from the porcine uterus flourish in medium 199 containing D- rather than L-valine. Presumably, they contain D-amino acid oxidase which allows the conversion of D-valine to L-valine via the intermediate 2-ketoisovaleric acid.

4. Cell Transfer

Epithelial cells generally attach more firmly to the substratum and to each other than fibroblasts, so that trypsin treatment alone is often insufficient to detach them. Trypsinization can often be used successfully if the reagent is prepared in $Ca^{2+}-Mg^{2+}-$free Hanks' salt solution or in presence of low concentrations (0.01%) of the chelating agent disodium EDTA, since divalent cations seem to play a significant role in cell–cell adhesion of epithelia, and their sequestration or removal aids cell loosening.

5. Steroid Responsiveness and Production of Secretory Protein

In the limited number of cases tested, estrogens appear to promote division of endometrial cells, while progesterone inhibits proliferation (Gerschenson *et al.*, 1974; Whitson and Murray, 1974). Similar results have been observed with short-lived cultures from chick oviducts (O'Malley and Kohler, 1967). In this sense, the response of the cells to sex steroids is similar to that *in vivo*. There has been only one published report on cultured endometrial cells producing a protein characteristic of uterine secretions. Thus, in the presence of progesterone, cells derived from the rabbit endometrium secreted significant quantities of blastokinin (uteroglobin) which was identified by its characteristic electrophoretic properties and cross-reactivity with anti-blastokinin antibody (Whitson and Murray, 1974). In our laboratory, we have been able to purify small quantities of the uterine-specific purple phosphatase from the medium supporting the growth of porcine endometrial cells which had been provided with ^{3}H-D-glucosamine and ^{14}C-L-leucine (R. M. Roberts and S. M. M. Basha, unpublished results). The double-labeled product was identical in all respects to the material from intact animals. It should be emphasized that, in such studies, the secretory products are always diluted with a large quantity of foreign protein derived from the serum in the culture medium. This complicates purification and the eventual identification of the secretory protein in question. This problem will not be circumvented until tissue culture media are developed in which hormones and other co-factors replace the need for serum.

III. METHODS FOR ANALYSIS OF FEMALE GENITAL TRACT SECRETIONS

A. General Approach

In this section, we shall describe some approaches that have been used to analyze and study macromolecules present in female genital tract secretions and to distinguish those whose appearance is hormonally controlled from those which are present whatever the hormonal state of the animal. It should be emphasized at the outset that most of these secreted macromolecules have been recognized, not by their biological properties, because, for the most part, their functions are obscure, but by their particular physical properties such as size, electrophoretic mobility, or isoelectric point. This section, therefore, will deal largely with separative techniques which exploit such physical characteristics of macromolecules. For the most part, such procedures are widely used by biologists and need not be discussed in detail. However, the authors feel that the function of this section is not simply to review methodology, but to suggest approaches that might prove useful in future work on the analysis of uterine secretions.

B. Preparation of Sample

Since the secretions are obtained by flushing the oviductal, uterine, or vaginal lumen with a buffered aqueous salt solution, they are dilute with respect to protein content. Moreover, whole cells and debris may be present. Much of this particulate material can be removed by passing the fluid under a vacuum through a filter of appropriate pore size (e.g., 0.45 μm), a procedure which also serves to sterilize the solution. Alternatively the preparation should be centrifuged at high speed (100,000 g).

The dilute protein solution can be concentrated in a number of ways. Probably the most practical is vacuum filtration, either through dialysis tubing or through special membranes that retain molecules only above certain specified size limits, but which are freely permeable to water and ions (Blatt, 1971). Various commercial concentrators employing filtration systems over a range of molecular weight cutoffs are available from companies such as Dow, Corning, and Amicon (Diaflo). This method of concentration is rapid and usually leads to minimal denaturation of protein. Care has to be taken, however, not to discard small peptides that might pass through the filters.

As an alternative to vacuum filtration, the proteins may be "salted out" using solid ammonium sulfate (Green and Hughes, 1955) or freeze-dried (Everse and Stolzenbach, 1971). Both methods tend to result in some denaturation, but are useful as concentration methods.

C. Gel Filtration

Gel filtration or molecular permeation chromatography has had wide application in fractionating different size proteins. The reader is referred to reviews that discuss the theoretical aspects of gel chromatography, as well as some of the technical details associated with its application (Fischer, 1970; Reiland, 1971). This technique has had wide application in the fractionation of female genital tract secretions either to identify new size classes of protein appearing in the fluids (Krishnan and Daniel, 1967; Beier, 1968; Murray *et al.*, 1972a; Squire *et al.*, 1972; Knight *et al.*, 1973; Roberts and Parker, 1974b), or to serve as a purification step (Krishnan and Daniel, 1967; Beier, 1968; Murray *et al.*, 1972b; Bullock and O'Connell, 1973; Chen *et al.*, 1973). In most instances, other analytical methods must be employed in combination with gel filtration in order to purify a protein completely.

D. Methods Depending upon Protein Charge

1. General Methods

Ion-exchange chromatography, electrophoresis, and isoelectric focusing are methods that take advantage of the charge on molecules to effect a separation. All three have been widely used in enzyme purification and will continue to have major application in the study of genital tract secretions.

2. Ion-Exchange Chromatography

This is usually carried out in columns that are filled with an ion-exchange support matrix (Himmelhoch, 1971; Rendina, 1971). The most commonly used materials are derivatives of cellulose or dextran. Diethylaminoethyl (DEAE) substituents on the polysaccharides contain a positive charge within physiological pH ranges, and can be used to bind negatively charged proteins. A counter ion (usually Cl^-, $CH_3 \cdot COO^-$ or HPO_4^{2-}) is exchanged in this process. Carboxymethyl (CM) or phospho-substituted polymers are cation exchangers and are useful for separating positively charged proteins. The counter ion is usually Na^+ or K^+. The highly basic purple protein from the porcine uterus, for example, binds to CM cellulose at pH 8.5 even in presence of 0.1 M NaCl, while the majority of the proteins in the flushings do not do so. Advantage is taken of this high basicity in order to effect an extensive purification (Chen *et al.*, 1973; Schlosnagle *et al.*, 1974).

The proteins bound to ion exchangers are eluted either by increasing the concentration of salt in the buffer or by altering the pH in order to reduce the charge interaction. For salt elution, either a continuous or stepwise elution gradient may be employed. As with gel filtration, the proteins appearing in the eluate may be detected optically by their absorption of 280 nm light or by a suitable colorimetric procedure. For preparation of the ion-exchange materials and details of their application to protein purification, the reader is referred to two reviews (Himmelhoch, 1971; Rendina, 1971).

3. Electrophoresis

It is frequently possible to fractionate mixtures of globular proteins on the basis of their net rate of migration in an electrical field. Since this depends on the net charge on the proteins, which are amphoteric molecules, the rate of migration is also a function of pH. The method of protein electrophoresis now most widely employed, and the one which has probably had widest application in detecting novel protein species in genital tract secretions is polyacrylamide gel electrophoresis (PAGE) in which gels cast of cross-linked polyacrylamide provide a solid support for the buffer containing the protein (see Gordon, 1970; Gabriel, 1971). PAGE has gained such favor largely because of the mechanical stability of the gels and their chemical inertness and purity. Moreover, the methodology is simple, fast, and provides extremely reproducible results. Since the concentration of polyacrylamide and its degree of cross-linking can be varied, the migration of a protein is determined by its size as well as its net charge. The system is applicable over a wide pH range and in presence of a variety of denaturants (e.g., urea). Such pretreatment may be necessary to maintain the proteins in solution during the separation. Following electrophoresis, the protein pattern is preserved in the gel by appropriate fixation and staining.

An example of the separation of proteins present in uterine secretions of ovariectomized sows that had received various hormonal treatments has been reported by Knight et al. (1973). The proteins were separated under nondenaturing conditions (i.e., they were not exposed to denaturants such as urea or detergents such as sodium dodecyl sulfate). Because of this, their native conformation and functional properties such as enzyme activity, are largely preserved. Knight et al. (1973) show gels run toward the anode to separate proteins bearing a net negative charge and indicated several bands present in progesterone-treated gilts; the bands were not evident in corn oil-treated pigs. Similarly, in gels run towards the cathode, a positively charged band was evident in animals receiving progesterone; this band was later identified as the purple phosphatase (Schlosnagle et al., 1974).

It is sometimes an advantage to separate proteins under denaturing conditions. For example, protein aggregates or large multi-subunit molecules can usually be dissociated and solubilized in solutions containing the detergent sodium dodecyl sulfate (SDS). Provided disulfide bonds are also reduced, the globular polypeptide chains uncoil completely and assume the shape of doubled-over helical rods whose length is directly proportional to their polypeptide chain length (Reynolds and Tanford, 1970). In addition, the strongly anionic SDS confers a similar charge density to each protein. Because of this, the electrophoretic mobility of the proteins in SDS–PAGE systems is inversely proportional to the logarithm of their molecular weights, much the same as in gel filtration. This is an extremely valuable aid in protein characterization and has been used in determining the molecular weights of proteins such as blastokinin (Murray *et al.*, 1972b; Bullock and O'Connell, 1973) and the porcine purple phosphatase (Chen *et al.*, 1973), as well as for detecting new or unusual polypeptides in secretions (G. P. Roberts *et al.*, 1976a,b).

4. Isoelectric Focusing

This method is being increasingly used for separating proteins and other amphoteric macromolecules, although it has not been widely employed in the analysis of genital tract secretions (Roberts and Parker, 1974a; G. P. Roberts *et al.*, 1976b). The substances under investigation are segregated according to their isoelectric points (pI) in pH gradients which are formed by electrophoresis of amphoteric buffer substances. The latter are known as ampholytes, and they may be purchased for a number of different pH ranges. When an electric field is applied, the proteins migrate to zones in the gradient where their net charge is zero. In this way, different proteins can be concentrated in sharp bands. For details of the theoretical background and practical application of the method, the readers are referred to two excellent reviews (Vesterburg, 1971; Righetti and Drysdale, 1974).

E. Fluorescent Antibody Techniques

Fluorescent antibody techniques have been reviewed adequately in another volume (Glass, 1971). The method has been used successfully to demonstrate the site of synthesis of the porcine purple phosphatase during pregnancy and through the estrous cycle (Chen *et al.*, 1975), and the localization of blastokinin in the uterus of the pregnant and pseudo-pregnant rabbit (Johnson, 1972) and rabbit blastocysts (Kirchner, 1972).

F. Labeling Techniques

1. Iodination

Iodination is widely used for introducing radioactive iodine (^{125}I or ^{131}I) into tyrosine residues on intact proteins. The resulting label is relatively stable and can be of extremely high specific activity. The modification of tyrosyl groups seems to result in a minimum of conformational change in the protein. For methodology, the reader is referred to two references which give detailed descriptions of the procedure (Greenwood *et al.*, 1963; Thorell and Johansson, 1971).

2. Acetylation

Acetic anhydride reacts readily in aqueous solution with nucleophilic R groups of low pKa on amino acid side chains of proteins (see Means and Feeney, 1971). At pH 7.0, most of the acetyl groups are introduced into ϵ-amino groups of lysine residues. Since acetic anhydride is also readily hydrolyzed in aqueous solution, it is quickly consumed so that the reaction is completed in a few minutes. Our normal procedure is to buy the radioactive reagent in dry benzene. This may be diluted if necessary and dispensed into a series of sublots for storage. We use ^{3}H-acetic anhydride at a dilution of about 10 μCi/μl benzene. The protein is dissolved in 0.1 M phosphate buffer at pH 7.0 at a concentration of about 5 mg/ml, and the benzene–acetic anhydride solution is added to this directly and mixed. We usually use about 20 μCi ^{3}H-acetic anhydride for each milligram of protein, but the amount may be decreased or increased, depending upon the extent of the labeling desired. Normally, about 1% of the radiolabel is incorporated. It should be realized that acetylation modifies the net charge on a protein, thus altering its isoelectric point. It also introduces a nonpolar substituent to what was a polar group. Therefore, acetylation may lead to changes in protein conformation and biologic activity (Thorell and Johansson, 1971).

3. Galactose Oxidase

Labeling of carbohydrate side chains by the galactose oxidase technique was originally described by Ashwell and Morell (1976). It depends upon the oxidation of exposed hydroxymethyl groups on D-galactose and N-acetyl D-galactosamine residues on the carbohydrate side chains of glycoproteins, using the commercially available fungal enzyme D-galactose oxidase.

We have used this method to label the pig purple protein. Approximately 2 mg of protein (in 1 ml of 0.5 M phosphate buffer, pH 7.0, containing 0.05 M NaCl) was treated with 40 μl of galactose oxidase solution (1 mg/ml). The solution was layered with 20 μl of toluene to reduce bacterial growth and incubated in a closed tube for 24 hours at 37C. A control was run without galactose oxidase. Five milliliters of 0.05 M phosphate buffer pH 7.8 were added to each, followed by a small amount (approximating about 500 μCi) of solid ^{3}H-borotritide. After 30 minutes at room temperature, the mixture was passed through a column of CM cellulose to bind the purple protein. After washing, this protein could be eluted with 0.05 M NaCl. Alternatively, dialysis followed by Bio-Gel P-100 gel filtration is suitable to separate the modified protein from radioactive contaminants. Using this method, the galactose oxidase-pretreated protein had a specific radioactivity of approximately 0.5 μCi/mg and retained its phosphatase activity. The control incorporated about one-twentieth this level of ^{3}H.

G. Enzyme Analyses

In initial survey work, it is clearly tempting to test for enzymes that are easy to assay, such as hydrolases which cleave glycosidic, peptide, or ester linkages, since a wide variety of artificial substrates that give rise to colored reaction products are available commercially. Thus, a series of enzymes which hydrolyze p-nitrophenylglycosides have been detected in uterine luminal fluids of the bovine (Roberts and Parker, 1974a,b), sheep (Roberts *et al.*, 1976a), and human (G. P. Roberts *et al.*, 1976b) uterus.

Our approach has been to assay for a wide variety of enzymes that have been reported to be active in the uterus or placenta. Most results have been negative, including attempts to detect carbonic anhydrase (which is known to function in CO_2 exchange) and steroid-metabolizing enzymes. Lysozyme, which is present in many exocrine secretions and probably induced by progesterone in the human vagina and uterus (Schumacher, 1974), was detectable. It can be isolated in milligram quantities from pigs administered progesterone. In the assay, the rate of clearing of a suspension of *Micrococcus luteus* cells is followed spectrophotometrically (Shugar, 1952; Worthington Biochemical Corp., 1972; Schumacher, 1974). Lysozyme has presumably a bacteriostatic role in reducing the risk of infection in the genital tract.

A number of protease activities, including the cathepsins B, C, and D, and leucine aminopeptidase were also induced by progesterone in the pig uterus (R. M. Roberts *et al.*, 1976b). Detailed methods for assaying these typically lysosomal enzymes have been described in detail elsewhere (Barrett, 1972).

In summary, therefore, it seems fair to conclude that little is known about the polypeptide components of genital tract secretions. Most future work will probably depend upon techniques already used successfully to purify proteins from other tissues, since in many cases it will be essential to isolate specific components in homogeneous form before their functional characteristics can be established. This work will be particularly difficult because only small amounts of protein can be recovered from these secretions. For more than 2000 years, it has been assumed that the uterine fluids were the nutritive material from which the fetus was formed. In the pig, at least, this may be close to the truth. Nevertheless, certain key questions remain. What mechanisms, for example, regulate the amount and composition of the fluid, and what is the role of each of its constituents in the growth and development of the placenta and fetus? We are a long way from answering these questions.

ACKNOWLEDGMENTS

Data obtained and referred to by authors of this chapter are from studies supported by the National Science Foundation (Grant DMF 741A016 to R. M. R.), National Institute of Health (Grant

HD08560 to F. W. B. and R. M. R.), and U.S. Department of Agriculture Cooperative Agreement (12-14-1001-402) with F. W. B. Dr. R. M. Roberts is recipient of USPHS Career Development Award K4AM70389.

REFERENCES

Amoroso, E. C. (1952). In "Marshall's Physiology of Reproduction" (A. S. Parkes, ed.), 3rd ed., Vol, 2, pp. 127–311. Longmans, Green, New York.
Anderson, L. L., Bland, K. P., and Melampy, R. M. (1969). Recent Prog. Horm. Res. 25, 57.
Ashwell, G., and Morell, A. (1976). Adv. Enzymol. 41, 99.
Austin, C. R. (1972). In "Reproduction in Mammals" (C. R. Austin and R. V. Short, eds.), Book 1, pp. 103–133. Cambridge Univ. Press, London and New York.
Barrett, A. J. (1972). In "Lysosomes. A Laboratory Handbook" (J. F. Dingle, ed.), pp. 46–135. Am. Elsevier, New York.
Bazer, F. W. (1975). J. Anim. Sci. 41, 1376.
Beier, H. M. (1968). Science 158, 490.
Beier, H. M., Kühnel, W., and Petry, G. (1971). Adv. Biosci. 6, 165.
Biggers, J. D., and Borland, R. M. (1976). Annu. Rev. Physiol. 38, 95.
Biggers, J. D., Gwatkin, R. B. L., and Brinster, R. L. (1962). Nature (London) 194, 747.
Bishop, D. W. (1956). Am. J. Physiol. 187, 347.
Black, D. L., Duby, R. T., and Reisen, J. (1963). J. Reprod. Fertil. 6, 257.
Black, D. L., Kumar, A., Crowley, L. V., Duby, R. T., and Spilman, C. H. (1970). J. Reprod. Fertil. 22, 597.
Blatt, W. F. (1971). In "Methods in Enzymology" (W. B. Jakoby, ed.), Vol. 22, pp. 39–49. Academic Press, New York.
Bond, C. J. (1898). J. Physiol. (London) 22, 296.
Bonnet, R. (1882). "Die Uterinmilch und ihr Bedeutung fa03ur die Frucht." Stuttgart.
Bouillant, A., Greig, A. S., and Genest, P. (1973). In Vitro 9, 92.
Brackett, B. G., and Mastroianni, L. (1974). In "The Oviduct and Its Function" (A. D. Johnson and C. W. Foley, eds.), pp. 134–153. Academic Press, New York.
Bullock, D. W., and O'Connell, K. M. (1973). Biol. Reprod. 9, 125.
Carlson, D., Black, D. L., and Howe, G. R. (1970). J. Reprod. Fertil. 22, 549.
Chen, T. T., Bazer, F. W., Cetorelli, J. J., Pollard, W. E., and Roberts, R. M. (1973). J. Biol. Chem. 248, 8560.
Chen, T. T., Bazer, F. W., Gebhardt, B. M., and Roberts, R. M. (1975). Biol. Reprod. 13, 304.
Chytil, F., Page, D. L., and Ong, D. E. (1975). Int. J. Vitam. Nutr. Res. 45, 293.
Clewe, T. H., and Mastroianni, L. (1960). J. Reprod. Fertil. 1, 146.
Daniel, J. C. (1972). J. Reprod. Fertil. 31, 303.
David, A., Brackett, B. G., Garcia, C. R., and Mastroianni, L. (1969). J. Reprod. Fertil. 19, 285.
Denker, H. W. (1972). Acta Endocrinol. (Copenhagen) 70, 591.
Edgerton, L. A., Martin, C. E., Troutt, H. F., and Foley, C. W. (1966). J. Anim. Sci. 25, 1265.
Engle, C. C., Witherspoon, D. M., and Foley, C. W. (1970). Am. J. Vet. Res. 31, 1889.
Everse, J., and Stolzenbach, F. F. (1971). In "Methods in Enzymology" (W. B. Jakoby, ed.), Vol. 22, pp. 33–39. Academic Press, New York.
Fahning, M. L., Schultz, R. H., and Graham, E. F. (1966). Vet. Rec. 79, 230.
Feigelson, M., and Kay, E. (1972). Biol. Reprod. 6, 244.
Fischer, L. (1970). Lab. Tech. Biochem. Mol. Biol. 1, 151–396.

Gabriel, O. (1971). *In* "Methods in Enzymology" (W. B. Jakoby, ed.), Vol. 22, pp. 565-578. Academic Press, New York.

Gamow, E., and Daniel, J. C. (1970). *Wilhelm Roux' Arch. Entwicklungsmech. Org.* **164,** 261.

Garcia, N., Caruso, A., Campo, S., Milano, L., and Bompiani, A. (1970). *Fertil. Steril.* **27,** 442.

Gerschenson, L. E., Berliner, E., and Yang, J.-J. (1974). *Cancer Res.* **34,** 2873.

Gilbert, S. F., and Migeon, B. R. (1975). *Cell* **5,** 11.

Glass, L. E. (1971). *In* "Methods in Mammalian Embryology" (J. C. Daniel, ed.), Vol. 1, pp. 355-377. Freeman, San Francisco, California.

Glenister, T. W. (1971). *In* "Methods in Mammalian Embryology" (J. C. Daniel, ed.), Vol. 1, pp. 320-330. Freeman, San Francisco, California.

Goding, J. R. (1974). *J. Reprod. Fertil.* **38,** 261.

Goldstein, M. H., Bazer, F. W., Spellacy, W. N., and Buhi, W. C. (1976). *Gyneol. Invest.* **7,** 58.

Gordon, A. H. (1970). *Lab. Tech. Biochem. Mol. Biol.* **1,** pp. 1-155.

Gore-Langton, R. E., and Surani, M. A. H. (1976). *J. Reprod. Fertil.* **46,** 271.

Green, A. A., and Hughes, W. L. (1955). *In* "Methods in Enzymology" (S. P. Colowick and N. O. Kaplan, eds.), Vol. 1, pp. 67-90. Academic Press, New York.

Greenwood, F. C., Hunter, W. M., and Glover, J. S. (1963). *Biochem. J.* **89,** 114.

Gwatkin, R. B. L. (1973). *In* "Tissue Culture Methods and Applications" (P. Kruse, Jr., and M. K. Patterson, eds.), pp. 3-5. Academic Press, New York.

Hafez, E. S. E. (1974). *In* "Reproduction in Farm Animals" (E. S. E. Hafez, ed.), pp. 123-142. Lea & Febiger, Philadelphia, Pennsylvania.

Hamner, C. E. (1971). *Adv. Biosci.* **6,** 143.

Hamner, C. E., and Williams, W. L. (1965). *Fertil. Steril.* **16,** 170.

Heap, R. B. (1962). *J. Endocrinol.* **24,** 367.

Heap, R. B., and Perry, J. S. (1974). *Br. J. Hosp. Med.* **12,** 8.

Heap, R. B., Perry, J. S., Gadsby, J. E., and Burton, R. D. (1975). *Biochem. Soc. Trans.* **3,** 1183.

Hilter, S. R. (1973). *In* "Tissue Culture Methods and Applications" (P. Kruse, Jr., and M. K. Patterson, eds.), pp. 16-20. Academic Press, New York.

Himmelhoch, S. R. (1971). *In* "Methods in Enzymology" (W. B. Jakoby, ed.), Vol. 22, pp. 273-286. Academic Press, New York.

Holmdahl, T. H., and Mastroianni, L. (1965). *Fertil. Steril.* **16,** 587.

Homberger, F., and Tregier, A. (1957). *Endocrinology* **61,** 627.

Homberger, F., Tregier, A., and Grossman, M. S. (1957). *Endocrinology* **61,** 634.

Iritani, A., Gomes, W. R., and Van Demark, N. L. (1969). *Biol. Reprod.* **1,** 72.

Iritani, A., Nishikawa, Y., Gomes, W. R., and Van Demark, N. L. (1971). *J. Anim. Sci.* **33,** 829.

Johnson, M. H. (1972). *Fertil. Steril.* **23,** 929.

Joshi, S. G., and Ebert, K. M. (1976). *Fertil. Steril.* **27,** 730.

Kirchner, C. (1972). *Fertil. Steril.* **23,** 131.

Kirchner, C., Hirschhäuser, C., and Kionke, M. (1971). *J. Reprod. Fertil.* **27,** 259.

Knight, J. W., Bazer, F. W., and Wallace, H. D. (1973). *J. Anim. Sci.* **36,** 546.

Krishnan, R. S., and Daniel, J. C. (1967). *Science* **158,** 490.

Kuramoto, H., Tamura, S., and Notake, Y. (1972). *Am. J. Obstet. Gynecol.* **114,** 1012.

Lippes, J., Enders, R. G., Progay, D. A., and Bartholomew, W. R. (1972). *Contraception* **5,** 85.

McCracken, J. A. (1971). *Ann. N. Y. Acad. Sci.* **180,** 456.

McCracken, J. A., Carlson, J. C., Glew, M. E., Goding, J. R., and Baird, D. T. (1972). *Nature (London)* **238,** 129.

Marco, R. D. (1930). *Arch. Fisiol.* **29,** 181.

Mastroianni, L., and Wallach, R. C. (1961). *Am. J. Physiol.* **200,** 815.

Mastroianni, L., Urmila, S., and Raja, A. K. (1961). *Fertil. Steril.* **12,** 417.

Means, G. E., and Feeney, R. E. (1971). "Chemical Modifications of Proteins." Holden-Day, San Francisco, California.

Moghissi, K. S. (1970). *Fertil. Steril.* **21**, 821.

Murray, F. A., Bazer, F. W., Wallace, H. D., and Warnick, A. C. (1972a). *Biol. Reprod.* **7**, 314.

Murray, F. A., McGaughey, R. W., and Yarus, M. J. (1972b). *Fertil. Steril.* **23**, 69.

Ogra, S. S., Kirton, K. T., Tomasi, T. B., and Lippes, J. (1974). *Fertil. Steril.* **25**, 250.

O'Malley, B. W., and Kohler, P. O. (1967). *Proc. Natl. Acad. Sci. U. S. A.* **58**, 2359.

Pack, B. A., and Brooks, S. C. (1970). *Endocrinology* **87**, 924.

Patek, C. E., and Watson, J. (1976). *Prostaglandins* **12**, 97.

Perkins, J. L., Goode, L., Wilder, W. A., and Henson, D. B. (1965). *J. Anim. Sci.* **24**, 383.

Reiland, J. (1971). *In* "Methods In Enzymology" (W. B. Jakoby, ed.), Vol. 22, pp. 287–321. Academic Press, New York.

Rendina, G. (1971). *In* "Experimental Methods in Modern Biochemistry" (G. Rendina, ed.), pp. 174–191. Saunders, Philadelphia, Pennsylvania.

Restall, B. J. (1966). *Aust. J. Biol. Sci.* **19**, 181.

Restall, B. J., and Wales, R. G. (1966). *Aust. J. Biol. Sci.* **19**, 687.

Reynolds, J. A., and Tanford, C. (1970). *J. Biol. Chem.* **245**, 5161.

Righetti, P. G., and Drysdale, J. W. (1974). *J. Chromatogr.* **98**, 271.

Roberts, G. P., and Parker, J. M. (1974a). *J. Reprod. Fertil.* **40**, 291.

Roberts, G. P., and Parker, J. M. (1974b). *J. Reprod. Fertil.* **40**, 305.

Roberts, G. P., Parker, J. M., and Symonds, H. W. (1976a). *J. Reprod. Fertil.* **48**, 99.

Roberts, G. P., Parker, J. M., and Henderson, S. R. (1976b). *J. Reprod. Fertil.* **48**, 153.

Roberts, R. M., Bazer, F. W., Baldwin, N., and Pollard, W. E. (1976). *Arch. Biochem. Biophys.* **174**, 499.

Schlosnagle, D. C., Bazer, F. W., Tsibris, J. C. M., and Roberts, R. M. (1974). *J. Biol. Chem.* **249**, 7574.

Schmacher, G. F. B. (1974). *In* "Lysozyme" (E. F. Osserman, R. E. Canfield, and S. Beycholk, eds.), pp. 427–447. Academic Press, New York.

Shapiro, S. S., and Van Der Schouw, M., and Hayerman, D. D. (1975). *Am. J. Obstet. Gynecol.* **121**, 570.

Shirai, E., Iizuka, R., and Notake, Y. (1972). *Fertil. Steril.* **23**, 522.

Shugar, D. (1952). *Biochim. Biophys. Acta* **8**, 302.

Squire, G. D., Bazer, F. W., and Murray, F. A. (1972). *Biol. Reprod.* **7**, 321.

Sturgis, S. H. (1942). *Endocrinology* **31**, 664.

Sturgis, S. H. (1957). *Fertil. Steril.* **8**, 1.

Surani, M. A. H. (1976). *J. Reprod. Fertil.* **48**, 141.

Thorell, J. I., and Johansson, G. B. (1971). *Biochim. Biophys. Acta* **251**, 363.

Van Wagenen, G., and Morse, A. H. (1940). *Endocrinology* **27**, 268.

Vesterburg, O. (1971). *In* "Methods In Enzymology" (A. San Pietro, ed.), Vol. 23, pp. 389–412. Academic Press, New York.

Vishwakarma, P. (1962). *Fertil. Steril.* **13**, 481.

Whitson, G. L., and Murray, F. A. (1974). *Science* **183**, 668.

Wolf, D. P., and Mastroianni, L. (1975). *Fertil. Steril.* **26**, 240.

Worthington Biochemical Corp. (1972). "Worthington Enzyme Manual." Freehold, New Jersey.

Woskressensky, M. A. (1891). *Zentralbl. Gynaekol.* **15**, 849.

24

Experimental Approaches for Elucidating the Antifertility Action of Intrauterine Devices in Monkeys and Rodents

P. ECKSTEIN AND P. R. HURST

I. INTRODUCTION

The emergence of the modern plastic intrauterine devices (IUD's) in the early 1960's has led to intensive research into their biologic effects and mode of action in women and lower mammals (see El-Sahwi and Moyer, 1970; Eckstein, 1970, 1972; Moyer and Shaw, 1973; Duncan and Wheeler, 1975).

There is near-consensus that the principal contraceptive action of IUD's is within the uterus, rather than in the tube, the ovary, or systemically. The block to pregnancy induced by the IUD's, therefore, must be exerted after the embryo has left the oviduct and before or during its attachment to the endometrium, whether by creating an ovotoxic environment or by inhibiting nidation or by a combination of both.

Opinions differ, however, about the actual mechanism(s) responsible for the antifertility action. More specifically, it has been proposed that the device: (1) stimulates tubouterine motility, leading to premature expulsion of ova and blastocysts from the reproductive tract; (2) reduces the life span and function of the corpus luteum, thereby depriving the conceptus of progesterone essential for implantation; (3) inhibits or modifies the decidual transformation of the endometrium in preparation for nidation; (4) acts as a foreign body and provokes a sterile inflammatory reaction in the endometrium which in some, as yet unknown, way renders the uterine cavity toxic to preimplantation embryos. In addition, the phagocytic elements in the cellular exudate may trap sperm and reduce their number to the point of interfering with fertilization.

The following account does not attempt to survey all the available evidence for or against the first three of these concepts (cf. Eckstein, 1970; Duncan and Wheeler, 1975), but accepts the fourth as a useful working hypothesis. The presence of large numbers of inflammatory cells, mainly polymorphonuclear leukocytes (polymorphs) and monocytes (macrophages), is a typical and constant feature of the endometrial reaction to the presence of an IUD in all species studied so far, from women and lower primates to rodents (cf. Parr *et al.*, 1967; Parr, 1969; Kelly *et al.*, 1969; Peplow *et al.*, 1973; Parr and Shirley, 1976; Hurst *et al.*, 1977a). A positive correlation between the number of leukocytes in the uterine fluid and the suppression of implantation has been found in rabbits fitted with various intrauterine devices (El-Sahwi and Moyer, 1971). In rats, it is known that a completely intramural uterine suture is ineffective, and, in order to become contraceptive, it has to enter the uterine cavity and induce an infiltration by polymorphs of its wall and lumen (Greenwald, 1965). Again, in germfree rats, the leukocytic infiltration and antifertility action is confined to the area in physical contact with the IUD, while the adjacent segment of the uterus remains fertile (Parr *et al.*, 1967). There is, thus, good reason to think that an IUD provokes a chronic inflammatory response in the endometrium, and that the resulting cellular exudate is contraceptive by virtue of its embryotoxic and/or antinidatory activity.

Accordingly, with this view of the mechanism of action of IUD's in mind, we have concentrated on the condition of the "free" uterine embryo and its cellular and hormonal environment, and on the changes brought about in them by the presence of a device.

Consequently, techniques have been developed for: (a) recovering preimplantation embryos from normal and IUD-fitted rhesus monkeys; (b) detecting tubal and uterine embryos in IUD-bearing and control mice by serial sectioning of the reproductive tract; and (c) demonstrating the involvement of polymorphs, and elucidating their specific role, in the antifertility action of IUD's in both mice and monkeys.

It is the purpose of this chapter to describe these techniques, as well as our surgical procedures for inserting IUD's in experimental primates and lower mammals, to list the results so far obtained in using these methods, and to discuss ways in which they might be extended or adapted for future research.

II. INSERTION OF IUD'S

A. Rodents and Rabbits

Insertion of IUD material in the form of a thread, is best accomplished in mice, rats, and rabbits by exposing the uterine horns at midventral laparotomy. A 1 to

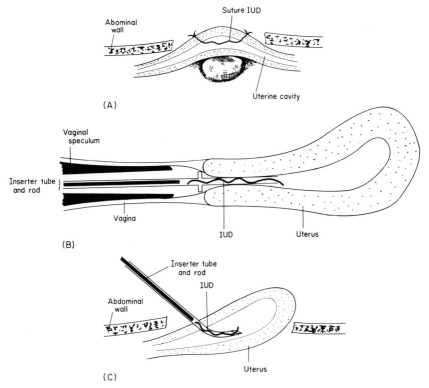

Fig. 1. Technique of inserting IUD's (diagrammatic). (A) Mouse and rat (suture IUD). (B) Baboon (plastic IUD). (C) Rhesus monkey (plastic IUD).

2-cm incision is usually sufficient to allow grasping of either horn and gently pulling it up to the incision site, where sterile gauze or cotton wool is used to support the organ and absorb any blood. A length of fine silk ["6.0" (0.75 metric) gauge] or nylon threaded to a round-bodied needle is passed into the chosen horn after piercing the uterine lumen with the needle near the cervical pole. If silk is used, knotting both ends outside the antimesometrial surface prevents loss of the IUD, but it is essential to allow the thread to be slack *in utero* so as to avoid tearing of tissue during myometrial activity (see Fig. 1A).

To obtain complete sterility in IUD-bearing uteri of rats and mice, at least one-third of the horn must be in contact with the device. Before repairing the abdomen, bleeding from either the incision site or the uterus should be stopped if peritoneal adhesions are to be avoided.

In the rabbit, implantation can occur in regions not in immediate contact with the IUD, although the resulting fetuses generally die before term (Adams and Eckstein, 1965). Therefore, if complete suppression of implantation is to be achieved, the IUD should occupy the entire length of the horn.

B. Primates

In experimental primates, such as rhesus monkeys and baboons, plastic devices, similar to those used in human contraception, but smaller, are normally employed. We have found shortened tailless Margulies coils, measuring 15–20 mm in diameter, suitable for average sized baboons and slightly smaller versions of these coils for rhesus monkeys. Almost any other kind of human device (including the copper-T and copper-7 types) can, however, be fitted after appropriate reduction in size.

1. Baboons

In this species, the cervical canal is almost straight and permits nonsurgical insertion of IUD's in a manner similar to that followed in women by using a slightly modified metal or polyethylene inserter (see Fig. 1B).

Location and gentle probing of the cervical canal with a fine probe is usually necessary before the device can be inserted. A pediatric vaginal speculum aids in identification of the external os of the cervix. In our experience, some individuals have a very tight os, especially in the luteal phase of the cycle, and attempts to pass either a probe or the inserter are liable to perforate the uterus. Perforations of this kind usually heal perfectly, and they rarely require surgical or medical treatment. After such an occurrence, IUD's are best inserted at laparotomy in a manner similar to that used in rhesus monkeys.

2. Rhesus Monkeys

The narrow and tortuous cervix of these and other macaques usually necessitates surgical insertion of the IUD by hysterotomy. A 6- to 8-cm midline incision of the lower abdomen gives adequate access to the uterus. The cervix is grasped with either Allis or Littlewood's forceps and the uterus raised to the incision site. IUD's are best inserted from either the fundal pole or the supracervical region by puncturing the organ with a sharpened steel tube of about 3-mm external diameter, containing the IUD. A piece of steel rod is introduced into the tube, and, in this way, the IUD is displaced into the lumen of the uterus (Fig. 1C). Some bleeding may be seen at the puncture site, but, with polyethylene coils, no perforations into the abdomen have occurred.

It is our practice to X-ray monkeys 1–2 weeks after insertion of an IUD to confirm the presence and correct conformation of the device in the uterine cavity. It is also advisable to repeat such X-rays subsequently before attempting embryo recovery or other manipulative procedures relating to the investigation of IUD action.

In recently delivered females, small plastic devices can sometimes be inserted by the cervical route. Their correct position within the uterine cavity must, however, be carefully checked by X-rays; they are also prone to be spontaneously expelled.

III. PROCEDURE FOR EMBRYO RECOVERY FROM PRIMATE UTERI

The following technique is based mainly on our experience with rhesus monkeys (*Macaca mulatta*) (Hurst *et al.*, 1976), although the procedure has also been used successfully in flushing baboon uteri.

Healthy, sexually mature monkeys are inspected daily for visible vaginal bleeding in order to determine their menstrual cyclicity. Newly imported animals should have at least two regular menstrual cycles before being considered for attempts at embryo recovery. We have used animals with cycles lasting from 24 to 33 (mean 28) days, but the majority ranged from 26 to 30 days.

Females are placed with males from days 10 to 14 of the cycle, counting the 1st day of overt vaginal bleeding as day 1 (see Fig. 2). Pairs should be watched for copulation; occasional vaginal lavage should be performed and examined for motile sperm.

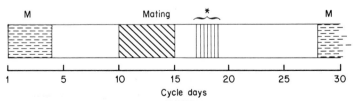

Fig. 2. Procedure for recovery of uterine embryos in rhesus monkeys: M, menstruation; *, laparotomy and uterine flush on one of these days.

Days 16, 17, or 18 appear to be the most favorable for successful recovery (see Table I). On the selected day, animals are tranquilized with 0.5 ml ketamine hydrochloride (Parke Davis) (100 mg/ml; im), and the abdomen shaved. General anesthesia is maintained with oxygen/fluothane delivered through a face mask. Laparotomy is performed in the midline of the abdomen; the incision need not exceed 8–10 cm in length, and should terminate about 1 cm above the symphysis pubis to avoid possible injury to the bladder. We favor the use of a cautery for incisions, since this minimizes bleeding into the abdomen. The wound margins are opened with retractors to allow clear visualization of the whole of the reproductive tract. The ovaries are inspected for signs of recent ovulation; unless these are present, no attempt at flushing is made. The cervix is carefully clamped with Littlewood's or Allis tissue forceps. This permits raising of the uterus to the incision site and provides the resistance necessary to insert the flushing needles. It also occludes the internal cervical os, thereby preventing loss of uterine fluid. The flushing needles are made by shortening 4½-inch 17-gauge stainless steel needles (Downbro Surgical) to about 1¼ inch and boring two fenestrations close

TABLE I
Flushing Data and Embryo Recoveries in
Rhesus Monkeys

Day of flush	No. of flushes attempted	No. of embryos recovered
Without IUD's		
16	3	2
17	33	18
18	14	7
19	4	1
	54	28
	Percentage recoveries:	52
With IUD's		
15	3	1
16	10	2
17	16	1[a]
18	7	0
19	8	2
20	2	1
	46	7
	Percentage recoveries:	15

[a] Degenerating morula (about 30 cells); X-ray showed IUD located in cervix.

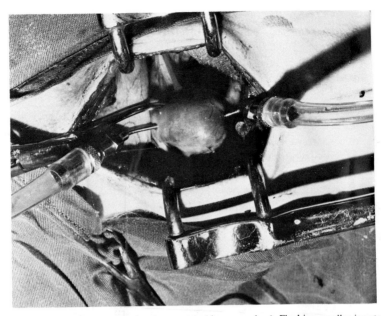

Fig. 4. Uterine flushing procedure in progress (rhesus monkey). Flushing needles inserted into supracervical region (left) and fundus (right) of uterus.

Removal of the needles from the uterus is usually accomplished without excessive bleeding; any bleeding that occurs must be stopped and clots removed to minimize potential adhesions. With suitable care, uteri can be flushed for at least six times before adhesions or scarring prevent any further operations of this kind. We usually allow a "recovery" menstrual cycle to occur before repeating the procedure.

In applying the method described above, we attempt to recover embryos generally between days 16 and 18, in normally cyclic females. This is based on the knowledge that, as a rule, ovulation in rhesus monkeys occurs on days 12–13 of the cycle (e.g., Hartman, 1932), and that eggs enter the uterus approximately 72–96 hours after ovulation (Jainudeen and Hafez, 1973; Eddy *et al.*, 1975). A recovery rate of over 50% of uterine eggs and embryos has been achieved by us in normal, non-IUD monkeys (Table I). Two representative blastocysts, one considered normal and the other abnormal, flushed out of non-IUD uteri, are illustrated in Fig. 5. By contrast, 46 attempts, made on corresponding cycle days, in IUD-fitted females have so far yielded seven embryos, but in one animal the IUD was found to be displaced into the cervix (Table I).

The fact that far fewer embryos have been recovered from the uteri of females with devices is striking and appears significant. Among possible causes of this to the sharpened tip. A bend is made about ¼ inch from the base of the needle (Fig. 3). The needles are connected to suitable lengths of polyethylene tubing which, in turn, are jointed to 5-ml disposable syringes. One syringe is loaded with flushing fluid (see below), and the needle is carefully forced into the uterine lumen just above the upper end of the cervix. The other needle, with attached empty syringe, is immediately pushed, preferably by an assistant, through the fundus and fluid flushed from one syringe to the other (Fig. 4). We generally use between 4 and 5 ml of fluid, at a delivery rate of about 1 ml/second. It is usually possible to achieve at least a 90% recovery of the flushing fluid, provided both needles are properly positioned in the lumen of the uterus (see Table I; Hurst *et al.*, 1976). The flush is rarely bloody or contaminated with excess endometrial debris. This greatly facilitates searching the flush for ova or embryos, in a watchglass, using a stereomicroscope.

For use as a flushing fluid we find that Hanks' 199 medium (Flow Labs, Irvine, Scotland) is preferable to Dulbecco's phosphate-buffered saline (Oxoid), which tends to cause shrinkage of the embryonic trophoblast within about 10 minutes. Use of physiological saline brings about rapid collapse of the trophoblast, and is not recommended.

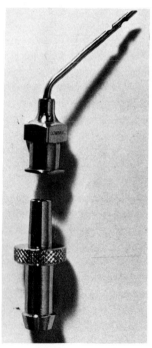

Fig. 3. Flushing needle and connector. (Reproduced from Fig. 1 in Hurst *et al.*, 1976.)

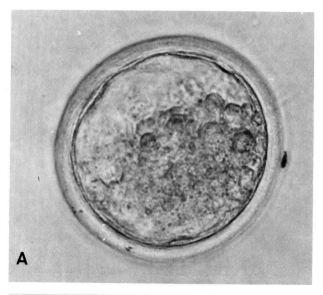

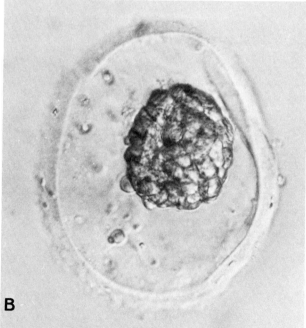

Fig. 5. Uterine blastocysts of rhesus monkeys without IUD's. Photographed after recovery from flush. (A) Normal, day 18 of cycle; unfixed (× 435). (B) Abnormal, day 17 of cycle; fixed in 2.5% glutaraldehyde (× 435). (Reproduced from Hurst *et al.*, 1976.)

disparity is that, in the presence of a uterine device, embryos might be "locked" in the oviduct; such a delay is known to occur in rats and mice (e.g., Doyle and Margolis, 1966; Marston and Kelly, 1969; Mackay, 1972; Hurst *et al.*, 1977a).

In order to explore this possibility, egg recovery from the oviduct can be attempted in rhesus monkeys by inserting a fine needle into the tubal lumen near the uterus and injecting flush fluid in a retrograde direction towards the ovary. The flush can be collected in a watchglass or other suitable container from the abdominal ostium of the tube (cf. Hendrickx and Kraemer, 1968; Hendrickx and Houston, 1971). A disadvantage of this approach is that the segment of the oviduct near the uterus is difficult to irrigate, and needle puncture is liable to cause tubal damage and localized stenosis or adhesions.

We, therefore, have evolved a different procedure which appears to produce complete flushing of the oviduct and not to carry such risks. It consists of introducing a blunted 21-gauge needle through the fimbriated end of the oviduct until the end of the needle lies about 1.5 cm along the tubal lumen. Gentle clamping with rubber-coated forceps is necessary to secure the needle in place (Fig. 6). After inserting a uterine flushing needle (see Section III, above) into either pole of the uterus, flush fluid (1.0 ml) is gently forced along the complete

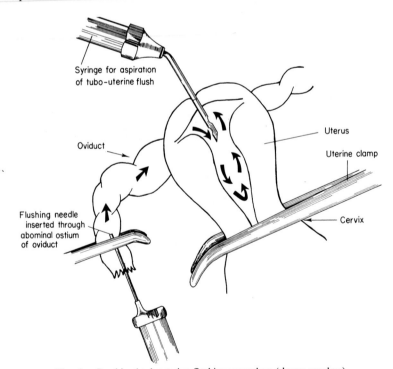

Syringe for aspiration
of tubo-uterine flush

Oviduct

Uterus

Uterine clamp

Flushing needle
inserted through
abominal ostium
of oviduct

Cervix

Fig. 6. Combined tubouterine flushing procedure (rhesus monkey).

length of the tube from the fimbriated end and collected via the uterine needle. The delivery rate is about 1 ml/10 seconds, and complete recovery of the infused fluid can normally be achieved. This procedure does not cause bleeding or adhesions of the oviduct, and the whole length of the tube is irrigated. In recent preliminary studies, we have used this technique immediately after a uterine flush in five IUD animals operated between days 19 and 20 of the cycle. So far, however, only one embryo has been recovered from the uterus in the way described. It, therefore, may be necessary to explore other time intervals following ovulation to establish the location and fate of the conceptus in monkeys fitted with IUD's.

IV. EMBRYO RECOVERY IN MICE

The flushing procedures outlined below are standard ones and probably differ little from those currently used in other laboratories.

Following removal of the entire reproductive tract, the uterus and fallopian tubes are divided at the tubouterine junction. A blunt 30-gauge needle is inserted into the abdominal ostium of the tube and 0.2 ml of flush medium gently injected along the tube. For uterine flushes, a 27-gauge needle is suitable, and flushes are collected directly into watchglasses. In the IUD horns of mice and rats, the presence of masses of polymorphonuclear leukocytes (PMNL's) complicates the search for embryos, especially if the accumulated leukocytes "clot." This can be prevented by using heparin in the flush medium at a concentration of 100 IU/ml.

Using this approach, we find that mouse embryos are difficult to recover from the IUD uterine horns, probably because they tend to be surrounded by large masses of PMNL's (Table II). Those that can be seen in the flushes have fewer

TABLE II

Mouse Embryos Recovered by Flushing Reproductive Tract at 72 and 96 Hours
Postcoitum

	Sham-oper. side		IUD side		Contralateral side	
	72 Hours	96 Hours	72 Hours	96 Hours	72 Hours	96 Hours
No. of mice	7	6	7	7	7	7
No. of corpora lutea	42	34	38	41	43	42
No. of embryos in oviducts	2	0	9	3	10	8
No. of embryos in uterine horns	34	30	4	6	18	12
Total embryo recoveries (%)	85.7	88.2	34.7	21.2	65.1	47.6

PMNL's attached to them, but, even so, their gross appearance and stage of development is difficult to evaluate. Occasionally, in particular, when animals are killed at about the time embryos enter the uterus (approximately 60–70 hours *postcoitum* in the LACA strain), it is possible to dislodge the attached PMNL's by repeated manipulation with micropipettes. If this fails to separate the leukocytes from the embryos, it is advisable to process the latter for transmission electron microscopy (T.E.M.), and examine 1-μm sections with a light microscope after staining with 1% toluidine blue. Embryos recovered by the flushing procedure outlined above can be further investigated, for instance by *in vitro* or transfer studies.

A. Identification of Embryos *in Situ*

Since, as referred to, the yield of uterine embryos is relatively low after flushing procedures in mice (and rats; unpublished observations) fitted with IUD's, histological processing of the whole reproductive tract is required to visualize the embryos *in situ* (Table III; see also Hurst *et al.,* 1977a). Ordinary histological techniques are employed, but it is essential to cut serial longitudinal sections through the entire horn. Since the lumen is inevitably distended by the IUD and the associated massive accumulation of PMNL's, it is generally necessary to prepare, and search through, about 300 sections per reproductive tract. The latter, consisting of both the dissected oviduct and uterine horn, should be pinned out before and during fixation. When the IUD concerned consists of silk or similar suture material, an ordinary rotary microtome is adequate, but harder

TABLE III
Mouse Embryos Observed in Serial Sections of Reproductive Tract at 72 and 96 Hours *Postcoitum*

	Sham-oper. side		IUD side		Contralateral side	
	72 Hours	96 Hours	72 Hours	96 Hours	72 Hours	96 Hours
No. of mice	3	4	6	6	6	6
No. of corpora lutea	17	26	40	36	37	34
No. of embryos in oviducts	0	0	9	5	0	0
No. of embryos in uterine horns	14	20	18[a]	11[a]	31[a]	22[a]
Total embryo recoveries (%)	82.3	76.9	67.5	44.4	83.7	64.7

[a] All embryos in IUD horns and most of those in contralateral horns surrounded by masses of PMNL's.

IUD's, such as nylon or polyethylene ones, require sections through the uterus to be cut with a "sledge" type of microtome.

V. ANALYSIS OF THE CELL CONTENT OF UTERINE FLUSHES FROM MONKEYS AND RODENTS

The flushing procedures for embryo recovery described in Sections III and IV, above, also yield material containing the cellular components of uterine fluid. The numbers, type, and viability of these cells have to be ascertained, but this is frequently complicated by contamination of the flush with blood and endometrial epithelial and stromal cells resulting from the slight trauma inevitably associated with the flushing techniques. This difficulty can be overcome when performing cell count and characterization, although the problem of determining cell viability remains to be solved. The following approach, based on methods evolved in our laboratory by Karin Dawson (unpublished), is confined to cell counting and characterization.

The flushed fluid is centrifuged in siliconized tubes at 400 g for 5–10 minutes. The supernatant fluid is decanted and stored frozen for further biochemical assay if so desired. The cell pellet is resuspended by vortex mixing with 1.0 ml of 0.9% phosphate-buffered saline, and an aliquot withdrawn with a plastic cannula for counting either in a hemocytometer or optical counting device. To obtain a total leukocyte and uterine-derived cell count, 0.1 ml of the suspension is added to 0.1 ml of Turk's solution (1% acetic acid). This lyses red cells within 1 minute, and an aliquot is withdrawn for cell counting.

To determine the differential distribution of cells, the suspension is fixed in formol saline and slides prepared with a cytocentrifuge (Shandon Southern Ltd.). This provides consistently good slide preparations which are superior to smears or air-dried drops of cells. If the flush is contaminated with erythrocytes, it is best to lyse them after fixing the suspension for 3 minutes to give a better preparation of white cells.

VI. FUTURE RESEARCH

The technique described in Section III has yielded a higher recovery rate of conceptuses and more advanced embryologic stages of *Macaca mulatta* than reported by other workers (e.g., Eddy *et al.*, 1975). It is also repeatable and basically simple. It should be fully within the competence of other workers, and may become the method of choice for the collection of uterine embryos in this and allied species, and perhaps also in other primates, including women, with a straight cervical canal.

In addition, it possesses considerable potential for future research, some of which could not previously be contemplated because of the dearth of living primate eggs and embryos. Among its possible application are investigations into the morphological and karyotypic normality (or abnormality) of embryos at the crucial "free" uterine stage of development and of the hormonal conditions present immediately before their attachment and implantation. In this context, it is of interest that several of the embryos collected by us from normal females during this phase have displayed clear signs of cell degeneration. With regard to the mode of action of IUD's, our latest findings show that embryos can be recovered from IUD-bearing monkeys, but that such embryos are invariably abnormal or degenerating as well as invaded by leukocytes (Hurst *et al.,* 1977b). Also, far fewer embryos can be recovered from such females, compared with normal (non-IUD) monkeys, studied on corresponding cycle days. Only a more accurate determination of ovulation times can establish whether, following normal fertilization and early cleavage, some embryos of IUD-fitted monkeys remain "blocked" within the tube, and are therefore not recoverable by uterine flushing. Nonetheless, the demonstrated association between degenerating uterine embryos and their invasion by leukocytes in IUD-monkeys is so constant and pronounced as to suggest that it is more than coincidental (Hurst *et al.,* 1977b).

Again, the increased availability of preimplantation embryos should permit their *in vitro* culture and possible transfer to host uteri, and, in this way, lead to a better understanding of early primate embryonic development and differentiation.

Similar considerations apply also to the study of embryos obtained from normal and IUD-fitted rodents. The technique outlined in Section IV should permit the development of test systems employing purified cultures of mouse PMNL's and the exposure of rodent and other mammalian embryos to PMNL's derived from both rodent and primate sources.

ACKNOWLEDGMENT

We wish to thank Mr. John D. Petty (Dept. of Anatomy) and Mr. Paul Morby (T. V. and Film Unit, University of Birmingham) for their help with the illustrations, and Mrs. Gladys Macbeth for her secretarial assistance.

The support of the Ford Foundation of New York(Grant 630-0576B) in the conduct of the work described in this chapter is gratefully acknowledged.

REFERENCES

Adams, C. E., and Eckstein, P. (1965). *Fertil. Steril.* **16,** 508–521.
Doyle, L. L., and Margolis, A. J. (1966). *J. Reprod. Fertil.* **11,** 27–32.

Duncan, G. W., and Wheeler, R. G. (1975). *Biol. Reprod.* **12**, 143–175.

Eckstein, P. (1970). *Br. Med. Bull.* **26**, No. 1, 52–59.

Eckstein, P. (1972). *Acta Endocrinol. (Copenhagen), Suppl.* **166**, 364–380.

Eddy, C. A., Garcia, R. G., Kraemer, D. C., and Pauerstein, C. J. (1975). *Biol. Reprod.* **13**, 363–369.

El-Sahwi, S., and Moyer, D. L. (1970). *Contraception* **2**, 1–28.

El-Sahwi, S., and Moyer, D. L. (1971). *Fertil. Steril.* **22**, 398–408.

Greenwald, G. (1965). *J. Reprod. Fertil.* **9**, 9–17.

Hartman, C. G. (1932). *Contrib. Embryol. Carnegie Inst.* **23**, 1–161.

Hendrickx, A. G., and Houston, M. L. (1971). *In* "Comparative Reproduction of Non-Human Primates" (E. S. E. Hafez, ed.), Chapter 13. Thomas, Springfield, Illinois.

Hendrickx, A. G., and Kraemer, D. C. (1968). *Anat. Rec.* **162**, 111–120.

Hurst, P. R., Jefferies, K., Eckstein, P., and Wheeler, A. G. (1976). *Biol. Reprod.* **15**, 429–434.

Hurst, P. R., Jefferies, K., Eckstein, P., and Wheeler, A. G. (1977a). *J. Reprod. Fertil.* **50**, 187–189.

Hurst, P. R., Jefferies, K., Eckstein, P., Dawson, K. and Wheeler, A. G. (1977b). *Nature (London)* **269**, 331–333.

Jainudeen, M. R., and Hafez, E. S. E. (1973). *Biol. Reprod.* **9**, 305–308.

Kelly, W. A., Marston, J. H., and Eckstein, P. (1969). *J. Reprod. Fertil.* **19**, 331–340.

Mackay, S. (1972). B.Sc. Thesis, University of Birmingham.

Marston, J. H., and Kelly, W. A. (1969). *J. Endocrinol.* **43**, 83–93.

Moyer, D. L., and Shaw, S. T. (1973). *In* "Human Reproduction: Conception and Contraception" (E. S. E. Hafez and T. N. Evans, eds.), pp. 309–334. Harper & Row, Maryland.

Parr, E. L. (1969). *J. Reprod. Fertil.* **18**, 221–226.

Parr, E. L., Schaedler, R. W., and Hirsch, J. G. (1967). *J. Exp. Med.* **126**, 523–538.

Parr, E. L., and Shirley, R. L. (1976). *Fertil. Steril.* **27**, 1067–1077.

Peplow, V., Breed, W. G., Jones, C. M. J., and Eckstein, P. (1973). *Am. J. Obstet. Gynecol.* **116**, 771–779.

25

Surgical Induction of Endometriosis

JOSEPH C. DANIEL, JR. AND PATSY K. WILLIAMS
BOYCE

I. INTRODUCTION

Endometriosis is defined as the condition in which tissue resembling the uterine mucous membrane, or endometrium, occurs outside of the uterus. It has been found in many locations, of which the following are the most common: the ovaries, the uterine ligaments, rectovaginal septum, the pelvic peritoneum, covering the uterus, tubes, rectum, sigmoid, or bladder, umbilicus, laparotomy and episiotomy scars, hernial sacs, appendix, vagina, vulva, cervix, tubal stumps, and lymph glands. It may also be found in extraabdominal areas such as the arm, the thigh (Mankin, 1935; Schlicke, 1946; Nunn, 1940), the pleural (Counsellor, 1939) and pericardial cavities (Sensenig et al., 1966), the lung (Assor, 1972; Lattes et al., 1956; Hartz, 1956; Jelihovsky and Grant, 1968), sheath of the sciatic nerve (Baker et al., 1966), and the spinal canal (Lombardo et al., 1968), and has even been reported in the male bladder (Oliker and Harris, 1971). It can be a severe pathological condition in women during their reproductive years. Sampson (1921, 1922, 1927) presented the first significant studies of endometriosis, but, according to Novak *et al.* (1975), it was first described in 1899. Endometriosis tissue has been shown to cycle with the normal endometrium, to slough with menstruation, yielding additional cells for endometrial cultures elsewhere, to be sensitive to injected hormones in the castrated rhesus monkey (Scott and Wharton, 1957) and to bind estrogen (Eisenfeld *et al.*, 1971).

There has been a continuing interest in developing methods of experimentally producing endometriosis in laboratory mammals to be used as basic techniques in studies of (1) contraception, (2) implantation, (3) ectopic pregnancy, (4) blockage of the immune response, (5) growth promotion, (6) the proliferative and secretory response of endometrial tissue to circulating hormones, and also (7) as a potential procedure for gaining exposure of and manipulative access to fetal stage embryos. Such a technique might also facilitate work to develop clinical applications because the majority of human patients suffering from endometriosis are sterile. Novak *et al.* (1975) describe studies where 75% of the patients were sterile and 20% had fecundity limited to one child. The possible correlation of endometriosis with ovarian cysts and certain kinds of cancer, namely, endometrioid carcinoma, adenoacanthoma, and mesonephroma, also justifies attempts to gain experimental facility with this aberrantly growing tissue.

As a naturally occurring phenomenon, endometriosis is known primarily in humans, but this may reflect the fact that this is the only species that can complain. There is considerable disagreement as to how it originates, but Novak *et al.* (1975) reviewed four possible ways: (1) transtubal regurgitation of menstrual blood, (2) abnormal differentiation of germinal epithelium or pelvic peritoneum, (3) lymphatic dissemination, and (4) hematogenous spread. It seems probable that all of these may indeed be effective, and different ones may be operational in different cases. For clinical purposes, four stages may be classified according to the amount of tubo-ovarian distortion and the extent of pelvic or adnexal adhesions (Kistner *et al.*, 1977).

Endometriosis was produced experimentally as early as 1926, when Jacobson successfully transplanted uterine mucosa to peritoneal surfaces of rabbits and monkeys. Levander and Norman (1955) and Bernhard (1959) induced subcutaneous tissue growth in rabbits by injection of endometrial fragments. Ridley (1968) produced endometriosis in humans and monkeys by interperitoneal injection of their own exfoliated endometrium and by plantation of endometrium into the abdominal wall. It can also be made to develop in the pleural pericardium of dogs by surgically implanting endometrial tissue obtained after hysterectomy, followed by hormonal support (1.5 mg DES daily) (Sensenig *et al.*, 1966). The work of Levander and Norman (1955) and of Bernhard (1959), noted above, provided support for the hypothesis that endometrium contains a factor which induces growth and/or differentiation of connective tissue or undifferentiated mesenchyme. In an effort to demonstrate the existence of an inducing agent, Merrill (1966) enclosed endometrium in a filter capsule from which it could not escape but its products could diffuse, and after transplanting the capsule to the peritoneal wall caused proliferation in the adjacent connective tissues.

A simple reliable method for achieving an endometrial graft at a specific site in rabbits follows below. With modifications to accommodate for size, it can also be used on most laboratory rodents.

II. ANIMALS

We use young, mature, New Zealand does. The animals are checked for stage of estrus by visually inspecting the vagina, using a deep purple vascularization and swollen lips as indicators of high estrus. Generally, accompanying the color indication, there is also a specific odor that is detectable when the vagina is checked. (Our greatest breeding success has been with does having all three characteristics.)

III. SURGERY

After weighing, the doe is placed in an animal retainer. The area around one marginal ear vein is wet with 70% EtOH and the vein area "thumped" with the fingers to initiate dilation. Nembutal (sodium pentobarbital) 27 mg/kg body weight is injected into the vein, quickly at first to expedite the rabbit's rapid passage through the excitatory phase of anesthesia and then more slowly to prevent cardiac arrest. The anesthetized animal is placed, abdomen up, on a surgical table and restrained with cotton cords attached to each limb, shaved, and draped. Ether or pentothrane is used via a nose cap to maintain the desired state of anesthesia during the surgery.

A midline incision of approximately 7 cm is made through the skin of the lower abdomen, followed by another incision through the body wall along the linea alba. If necessary, the bladder may be emptied manually by finger pressure to the outer surface. The opposing abdominal walls are retracted and the uterus exposed. For research, we routinely use the right uterine horn for experimental purposes and reserve the left horn intact to provide a control, if needed. A 3.5–4.0 cm incision is made longitudinally in the right uterine horn along the antimesometrial border (Fig. 1A and B). The side of the horn adjacent to the peritoneal wall is stitched with 000 silk suture, and then the opposing open edge is pulled over so as to flatten the graft region and then stitched in a like manner to the wall (Fig. 1C and D). Figure 2 shows the appearance of the uterus attached to the wall with the mesometrium removed.

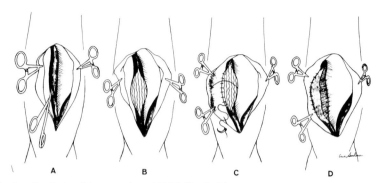

Fig. 1. Surgical grafting procedure. (A) Midline incision; uterus exposed; (B) right horn opened along antimesometrial border; (C) one side of cut edge sutured to peritoneal wall; (D) second side sutured to wall.

The abdominal musculature is closed by a loop lock stitch with 0 silk suture and a topical antibiotic (Furacin, Eaton Laboratories, Norwich, New York) is sprayed on the sutured area. The skin is then closed, using single stitches and placing wound clips between adjacent stitches. A surgical spray dressing with an antibacterial agent (Rezifilm, E. R. Squibb and Sons, Inc., New York) is applied to the dermal sutured area. The animal is then given 100,000 units/kg of antibio-

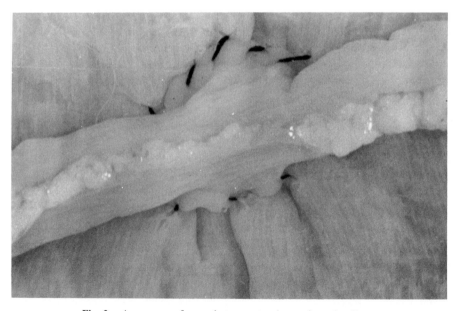

Fig. 2. Appearance of opened uterus sutured to peritoneal wall.

tic; we use an intramuscular benzathine penicillin, which is absorbed slowly into the blood.

Rabbits are proficient suture removers, and, thus, it is necessary to check the animals daily for the first 4 days after surgery and repair any openings. The animals are maintained on a normal colony schedule of food, photoperiod, and treatment for 2 weeks, which is the time allotted for good tissue adherence to the peritoneal wall. At the end of the 2-week period, the animals are again anesthetized and reopened along the left margin of the primary incision. The uterus is removed from the wall gently by cutting the original sutures and then separating the endometrium, so that the endometrial graft is left adhering to the peritoneal wall. The opened uterine horn is repaired if possible, or simply excised after the uterine vessels in the mesometrium are ligatured. The animals are closed as before. After a period of 1–3 weeks, allowing for adherence of the endometrial graft without the supporting influence of the intact uterus, the animals are ready for further study.

IV. GRAFT IDENTITY

We have used two criteria to establish that the tissue grafted by this procedure is truly of endometrial origin: (1) histological appearance and (2) the secretory response during pregnancy and to exogenous hormones.

(1) To examine the histological structure of the graft and its relationship to other tissues, small pieces (about 5 mm) of graft along with the underlying peritoneum and bound muscle layer were cut from the wall, fixed in Bouin's solution, dehydrated in an alcohol series, cleared in xylene, and embedded in paraffin. Sections were cut at 8 μm and stained with hematoxylin–eosin. Figure 3A shows a typical section through the tissue junction. The grafted tissue clearly has the secretory–epithelial character of endometrium; skeletal muscle and adipose and connective tissue layers are present on the peritoneal side. There is, however, an especially thick layer of dense irregular fibrous connective tissue, not unlike that described by Merrill (1966), which develops at the junction. We presume this has proliferated from the peritoneum, but we are still uncertain about its origin. Figure 3B shows an enlarged region of an adjacent graft area to demonstrate the glandular composition of the tissue. This particular sample was taken from a progesterone-treated animal as noted below.

(2) Methods were used to determine if the induced endometrioma demonstrate the same hormone regulation as intact endometrium, namely, during pregnancy and steroid hormone supplementation. At the appropriate time, homogenates were made of endometrial scrapings from the intact horn and of scrapings from the peritoneal wall, both in the region of the endometrial graft and in an adjacent region of wall for comparison. Uterine flushings from the intact horn were also

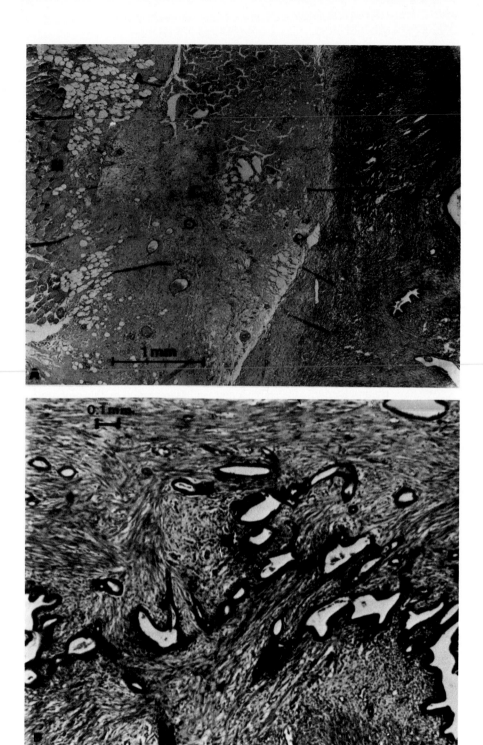

Fig. 3.

used. With each system, our criterion for normal function was the presence of the uterine protein, blastokinin (Krishnan and Daniel, 1967).

A. Pregnancy

Three weeks after the excision of the uterus from the peritoneal wall, the animals were bred. They were killed by cervical dislocation 5 days later. This time was selected because the blastokinin level in rabbit uterine fluids reaches its peak on the 5th and 6th day of pregnancy.

The method preferred in this laboratory for killing rabbits involves separation of the cervical vertebrae. It is done by using one hand to hold the head which is twisted suddenly upward into an arc while the rest of the body is being stretched by the other hand holding the hind legs (see Fig. 4). The animal's body can be rested against the operator's upper leg for added support. Properly performed, this method results in an almost instantaneous, painless and bloodless death. A few mild reflexive movements may precede complete cessation of activity.

B. Hormone Regimen

To determine if the endometrial graft is sensitive to injected hormones, the following regimen was followed. At the time when the uterine horn was removed from the wall to separate it from the graft, the animals were also ovariectomized. The ovariectomy was performed by ligating the ovarian vessels and cutting the ovary from its mesentery. After 10 days, allowed for healing, the animals were daily injected subcutaneously with either (1) 1 ml corn oil carrier, (2) 3 mg progesterone in corn oil/kg body weight, or (3) 10 μg 17β-estradiol/kg, for a period of 4 days. They were then killed on the afternoon of the 4th day and the tissues collected.

Tissue Collection

The control horn was flushed with 5 ml of 0.01 M sterile phosphate-buffered saline, pH 7.1, and 5 ml air and the flushings checked for embryos to confirm pregnancy. The flushing was decanted and centrifuged at 2000 g at 4°C for 20 minutes to remove cellular debris. The supernatant was concentrated and subjected to gel filtration at 4°C through a Sephadex G-200 chromatography column according to the procedure of Murray et al. (1972). The eluant was 0.01 M PBS, pH 7.1, with 25-drop fractions collected, and the protein concentration determined by the method of Lowry et al. (1951). From

---

Fig. 3. (A) Histological cross section of endometrial graft junction showing adherence to the peritoneal wall. M, Skeletal muscle; A, adipose tissue; C, connective tissue; S, secretory endometrial tissue. (The dark lines are tissue folds commonly seen in these preparations.) (B) Adjacent tissue section of glandular region of endometrial graft.

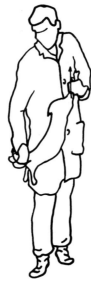

Fig. 4. Procedure for killing rabbits by cervical dislocation.

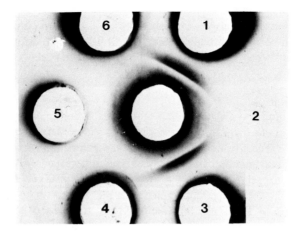

Fig. 5. Immunodiffusion test for blastokinin in endometrial grafts. Homogenates of scrapings from well 1: graft site—progesterone-treated animal; well 2: adjacent body wall—progesterone-treated animal; well 3: graft site—5-day pregnant animal; well 4: adjacent body wall—5-day pregnant animal; well 5: graft site—estrogen-treated animal; well 6: adjacent body wall—estrogen-treated animal. Center well contains anti-blastokinin serum.

the elution graph we identified the blastokinin peak, the fractions of which were then pooled and concentrated as were the initial flushings. The supernatants of the homogenates were treated in exactly the same manner as the flushings, or were simply concentrated to approximately 1 ml. The blastokinin content of the concentrates from the flushings and scrapings was confirmed by immunodiffusion and immunoelectrophoresis with antisera produced in goats against rabbit uterine fluids, and then absorbed with serum and liver powder so as to be essentially monospecific for blastokinin (Johnson *et al.*, 1972). In both systems, as shown in Figs. 5 and 6, there appears a blastokininlike precipitation band with the endometrial graft scraping, the uterine scraping, and the flushings from the pregnant and the progesterone-treated animals, but not in the estrogen- or carrier-treated animals. The peritoneal wall samples of the pregnant or progesterone-treated animals also had no detectable blastokinin. As shown in Fig. 6, the immunoelectrophoresis precipitation bands appear only in the pregnant and progesterone-treated animals under the two precipitation arcs of blastokinin.

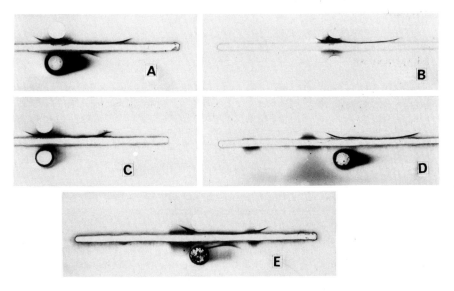

Fig. 6. Immunoelectrophoresis of homogenates of endometrial grafts and peritoneal wall scrapings compared to purified blastokinin (BKN). Top well of each slide contains BKN. Center well contains anti-BKN serum. Bottom well contains (A) graft—progesterone-treated animal; (B) wall—progesterone-treated animal; (C) graft—estrogen-treated animal; (D) graft—corn oil-injected control; (E) graft—5-day pregnant doe. BKN typically gives two bands in this system (i.e., 1,2). As in Fig. 5, only grafts from progesterone-treated and pregnant does give corresponding bands against anti-BKN.

From the above experiments, we conclude that the secretory response of the endometrial tissue grafted to the peritoneal wall by the procedure described here mimics that of normal uterine endometrium during early pregnancy or after exposure of the animal to exogenous ovarian steroids.

With this system, we hope to provide a simulated uterine environment where an embryo might find a supportive ectopic site for development and, thereby, test the hypothesis that the uterus is an immunologically privileged organ. While the embryo will have a normal endometrium in which to implant, there will be no uterine enclosure to offer protection from the mother's antibodies in the peritoneal cavity. With the tissue so placed on the wall, viewing of embryonic growth and interaction will also be enhanced and possibly manipulation facilitated for immunologic, teratogenic, genetic, induction, and grafting experiments. "Endometriosis, recognized over 50 years ago . . . has defied verification of its etiology, its pathogenesis, its functional capacities (especially its disturbance of menstrual disorders), its relationship to fertility, and its capacity for malignant degeneration." (Weed and Holland, 1977). We would hope that the method described above will offer a system for studying the relationship between sterility and endometriosis and potentially the prevention cure of this affliction.

REFERENCES

Assor, D. (1972). *Am. J. Clin. Pathol.* **57,** 311–315.
Baker, G. S., Parsons, W. R., and Welch, J. S. (1966). *J. Neurosurg.* **25,** 652–655.
Bernhard, J. (1959). *Z. Geburstshilfe Gynaekol.* **153,** 112–136.
Counseller, V. (1939). *Am. J. Obstet. Gynecol.* **37,** 788–794.
Eisenfeld, A. J., Gardner, M. U., and Van Wagenen, G. (1971). *Am. J. Obstet. Gynecol.* **109,** 124–130.
Hartz, P. H. (1956). *Am. J. Clin. Pathol.* **26,** 48–51.
Jacobson, V. C. (1926). *Arch. Pathol. Lab. Med.* **1,** 169–174.
Jelihovsky, T., and Grant, A. T. (1968). *Thorax* **23,** 434–437.
Johnson, M. H., Cowan, B. D., and Daniel, J. C. (1972). *Fertil. Steril.* **23,** 93–100.
Kistner, R. W., Siegler, A. M., and Behrman, S. J. (1977). *Fertil. Steril.* **28,** 353.
Krishnan, R. S., and Daniel, J. C. (1967). *Science* **185,** 490–492.
Lattes, R., Shephard, F., Tovell, H., and Wylie, R. (1956). *Surg., Gynecol. Obstet.* **103,** 552–558.
Levander, G., and Norman, P. (1955). *Acta Obstet. Gynecol. Scand.* **34,** 366–398.
Lombardo, L., Mateos, J. H., and Barroeta, F. F. (1968). *Neurology* **18,** 423–426.
Lowry, O. H., Rosebrough, N. J., Farr, A. L., and Randall, R. J. (1951). *J. Biol. Chem.* **193,** 265–275.
Mankin, Z. W. (1935). *Arch. Gynaekol.* **159,** 671–688.
Merrill, J. A. (1966). *Am. J. Obstet. Gynecol.* **94,** 780–790.
Murray, F. A., McGaughey, R. W., and Yarus, M. J. (1972). *Fertil. Steril.* **23,** 69–77.
Novak, E. R., Jones, G. S., and Jones, H. W. (1975). "Novak's Textbook of Gynecology," 9th ed. Williams & Wilkins, Baltimore, Maryland.

Nunn, L. L. (1940). *Northwest Med.* **48,** 474.
Oliker, A. J., and Harris, A. E. (1971). *J. Urol.* **106,** 858–859.
Ridley, J. H. (1968). *Obstet. & Gynecol. Surv.* **23,** 1–35.
Sampson, J. A. (1921). *Arch. Surg. (Chicago)* **3,** 245–323.
Sampson, J. A. (1922). *Am. J. Obstet. Gynecol.* **4,** 451–470.
Sampson, J. A. (1927). *Am. J. Obstet. Gynecol.* **14,** 422–469.
Schlicke, C. P. (1946). *J. Am. Med. Assoc.* **132,** 445–446.
Scott, R. B., and Wharton, L. R., Jr. (1957). *Am. J. Obstet. Gynecol.* **74,** 852–865.
Sensenig, D. M., Serlin, O., and Hawthorne, H. R. (1966). *J. Am. Med. Assoc.* **198,** 645–647.
Weed, J. C., and Holland, J. B. (1977). *Fertil. Steril.* **28,** 135–140.

Index

A 8
B 9
C 0
D 1
E 2
F 3
G 4
H 5
I 6
J 7